Electrotherapy

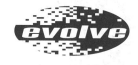

Evolve Learning Resources for Students and Lecturers:
The complete collection of over 300 images from this book in JPEG and PDF format.
Suitable for downloading and importing into applications such as Powerpoint and Word

See the instructions and PIN code panel on the inside cover for access to the web site and your image bank.

Think outside the book...evolve

For Churchill Livingstone

Publisher: Heidi Harrison
Commissioning Editor: Rita Demetriou-Swanwick
Associate Editor: Siobhan Campbell
Development Editor: Veronika Watkins
Project Manager: Anne Dickie
Design: George Ajayi
Illustration Buyer: Bruce Hogarth
Illustrator: Robert Britton

Electrotherapy:
Evidence–Based Practice

TWELFTH EDITION

Edited by
Tim Watson

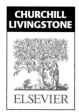

EDINBURGH LONDON NEW YORK OXFORD PHILADELPHIA ST LOUIS SYDNEY TORONTO 2008

CHURCHILL
LIVINGSTONE
ELSEVIER

© 2008, Elsevier Ltd

No part of this publication may be reproduced, stored in a retrieval system, or
transmitted in any form or by any means, electronic, mechanical, photocopying,
recording or otherwise, without the prior permission of the Publishers.
Permissions may be sought directly from Elsevier's Health Sciences Rights
Department, 1600 John F. Kennedy Boulevard, Suite 1800, Philadelphia,
PA 19103-2899, USA: phone: (+1) 215 239 3804; fax: (+1) 215 239 3805; or,
e-mail: healthpermissions@elsevier.com. You may also complete your request
on-line via the Elsevier homepage (http://www.elsevier.com), by selecting
'Support and contact' and then 'Copyright and Permission'.

First published 1948 as Clayton's Electrotherapy and Actinotherapy
Eight edition 1981 as Clayton's Electrotherapy
Eleventh edition 2002 as Electrotherapy: Evidence-Based Practice
Twelfth edition 2008

ISBN: 978-0-443-10179-3

British Library Cataloguing in Publication Data
A catalogue record for this book is available from the British Library.

Library of Congress Cataloging in Publication Data
A catalog record for this book is available from the Library of Congress.

Note
Neither the Publisher nor the Authors assume any responsibility for any loss or
injury and/or damage to persons or property arising out of or related to any use
of the material contained in this book. It is the responsibility of the treating
practitioner, relying on independent expertise and knowledge of the patient, to
determine the best treatment and method of application for the patient.

Working together to grow
libraries in developing countries

www.elsevier.com | www.bookaid.org | www.sabre.org

ELSEVIER   BOOK AID
            International   Sabre Foundation

your source for books,
journals and multimedia
in the health sciences
www.elsevierhealth.com

The
publisher's
policy is to use
paper manufactured
from sustainable forests

Printed in China

Contents

Preface

The important thing in science is not so much to obtain new facts as to discover new ways of thinking about them

[Sir William Bragg]

Evidence Based Practice (EBP) has become a cornerstone of contemporary therapeutics, and whilst the phrase has become widespread in the last 10 years or so, the underlying philosophy has been a part of therapy for a lot longer than that. Sackett et al (1996) have provided probably the most widely cited sound bite in relation to EBP which is: "the conscientious, explicit and judicious use of current best evidence in making decisions about the care of the individual patient. It means integrating individual clinical expertise with the best available external clinical evidence from systematic research".

The issues surrounding EBP are myriad and widely discussed in the literature, and this text is not about disseminating the philosophy of EBP. What this book does aim to consider is the range and the quality of the evidence, pertinent to current electrotherapy practice. The term Electrotherapy is used here in its widest (historical) sense, and the emergent, and probably more proper term, Electro Physical Agents (EPA's) is likely to supersede it in the not too distant future.

It is widely suggested that Electrotherapy 'lacks evidence'. If you look through the reference lists at the end of each chapter, you will see this is patently untrue. There are gaps in this evidence base – as there are for all areas of practice – and identifying and filling these gaps is a major component of the workload for many of us. A lack of awareness of the existing evidence is, in my view, a much more common problem. Certainly, some of this evidence is not easy to access, and some is difficult to comprehend and integrate into our existing framework of knowledge. This text is therefore a consideration, by experts in their field, of the current evidence base for the key electrotherapy modalities, and an analysis of how this existing evidence can be integrated into practice.

My own interest in Electrotherapy started from my student days, but more seriously, from the earlier part of my teaching career when 'given' Electrotherapy to teach. Looking through the existing texts, I was unconvinced of the accounts proffered to explain how the various modalities achieved their effects, what those effects were and how to apply the treatments. I set out to try and debunk some of the dubious claims made – for my own sake if nothing else – so that at least I could be more convinced about the subject I was charged with presenting. This debunking process is incomplete. Despite reading many books, papers and articles, and discussing issues at considerable length with many people, I have still to fully understand all that is happening – and in fact, I doubt that I ever will. Applying energy to the body inevitably has an effect on that body, and my own fascination is in the relationship between the applied energy, the physiological changes that result, and how these might be harnessed for therapeutic gain. This is the essential tenet of this form of therapy and the discovery process is ongoing.

There is a fundamental difference between a 'lack of evidence' and an 'evidence of lack'. By that I mean that there are some areas where we simply do not have the level of evidence that we would wish for. There are some areas where we have evidence of a lack of effect. They are clearly not one and the same. Some people use a different version of the same phrase – 'absence of evidence versus evidence of absence', but the overall meaning is the same. Adding to the evidence base is an ongoing task. Identifying gaps in the evidence and attempting to fill them is something that many of us undertake by research. Research attempts to answer questions, but inevitably generates more questions as a consequence of that process. Taking the evidence that we already have, and using it to best effect is something that all practitioners are charged with. Sir William Bragg, Nobel Laureate in Physics in 1915, provided the quote at the start of this preface. He was not a medical man, a therapist, nor, so far as I am aware, did he have any interest in Electrotherapy. He did recognise however that doing things with facts is paramount. He does not suggest that finding out new facts is unimportant, but using the existing material is critical.

This book provides a substantive volume of facts, based on the current evidence, analysed and evaluated by the authors. Gaps in the evidence have been identified, but the authors have tried to make sense of the facts as we know them, and in doing so, have attempted to integrate them into an existing body of knowledge, thus augmenting our understanding of electrotherapy and enhancing patient care. Electrotherapy is no more important than other therapeutic tools. It is an effective form of intervention when used appropriately and deserves a place in current practice. That it should be dismissed as 'without evidence' is inappropriate. I trust that what follows will serve to enhance knowledge and understanding in this field.

Tim Watson
www.electrotherapy.org

Reference

Sackett DL, Rosenberg WM, Gray JA et al (1996). "Evidence based medicine: what it is and what it isn't." BMJ 312(7023): 71–72.

Acknowledgements

As with any text of this size and complexity, there are a host of people who have made significant effort and whose efforts need to be acknowledged, and at the risk of making this sound like an acceptance speech at a film awards ceremony, I would like to identify the following.

Firstly, the authors and contributors of the chapters, without whom, the whole venture could not have been achieved. Sheila Kitchen, editor of the previous edition additionally provided encouragement and support for which I am indebted.

At Elsevier, there have been many individuals who have assisted greatly in getting the publication into its final form, but in particular, I am very grateful to Siobhan Campbell, Heidi Harrison, Jack Geddes and Veronika Watkins who have supported, and assisted in the planning process and facilitated production.

Hazel Hindes provided considerable effort and skill when it came to proofing, reference checking and other editorial duties.

Lastly, but by no means least, all the students, post grads, PhDs, researchers, colleagues and patients who have, over the years asked questions which have (maybe unbeknown to them) prompted me to go away and find out something more, something new or set up another research programme. Paul Standing and Jimmy Guest (Mr Guest to almost all of us!), both of West Middlesex Physiotherapy, and both sadly, no longer with us, were instrumental in my passion for the subject and tolerated my early inane questions and repeated abstract discussions. Professor John Mellerio at University of Westminster who woke up the researcher in me and encouraged a style of thinking that I value to this day.

There are, I have no doubt, many others who could be mentioned, and my apologies if your being omitted by name causes offence – none is intended.

Contributors

Maryam M. Al-Mandeel BSc, MSc, PhD
Assistant Professor, Faculty of Allied Health Sciences, Physical Therapy Department, Kuwait University, Kuwait

G. David Baxter TD, BSc (Hons), DPhil, MBA, MCSP, MNZSP
Professor and Dean, School of Physiotherapy, University of Otago, Dunedin, New Zealand

Mary Cramp PhD, MCSP
Senior Lecturer, School of Health and Bioscience, University of East London, London

Sally Durham MCSP
Clinical Specialist Physiotherapist, Gait Laboratory, Douglas Bader Rehabilitation Centre, Queen Mary's Hospital, London

Mary Dyson BSc, PhD, FCSP(Hons), FAIUM(Hons), LDH(Hons)
*Emeritus Reader in the Biology of Tissue Repair, King's College, University of London, London
Executive Vice President, Longport Inc., Glen Mills, PA, USA*

David Ewins PhD, BSc, CEng, MIET, MIPEM, SRCS
*Reader in Biomedical Engineering, Centre for Biomedical Engineering, University of Surrey, Guildford
Consultant Clinical Scientist, Douglas Bader Rehabilitation Centre, Queen Mary's Hospital, London*

Mark I. Johnson PhD, BSc, PGCHE
Professor of Pain and Analgesia, Faculty of Health, Leeds Metropolitan University, Leeds

Sheila Kitchen MSc, PhD, MSCP, DipTP
Professor of Physiotherapy, Academic Department of Physiotherapy, School of Biomedical and Health Sciences, King's College London, London

John Leddy BSc, BSc, PgD
*Musculoskeletal Physiotherapist, Royal Berkshire Hospital, Reading
Sonographer, Department of General Practice and Primary Care, King's College, London*

Denis Martin DPhil, MSc, BSc (Hons)
Director, Centre for Rehabilitation Science, University of Teesside, Middlesbrough

Suzanne McDonough PhD, BSc (Hons), HDip
Professor of Health and Rehabilitation, School of Health Sciences, University of Ulster, Newtownabbey, Co. Antrim

Shea Palmer PhD, BSc (Hons)
Principal Lecturer in Physiotherapy, Faculty of Health and Life Sciences, University of the West of England, Bristol

Oona Scott PhD, FCSP
Professor Emeritus in Neurophysiology, School of Health and Bioscience, University of East London, London

Gail ter Haar MA (Oxon) PhD, DSc (Oxon)
Reader in Therapeutic Ultrasound, Joint Physics Department, Institute of Cancer Research: Royal Marsden Hospital, Sutton

Deirdre M. Walsh DPhil, B. Physio, PgCUT, MCSP
*Professor of Rehabilitation Research, Health and
Rehabilitation Sciences Research Institute,
University of Ulster, Newtownabbey, Co. Antrim*

Tim Watson PhD, BSC (Hons), MCSP, DipTP
*Professor of Physiotherapy, School of Health and
Emergency Professions, University of Hertfordshire,
Hatfield*

Leslie Wood BSc, PhD
*Senior Lecturer in Physiology, Department of Biological
and Biomedical Sciences, Glasgow Caledonian
University, Glasgow*

Stephen R. Young Bsc, PhD
*Formerly Senior Lecturer, Tissue Repair Research Unit,
Guy's Hospital, London*

SECTION 1

Introduction and scientific concepts

SECTION CONTENTS

Chapter 1

Introduction: current concepts and clinical decision making in electrotherapy

Tim Watson

INTRODUCTION

Electrotherapy has a long-established place in therapy practice, being one of the mainstays of professional activity over many years. The emphasis on this mode of intervention has gone through significant changes over time and, in current practice, it is seen for the most part as an adjunct to treatment rather than as a means to an end in isolation. There are instances where it can be rightly considered to be the focus of the treatment but this is unusual and, arguably, the exception rather than the rule.

Given that many of the modalities that have been used in the past have waned in popularity, and that every year new machines and new 'treatments' come to the marketplace, it can be difficult for the therapist to know whether this 'new' treatment is in fact new or just a revamped version of an already existing intervention. There are undoubtedly new interventions and certainly new approaches to existing treatments, driven by a demand from patients, from manufacturers and from research. To claim that all current electrotherapy practice is 'evidence based' would be naïve, although there is room for debate as to what actually constitutes evidence-based practice, from where the evidence is sourced and the role of individual experience and that of colleagues in that process. Some of these issues will be explored in this introductory chapter.

From the published and experiential evidence, it appears that electrotherapy can be clinically effective and need not be written off as something that is 'old fashioned' and that no longer deserves a place in the therapeutic tool kit. That it can be applied in a clinically effective manner is evidenced in the chapters that follow. That it can also be delivered in an ineffectual manner is something that will be recognised by practitioners from many disciplines. The evidence would suggest that when the appropriate modality is applied at the 'right' dose for the presenting problem, it can make a significant contribution to the improvement and well being of the patient. The fact that it does not work in all cases is not surprising at all. This would be a common feature of any therapy – whether manual therapy, exercise or drug therapy. If one were to use a particular manual therapy technique for patient X, and the next day or the next week, when X returns, there was no improvement, it would not mean that all manual therapy was a waste of time, or even that the therapist was incompetent. There are patients who fail to respond to therapy A, but do very well with therapy B. The reasons for these individual differences are poorly understood, but certainly add to the richness of clinical experience. If therapy was simply a matter of applying the right recipe to the patient presenting with a given problem, clinical practice would lose a deal of its attractiveness. For any therapeutic intervention to be effective there is the need for a clear assessment, a rationalisation of the problem(s), and the construction of a proposed treatment plan that matches the needs of the individual taking into account their holistic circumstances, not just their presenting signs and symptoms. The applied intervention is that which is deemed to be most likely to be effective. This is no guarantee that there will be 100% success, but the best odds for a beneficial outcome. The thinking therapist then re-evaluates the outcomes as the treatment progresses, modifying the treatment package in the light of these results.

One of the problems with the application of research in electrotherapy, as well as in other fields, is that the research tends to be somewhat reductionist in approach. A clinical trial that evaluates, for example, the effect of ultrasound for patients with a tear of the medial collateral ligament of the knee, aims to construct a methodology that readily identifies the contribution that ultrasound makes to the clinical outcome. By keeping all other treatment parameters 'constant' – the advice, exercise, manual therapy, environment, number of treatment and treatment intervals – the real effect of the ultrasound therapy can be evaluated.

The clinical reality is that it is the *package* of care that is clinically effective (or not), rather than any one individual component of it. If a patient has received several forms of intervention (e.g. some advice, electrotherapy, manual therapy and exercise coupled with appropriate advice and education) and comes back for the next session with an improvement, it is extraordinarily difficult to know which elements of the treatment package (if any) were responsible for the change. It could be that all were necessary in that particular combination; it could be that one could have been safely omitted and the equivalent outcome would have been achieved.

When making a clinical decision, practitioners will put together the package that in their opinion is most likely to be effective for that patient. Some patients will not take advice well, others will almost certainly not undertake the exercises that are suggested, and others might have a strong aversion to the idea of electrical stimulation. The effective package is the one that matches the patient's presentation and the treatment context. Some patients might be treated several times a week whereas others can only be seen once every 2 or 3 weeks on a 'check-up' basis. Package tailoring is an essential skill for any therapist.

The current stage of research in electrotherapy and many other therapeutic fields is still at the point where the building blocks of these packages are being evaluated. We might know, in absolute terms, the effect of this particular treatment, at this particular dose on a specific problem in a controlled research environment. We might not know what happens when the same therapy is used in a different combination – there are almost too many variables to evaluate at the current time.

The research evidence suggests that electrotherapy can be effective as an element of treatment. Further work is needed to evaluate the combinations – or treatment packages – that are most effective. Practitioners will have, from their own experience, ideas about combinations that are more or less effective. This is the source of the richness of therapeutic experience and until substantially more work has been completed – both in the laboratory and in clinical practice, using reductionist, holistic and pragmatic methodologies – the full story is unlikely to emerge.

The intention of this publication is to provide a review of the background, evidence and clinical applicability of various modalities in use. The authors of each chapter are writing because they know their subject and, although there might be gaps in the knowledge that deserve to be filled, there is sufficient evidence out there from which clinical decision making can be enhanced and further developments achieved.

CURRENT CONCEPTS IN ELECTROTHERAPY

No matter which classification one uses, there is no one correct way to divide and categorise the range of electrotherapy modalities available. One could for example use a thermal/non-thermal division, but reading the literature on thermal vs. non-thermal vs. microthermal will soon demonstrate that this is an almost certainly flawed proposition. One could attempt to categorise by type of applied energy: light (e.g. laser, ultraviolet) versus electrical stimulation (e.g. transcutaneous electrical nerve stimulation [TENS], interferential) versus the high-frequency radiations (shortwave, microwave). Ultrasound would have to sit in a category of its own and biofeedback would not belong anywhere in that, for the most part, it does not involve the delivery of energy but enables the patient to respond to the behaviour of his or her body. This division could also be challenged in that, for example, the effects of continuous shortwave are similar but clinically different from those of pulsed shortwave. The fundamental energy might be the same but the mode of delivery makes a substantial difference to the treatment outcome.

Furthermore, there is an issue with the inclusion of 'new' therapies into the classification. Magnetic therapy is a swiftly developing field although, one would suggest, still in its clinical infancy. Should it have a category of its own or should it be incorporated with some forms of shortwave that employ and electromagnetic field?

The modalities covered in this text include those that are in common clinical use, and have been divided into sections that reflect the type of energy employed, for example, the thermal energies are grouped as are various forms of electrical stimulation. The grouping of laser, ultrasound and biofeedback does not imply a common energy type or mode of action, but rather their individuality.

MODELS OF ELECTROTHERAPY

All electrotherapy modalities – whether in current use, abandoned from the past or yet to be 'invented' – actually follow a very straightforward model that is presented below. It is sufficiently robust to explain current practice, yet sufficiently flexible to incorporate future developments. It has been refined over the years and will almost certainly be subject to further refinement in the future.

In principle, the model identifies that the delivery of energy from a machine or device is the start point of the intervention (Fig. 1.1). The energy entry to the tissues results in a change in one or more physiological events. Some are very specific whereas others are multifaceted. The capacity of the energy to influence physiological events is key to the processes of all electrotherapy modalities and will be reflected throughout this publication. The physiological shift that results from the energy delivery is used in practice to generate what is commonly referred to as a therapeutic effect.

This is a fairly classical learning sequence for many therapists. One learns what the energy is, where it goes, what it does when it gets there and

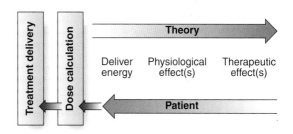

Figure 1.1 A simple model of electrotherapy.

what the outcome might be. One has to learn the material somehow, and this is possibly as good a way as any.

The clinical application of the model is best achieved by what appears to be a reversal of this process. Start with the patient and his or her problems, which are identified from the clinical assessment. Once the problems are known, the treatment priorities can be established and the rationale for the treatment determined. Knowing what it is that is intended to be achieved generates the target for the intervention. Moving one step back through the model, the question then arises: 'If that is the intended outcome or therapeutic effect, which physiological process(es) need to be stimulated, modified or affected in order for the outcome to be achieved?' Once the physiological changes are established, one further step back through the model will enable the determination of the most appropriate modality that can be used to achieve this effect, based on the best available evidence. If, for example, the patient presents with a chronic hamstring muscle tear, with pain, disturbed movement patterns and functional difficulty, then what needs to be changed, stimulated or activated to get a clinically beneficial outcome? Once this is decided, it is a matter of deciding from the evidence which modality, if any of them, is best able to achieve these results? If there is no electrotherapy modality capable of stimulating this/these physiological change(s) in the tissue in question, then what place does electrotherapy have in the management of this particular patient?

The effects of electrotherapy appear to be modality dependent. The primary decision that has to be made is critical, in that some modalities have a limited subset of effects that are fundamentally different from another modality. They are not necessarily interchangeable, although they might be.

Having identified the modality that is best able to achieve the effects required, the next clinical stage is to make a 'dose' selection. Not only is it critical to apply the right modality, but it needs to be applied at the appropriate 'dose' for maximal benefit to be achieved. There is a substantial and growing body of evidence that the same modality can be applied at different doses and the results will not be the same. An obvious example might be laser therapy. Applied at a low dose, laser

has effects that are harnessed by therapists when treating a variety of open wounds and musculoskeletal tissue problems. Applied at a higher dose, the same light energy is used by the surgeon as a means to ablate or vaporise tissue. The energy might be the same, but the dose is different and the outcome is easily distinguished.

One might argue that this is an extreme example, which in some ways it is, but the point is that the effects of the therapy are both modality and dose dependent. There are 'therapeutic windows' in electrotherapy (as there are in almost all therapeutic interventions) and, to achieve the 'best' outcome, it is essential to get as close to this window as one possibly can. The theory of these windows will be briefly explored in the next section, but the principle is introduced here (see the section 'Electrotherapeutic windows', below).

This fundamental model of electrotherapy could be applied to many interventions: drug therapy, manual therapy, exercise therapy. All involve the use of an intervention to achieve a physiological shift or change. It is this change that is the therapeutic tool. The treatment – whether a drug and exercise, or the energy from a machine – is just a tool to stimulate the physiological change. Electrotherapy is therefore little different from manual therapy or anything else in the treatment realm. It is a tool that, when applied at the right time, at the right dose and for the right reason, has the capacity to be beneficial. Applied inappropriately, it is not at all surprising that is has the capacity to achieve nothing or in fact to make things worse. The skilful practitioner uses the available evidence combined with experience to make the best possible decision taking into account the psychosocial and holistic components of the problem – it is not a simple reductionist solution.

ELECTROTHERAPEUTIC WINDOWS

Windows of opportunity are topical in many areas of medical practice and are not a new phenomenon at all. It has long been recognised that the 'amount' of a treatment is a critical parameter. This is no less true for electrotherapy than for other interventions. Literally hundreds of research papers illustrate that the same modality applied in the same circumstances, but at a different 'dose', will produce a different outcome. The illustrations used in this section are deliberately taken from cell, animal and clinical research studies with various modalities to illustrate the breadth of the principle. Furthermore, the examples used are not intended to criticise the researchers reporting these results. Knowing where the window 'is not' is possibly as important as knowing where it is.

Given the research evidence, there appear to be several aspects to this issue. Using a very straightforward model, there is substantial evidence, for example, that there is an *amplitude window* or *strength window*. An energy delivered at a particular amplitude has a beneficial effect, whereas the same energy at a lower amplitude might have no demonstrable effect. The laser example above is a simple extension of this case – one level will produce a distinct cellular response whereas a higher dose can be considered to be destructive. Karu (1987) demonstrated and reported these principles related to laser energy and the research produced since has served to reinforce the concept (Vinck et al 2003).

There are many examples of amplitude windows in the electrotherapy-related literature, and in some instances, the researchers have not set out to evaluate window effects but have none the less demonstrated their existence. Papers by Larsen et al (2005) measuring ultrasound parameter manipulation in tendon healing, Aaron et al (1999) investigating electromagnetic field strengths, Goldman et al (1996) considering the effects of electrical stimulation in chronic wound healing, Rubin et al (1989) investigating electromagnetic field strength and osteoporosis and Cramp et al (2002) comparing different forms of TENS and its influence on local blood flow all provide evidence in this field.

Along similar lines, *frequency windows* are also apparent. A modality applied at a specific frequency (pulsing regimen) might have a measurable benefit, whereas the same modality applied using a different pulsing profile might not appear to achieve equivalent results.

Electrical stimulation frequency windows have been proposed and there is clinical and laboratory evidence to suggest that there are frequency-dependent responses in clinical practice. TENS applied at frequency X appears to have a different

outcome to TENS applied at frequency Y in an equivalent patient population. Studies by Han et al (1991), Kararmaz et al (2004) and Sluka et al (2005) are among the many that have demonstrated frequency-dependent effects of TENS. Several authors have appeared to demonstrate that frequency parameters are possibly less critical, especially in clinical practice, and Chapters 16 and 17, on TENS and interferential therapy, include useful discussion on these issues. Frequency windows are not confined to TENS treatments and there are examples from other areas, including electromagnetic fields (Blackman et al 1988), ultrasound (Schafer et al 2005) and interferential (Noble et al 2000).

A simple therapeutic windows model is illustrated in Figure 1.2, using amplitude and frequency as the critical parameters. The figure shows that the 'ideal' treatment dose would be that combination of modality amplitude and frequency that focuses on the central effective zone. It can be suggested (from the evidence) that if the right amplitude and the right frequency are applied at the same time, then the maximally beneficial effect will be achieved. Unfortunately, there are clearly more ways to get this combination 'wrong' than 'right'. A modality applied at a less than ideal dose will not achieve best results. Again, this does not mean that the modality is ineffective, but more likely, that the ideal window has been missed. The same principle can be applied across many, if not all areas of therapy.

In Figure 1.3, the most effective treatment window (black box, lower central) has clearly been

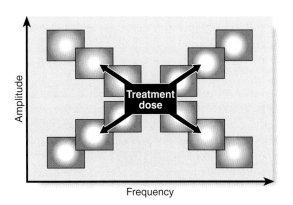

Figure 1.2 Basic windows of opportunity.

missed by the delivered treatment (upper left) and hence whatever the effect of the therapy, it will fail to be maximally effective.

The situation is complicated by the apparent capacity of the windows to 'move' with the patient's condition. The position of the therapeutic window in the acute scenario appears to be different from the window position for the patient with a chronic version of the same problem. A treatment dose that might be very effective for an acute problem may fail to be beneficial with a chronic presentation.

In Figure 1.4, the effective 'acute window' shown in the left-hand picture is in a different position to the most effective 'chronic window' shown in the right-hand picture.

Given the rapidly increasing complexity seen in this simple two-parameter model (amplitude and frequency) with two levels of condition (acute and chronic), it is easy to see how difficult clinical reality might be. As the volume of published work continues to increase, new results can be included in the existing framework, and this helps to identify where the windows are (positive research outcomes) and where they are not (negative outcomes). If this methodology is pursued, it is interesting to note how the effective treatments cluster when plotted, adding weight to the therapeutic windows theory.

Assuming that there are likely to be more than two variables to the real-world model, some complex further work needs to be invoked. There is almost certainly an energy- or time-based window (e.g. Hill et al 2002) and then another factor based on treatment frequency (number of sessions a week or treatment intervals). Work continues in our own, and other, research units to identify the more and less critical parameters for each modality across a range of clinical presentations.

One research style that has proved to be helpful in this context is to test a treatment on non-injured subjects in the laboratory using a variety of doses, and then to take the same protocol out into the clinical environment and repeat the testing procedure with real patients with particular clinical problems. Preliminary results indicate that there are distinct differences between the responses on 'normal' and 'injured' tissues at equivalent doses and further work is essential to maximise our understanding of these behaviours. Research that demonstrates significant effect in a laboratory study might, or might not, transfer directly to

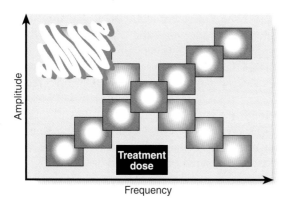

Figure 1.3 Treatment dose 'missing' the window.

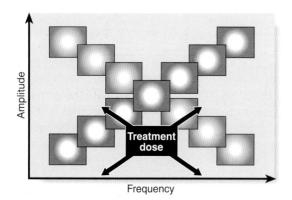

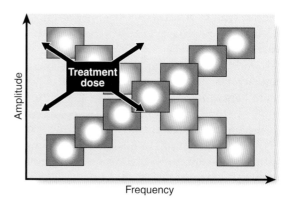

Figure 1.4 Moving acute (A) and chronic (B) windows.

the clinical environment. Recent work with pulsed shortwave therapy (Al Mandil & Watson 2006) clearly demonstrated a different magnitude of physiological effect when the same 'treatment' was delivered to asymptomatic subjects in the laboratory and real patients in a clinical setting: the physiological changes were similar, but of a different magnitude.

CLINICAL DECISION MAKING IN ELECTROTHERAPY

When it comes to making a clinical decision with regard to electrotherapy as a component of treatment (and taking into account the preceding sections), it can be seen that the effects of the intervention appear to be both modality and dose dependent (at least to some extent), and thus both elements need to be taken into account. The first decision needs to be with regards to the modality, as this is the primary concern; the secondary decision, although still of importance is that of dosage.

This having been said, it is important to remember that the use of electrotherapy in clinical practice is a matter if its integration into the whole treatment programme. Rarely is electrotherapy alone the most beneficial way forward. There are times when this might be the case, but they are the exception rather than the rule. Some patients would gain nothing significant from the addition of a modality into their treatment programme, whereas others would derive considerable gains. Electrotherapy has, in the past, probably been an overused intervention. Its current incorporation into clinical practice is more evidence based and selective, and hence should be more effective.

The detailed chapters in this text examine the evidence base for each of the modalities covered and, within that evidence, the areas where the modality has the capacity to be effective and those where there is insufficient evidence at the present time. A commonly cited phrase that is important in this context relates to the difference between a *lack of evidence* as opposed to an *evidence of lack*; in other words, there are many areas of practice, including several areas in electrotherapy, where there is a substantial lack of evidence – it is simply not there – whereas in other areas there is evidence that demonstrates a lack of effect. In the former circumstance, the clinician might have to make a clinical decision based on experience and expert opinion in the absence of published research. In the latter circumstances, the clinician who takes account of the available evidence would refrain from adopting that particular clinical approach in favour of another.

If it were simply a matter of learning a set of rules or guidelines, the use of electrotherapy in practice might appear to be somewhat simpler but, in reality, there are (at present at least) no rule sets that would govern any possible clinical scenario, and therefore clinical decision making remains an art with a scientific bias, or a science with an integrated art, depending on which philosophy you follow. Whichever one of these it is, the employment of electrotherapy into current clinical practice cannot be reduced to a simple rule set, and possibly it never will. The evidence will continue to close the gaps, although, inevitably, by closing down one gap, another will become apparent, and hence further research will be needed.

The individual chapters in this text aim to identify the key issues about each modality, examine the evidence for their effects and relate this to clinical practice. None of the chapters aims to provide clinical recipes, but will enable practitioners to evaluate the available evidence in order to facilitate their clinical decision making.

CONCLUSION

Incorporation of electrotherapy modalities into clinical intervention programmes can result in significant benefit for the patient. Used unwisely, it is at best an inefficient use of resources and at worst, can easily have effects that are neither wanted nor beneficial. Critical clear thinking, an understanding of the capacity of the various modalities to influence the tissues combined with the joined-up thinking that links this aspect of practice with others such as manual therapy and exercise therapy can result in gains for the patient. Patients who are routinely denied electrotherapy because the clinician does not believe it to be effective would seem, based on the evidence presented in this text, to be denied potential benefit.

References

Aaron RK, Ciombor DM, Keeping H et al (1999) Power frequency fields promote cell differentiation coincident with an increase in transforming growth factor-beta(1) expression. *Bioelectromagnetics* **20**(7): 453–458.

Al Mandil M, Watson T (2006) An evaluative audit of patient records in electrotherapy with specific reference to pulsed short wave therapy (PSWT). *Int J Ther Rehab* **13**(9): 414–419.

Blackman CF, Benane SG, Elliott DJ et al (1988) Influence of electromagnetic fields on the efflux of calcium ions from brain tissue in vitro: a three-model analysis consistent with the frequency response up to 510 Hz. *Bioelectromagnetics* **9**(3): 215–227.

Cramp FL, McCullough GR, Lowe AS et al (2002) Transcutaneous electric nerve stimulation: the effect of intensity on local and distal cutaneous blood flow and skin temperature in healthy subjects. *Arch Phys Med Rehab* **83**(1): 5–9.

Goldman R, Pollack S (1996) Electric fields and proliferation in a chronic wound model. *Bioelectromagnetics* **17**(6): 450–457.

Han JS, Chen XH, Sun SL et al (1991) Effect of low- and high-frequency TENS on Met-enkephalin-Arg-Phe and dynorphin A immunoreactivity in human lumbar CSF. *Pain* **47**(3): 295–298.

Hill J, Lewis M, Mills P et al (2002) Pulsed short-wave diathermy effects on human fibroblast proliferation. *Arch Phys Med Rehab* **83**(6): 832–836.

Kararmaz A, Kaya S, Karaman H et al (2004) Effect of the frequency of transcutaneous electrical nerve stimulation on analgesia during extracorporeal shock wave lithotripsy. *Urolol Res* **32**(6): 411–415.

Karu TI (1987) Photobiological fundamentals of low power laser therapy. *J Quant Electron QE* **23**(10): 1703–1717.

Larsen A, Kristensen G, Thorlacius-Ussing O et al (2005) The influence of ultrasound on the mechanical properties of healing tendons in rabbits. *Acta Orthopaed* **76**(2): 225–230.

Noble JG, Henderson G, Cramp AF et al (2000) The effect of interferential therapy upon cutaneous blood flow in humans. *Clin Physiol* **20**(1): 2–7.

Rubin CT, McLeod KJ, Lanyon LE et al (1989) Prevention of osteoporosis by pulsed electromagnetic fields. *J Bone Joint Surg* (Am) **71**(3): 411–417.

Schafer S, Kliner S, Klinghammer L et al (2005) Influence of ultrasound operating parameters on ultrasound-induced thrombolysis in vitro. *Ultrasound Med Biol* **31**(6): 841–847.

Sluka KA, Vance CG, Lisi TL et al (2005) High-frequency, but not low-frequency, transcutaneous electrical nerve stimulation reduces aspartate and glutamate release in the spinal cord dorsal horn. *J Neurochem* **95**(6): 1794–1801.

Vinck EM, Cagnie BJ, Cornelissen MJ et al (2003) Increased fibroblast proliferation induced by light emitting diode and low power laser irradiation. *Lasers Med Sci* **18**(2): 95–99.

Chapter 2

Electrophysical and thermal principles

Gail ter Haar

INTRODUCTION

Electrophysical agents are used by physiotherapists to treat a wide variety of conditions. These agents include both electromagnetic and sound waves, in addition to muscle- and nerve-stimulating currents. In part, these techniques are used to induce tissue heating. This chapter contains, in simple terms, an introduction to the effects of heat on tissue and the basic physics necessary for the understanding of the remainder of the book. The electrical properties of cells and the implications for electrotherapy are described in Chapter 3.

For centuries, early philosophers have speculated on the nature of heat and cold. Opinions have been divided as to whether heat was a substance or an effect of the motion of particles, but in the eighteenth century, physicists and physical chemists came to the conclusion that what gave our senses the impression of heat or cold was the speed of motion of the constituent molecules within the body or object. An accurate investigation of the relationship between the work done in driving an apparatus designed to churn water, and the heat developed while doing so, was undertaken by Dr JP Joule of Manchester in the year 1840. He showed quite clearly that the amount of heat produced by friction depended on the amount of work done. Subsequently, his work also contributed to the theory of the correlation of forces and, in 1847, he stated the law of the conservation of energy (the basis of the first law of thermodynamics).

It became the accepted view that heat can be regarded as a form of energy which is interchangeable with other forms such as electrical or mechanical energy. The theory supposed that, when a body is heated, the rise in temperature is due to the increased energy of motion of molecules in that body. The theory went further and explained the transmission of radiant energy from one body to another, as from the sun to an individual on earth. Evidence was found in favour of the supposition that light is an electromagnetic wave, and exactly the same evidence was adduced with regard to radiant energy. Apart from the fact that radiant heat waves (e.g. infrared radiations) have a longer wavelength than light waves, their physical characteristics are the same. It was therefore suggested that molecules of a hot body are in a state of rapid vibration, or are the centre of rapid periodic disturbances, producing electromagnetic waves, and that these waves travel between the hot body and the receiving body, causing a similar motion in the molecules. The sensation of heat may thus be excited in an organism by waves of radiant heat energy which emanate from a hot object, just as the sense of sight is excited by waves of light which arise from a luminous object.

An understanding of wave motion is central to getting to grips with the physics of any form of therapy that uses either electrical or mechanical energy. A general description of wave motion therefore precedes more detailed treatment of electricity and magnetism, and of ultrasound here.

WAVE MOTION

Wave motion transfers energy from one place to another. Think of a cork floating in a pond into which a stone is dropped. Ripples move out from where the stone enters the water and some of the stone's energy is transferred to the pond's edge. The cork bobs up and down but does not move within the pond.

An easy way to demonstrate wave motion is to use a Slinky spring toy. Two types of wave exist: *transverse waves*, which can be mimicked by raising and lowering one end of the spring rapidly, as shown in Figure 2.1, and *longitudinal waves*, which can be demonstrated by extending the spring along its length and then letting it go (Fig. 2.2). Water waves, the motion of a violin string and electromagnetic waves – as used in short-wave

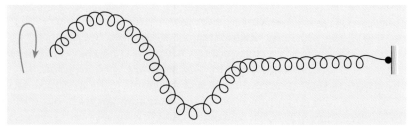

Transverse wave

Figure 2.1 If a spring that is attached at one end is flicked up and down, a transverse wave is produced.

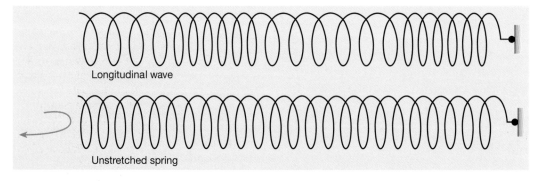

Longitudinal wave

Unstretched spring

Figure 2.2 Extending a spring along its length and letting it go again produces a longitudinal wave.

diathermy, infrared and interferential current therapy – are examples of transverse waves. Sound, as used in ultrasound therapy, propagates mainly as longitudinal waves.

It is much more difficult to picture a longitudinal wave than a transverse wave. If the spring with the wave travelling down it (Fig. 2.2) is compared with an unstretched spring, some regions can be seen where the coils are closer together, and other regions where the coils are further apart. The part of the spring where the coils are closely spaced is called a region of *compression*, and the region where they are separated more widely, is the *rarefaction* region.

Waves on the sea are generally described in terms of peaks and troughs. The movement up to a wave crest, down to a trough, and back up to the crest again is known as a *cycle of oscillation*. A cork floating in the sea bobs up and down as the waves go past. The difference in height of the cork between a crest and a trough is twice the *amplitude*. Perhaps a simpler way of visualising the amplitude is as the difference in water height above the seabed between a flat, calm sea and the crest of the wave. The number of wave crests passing the cork in a second is the wave *frequency* (f). Frequency is measured in *hertz* (Hz), where 1 Hz is 1 cycle/second. The time that elapses between two adjacent wave crests passing the cork is the *period* (τ) of the oscillation. This has units of time: if each cycle takes t seconds, there must be 1/t cycles in each second. The number of cycles that occur in a second has already been defined as the frequency, and so can be written as follows:

$$f = 1/\tau \qquad [1]$$

$$\tau = 1/f \qquad [2]$$

The distance between two adjacent wave crests is the *wavelength* (λ).

Figure 2.3A and B show a wave frozen at two moments, a short time apart. It can be seen that the different points on the wave have changed position relative to the central line but have not moved in space. In fact, if you tracked the motion of point A over several periods, the movement up and down would look like the picture shown in Figure 2.3C. The speed at which the wave crests move is known as the wave *speed*. As the wave moves a wavelength (λ) in one cycle, and as one cycle takes a time equal to the period t, then the wave speed (c) is given by the equation:

$$c = \lambda/t \qquad [3]$$

It is known that 1/t is the same as the frequency f, and so:

$$c = f\lambda \qquad [4]$$

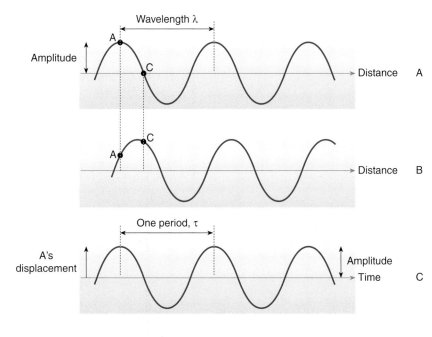

Figure 2.3 A and B, the position of two points A and C in the path of a wave as it passes through. The displacements shown are frozen at two different times, between which the wave has moved on a fraction of a wavelength. C, the displacement of the point during two cycles.

In Figure 2.4, points A and B on the wave (or, equally, A^1 and B^1) are moving in the same way and will reach the crest (or trough) together. These points are said to be in *phase* with each other. The

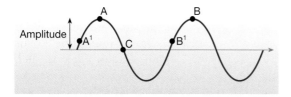

Figure 2.4 Points A and B, and also A^1 and B^1, are always in the same relative position in the wave. They are in phase. Points A and C are out of phase.

movement from A to B (or A^1 to B^1) represents one cycle of the wave motion. A and C, however, are not in phase: C is a quarter of a cycle ahead of A and they are said to have a *phase difference* (ϕ) of a quarter cycle. Phase is usually expressed as an angle, where a complete cycle is 2π radians (or 360°). A quarter cycle therefore represents a phase difference of $\pi/2$ radians (90°). This is illustrated in Figure 2.5.

REFLECTION AND REFRACTION OF WAVES

When waves travelling through a medium arrive at the surface between two media, some of the energy is reflected back into the first medium and some is

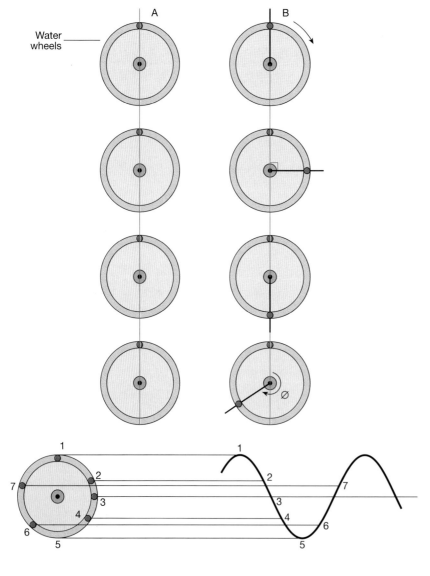

Figure 2.5 The phase angle can be likened to the turning of a water wheel. Imagine two wheels, A and B, both with a mark on their rim.
A does not move but B turns and, as it does, the rim mark executes the circles, each complete turn representing one *cycle*. The angle through which the mark turns in one cycle is 360° (2π radians). Thus, for example, compared with A, when the mark on B's rim has moved around a quarter of a turn (cycle), the angle between the two marks is a quarter of 360° (90° or $\pi/2$ radians); after half a turn, the angle between the two marks is 180° or π radians. This angle between the two marks is analogous to the *phase difference*. As B rotates, the height of the mark above the wheel's hub varies. If the wheel turns at a constant speed, then the mark's height traces out a *sine wave* when plotted against time.

transmitted through into the second medium. The proportion of the total energy that is reflected is determined by the properties of the two media involved. Figure 2.6 shows what happens when waves are reflected by a flat (plane) surface. An imaginary line that is perpendicular to the surface is called the *normal*. The *law of reflection* states that the angle between the incident (incoming) wave and the normal is always equal to the angle between the reflected wave and the normal. If the incident wave is at normal incidence (perpendicular to the surface), the wave is reflected back along its path.

The waves that are transmitted into the second medium may also undergo *refraction*. This is the bending of light towards the normal when it travels from one medium into one in which the wave speed is lower, or away from the normal when the wave speed in the second medium is higher (Fig. 2.7). For example, light bends towards the normal as it enters water from air since it travels more slowly in water than in air, and so a swimming pool may appear shallower than it really is.

As has been discussed earlier, waves carry energy. There are conditions, however, in which the transport of energy can be stopped, and the energy can be localised. This happens in a *standing (stationary) wave*. A standing wave is produced when an incident wave meets a returning reflected wave with the same amplitude. When the two waves meet, the total amplitude is the sum of the two individual amplitudes. Thus, as can be seen in Figure 2.8A, if the trough of one wave coincides with the crest of the other, the two waves cancel each other out. If, however, the crest of one meets the crest of the other, the wave motion is reinforced (Fig. 2.8B) and the total amplitude doubles. In the reinforced standing wave there are points that always have zero amplitude; these are called *nodes*. Similarly, there are points that always have the greatest amplitude, and these are called *antinodes*. Nodes and antinodes are shown in Figure 2.8B. The distance between adjacent nodes, or adjacent antinodes, is one-half of the wavelength ($\lambda/2$).

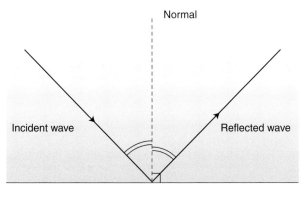

REFLECTION

Figure 2.6 The law of reflection states that the angle of incidence equals the angle of reflection.

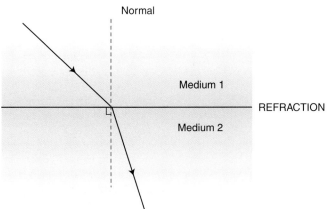

REFRACTION

Figure 2.7 When a beam passes from one medium to another it can be refracted (i.e. it changes its direction).

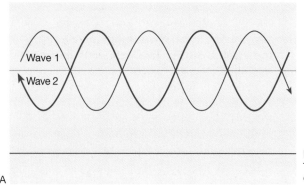

Resultant wave –
The two waves have
cancelled each other ou

A

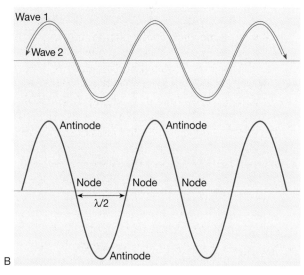

Resultant wave –
The two waves reinforce
each other

B

Figure 2.8 A standing wave is formed when two waves of equal amplitude travelling in opposite directions meet. A, the two waves cancel each other out; B, the two waves add to reinforce each other.

POLARISATION

When flicking the Slinky spring up and down to produce a transverse wave, one has an infinite number of choices as to the direction in which to move it, so long as the motion is at right angles to the line of the spring. If the spring is always moved in a fixed direction, the wave is said to be *polarised* – the waves are in that plane only. However, if the waves (or directions in which the spring is moved) are in a number of different directions, the waves are *unpolarised*. It is possible to polarise the waves by passing them through a filter that allows only waves that are in one plane through. This can be visualised by envisaging a piece of card with a long narrow slit in it. This will allow the waves formed in the plane of the slit to go through, but no others – the card therefore acts as a polarising filter.

ELECTRICITY AND MAGNETISM

Everyone is familiar with effects of electrical charges, even if they are not aware of their causes. The 'static' experienced when brushing newly washed hair, or undressing, and the electrical discharge obvious in lightning are examples of the effects of charges.

ELECTRICITY

Matter is made up of atoms, an atom being the smallest particle of an element that can be identified as being from that element. The atom consists of a positively charged central nucleus (made up of positively charged *protons* and uncharged *neutrons*), with negatively charged particles (*electrons*) orbiting around it, resembling a miniature solar system. An atom contains as many protons as there are electrons, and so has no net charge. If this balance is destroyed, the atom has a non-zero net charge and is called an *ion*. If an electron is removed from the atom it becomes a *positive ion*, and if an electron is added the atom becomes a *negative ion*.

Two particles of opposite charge attract each other, and two particles of the same charge repel each other (push each other away). Hence, an electron and a proton are attracted to each other, whereas two electrons repel each other.

The unit of charge is a *coulomb* (C). An electron has a charge of 1.6×10^{-19} C, so it takes a very large number (6.2×10^{18}) of electrons to make up one coulomb.

The force between two particles of charge q_1 and q_2 is proportional to the product of q_1 and q_2 ($q_1 \times q_2$), and inversely proportional to the distance between them (d) squared (Fig. 2.9). Thus, the force is proportional to $q_1 q_2 / d^2$. The constant of proportionality (i.e. the invariant number) necessary to allow one to calculate the force between two charges is $1/4\pi\varepsilon$, where ε is the *permittivity* of the medium containing the two charges:

$$F = q_1 q_2 / 4\pi\varepsilon d^2 \qquad [5]$$

If one of the charges is negative, then the force is attractive. If the particles are in a vacuum, the permittivity used is ε_0; this is known as the *permittivity of free space*. For a medium other than a vacuum, the permittivity is often quoted as a multiple of ε_0, where the multiplying factor, κ, is known as the *relative permittivity* or *dielectric constant*. So:

$$\varepsilon = \kappa\varepsilon_0, \text{ or} \qquad [6a]$$

$$\kappa = \varepsilon / \varepsilon_0 \qquad [6b]$$

Electric fields

An *electric field* exists around any charged particle. If a smaller charge that is free to move is placed in the field, the paths it will move along are called *lines of force* (or *field lines*). Examples of fields and their patterns are shown in Figure 2.10.

The *electric field strength*, *E*, is defined as the force per unit charge on a particle placed in the field. A little thought shows that $E = F/q$, where F

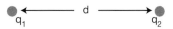

Figure 2.9 Two particles of charge q_1 and q_2 a distance of *d* apart experience a force between them that is proportional to $q_1 q_2 / d^2$.

is the force and q is the particle's charge. The units used to describe E are newtons/coulomb (N/C).

If E is the same throughout a field, it is said to be uniform. In this case, the field lines are parallel to each other as shown in Figure 2.10D. If a charged particle is moved in this field, work is done on it, unless it moves perpendicular to the field lines. This is somewhat analogous to moving a ball around on Earth. If the ball is always kept at the same height, and moved horizontally, its potential energy remains constant. If the ball is raised or lowered, its potential energy is changed. The ball has no potential energy when it lies on the ground. In a non-uniform field where the lines are not parallel, moving a charged particle always results in a change of potential energy. The *electric potential, V,* is defined as the potential energy per unit charge of a positively charged particle placed at that point. Electric potential is measured in units of *volts*. As the position at which the electric potential energy is zero is taken as infinity, another way of thinking of the electrical potential at a point is as the work done in moving the charge to that point from infinity. In practice it is easier to compare the electrical potential at two points in the field than to consider infinity. The difference in the work required to move a charge from infinity to a point, A, and that required to move it to another point, B, is called the *potential difference* (p.d.) between the two points; this is also measured in *volts*. The p.d. is best thought of as a kind of pressure difference. Between the two points there will be a gradient in potential (just as there is a pressure gradient between the top and bottom of a waterfall). This gradient is described in units of volts/metre. In a uniform field between parallel plates with potential difference V, and separation d, the potential gradient is given by V/d. If a particle of charge q is moved from one plate to another, the work done is qV. Work is force × distance, and so the force, F, is given by:

$$F = qV/d \qquad [7]$$

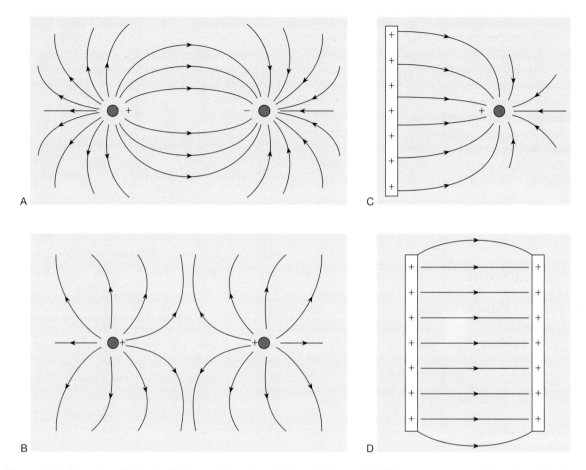

Figure 2.10 Examples of electric fields near charged particles and plates. A, field between two particles of equal and opposite charges; B, field between two positively charged particles; C, field between a charged particle and an oppositely charged plate; D, field between two oppositely charged plates.

As the electric field strength, E, is given by:

$$E = F/q \qquad [8]$$

it follows that:

$$E = V/d \qquad [9]$$

Remember that V/d is the potential gradient. From equation [9] we can see that the electric field strength can be increased by bringing the two plates closer together. Although the derivation is more complicated, the electric field strength at any point in a non-uniform field can also be shown to be the same as the potential gradient at that point.

Any electric circuit needs a supply of power to drive the electrons around the conductors. A power source has one positive and one negative terminal, and the source forces the electrons out from its negative terminal. Electrical energy can be produced within the source by a number of means. Dynamos convert mechanical energy into electrical energy, solar cells convert the sun's energy into electrical energy, and batteries convert chemical energy into electrical energy. The force acting on the electrons is called the *electromotive force* (e.m.f.). This is defined as the electrical energy produced per unit charge inside the source. The unit in which e.m.f. is measured is the volt, because 1 volt is 1 joule/coulomb.

Electric current

An *electric current* is the flow of electric charge (usually electrons). In some materials (e.g. metals) where the atoms are bound into a lattice structure, the charge is carried by electrons. In materials in which the atoms are free to move, the charge is carried by ions. A liquid in which the ions are the charge carriers is called an *electrolyte*. An *insulator* is a material that has no free charge carriers, and so is unable to carry an electric current. Current is measured using an ammeter, and the unit in which it is given is the *ampere*. An ampere represents 1 coulomb of charge flowing through a point in 1 second.

There are two types of electric current. A *direct current* (DC) is one in which the flow of electrons is in one direction only, and an *alternating current* (AC) is one in which the current flows first one way and then another. In considering electric circuits, it is easiest to think first of direct currents. A later section points to the differences between AC and DC circuits.

Resistance and Ohm's law

The flow of electric charge through a conductor is analogous to the flow of water through pipes. If water is pumped round the system, narrow pipes put up more resistance to flow than wide ones. Electrical conductors also put up a *resistance* to the flow of charge. As the charged particles move through a conductor they collide with other charge carriers and with the resident atoms; the constituents of the conductor thus impede the current flow.

Georg Ohm was able to demonstrate that the current flowing in a circuit is proportional to the potential difference across it. His law (*Ohm's law*), formally stated, is:

> The current flowing through a metallic conductor is proportional to the potential difference that exists across it, provided that all physical conditions remain constant.

So, $I \propto V$; this can also be written as $V \propto I$, where the constant of proportionality is the *resistance*, R. The equation resulting from Ohm's law is therefore:

$$V = IR \qquad [10]$$

R is measured in ohms (Ω). The ohm is defined as the resistance of a body such that a 1-volt potential difference across the body results in a current of 1 ampere through it.

The resistance of a piece of wire increases with its length, and decreases as its cross-sectional area increases. A property, the *resistivity*, is defined which is a property of the material only, and not of the material's shape. The resistance R of a piece of wire with resistivity ρ, length L and area A is given by:

$$R = \rho L / A \qquad [11]$$

When electrons flow through a conductor, they collide with the atoms in the conductor material and impart energy to those atoms. This leads to heating of the conductor. The unit used for measuring energy is the *joule*. It has been seen earlier (see equation [7]) that the potential difference measured in volts is the work done in moving a unit charge between two points. So it follows from this that since the potential difference is the work done per unit charge:

$$\text{volt} = \text{joule}/\text{coulomb} \qquad [12a]$$

and so:

$$\text{joule} = \text{volt coulomb} \qquad [12b]$$

The unit of power measurement is the *watt*. Power is the rate of doing work, so a watt is a joule/second. It follows from the equation above that:

$$1 \text{ watt} = 1 \text{ joule}/\text{second} \qquad [13a]$$
$$= 1 \text{ volt coulomb}/\text{second} \qquad [13b]$$

From the definition given it is known that a coulomb/second is an ampere. So, therefore:

$$1 \text{ watt} = 1 \text{ volt} \bullet \text{ampere} \qquad [14]$$

In other words, the electrical power developed in a circuit is given by:

$$\text{Power} = VI \qquad [15]$$

where V is in volts, I is in amperes, and the power is in watts.

From Ohm's law, substitutions can be made in this equation to express power in terms of different combinations of V, I and R. So:

$$W = VI \qquad [16a]$$
$$W = I^2 R \qquad [16b]$$
$$W = V^2 / R \qquad [16c]$$

are equivalent equations, where W is in watts, V is in volts and R is in ohms.

Capacitance

Any passive device capable of storing electric charge is called a *capacitor*. This is the electrical equivalent of a compressed spring, which stores energy until it is allowed to expand. A capacitor stores charge until it can release it by becoming part of a completed electrical circuit. If you apply an electric potential, V, between two plates of a capacitor, one plate becomes positively charged and the other becomes charged with an equal but opposite negative charge. If an insulating material, known as a *dielectric*, is placed between the plates, the capacity to store charge is increased. The *relative permittivity*, or *dielectric constant* mentioned earlier, has another definition: it is also the ratio of the charge that can be stored between two plates with a dielectric material between them, to that which can be stored without the dielectric.

A capacitor is drawn in a circuit diagram as a pair of vertical parallel lines. Its *capacitance, C,* is defined as the charge (Q) stored per unit potential difference across its plates.

$$C = Q/V \qquad [17]$$

As Q is measured in coulombs, and V is measured in volts, the unit for capacitance is the coulomb/volt, known as the *farad*. Commonly, the capacitance of a capacitor found in an electric circuit is a few micro- (10^{-6}) or pico- (10^{-12}) farads.

A capacitor is *charged* by applying a potential difference across its plates. It is *discharged* (i.e. the charge is allowed to flow away from the plates) by providing an electrical connection between the plates.

Electric circuits

The symbols used to denote different components used in electrical circuits are shown in Figure 2.11. Two electrical components are said to be in *series* if they carry the same current. The potential difference across a series of components is the sum of the potential differences across each one. The components are in *parallel* if they have the same potential difference across them. The current is then the sum of the currents flowing through them.

Resistors in series If several resistors are joined in series with each other, the same current flows

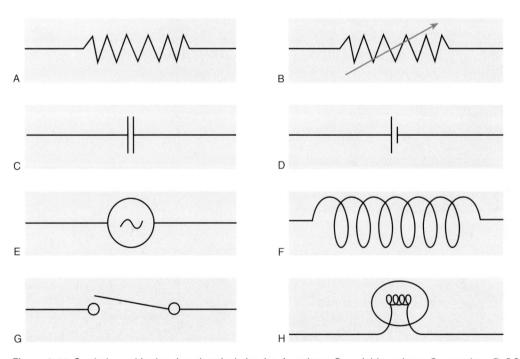

Figure 2.11 Symbols used in drawing electrical circuits. A, resistor; B, variable resistor; C, capacitor; D, DC source; E, AC source; F, inductance; G, switch; H, bulb.

through them all, since electrons cannot be lost on the way through. From Ohm's law, the potential, V_i across each resistance in Figure 2.12A, is given by:

$$V_i = IR_i \qquad [18]$$

If the total potential across the whole string is V, then:

$$V = V_1 + V_2 + V_3 + \cdots + V_i \qquad [19]$$

So:

$$V = IR_1 + IR_2 + IR_3 + \cdots + IR_i$$
$$= I[R_1 + R_2 + R_3 + \cdots + R_i] \qquad [20]$$

Thus the single resistance needed to have the same effect as the string of resistors, R_{total}, is the sum of all the resistances:

$$R_{total} = R_1 + R_2 + R_3 + \cdots + R_i \qquad [21]$$

For example, in the string shown in Figure 2.12B, the total resistance, R_{total}, is $2 + 5 + 10\,\Omega = 17\,\Omega$.

Resistors in parallel Resistors can also be wired up in parallel, as shown in Figure 2.13A. The electron flow splits up at A, electrons taking different routes to B where they join up again. The total flow of current through all resistors, I, is the same as the sum of the currents through each resistor:

$$I = I_1 + I_2 + I_3 + \cdots + I_i \qquad [22]$$

The potential difference across each resistor is identical. Using Ohm's law in the above equation, we can write:

$$I = V/R_1 + V/R_2 + V/R_3 + \cdots + V/R_i$$
$$= V[1/R_1 + 1/R_2 + 1/R_3 + \cdots + 1/R_i] \qquad [23]$$

Therefore the single resistance that could replace these parallel resistors has a value:

$$1/R_{total} = 1/R_1 + 1/R_2 + 1/R_3 + \cdots + 1/R_i \qquad [24]$$

For example, if three resistors of 2, 5 and 10 Ω are in parallel, as shown in Figure 1.13B, the equivalent

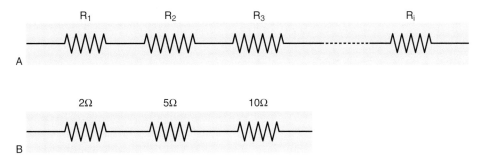

Figure 2.12 Resistors in series.

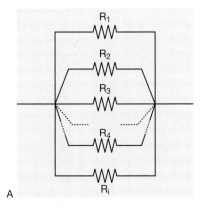

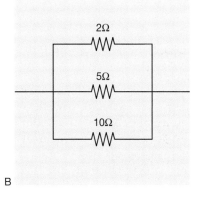

Figure 2.13 Resistors in parallel.

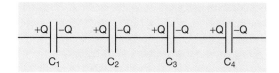

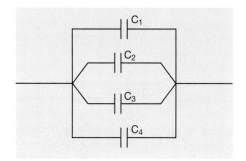

Figure 2.14 Capacitors in series.

Figure 2.15 Capacitors in parallel.

resistor to replace these is $1/(\{1/2\} + \{1/5\} + \{1/10\})$, which is $1/(0.5 + 0.2 + 0.1) = 1/0.8 = 1.25\,\Omega$.

Capacitors in series A voltage applied across four capacitors in series induces charges of $+Q$ and $-Q$ on the plates of each (Fig. 2.14). Using equation [17] we know that:

$$1/C = V/Q$$

The potential difference across the series row is the sum of the potentials across each capacitor, and so the single capacitance, C, equivalent to the four capacitors C_1, C_2, C_3 and C_4 is given by:

$$1/C = [V_1 + V_2 + V_3 + V_4]/Q \qquad [25]$$

$$= V_1/Q + V_2/Q + V_3/Q + V_4/Q$$

$$= 1/C_1 + 1/C_2 + 1/C_3 + 1/C_4 \qquad [26]$$

If the capacitances are 2, 1, 5 and 10 µF, then $C = 0.56\,\mu F$.

Capacitors in parallel If capacitors are connected in parallel (Fig. 2.15), the total charge developed on them is the sum of the charges on each of them. The current is never negative. The potential difference is the same across all the capacitors.

The effective capacitance of all the capacitors put together is given by the expression:

$$C = Q/V$$

where:

$$Q = Q_1 + Q_2 + Q_3 + Q_4$$

and so:

$$C = Q_1/V + Q_2/V + Q_3/V + Q_4/V \qquad [27]$$

$$= C_1 + C_2 + C_3 + C_4 \qquad [28]$$

If the capacitances are 1, 2, 5 and 10 µF, then C is 18 µF.

Direct and alternating current

As discussed earlier, two types of electric current exist: direct current (DC) and alternating current (AC). The most common type of alternating current has a sinusoidal waveform, such as that found in the electricity mains. For sinusoidal AC, the relationships between frequency and period, etc., defined in the first section hold true. The variation of current can be described by the relationship:

$$I = I_0 \sin[2\pi ft] \qquad [29]$$

and, similarly, the voltage is described by:

$$V = V_0 \sin[2\pi ft] \qquad [30]$$

where $\sin[2\pi ft]$ is the expression that tells you that the wave form is a sine wave of frequency f, and I_0 and V_0 are the maximum values of current and voltage (the amplitude of the oscillation). Clearly, the average current over one cycle in Figure 2.16 is zero – the current is positive as much as it is negative – and the same applies to the voltage.

In some instances, an alternating current may be *rectified*, as shown in Figure 2.16B and C. Here, the average current is clearly not zero. For *half-wave rectification*, the average current is $0.318I_0$, and for *full-wave rectification* the average current is $0.636I_0$.

If an alternating current flows through a resistor the average current is zero, but the heating effect is not. On each pass through the resistor, the electrons heat it slightly, whatever the direction of flow. Clearly, despite the zero net current, some energy is expended in the circuit, and an *effective current* is defined to account for this. The effective current (also known as the *root mean square (RMS) current*, I_{RMS}), is the value of the constant current that if allowed to flow for the same length of time would expend the same amount of electrical energy for a fixed voltage as the alternating current. An *effective*

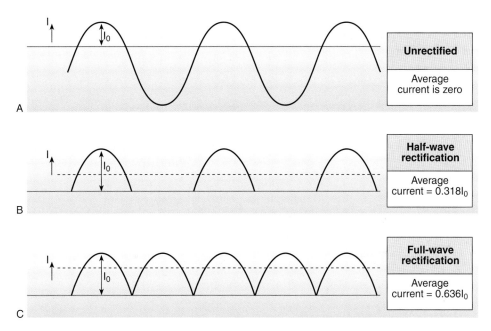

Figure 2.16 Rectification of an alternating current. A, unrectified wave; B, half-wave rectification; C, full-wave rectification.

voltage (*root mean square* (*RMS*) *voltage*, V_{RMS}) is defined in a similar way as the constant voltage that, if present for the same length of time, would expend the same amount of electrical energy for a fixed voltage as the alternating voltage.

From equation [16] the power, W, in DC circuits is given by:

$$W = VI$$

where W is in watts, V is in volts, and I is in amperes. Similarly, in an AC circuit:

$$W = V_{RMS}I_{RMS} \tag{31}$$

Ohm's law can be used if the effective currents and voltages are used. Thus the power may also be written:

$$W = I_{eff}^2 R \tag{32}$$

or

$$W = V_{eff}^2/R \tag{33}$$

It can be shown that $I_{eff} = I_0/\sqrt{2} = 0.707I_0$ and that $V_{eff} = V_0/v2 = 0.707V_0$.

Capacitors allow alternating currents to flow. The resistance across capacitor plates is known as *impedance* (*Z*). This is defined as the ratio of the amplitudes of the voltage and current in the same way as resistance is given by V/R for direct current. It can be shown that:

$$Z = 1/\omega C \tag{34}$$

where C is the capacitance and ω (the *angular frequency*) $= 2\pi f$.

MAGNETISM

Most of us have used a compass, and know that the needle swings around to point North–South. The compass is a permanent bar magnet that aligns itself with the earth's magnetic field.

There are two magnetic poles: the North pole and the South pole. In many ways, the two poles of a magnet act in the same way as opposite electric charges. Like magnetic poles repel each other, and unlike poles attract. There is a force between two magnets a distance d apart from each other, and the equation describing this force is very similar to that in equation [5]:

$$F = m_1 m_2/4\pi\mu d^2 \tag{35}$$

Here, μ is the *permeability* of the medium, μ_0 (the permeability of free space) is used when the magnets lie in a vacuum. The strength of a magnet is measured in units of *webers* (Wb). The unit of permeability is the *henry/metre* (H/m). *Relative permeability, m_r,* is defined by the relationship:

$$\mu_r = \mu/\mu_0 \qquad [36]$$

A *magnetic field* exists at a point if a small magnet put there experiences a force. It will line up along the *magnetic field lines*. The fields around some permanent magnets are shown in Figure 2.17.

The number of magnetic lines of force passing through an area, A, is known as the *magnetic flux* (N). The magnetic flux going through a unit area that is aligned perpendicular to the field is the *magnetic flux density* (B). Magnetic flux density is measured in units of *teslas* (T); 1 tesla = $1\,\text{Wb}/\text{m}^2$.

Electromagnetism

Wires carrying an electric current produce magnetic fields around them. The magnetic field around a long straight wire forms a series of concentric circles with the wire at their centre. A solenoid (i.e. a coil of wire) creates a field somewhat similar to that produced by a permanent bar magnet, the main difference being that there is a uniform field inside it. This uniformity of field is used to advantage in short-wave diathermy applications. Figure 2.18 illustrates these fields.

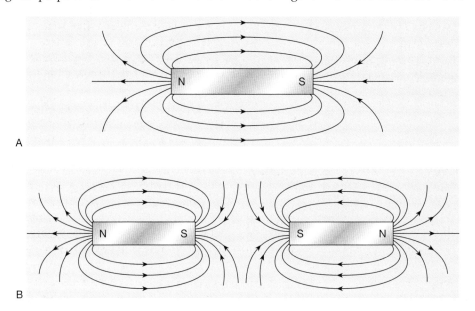

Figure 2.17 A, magnetic field around a single permanent bar magnet; B, magnetic field around two bar magnets.

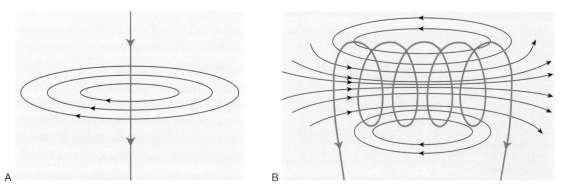

Figure 2.18 A, magnetic field around a long straight wire carrying an electric current; B, magnetic field around a coil carrying an electric current.

The electromagnetic spectrum Light is a form of electromagnetic radiation. It can be split up into its different component parts using a prism, with each colour of the 'rainbow' having a different wavelength. Electromagnetic waves are electrical and magnetic fields that travel together through space without the need for a carrier medium (Fig. 2.19). They travel at a speed of 33.10^8m/s in a vacuum. There is a whole spectrum of such waves of which light is only a small part. Other radiations in the electromagnetic spectrum include radio waves, microwaves and X-rays; the spectrum is shown in Figure 2.20. The behaviour of electromagnetic radiation can be usefully described, not only in terms of wave motion, but also in terms of 'particles'. It can be thought of as discrete 'packets' of energy and momentum, sometimes referred to as *quanta*. The energy in joules of a quantum of radiation is determined by its frequency, v, and is given by the equation:

$$E = hv \hspace{4cm} [37]$$

where h is *Planck's constant* ($h = 6.62 \times 10^{-34}$J). It is more usual to quote electromagnetic energies in *electron-volts* (eV); 1 eV $= 1.6 \times 1.10^{-13}$ J. It can be seen from Figure 2.20 that energies at the long-wavelength end of the spectrum are very small. It is generally thought that energies at excess of 30 eV are required to ionise atoms, and so this allows the spectrum to be classified into two bands: ionising and non-ionising radiation.

The wavelength of the radiation determines the size of objects with which it will interact. A wave with a wavelength of 100 m (a radio wave) will not 'see' something of the size of an atom and will pass by undisturbed. However, a wave with a wavelength of 10^{-12}m (a gamma ray) will interact with the atomic nucleus, with which it is a comparable size. Infrared radiation is a wavelength comparable to the size of atoms or molecules and so can interact with them, imparting kinetic energy (heat).

Electromagnetic induction The dynamo on a bicycle wheel that is used to power the bicycle's lights makes use of electromagnetic induction. Electromagnetic induction is in many ways the reverse of electromagnetism. When a magnet and a conducting wire move relative to one another, a current is induced in the wire. In the bicycle wheel, a magnet is made to rotate near a fixed coil of wire that forms part of a circuit that includes the lamp bulb. Current is induced in the wire and the lamp is lit.

The electrons in the wire approaching (or being approached by) a magnetic field experience a force as they enter the field. All of the electrons are displaced towards one end of the wire, and so that end becomes negatively charged. Conversely, the other end takes up a positive charge. An electromotive force is therefore induced between the two ends, and, if the circuit is completed, a current will flow. If the wire is coiled, the induced current is increased. A coil of conducting wire used in this way is called an *inductor*. The e.m.f. induced in the conductor equals the rate of change of flux linkage – this is *Faraday's law* of electromagnetic induction. The

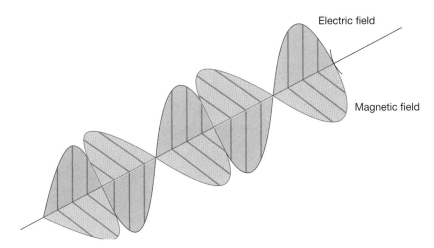

Electric field

Magnetic field

Figure 2.19 An electromagnetic wave; the electric and magnetic fields travel together.

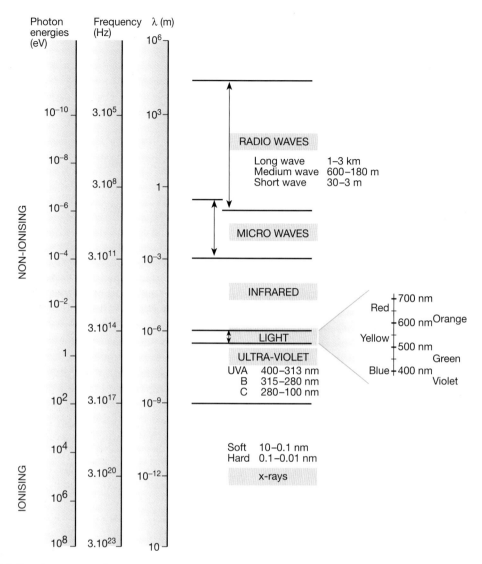

Figure 2.20 The electromagnetic spectrum.

direction of the induced current is always such that it opposes the change that caused it: *Lenz's law*. In this sense, inductors act as resistances in circuits; they are often used to block changing voltages while allowing steady (DC) voltages through.

An inductor (L) and capacitor (C) are sometimes used in series or in parallel to produce *LC-tuned* circuits (Fig. 2.21). It can be shown that these circuits have a resonant frequency, *f*, such that series LC-tuned circuits offer a very low impedance to waves of that frequency, but an extremely high impedance to everything else, whereas parallel LC-tuned circuits offer a very high resistance to waves of frequency *f* and allow other frequencies through. They therefore act as filters. The resonant frequency is given by the equation:

$$f = 1/2\pi r(LC)$$ [38]

Mutual induction

A changing magnetic field from a current-carrying conductor can induce an e.m.f. and current in a second conductor nearby. This current will vary, and in its turn can produce its own varying magnetic

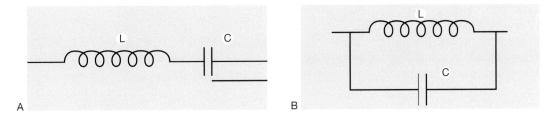

A

B

Figure 2.21 LC-tuned circuits. A, series LC circuit; B, parallel LC circuit.

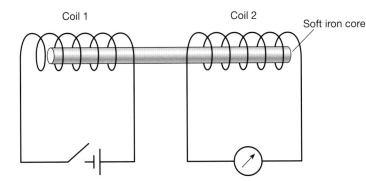

Figure 2.22 Mutual induction. The changing magnetic field in one coil can induce a current in a second coil. The magnetic field thus created will create a current in the first coil. A soft iron core enhances this effect.

field that induces an e.m.f. and current in the first conductor. Each conductor therefore induces a current in the other (Fig. 2.22). This is called *mutual inductance*. The mutual inductance is 1 henry if 1 volt is induced in one conductor by a current change of 1 ampere per second in the other. An AC transformer makes use of mutual inductance.

Self-inductance

When a current is switched on in a coil, the growing current in the coil causes a change in magnetic flux in the coil. This, in turn, causes an e.m.f. that opposes the e.m.f. of the battery. This is called a *back e.m.f.* This effect is increased if there is a soft iron core in the coil.

A conductor has a self-inductance of 1 henry if a back e.m.f. of 1 volt is induced by a changing current of 1 ampere/second.

MECHANICAL WAVES

The most important mechanical wave used in physiotherapy is ultrasound. Sound waves differ from electromagnetic waves in one major way: the waves are a form of *mechanical energy* and, as such, cannot propagate through a vacuum. This is because energy passes through the medium by the movement of molecules, which transfer their momentum to their near neighbours in the direction of the wave. Sound is produced by a moving surface; this may be a diaphragm in a loudspeaker, for example, or a transducer front face in medical ultrasound. As the surface moves forward, it *compresses* the molecules immediately in front. These molecules in turn push forward against their neighbours in an attempt to restore their former arrangement, and these in turn push their neighbours. The compression therefore moves away from its source. If the surface now moves in the opposite direction, the density of the molecules is reduced next to it (a region of *rarefaction* is created), and so molecules move in to fill the space. This in turn leaves a low-density region which is immediately filled by more molecules, and so the rarefaction moves away from the source (Fig. 2.23). This type of wave is called a *longitudinal* wave because the displacement of the molecules is along the direction in which the wave moves.

ULTRASOUND

The velocity of sound in air is 330 m/s. The human ear can hear frequencies up to about 18 000 Hz

(18 kHz). The wavelength of audible sound (calculated using equation [4]) where the ear is most sensitive (about 1.6 kHz) is about 20 cm. At ultrasonic frequencies (above 18 kHz), the wavelength becomes so short that the sound does not travel far through air. (At 1.5 MHz, the wavelength is about 0.2 mm.) However, ultrasound will travel through water, a medium for which the sound velocity is 1500 m/s. At 1.5 MHz the wavelength in water is 1 mm. This fact is used in medicine since most body tissues are comprised mainly of water, and the millimetre wavelengths at the low megahertz frequencies used (0.75–10 MHz) are comparable with the size of the tissue structures with which interaction is required.

Ultrasound is generated from a *transducer*, i.e. a device that transforms one form of energy into another. The transducer most commonly used in ultrasound changes electrical energy into mechanical energy using the *piezoelectric effect*. A piezoelectric crystal has the property that if a voltage is applied across it, it will change its thickness, and alternatively if the crystal thickness is changed then a voltage develops across the crystal (this is the *inverse* piezoelectric effect). Thus, if an oscillating voltage is applied across the crystal it will alternately get thicker and thinner than its resting thickness, following the polarity of the voltage (see Fig. 2.23). As the front face of the transducer moves backwards and forwards, regions of compression and rarefaction move out from it, forming an ultrasonic wave. The piezoelectric material most commonly used for physiotherapy transducers is lead zirconate titanate (PZT).

The voltage across the ultrasound transducer may either be applied continuously over the whole treatment time (*continuous wave*, CW), or may be applied in bursts – on for a time, off for a time, and so on; this is known as *pulsed mode*. The wave trains for a continuous wave and a pulsed mode are shown in Figure 2.24.

In the pulsed mode, the pulsing regimen may be described in one of three ways (Figure 2.24B):

1. *x* seconds on; *y* seconds off

2. *m* : *s*, where *m* represents the 'mark' and *s* represents the 'space', where the ratio represents that of the on time to the off time; this is called the *mark* : *space ratio*. So, if the on-time is twice the off-time, *m* : *s* is 2 : 1. To discover the true

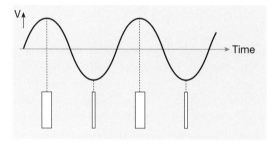

Figure 2.23 The piezoelectric effect. The crystal gets fatter and thinner, depending on the polarity of the voltage.

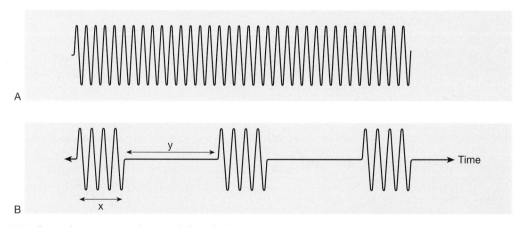

Figure 2.24 A, continuous wave ultrasound; B, pulsed ultrasound. In this example, the sound is on for *x* seconds and off for *y* seconds.

pulsing regimen, it is also necessary to know the pulse length

3. the *duty cycle*: this is the pulse length as a percentage of the total on and off time, so it is given by $x/(x + y) \times 100\%$.

Take, for example, a common pulsing regimen as shown in Figure 2.25. This may be described as 2 ms on : 8 ms off, as 1 : 4 mark : space ratio, pulse length 2 ms, or as a 20% ({2/10} × 100%) duty cycle. It is worth noting that, at 1 MHz, a pulse of length 2 ms contains 2000 cycles.

Intensity

The energy in an ultrasound wave is characterised by *intensity*. This is the energy crossing a unit area perpendicular to the wave in unit time; the units used are *watts/m²*. However, for clinical applications, the square metre is an inappropriately large area in terms of regions of the human body to be treated, and so the unit used in medical ultrasound is watts/cm² ($1 \, \text{W/m}^2 = 10^4 \, \text{W/cm}^2$).

Several types of intensity are used to describe ultrasound exposures. The field from a circular piezoelectric disc is complex. Near the transducer there are many peaks and troughs, but as the beam moves further from the transducer the field pattern becomes more uniform. The region near the transducer is known as the *near field* or *Fresnel zone*; the region beyond that is called the *far field* or *Fraunhoffer zone*. The boundary between the two zones is at a distance given by r^2/λ where r is the transducer radius and λ is the wavelength of the ultrasound. This is the position of the peak of intensity on the beam axis that is furthest from the transducer. Physiotherapy ultrasound commonly operates at 0.75, 1.0, 1.5 or 3 MHz. The extent of the near field is shown in Table 2.1 for a number of frequencies and transducer sizes. This demonstrates

that most physiotherapy ultrasound exposures are carried out in the near field, which has many peaks of intensity. It also indicates that a number of intensities need to be identified.

The transverse field profiles shown in Figure 2.26 illustrate the problem. Both profiles have the same peak intensity, I_0, but the levels are rather different if they are averaged over the whole beam. Peak levels are the most significant parameter if the beam is held stationary over one tissue volume for a long time, but if the transducer is kept in continuous motion the average value becomes more important since this is more representative of what the tissue will experience. In a continuous wave field, therefore, two intensities are defined, the *spatial peak intensity* (I_{SP}) and the *spatial average intensity* (I_{SA}).

Things become more complicated in a pulsed field. Here, the analogy is of a boy standing up to his ankles in the sea. As the waves come in, the water

Table 2.1 Extent of near field for different ultrasound transducers

Frequency (MHz)	r (cm)	r^2/λ (cm)
0.75	0.5	1.25
	1.0	5
	1.5	11.25
1.0	0.5	0.6
	1.0	6.7
	1.5	15
1.5	0.5	2.5
	1.0	10
	1.5	22.5
3.0	0.5	5
	1.0	20
	1.5	45

λ, ultrasonic wavelength; r, transducer radius.

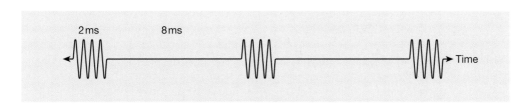

Figure 2.25 A typical physiotherapy pulsing regimen. λ, ultrasonic wavelength; r, transducer radius.

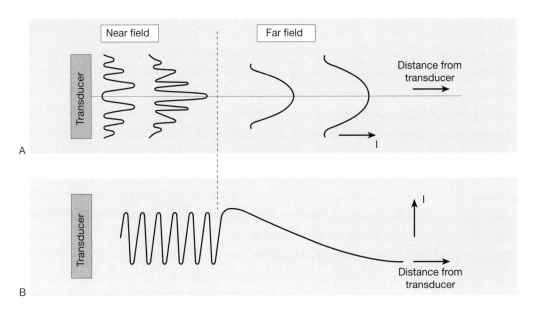

Figure 2.26 A, transverse intensity distributions at different distances from the transducer; B, intensity distribution on axis.

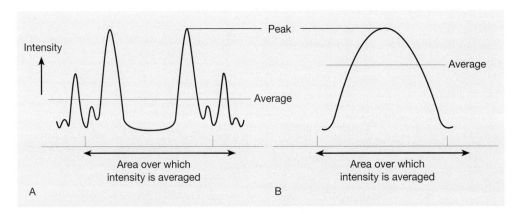

Figure 2.27 A, example of a transverse beam profile in the near field; B, transverse beam profile in the far field. This has the same peak intensity as the profile in A.

rises up his legs, and drops again as the wave moves past, only to come up again on the next wave. There is a high-water mark on the boy's legs, representing the highest point reached by the wave while he was standing there (the *temporal peak*) and there is an average water level experienced during the paddle (the *temporal average*). In the same way, a *temporal peak intensity* and a *temporal average intensity* can be identified as the highest intensity experienced at a point in tissue over a period of time, and the average intensity experienced at that point over a time, where the averaging is done over both on-times and

off-times. If these temporal intensities are measured at the point in tissue where the spatial peak intensity is found, then a *spatial peak temporal peak intensity* (I_{SPTP}) and a *spatial peak temporal average intensity* (I_{SPTA}) can be determined. If these temporal intensities are combined with spatial averaging, the *spatial average temporal average* (I_{SATA}) and *spatial average temporal peak intensities* (I_{SATP}) can also be defined. These are demonstrated in Figures 2.27 and 2.28.

For example, take a beam with $I_{SP} = 3\,W/cm^2$ and $I_{SA} = 2\,W/cm^2$ while the sound is on, pulsed 2 ms on, 8 ms off. Whatever the temporal peak, the

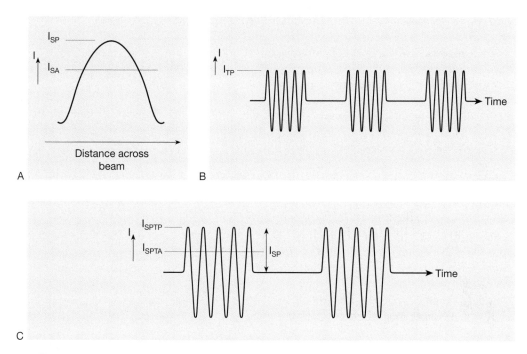

Figure 2.28 The different types of intensity. I_{SA}, spatial average; I_{SP}, spatial peak; I_{SPTA}, spatial peak-temporal average; I_{SPTP}, spatial peak-temporal peak; I_{TP}, temporal peak.

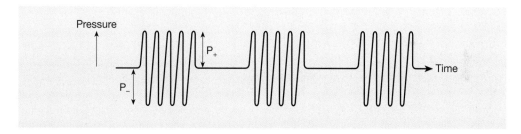

Figure 2.29 An ultrasound exposure can be described in terms of pressure. The peak positive pressure amplitude, P_+, and the peak negative pressure amplitude, P_-, are shown.

temporal average will be 20% of this since the sound is on for only a fifth of the time. Thus, $I_{SPTP} = 3\,W/cm^2$, $I_{SPTA} = 0.6\,W/cm^2$, $I_{SATP} = 2\,W/cm^2$, $I_{SATA} = 0.4\,W/cm^2$.

The ultrasound field can also be described in terms of the pressures involved. It can be seen from Figure 2.29 that the pressure oscillates around the ambient level of the medium through which it passes. The field can therefore also be characterised in terms of *pressure amplitude* (usually the *peak positive pressure amplitude*, p_1, and the *peak negative pressure amplitude*, p_2) found anywhere in the field.

Intensity and pressure are related in a plane wave by the expression:

$$I = p^2/2\rho c \qquad [39]$$

where ρ is the density and c is the speed of sound in the medium.

Ultrasound interacts with tissue in several ways. The two mechanisms thought to be most important are heat and cavitation. Cavitation is the activity of bubbles in an ultrasonic field. The oscillating pressure can cause bubbles to grow, and to oscillate. An oscillating bubble causes the liquids around it to stream, and considerable shear stresses may occur. In some instances they may become *resonant*, in which case they start to oscillate unstably and may undergo violent collapse, causing tissue damage in their vicinity. When the amount of tissue heating is being considered, spatially averaged intensities are the most relevant parameters. However, when cavitation is considered, it is the peak negative pressure that is the most relevant parameter.

Calibration

Ultrasound fields can be calibrated using a number of methods, depending on the information required. The pressure distribution can be mapped using a pressure-sensitive polyvinylidene difluoride (PVDF) membrane hydrophone, which makes use of the inverse piezoelectric effect. Field plotting is a lengthy and detailed process usually undertaken by manufacturers or medical physics departments. It is always advisable to have transducers calibrated in this way before use, and again when a fault is suspected; it provides an easy way of identifying damaged crystals. The calibration method of choice within a physiotherapy department should be a radiation pressure balance. When ultrasound hits a target in water, it exerts a force on the target (radiation pressure) and tries to move it. If this is suitably counterbalanced, the radiation force can be calculated. This device averages over the target area, and allows a rapid assessment of reproducibility of output from day to day. This is an important check that should be incorporated into any treatment routine.

Reflection of ultrasound waves

Tissue offers resistance to the passage of ultrasound. This resistance is called the *acoustic impedance, Z*, and may be calculated from the expression:

$$Z = \rho c \qquad [40]$$

where ρ is the density and c is the velocity of sound. The unit in which Z is reported is the *rayl*.

The amount of sound reflected from a plane surface between two materials of impedance Z_1 and Z_2 is $(Z_2 - Z_1)/(Z_2 + Z_1)$, and the amount of sound transmitted is $2Z_2/(Z_2 + Z_1)$. Water has an impedance of 1.5×10^6 rayl, fat has an impedance of 1.4×10^6 rayl, muscle of 1.7×10^6 rayl and bone of 7×10^6 rayl.

Attenuation

As ultrasound passes through tissue, some of the energy is reflected by the structures in the path (*scattering*), and some of the energy is absorbed by the medium itself, leading to local heating (*absorption*). *Attenuation* (the loss of energy from the beam) is due to these two mechanisms, with absorption accounting for 60–80% of the energy loss. If the intensity incident on tissue is I_0, and the intensity after travelling through x cm of tissue of attenuation coefficient a, is I, these are related by the expression:

$$I = I_0 e^{-ax} \qquad [41]$$

The way in which the intensity drops as it goes through tissue is shown in Figure 2.30; this is known as *exponential decay*.

Attenuation coefficient values are often quoted in dB/cm/MHz or nepers/cm/MHz (1 dB/cm = 4.34 nepers/cm). The decibel (dB) represents a ratio of intensity levels such that the intensity level quoted in decibels is $10 \log_{10} I_0/I$. It can be shown that when the intensity level is 3 dB the ratio of intensities is 2. The attenuation coefficient is quoted as a function of frequency, as they are approximately linearly related.

Table 2.2 shows relative attenuation coefficients for different biological tissues. Also shown are half-value thicknesses. This is the thickness of tissue needed to reduce the intensity by a factor of 2. It can be seen that bone and lung attenuate the sound very rapidly and very little energy gets into them. They are therefore not suited to physiotherapy ultrasound treatments. In fact, care should be taken when treating over such regions because the lost energy goes into heating the tissue locally. It can also be seen that the half-thickness layer decreases with increasing frequency and so, where deep treatments are required, low frequencies should be used.

Coupling agents

It can be seen from Table 2.2 that megahertz-frequency sound does not travel through air. Therefore, when a patient is being treated, it is essential for an effective treatment that no air comes between the transducer and the skin. There are a number of methods by which ultrasound is applied. The most common method is to use a 'contact' application, where a thin layer of oil or

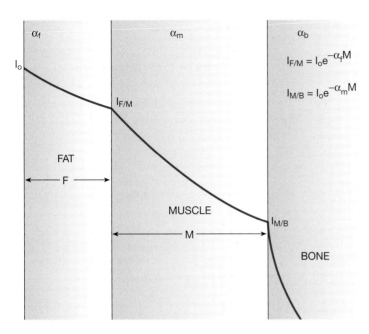

$$I_{F/M} = I_o e^{-\alpha_f M}$$

$$I_{M/B} = I_o e^{-\alpha_m M}$$

Figure 2.30 Ultrasound energy is attenuated exponentially as it travels through tissue. Bone attenuates most strongly.

Table 2.2 Tissue ultrasound attenuation coefficients and half-value layers

Tissue	Attenuation (dB/cm/MHz)	Half-value layer at 1 MHz	Half-value layer at 3 MHz
Blood	0.2	15 cm	5 cm
Fat	0.6	5 cm	1.6 cm
Liver	1.0	3 cm	1 cm
Muscle	1.3–3.3	1–2 cm	3–6 mm
Bone	20	1.5 mm	0.5 mm
Lung	41	0.7 mm	0.2 mm
Air	342 (1 MHz)	0.02 mm	
Water	0.002	1500 cm	500 cm

gel is applied to the skin prior to treatment. The requirement for the coupling medium is that it has a similar acoustic impedance to skin. Mineral oils and water-based gels are most commonly used. Awkward geometries can most readily be treated in a water bath, with both the limb to be treated and the transducer being immersed.

HEAT AND TEMPERATURE

The fact that when various forms of energy are converted into heat there is always a constant ratio between the amount of energy that is lost and the amount of heat produced, suggests that in all these processes, energy is neither created nor destroyed. This principle is a partial expression of the *first law of thermodynamics*: 'in all processes occurring in an isolated system, the energy of the system remains constant'. Electrical, chemical, magnetic and other forms of energy can be converted into heat energy with 100% efficiency, but it is not possible to achieve the reverse and transform all heat energy stored in the microstructure of matter to some other energy form. Again, if one form of energy is converted to another (e.g. chemical to mechanical) the process is not 100% efficient and some of the energy is always converted to heat. The tendency to randomise molecular motion into heat energy eventually suggests that heat is a primordial component in the structure of matter.

The concepts of *heat* and *temperature* are rigorously differentiated in physics and the distinction needs to be similarly maintained in the theory of electrotherapy. Supposing that the same quantity of heat (Q) is distributed over a large or a small volume of the same material, the larger volume will have a lower temperature (T_1) than the smaller volume (T_2). Thus, while the quantity of heat is a form of energy, the temperature of an object is a measure of the *average kinetic energy* of the constituent molecules. Because it is related to the 'average' movement of molecules, the concept of temperature can be applied only to bodies consisting of a large number of molecules.

The only term for temperature that allows consistent expression of all states of matter, solid, liquid and gas in accord with the laws of thermodynamics is the thermodynamic temperature, the base unit of which is the *kelvin* (K). In this system, introduced by Lord Kelvin in 1848, the linear scale starts at the absolute zero of temperature (0K). The thermodynamic *Celsius* scale is subdivided into the same intervals as the Kelvin scale but has a zero point displaced by 273.15. The Celsius scale is divided into 100 unit intervals between two fixed points: the condensing point of steam (100°C = 373.15K) and the melting point of ice (0°C = 273.15K). Absolute zero on the Celsius scale is −273.15°C. The *Fahrenheit* (F) scale does not conform to the International System (SI) of units but continues to be used in many regions of the world particularly for meteorological data; 0°C is 32°F, 100°C is 212°F, so 1° on the Celsius scale is equivalent to 1.8° on the Fahrenheit scale.

HEAT UNITS

Energy, work and the *amount of heat* are physical quantities with the same dimensions and ideally should be measured by a common unit. Traditional units such as the calorie are deeply rooted in technical as well as in dietary usage, but in accordance with SI strategy, the calorie is a 'non-coherent' unit. To conform with the SI, a quantity of heat should be expressed in *joules* (J). Heat exchanges are usually described in terms of *power* (energy per unit time), for example joules per second (51 watt or W). The watt is probably more familiar in everyday use as a measure of power consumption of electrical appliances, for instance in kilowatt hours (kWh), which is actually energy per unit time × time. Table 2.3

derives the relationship between the physical expressions of *force, energy* and *power*.

The amount of heat energy required to raise a unit mass of material by 1°C is known as the *specific heat* of the material. The specific heat of water is 4.185 J/g per °C. Far less heat is needed to raise the temperature of a gas (e.g. the specific heat of air is 1.01 J/g per °C). The human body comprises approximately 60% water and not surprisingly has a relatively high specific heat (3.56 J/g per °C). The specific heats of skin, muscle, fat and bone are respectively 3.77, 3.75, 2.3 and 1.59 J/g per °C. It is thus readily calculated that if the mean body temperature of a 65-kg person is increased by 1°C over a period of 1hour then an extra 231 kJ of heat has been stored in the body.

PHYSICAL EFFECTS OF HEAT

When heat is added to matter, a number of physical phenomena result from increasing the kinetic energy of its microstructure. These can be summarised as follows:

1. Temperature rise: the average kinetic energy of constituent molecules increases.

2. Expansion of the material: increased kinetic energy produces a greater vibration of molecules, which move further apart and expand the material. Gases will expand more than liquids, and liquids more than solids. If, for example, a gas is enclosed so that expansion cannot take place, a rise in gas pressure will occur instead.

3. Change in physical state: changing a substance from one physical state (phase) to another requires a specific amount of heat energy (i.e. latent heat). For example, the latent heat of fusion is the energy required for, or released by, 1 g ice at 0°C to convert it to 1 g water at 0°C (336 joules), and the latent heat of vaporisation

Table 2.3 Derivation of coherent heat units

Quantity	Physical definition	SI unit	Dimension
Force	Mass × acceleration	Newton (N) (kg × metres^{-2})	MLT^{-2}
Energy	Force × distance	Joule (J)	ML^2T^{-2}
Power	Energy/unit time	Watt (W)	ML^2T^{-3}

L, distance; M, mass; T, time.
Non-coherent units: 1 calorie = 4.185 joules; 1 kcal/hour = 1.16 watts.

is the energy needed to convert 1 g water at 100°C to 1 g steam at 100°C (2268 joules).

4. Acceleration of chemical reactions: van't Hoff's law states that 'any chemical reaction capable of being accelerated, is accelerated by a rise in temperature; the ratio of the reaction rate constants for a reaction occurring at two temperatures 10°C apart is the Q_{10} of the reaction'.

5. Production of an electrical potential difference: if the junction of two dissimilar metals (e.g. copper and antimony) is heated, an e.m.f. (electromotive force or electrical potential difference) is produced between their free ends (the Seebeck or thermocouple effect). Conversely, an e.m.f. applied to the junction of two metals can cause a rise in temperature at the junction (Peltier effect).

6. Production of electromagnetic waves: when energy is added to an atom (e.g. by heating) an electron may move out into a higher-energy electron shell. When the electron returns to its normal level, energy is released as a pulse of electromagnetic energy (a photon).

7. Thermionic emission: heating of some materials (e.g. tungsten) may cause such molecular agitation that some electrons leave their atoms and may break free of the metal. This leaves a positive charge which tends to attract electrons back. A point is reached where the rate of loss of electrons equals the rate of return, and a cloud of electrons then exists as a space charge around the metal. This process is known as thermionic emission.

8. Reduction in viscosity of fluids: dynamic viscosity is the property of a fluid (liquid or gas) of offering resistance (internal friction) to the non-accelerated displacement of two adjacent layers. The molecules in a viscous fluid are quite strongly attracted to one another. Heating increases the kinetic movement of these molecules, reducing their cohesive mutual attraction and making the fluid less viscous.

HEAT TRANSFER

The laws of thermodynamics govern processes involving the movement of heat energy from one point to another. Mention has previously been made of the first law, which deals with the conservation and interchange of different forms of energy.

The second law of thermodynamics states that 'heat cannot by itself, i.e. without performance of work by some external agency, pass from a colder to a warmer body'. These general laws establish the principles that govern heat exchanges (gain or loss) within the body and between the body and its environment. In electrotherapy we are concerned with the transfer of heat energy between the external environment and the body surface, and between the component tissues and fluids of the body itself as well as with the therapeutic effects of heat.

CONDUCTION

Conduction is the mechanism of energy exchange between regions of different temperature, from hotter to colder regions, which is accomplished by direct molecular collision. The energy thus transferred causes an increased vibration of molecules, which is transmitted to adjacent molecules. A simple example of this process is the metal bar heated at one end which, by heat conduction, eventually becomes hot at its other end. The application of a cold pack to the skin surface induces skin cooling by heat conduction from the warm skin, and vice versa for a hot pack. The rate of heat transfer depends on the difference in temperature between the regions in contact, the surface area of contact at the boundary and the thermal conductivity of the materials in contact. Thermal conductivity is a specific property of the material itself; for example metals are better conductors than wood, water a better conductor than air.

CONVECTION

Convection is the heat transfer mechanism that occurs in a fluid due to gross movements of molecules within the mass of fluid. If a part of a fluid is heated, the kinetic energy of the molecules in that part is increased, the molecules move further apart and the fluid becomes less dense. In consequence, the heated fluid rises and displaces the more dense fluid above, which in turn descends to take its place. The immediate process of energy transfer from one fluid particle to another remains one of conduction, but the energy is transported from one point in space to another primarily by convective displacement of the fluid itself. Pure conduction is rarely observed in a fluid, owing to the ease with which even small temperature differences initiate free convection currents.

THERMAL RADIATION

Heat may be transmitted by electromagnetic radiation emission from the surface of a body whose surface temperature is above absolute zero. The heating of certain atoms causes an electron to move to a higher-energy electron shell; as it returns to its normal shell, the energy is released as a pulse of electromagnetic energy. This radiation occurs primarily in the infrared band, with wavelengths of about 10^{-5}cm to 10^{-2}cm (0.1–100 mm, or 10^3–10^6 Å). A thermal radiation incident upon a surface can be:

1. reflected back from that surface
2. transmitted through it
3. absorbed.

In many everyday circumstances, objects are radiating and absorbing the same amount of infrared energy, thus maintaining a constant temperature. The amount of radiation from an object is proportional to the fourth power of the temperature (in kelvins). The rate of emission from a surface also depends on the nature of the surface, being greatest for a black body. A perfect black body absorbs all the radiation, whereas other surfaces absorb some and reflect the remainder.

EVAPORATION

Thermal energy is required to transform a liquid into vapour; the rate at which this proceeds is determined by the rate at which the vapour diffuses away from the surface. The rate depends on the power supplied and the vapour pressure of the air above the liquid. Evaporation follows laws very similar to those governing convection. When water vaporises from the body surface (e.g. during sweating) the latent heat required is extracted from the surface tissue, thereby cooling it. The converse process, condensation, entails latent heat gain at the surface as vapour is changed into liquid.

BODY HEAT TRANSFER

In thermoregulation, heat is exchanged by conductive, convective, radiative and evaporative transfer processes between the body surface and the environment so that the body's core temperature remains constant, and equilibrium is maintained between internal (metabolic) heat production and heat loss (or gain) from the skin's surface.

Heat transfer within tissues takes place primarily by conduction and convection. The temperature distribution will depend on the amount of energy converted into heat at a given tissue depth and the thermal properties of the tissue (e.g. specific heat, thermal conductivity). Physiological factors are important in determining tissue temperature: for example when a raised tissue temperature produces increased local blood flow, cooler blood reperfusing the heated tissue will selectively tend to cool the tissue by conduction. The technique of application of a treatment modality will also clearly modify the tissue temperature through variations in time and intensity, etc. When deep treatment is applied (e.g. short-wave diathermy, microwave, or ultrasound) conversion of the energy into heat occurs as it penetrates into the tissues. Heating modalities may be subdivided according to their primary mode of heat transfer during selective heating of superficial or deep tissues (Table 2.4).

In thermotherapy, the important properties concerned with heat conduction in tissues are thermal conductivity, tissue density and specific heat. Convection involves these properties also but, in addition, fluid viscosity becomes important. Understanding of the interaction of electromagnetic waves within biological media requires knowledge of the dielectric properties of tissues with different water contents.

Table 2.4 Heating modalities and their primary mode of heat transfer

Primary method	Modality of heat transfer
Conduction	Hot packs
	Paraffin wax baths
Convection	Hydrotherapy
	Fluidotherapy
	Moist air
'Conversion'	Radiant heat
	Laser
	Short-wave
	Ultrasound
	Microwave

After Lehmann JF (1990) *Therapeutic Heat and Cold*, 4th edn. Baltimore, MD, Williams & Wilkins.

Chapter 3

Electrical properties of tissues

Tim Watson

CHAPTER CONTENTS

INTRODUCTION

There is a substantial, and growing, evidence base to support the concept that biological tissues demonstrate electrical characteristics, and that this bioelectric activity is not just an epiphenomenon but is integral to both their form and function. It would appear that without these electrical characteristics, behaviour and response to adverse events (injury, pathology), the body would not be able to deal with the environment as efficiently as it does. That is not to say that the bioelectric systems are exclusively in control, but rather that their influence is both substantial and significant.

The concept of bioelectrics is certainly not new, and the links between bioelectrics and electrotherapy have been proposed on numerous occasions (e.g. Charman 1990, 2002). It is not surprising that these suggestions have attracted a degree of scepticism, but looking objectively at the research literature from several fields (physiology, bioengineering, biophysics, cell biology), the integration of existing knowledge into a new discipline (or at least a subdiscipline) is possibly the most logical way forward.

Not only does bioelectricity and bioelectric tissue activity have an influence on the practice of electrotherapy (Chapter 19 'Electrical stimulation for enhanced wound healing' is an example), but there is a strong case for its potential to influence manual and exercise therapies and a range of 'alternative' and 'complementary' therapies, which, although, beyond the remit of this chapter, and indeed this whole text, might be of significance in the future development of therapy.

The concepts presented here are founded on physiology and physics in order to ground them in the framework most familiar to the reader. Adequate reference material will be provided for those with a particular interest to investigate further. Even if you do not feel that this is likely to be a chapter for you, it is distinctly possible that a skim through its contents might be rather more thought-provoking than you anticipate, and if you then decide that the concepts as presented lack what is deemed to be credible evidence, at least it will have been rejected from a considered rather than a dismissive viewpoint.

THE BODY BIOELECTRIC

It is well recognised that many 'activities' in the body are electrically detectable, and it is not radical to propose that the electrocardiogram (ECG) provides an effective and accurate 'picture' of the activity of the heart. Similarly, an electromyogram (EMG) is deemed to be an informative reflection of activity in the nerve/muscle complex and the electroencephalogram (EEG) relative to brain activity. Many other examples of E*Gs are employed in specialist fields as a means to determine the activity of internal organs or tissues without the need for invasive evaluation.

The reason for the ECG, EMG, EEG and others being accepted in practice (other than their efficacy) relates to the fact that these tissues (heart, muscle, nerve, brain) are deemed to constitute the 'excitable' tissues. Indeed, they are, but this is a classification that leads one to consider other tissues to fall by default into the 'non-excitable' group. Nothing could be much further from the truth and a brief evaluation of what is to follow will demonstrate both the extent and the importance of bioelectric activity in 'other' tissues.

THE ELECTRIC CELL

The transmembrane potential, readily accepted as a normal phenomenon, is an example of bioelectric activity on a small scale, although there is evidence that bioelectric activity is present and important at smaller (subcellular) scales. This section will largely avoid bioelectrics at a subcellular level, not because it lacks importance or evidence but rather because the larger scale is more understandable as an introduction and is more easily appreciated in a therapeutic context. Those with an interest in subcellular bioelectrics are encouraged to consider material by Charman (1990, 2002) and Oschman (2005).

The electrical potential across the cell membrane will average several 10s of millivolts (typical values cited for nerve membrane for example would be in the order of 70 mV). This potential is actively generated rather than an accidental event and is dependent on the continued pump and ion transport system of the cell membrane for its maintenance. Ion concentrations are deliberately made unequal (against the tendency for diffusion gradients to generate ionic and thus a charge balance) and there are many different ionic transfer mechanisms across any cell membrane – from the now well-known and well-understood sodium–potassium pump (Na/K) through to the less well-known, but equally important, calcium ion gated channels (Charman 2002).

The electrical potential of the cell membrane might be small in absolute terms but it is actually very substantial when considered on a cellular scale. The membrane itself is on average between 7 and 10 nm thick (a nanometre is 10^{-9} metre, i.e. a thousandth of a millionth of a metre). This is a difficult dimension for most of us to appreciate. To give it some kind of scale, it means that considering a 'thick' membrane (at 10 nm), it would be possible to fit in the order of 100 000 membranes into a millimetre. Although this is still difficult to comprehend, it is a bit more manageable.

A transmembrane voltage (of, say, 70 mV) is difficult to imagine. A cell membrane thickness of a few nanometres is more difficult, so by scaling both measurements up by the same factor, it is possible to grasp the magnitude of this energy system on a more 'human' scale. If we were to make the cell membrane a metre thick, the equivalent voltage across that membrane would be in the order of 7 million volts. Given that this is the equivalent potential in every living cell in the body, it constitutes an impressive energy system, and one that will clearly 'cost' the body to maintain. It is important to stress that this is the *equivalent* rather than the *actual* voltage across the cell membrane – what it would be *if* the cell membrane was a metre thick – which clearly it is not. One could then multiply up this membrane potential by the number of cells in the body and come up with some very impressive large numbers and an impressive amount of electrical activity.

Leaving to one side the numbers, one has to consider why this energy level is needed in the cell membrane. The membrane electrical activity is key in terms of cellular activity levels. Cells can adjust their 'level of activity' very efficiently, and this rapid response mechanism is, for a large part, due to the influence of the membrane. A cell can increase its activity – not to change *what* it does, but to change the *amount* of work that it is doing. In physiological terms this is referred to as 'upregulation' and is an important and normal physiological phenomenon. Clearly the converse response will also be possible – a cell can reduce its work rate – downregulation.

The level of 'excitement' in the cell membrane is strongly linked to these physiological changes at a cellular level, and thus linked with many aspects of medical and therapeutic intervention. Cells can be forced, or encouraged, to increase activity levels – using drugs, heat or other energy sources such as ultrasound or laser light. Confining the argument here to the use of energy in the therapeutic environment, the absorption of energy at cell membrane level is partly, if not totally, responsible for the cellular upregulation seen with modalities such as ultrasound and laser, and almost certainly pulsed shortwave. Evidence that these modalities are able to exert their influence primarily at a cell membrane level (Cleary 1987, Karu 1987, Mortimer & Dyson 1988) supports a transduction mechanism by which the delivery of energy to the tissues is able to generate physiological (and thus therapeutic) effects (see Chapter 1).

Given, then, that the cell membrane potential is very substantial relative to the size of the cell, and given that the membrane potential is able to influence cell activity levels (by means of the up- and downregulation mechanisms), there is a substantive link between what happens in the membrane and therapeutic influence.

TISSUE BATTERIES

Bioelectric activity, however, operates at a scale that is larger than individual membrane potentials, and the concept of tissue batteries is supported by a growing body of evidence. Tissues demonstrate a 'gross' electrical characteristic that is greater than simply the sum of the individual parts, i.e. the individual cells that make up that tissue. There are many examples of tissue batteries and a couple will be examined here in some detail as a means to explain their existence and to draw the links between battery function and therapy.

THE BONE BATTERY

The bone battery is a well-documented physiological reality. In the 1950s, it was found that bone demonstrated a piezoelectric potential when subjected to physical (bending) stress (Fukada & Yasuda 1957); this work has since been extended by many researchers (reviewed in Black 1987, Guzelsu & Walsh 1993, Walsh & Guzelsu 1993). The demonstration of piezoelectric phenomena in bone is illustrated in Figure 3.1.

This work was extended in the 1960s by the demonstration of streaming potentials (Pollack et al 1984) and, more importantly than both of these (in the context of this chapter), in the late 1960s and 1970s by the steady potential (or battery potential) (reviewed in Black 1987). The streaming potentials are generated in bone when it is physically stressed and are a result of charged particles (ions) moving within the fluid-filled Haversian systems; more recently, they have also been demonstrated in cartilage (Legare et al 2002). Both the piezoelectric and streaming potentials are therefore stress related – they occur when bone (in this instance) is physically stressed. The steady potentials are measurable even when the bone is not physically stressed – they are there all of the time. It is these latter potentials that are derived directly from the 'bone battery'.

The magnitude of the electrical potentials generated by the bone battery will vary between individuals (in keeping with almost all physiological phenomena) but if one considers the overall electrical pattern of a long bone, the femur for example, the gross electrical charge pattern will be similar

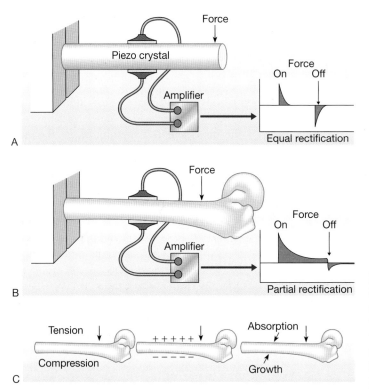

Figure 3.1 Apparent piezoelectricity in bone. A, typical piezocrystal response to momentary deformation. B, similar transducing response in bone. C, tension/compression surface potentials of opposite sign to resulting bone cell response (after Becker & Selden 1985, with permission of HarperCollins Publishers, Inc.).

between individuals, even if the actual values are variable (Rubinacci et al 1984).

The bone battery charge is physiologically relevant in that bone electricity varies when the bone is actively growing (Black 1987), when subjected to abnormal mechanical stress (e.g. Becker & Selden 1985) and when subjected to a pathological state (Borgens et al 1989, Marino 1988). Not only does the 'charge' generated by the battery vary under normal and pathological conditions, there is also a relationship between battery output and tissue injury/repair. When bone is subjected to injury, there is a physical discontinuity in the battery structure (the fracture) and a local electrical change will result. This local 'current of injury' has been demonstrated in many musculoskeletal tissues; bone in this instance is just an example.

It is argued that this local electrical current – or disturbance from the normal – is an essential driver for the process of fracture repair, and that without it, repair of the damaged bone will be inhibited or might indeed be absent (Black 1987). Becker (1974a, b) reports the experimental evidence

with regard to fracture healing and denervation. It was noted that there was retardation of fracture healing in peripherally denervated extremities and that, when the nerve transection gap is bridged by the supporting (Schwann) cells (but not yet by the neurons themselves), the fracture healing rate was returned to normal. This is considered to link the local bone injury potentials with the direct current (DC) control theory (see the section 'Direct current (DC) control theory', below).

It is further argued that for individuals in whom this electrical activity is for some reason absent or reduced, a delayed or non-union is an inevitable consequence. It would be presumptuous to suggest that the only reason for non- or delayed union relates entirely to this 'flat battery' function but there is substantial experimental and clinical evidence to support the link between the phenomena (Black 1987).

There are many further relevant issues related to the bone battery, its existence and behaviour, but the primary issue in the context of this chapter is that the bone battery – internally generated electrical potentials coming from the bone tissue rather than conducted there by some other tissue – has an integral and important influence on bone physiology in health and disease. Extensive reviews have been written in this area and some accessible work is available (Black 1987, Evans et al 2001, Singh & Katz 1989).

There are therefore some obvious correlates between the electrical activity in bone, the process of fracture healing and the role of various aspects of the rehabilitation process. Given that the level of electrical activity in bone changes as a result of physical stress, and that it has been shown that bone bioelectric activity is an essential element of a 'normal' repair process, there is a strong argument that active exercise, manual therapy and various forms of electrotherapy are able to influence fracture healing by their capacity to directly or indirectly influence the bioelectric environment. That is not to say that the only influence of exercise or manual therapy is as a 'battery' stimulant, but just to make the point that in addition to the established value of these interventions in terms of local blood flow, increased muscular and general limb activity, mobility and strength, part of their mechanism of action is very likely to relate to enhanced bioelectric function. This would certainly be the case in relation to skin and wound healing (see the next section) and is directly related to the promotion of this activity by means of electrical stimulation (see Chapter 19). The enhancement of bone healing has been demonstrated by several different types of electrotherapy intervention, including ultrasound (e.g. Gebauer et al 2005, Malizos et al 2006, Warden et al 2006), laser therapy (da Silva & Camilli 2006, Garavello-Freitas et al 2003, Luger et al 1998), magnetic fields (Bassett 1989, 1993, Ryaby 1998, Trock 2000) and electrical stimulation (Anglen 2003, Ciombar & Aaron 2005, Park & Silva 2004) and although these might not constitute a major aspect of the context of this text, they are important and emergent issues in current electrotherapy practice.

THE SKIN BATTERY

The skin has a battery that is at least as impressive and as extensive as the bone battery. The skin, as is well documented, is a particularly extensive organ, and the skin battery is therefore large in terms of extent.

The skin battery itself exists across the living layers of the epidermis and is oriented such that the external surface of the skin is always electrically negative in relation to the internal environment of the body (Barker et al 1982). The role of this battery function is similar in many respects to that of the bone battery already described. It is important as part of the maintenance of healthy skin function, and appears to be of critical importance in terms of the response of the skin to injury and the subsequent repair phases.

The mammalian skin potential work of Barker et al (1982) and Jaffe & Vanable (1984), using a skin injury model in guinea-pigs, has demonstrated that there is a current flow (movement of positive ions) out from a skin lesion due to an altered skin battery function. The skin potential at the wound site is zero because the battery has been short circuited, although, a few millimetres away, a normal transcutaneous potential exists. There is a lateral voltage gradient in the superficial tissues, the mean strength of which was 140 mV/mm in guinea-pig skin. The lateral gradient was not present if the wound was allowed to dry. The model predicts a current flow from the intact skin battery into the deep wound, with a return path through the wound and to the tissue layer between the dead and living layers of the epidermis. The wound current is illustrated in Figure 3.2. Close to the wound, the outer surface of the living layer would be electrically positive with respect to the outer surface of the same layer far from the wound.

The strength of the lateral voltage gradients associated with mammalian wounds is within the range of fields found to influence development (Jaffe & Vanable 1984). It is suggested that these wound currents could be responsible for stimulating wound cover by epithelial cells (Foulds & Barker 1983, Jaffe & Vanable 1984). The stimulation of skin lesions by externally applied electrical currents is gaining clinical acceptance and is in itself a considerable field of study (Vanable 1989, Watson 1996).

Illingworth & Barker (1980) have demonstrated local currents associated with amputated fingertips in children. The current density was on average $22\,\mu\mathrm{A\,cm^{-2}}$ and reached its peak approximately

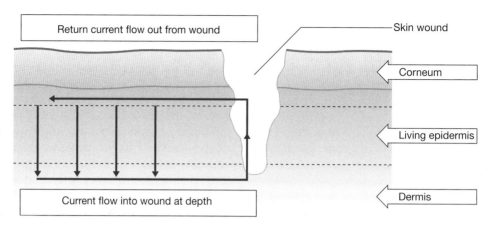

Figure 3.2   Current path with full-thickness wound in mammalian skin. The current represents the movement of positive ions (after Jaffe & Vanable 1984).

1 week after the injury. The fingertips regenerated if left unsutured and the battery function of the skin was found to be comparable to that involved in amphibian limb regeneration. The skin battery current driving capacity is in the order of $1 \, \mu A/mm$ of wound length (Borgens 1982, Jaffe & Vanable 1984, Vanable 1989).

An extensive literature has demonstrated the relationship between skin injury and changes in bioelectric activity (e.g. Vanable 1989, Watson 1995) and it would take at least a whole chapter to provide a minimal review. There is a strong relationship between this normal level of skin electrical activity and the levels of current/potential in wounds that are not healing. Just as was the case with the delayed or non-unions in bone, the equivalent in the skin is the chronic, non-healing or slowly healing ulcer or pressure sore.

In the same way that the repair process can be stimulated in bone by various means, including electrotherapy in the form of ultrasound, laser and electrical stimulation, it is also the case with chronic venous ulcers and equivalent skin lesions. Chapter 19 covers the use of electrical stimulation as a means to enhance the local bioelectric activity in open wounds, and Chapters 10, 11 and 12, concerned with pulsed shortwave, laser and ultrasound, make mention of their role in this context.

The use of electrical stimulation in wound management is not common practice in the UK,

although in some countries it has been adopted as a matter of routine and thousands of patients benefit from this intervention (Kloth 2005).

BATTERIES IN OTHER MUSCULOSKELETAL TISSUES

Musculoskeletal tissues other than skin and bone exhibit strong physiological bioelectric phenomena. Experimental work has demonstrated that this bioelectric activity is both normally present and altered following injury or disease, and during the repair process. Potentials have been demonstrated in muscle (Betz & Caldwell 1984, Betz et al 1986) and collagenous-based tissues (Anderson & Eriksson 1968, Athenstaedt 1970). Endogenous bioelectric activity has been demonstrated and deemed to be of importance in numerous musculoskeletal tissues (Grodzinsky 1983, Wachtel 1992).

DIRECT CURRENT (DC) CONTROL THEORY

An alternative consideration of the bioelectric potentials measured from the skin has been advanced by numerous researchers, including Burr and co-workers beginning in the 1930s (Burr et al 1938) and Becker and co-workers in the 1960s. Both groups developed a concept of the skin potential being a measurable phenomenon of a DC control system that plays an essential role in monitoring and controlling growth and healing. At the present time, no evidence has been identified to refute the basic concepts, and several research groups have used them as a fundamental theoretical underpinning for their own work (e.g. Shibib et al 1988, Wilber 1978). This appears to be particularly true in the area of electrical stimulation of skin and bone to enhance healing.

The essential difference between the transcutaneous electrical potentials and the DC potentials recorded by Burr and Becker is that the latter attribute the potentials to a nerve-related phenomenon, anatomically distributed, and not to local epidermal membrane or psychological episodes.

Measuring the DC potentials from the same level of the epidermis (i.e. both electrodes on the surface), Becker demonstrated that – both in amphibians and in man – a pattern of equipotential lines follows a predictable arrangement (Becker et al 1962a,b, 1990). These investigations demonstrated the presence of a complex electrical field with a spatial configuration that has a close relationship to the gross distribution of the central and peripheral nervous systems. In various species, including man, the cranial, brachial and lumbar neuraxes were found to be positive, with increasing negative potentials along the peripheral outflows (Becker 1962). On further investigation, it was proposed that the peripheral nerves were responsible for the distribution of this electric field, with DC gradients extending longitudinally

throughout the neural network. The dendrites (sensory components) were found to be distally positive and the axons (motor components) distally negative resulting in an axiodendritic polarisation model for the DC control system (Becker et al 1962a,b). A representation of Becker's polarisation concept is shown in Figures 3.3 and 3.4.

The role of the peripheral nerves in the transmission of these DC potentials was strengthened when it was observed that the potentials were reduced to zero after sectioning the nerves to the extremity (Becker et al 1962b).

The DC potentials were shown to be independent of the action potentials. They are related to a longitudinal continuous movement of charges in the nerve, whereas the action potential is a travelling wave of membrane depolarisation: a radial movement of ions in and out of the nerve fibre with no longitudinal transmission of electric charges (Becker 1962, 1974a,b).

Becker's experimentation suggested that the charge carriers were not ionic but were units the size of electrons, implying that a phenomenon such as semiconduction was occurring in the nerve fibre (Becker et al 1962b). Becker (1974a,b) cites numerous examples of semiconductor-like behaviour of biological tissues, including nerve (Becker 1961), collagen and bone (Becker & Brown 1965).

Becker (1974a,b) concludes that two data transmission and control systems coexist in most present-day animals. One is a sophisticated action potential, digital-type system; the second a more

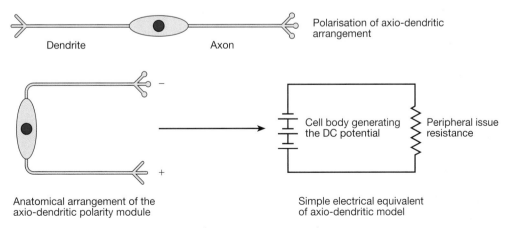

Figure 3.3   Axiodendritic polarisation of nerves (after Becker et al 1962).

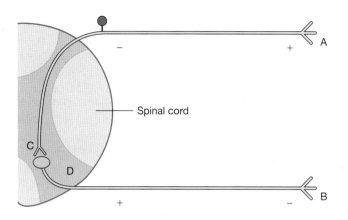

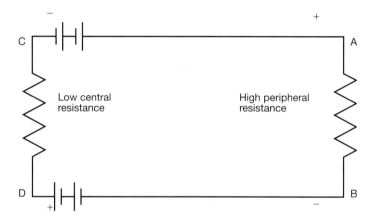

Figure 3.4 Physiological and electrical model of a neuron pair forming an elementary circuit (after Becker et al 1962).

basic/primitive analogue-type system that antedates the former and is thought to be solid state in nature. Becker (1974b) proposes that these currents are both generated and transmitted by the Schwann cells that surround the peripheral neurons and the glial cells in the central nervous system. This hypothesis is compatible with the demonstration (Lowestein 1981) of cell-to-cell conductances and junctional communications in glial and epithelial cells. Evidence is presented (Becker et al 1962b, O'Leary & Goldring 1964) to support the steady state of varying DC fields within the central and peripheral nervous systems and to suggest that these DC potentials have a controlling function over the general level of the digital (action) potential – that they act as a 'bias control' over the functions of the action-potential system (Becker 1974a,b). In addition to the modulation influence on the peripheral nervous system,

Becker's research group propose that the DC potentials exert a control over growth and repair processes (Becker et al 1962a).

The DC control theory has gained popularity with those concerned with the electrical stimulation of damaged tissues in order to facilitate or promote repair. Several significant studies have produced results that appear to support Becker's proposal (including Chakkalakal et al 1988a,b, Chang & Snellen 1982, Weiss et al 1990) and these are considered later in this chapter.

LOCAL INJURY CURRENT AND WHOLE BODY BIOELECTRIC INTERACTION

Becker (1967, 1974a,b) proposed a local model to explain the role of the bioelectrical 'current of injury' and the local tissue response to injury (Fig. 3.5).

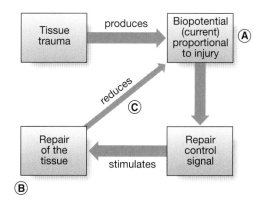

Figure 3.5   Bioelectric repair model.

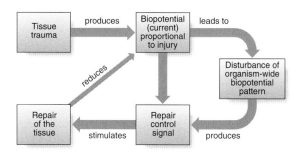

Figure 3.6   Bioelectric repair model – extended.

Essentially, the local injury generates the well-established current of injury (A). The local current of injury influences the local tissue-repair process (B) and thereby, as the extent of the damaged tissue diminishes, a feedback loop (C) results in a smaller current of injury, reduced driver for repair and so on. The evidence for this local arrangement is difficult to refute and extensive literature reviews cover this almost standard physiological activity (e.g. Nuccitelli 2003). Becker and others have proposed an extension to this local injury and repair model and this is also worthy of consideration, although it has to be said that the evidence is less strong in some respects, but certainly not lacking in others (Lafargue et al 2002).

The extended model (Fig. 3.6) does not result in the local arrangements being negated or their importance diminished. The extension (to the right in the figure) implies that the local bioelectric changes not only exert a local influence but that they also bring about a change in the 'whole body'

bioelectrical pattern. Becker (1990) and others suggest that there is a demonstrable whole-body bioelectric pattern that has a common theme amongst vertebrate (and in fact some invertebrate) species. According to Becker, this body-wide pattern is attributed to a complex duality of nerve function, whereas others (e.g. Nordenstrom 1983, 1994) attribute it to a blood-vessel-mediated function. The hypothetical arguments are too extensive to be considered here but, assuming that such a gross bioelectric, organism-wide potential pattern exists, it is rationalised that any local disturbance in this activity will result in a general change in body bioelectrics and, furthermore, that this whole-body change is important in terms of holistic therapy approaches and therapeutic intervention strategies that do not focus necessarily on local events. Examples might include acupuncture, reflexology and a wide range of 'energy'-based therapies (Charman 2000).

The fact that acupuncture applied at point X in the body appears to have the capacity to influence a local process at point Y in the body is difficult to explain in terms of classic Western medical philosophy with its patient-dependent medical model. The recognition of the validity of the psychosocial aspects of therapy practice, together with the growing evidence base that 'alternative' and/or 'complementary' therapies are capable of demonstrable effect, might be in part at least attributable to the body-wide bioelectric phenomenon.

BIOELECTRIC CHANGES FOLLOWING INJURY AND DURING REPAIR

The bioelectric disturbances that occur on injury persist for various lengths of time depending on the tissue involved and the extent of the injury. Barnes (1945), Burr (1938), Chakkalakal et al (1988a,b), Chang & Snellen (1982), Friedenberg & Brighton (1966), Illingworth & Barker (1980), Watson (1995) and Wilber (1978) are among those who have monitored the electrical activity of damaged tissues as they progress through their proliferative and healing processes. Each of these groups has reported progressive changes associated with the healing process and obtained results from mammalian tissue.

The greatest difference from the baseline potential occurs during the early proliferative phase and tails off during the subsequent reparative and remodelling phases. Bioelectric changes following injury have been demonstrated in several tissue types (predominantly, but not exclusively, bone, skin and nerve). The recorded potentials are different from those normally present in these tissues, although there does not appear to be any universally accepted explanation for the generation of such potentials (Watson 1995).

O'Leary and Goldring (1964) suggest that an injury potential will develop between injured and uninjured parts of a nerve, muscle, skin and – theoretically at least – of any living tissue or cell that presents a membrane vulnerable to depolarisation as a result of trauma.

Many workers have considered the bioelectric correlates of injury/repair/regeneration in amphibians and other lower vertebrates. Borgens (1982, 1984) has established clear patterns of electrical behaviour in amphibians following limb amputation and subsequent regeneration. Becker (1961) has demonstrated a difference in electrical behaviour between regenerating and non-regenerating species (Fig. 3.7). In regenerating systems (i.e. where the lost tissue is actually replaced with similar tissue), the initial injured positive polarity reverses to a high negative polarity and progressively

returns to normal when the regeneration process is complete. In non-regenerating systems, the initial positive polarity slowly returns to normal with no phase of negative polarity (Becker 1967). Whether this electrical activity is a consequence of local metabolic and physiological processes, or whether it acts as an initiator/control mechanism for the reparative process, has yet to receive unequivocal confirmation. Barker et al (1982), Becker (1974 a,b), Borgens & McCaig (1989), Kloth & McCulloch (1996), Vanable (1989), Watson (1995) and Weiss et al (1990) are among a growing body of researchers who present evidence for the latter view.

Further evidence to support the initiator/control theory is derived from studies (in animal models) where the natural electrical activity associated with tissue repair is inhibited or subjected to polarity reversal. The effect of this type of manipulation is either to slow down significantly or more usually to inhibit completely, the normal repair process (Borgens 1981).

Friedenberg & Brighton (1966, 1981) and Friedenberg et al (1973) are among those who have shown that there is an increased electronegativity on the bone surface in the vicinity of an injury. Borgens (1984) has measured current densities at the surface of injuries to mouse metatarsals *in vivo*. He concluded that there was a metabolic-powered ionic pump in the vicinity of the bone marrow, which was the source of the stable, persistent current (referred to as the plateau current). The experimental evidence rules out the periosteum as the source of the potential. It is suggested that these endogenous currents are actively involved in fracture repair, remodelling and possibly growth rather than just being an 'epiphenomenon'. The replication or simulation of the natural injury currents to induce/enhance fracture healing, when applied in the same direction and at appropriate magnitude, seems to substantiate this hypothesis (Ciombor & Aaron 2005, Evans et al 2001, Kesani et al 2006).

Chakkalakal et al (1988a,b) present evidence to support the hypothesis that musculoskeletal injuries in humans and in animals cause an increase in endogenous electrical activity in the injured region. The aim of the experimental work they carried out was to determine the source(s) of

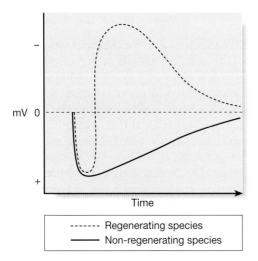

Figure 3.7 Varying bioelectric patterns during repair and regeneration.

the endogenous activity and to determine the distribution of the electric fields and currents in the injured limb. The research measured the change in voltage and current in dog forelegs during progressive stages of surgically created injury, ranging from skin incision to radial osteotomy. The results show that the skin injury activated an epidermal battery of an effective open-circuit voltage of 17–42 mV and that the bone injury activated an endosteal battery of 15–56 mV, which gave rise to a net outward flow of current through the osteotomy gap. The voltages and currents measured in the wound following the skin incision were significantly higher than the variable baseline values measured on the skin surface before injury. The variable baseline results were comparable to those found in animals and humans in other studies (Friedenberg & Brighton 1966, MacDonald & Watson 1982).

The endogenous currents noted in this study were comparable to or even greater than those induced by exogenous signals in electrical osteogenesis studies. It is expected, therefore, that the endogenous activity would be physiologically significant. Large currents on the soft tissue surface (10–32 μA) from the epidermal battery were detected and these support Barker et al's (1982) hypothesis that these are important for wound healing. It is suggested (Sevitt 1981) that endogenous electrical activity influences fracture healing and acts as a trigger for proliferation of osteogenic cells in the periosteum, with the bone surface acting as a pathway for currents arising from muscle injury potentials. The currents along the periosteal surface, in the medullary cavity and through the osteotomy gap are such that migration of negatively charged cells towards and into the gap would be enhanced.

The extensive experimentation by Chakkalakal et al avoided the problem of muscle damage by carefully dissecting between the muscle planes. Lokietek et al (1974), however, investigated the effects of several forms of soft tissue damage on the potentials measured from an undeformed tibia in rabbit. They conclude that muscle injury was the dominant factor in generating the voltage detected. It is hypothesised that the bone acts as a pathway for the injury currents produced in the damaged muscle.

An example of a soft tissue bioelectric injury current comes from the work of Wilber (1978), who measured direct current bioelectric potentials from normal and injured thighs. Using a differential skin surface electrode technique, with a reference electrode over the greater trochanter of the femur and an active mobile electrode along the lateral aspect of the thigh, a series of readings were made from normal and injured subjects to determine the surface potential pattern. The readings obtained from normal (i.e. non-injured) subjects followed four distinct patterns. Three injury groups were subsequently investigated: acute femoral fracture, delayed/non-union and contusion. The patient numbers in each group were small (seven, four and three, respectively) and the results tended to show differences between injured and non-injured limbs, although statistical analysis was problematic because of the small sample.

Numerous studies have produced results that compare favourably with those cited above. There would seem to be a general agreement that injury to bone or soft tissue causes a significant and relatively predictable alteration in the electrical state of the tissues. Most workers also state, with considerable confidence, that this increased endogenous electrical activity is most likely to have a role in stimulating and/or controlling the repair process itself.

BIOELECTRICITY AND ELECTROTHERAPY

Many links can be forged between the bioelectric environment of the body, the electrical responses of injured and repairing tissues, and the potential to influence these events with external (exogenous) energy sources, i.e. electrotherapy. The delivery of energy to the tissues brings about physiological responses (see Chapter 1) and these are known to have therapeutic value when applied at appropriate levels. The predominant explanation proffered in most instances relates to the interaction of the exogenous energy and physiological systems, and, on the whole, interaction with endogenous currents does not constitute a mainstream explanation. It remains a strong possibility, however, that the endogenous energy interaction is at least partly responsible for the effectiveness of the therapy – not as a replacement for existing theories and knowledge, but as an additional or supplementary explanation (Watson 2006).

Numerous areas of bioelectromagnetic research are demonstrating irrefutable links between internal and external energy systems, including effects at a cellular level (e.g. Gapayev & Chemeris 2000, Luchian et al 2002, Marino et al 2003, Pokorny 2001, Sonnier & Marino 2001, Zhao et al 1999) nerve tissue (Bervar 2005, De Pedro et al 2005, Zhang et al 2005) and bone (Chang et al 2003, Diniz et al 2002). Research linking bioelectric events with more general growth and development (Jaffe 1986, Juutilainen 2005, Saunders & McCaig 2005) opens up further possibilities with regard to electrotherapy and the continuing demonstration of the benefits of electrotherapy with skin wound healing (Kloth 2005, Nucitelli 2003, Ojingwa & Isseroff 2002) reinforces the relationship between skin bioelectricity, wound repair and therapy. New areas of therapy that overtly work the relationship between extremely small exogenous currents and tissue repair and recovery – microcurrent type therapies – are starting to generate research evidence in the clinical environment, which is a logical extension of the laboratory and animal-based research that has been available for the last 20 or 30 years (El Husseini et al 2006, Lambert et al 2002, McMakin 2004, Smith 2002, Watson 2006).

The majority of the chapters in this text focus on the 'standard' interaction between electrotherapy modalities and physiological responses of the tissues. The potential to extend these explanations into the bioelectric realm remains a strong possibility for the future.

SUMMARY

One is led to the conclusion that musculoskeletal tissues (not just muscle and nerve) are electrically active; that following injury, the behaviour of this electrical activity is modified, and that as the repair process proceeds there is a progressive return to a normal pattern of bioelectric behaviour. Although the generation mechanism of this bioelectricity is not yet fully explained, there is a growing body of evidence to support the concept that it has a strong relationship to normal tissue behaviour, tissue growth and development and importantly, to the response of the tissue to injury.

Some authors have suggested that this complex interaction provides an opportunity to 'measure' the repair process; others have taken this a step further and consider the bioelectric activity of the tissues to be a therapeutic pathway through which healing can be stimulated, and especially pertinent in clinical conditions whereby tissue repair is inhibited.

It is proposed that *part* of the mechanism through which electrotherapy acts is via this bioelectric system. It is recognised that different modalities have a demonstrable effect on various physiological processes (as detailed in subsequent chapters), and part of their mechanism of action relates to their interaction with the endogenous bioelectric environment, and therefore the possibility exists for a very subtle form of intervention, using very low-energy applications to facilitate/stimulate/enhance the 'natural' electrical environment. There is little doubt that electrotherapy 'doses' in modern practice are generally lower than 10 or 15 years ago (Watson 2000) and yet the demonstrated clinical effects appear to be stronger. Delivering less energy and achieving a stronger effect appears to go against the grain but, in the context of bioelectric behaviour, it is entirely consistent.

There are links between endogenous bioelectric activity, manual therapy and exercise in addition to the links with electrotherapy. This chapter has deliberately avoided the majority of these areas, although they are potentially just as important. When tissues are subjected to mechanical stress (e.g. manual therapy or exercise) there will be a change in the local bioelectric environment. The effects of these therapies were largely explained in terms or mechanical effects, and then, more recently, with an additional neurological explanation. It is suggested that an additional 'bioelectric' effect might be added to the list.

Endogenous bioelectricity is complex and, as yet, not fully understood. It has the potential to add to the existing explanations employed for various electrotherapy interventions and possibly other areas of therapy. That bioelectric activity exists is not in question. The relationship between it and therapy is an area of significant potential.

References

Anderson JC, Eriksson C (1968) Electrical properties of wet collagen. *Nature* **218**: 166–168.

Anglen J (2003) The clinical use of bone stimulators. *J South Orthop Assoc* **12**(2): 46–54.

Athenstaedt H (1970) Permanent longitudinal electric polarization and pyroelectric behaviour of collagenous structures and nervous tissue in man and other vertebrates. *Nature* **228**: 830–834.

Barker AT, Jaffe LF, Vanable JW (1982) The glabrous epidermis of cavies contains a powerful battery. *Am J Physiol* **242**: R358–R366.

Barnes TC (1945) Healing rate of human skin determined by measurement of the electrical potential of experimental abrasions. *Am J Surg* **69**: 82–88.

Bassett CA (1989) Fundamental & practical aspects of therapeutic uses of pulsed electromagnetic fields (PEMFs). *CRC Crit Rev Biomed Eng* **17**(5): 451–529.

Bassett CA (1993) Beneficial effects of electromagnetic fields. *J Cell Biochem* **51**(4): 387–393.

Becker RO (1961) The bioelectric factors in amphibian limb regeneration. *J Bone and Joint Surg* **43A**: 643–656.

Becker RO (1962) Some observations indicating the possibility of longitudinal charge-carrier flow in the peripheral nerves. *Biol Prototype Synthet Systems* **1**: 31–37.

Becker RO (1967) The electrical control of growth processes. *Med Times* **95**: 657–669.

Becker RO (1974a) The basic biological data transmission and control system influenced by electrical forces. *Ann N Y Acad Sci* **238**: 236–241.

Becker RO (1974b) The significance of bioelectric potentials. *Bioelectrochem Bioenerg* **1**: 187–199.

Becker RO (1990). *Cross Currents*. London, Bloomsbury Publishing.

Becker RO, Brown FM (1965) Photoelectric effects in human bone. *Nature* **206**: 1325–1328.

Becker RO, Selden G (1985). *The Body Electric: Electromagnetism and the Foundation of Life*. New York, William Morrow.

Becker RO, Bachman CH, Friedman H (1962a) The direct current control system: A link between environment and organism. *N Y State J Med* **62**: 1169–1176.

Becker RO, Bachman CH, Slaughter WH (1962b) Longitudinal direct current gradients of spinal nerves. *Nature* **196**: 675–676.

Bervar M (2005) Effect of weak, interrupted sinusoidal low frequency magnetic field on neural regeneration in rats: functional evaluation. *Bioelectromagnetics* **26**(5): 351–356.

Betz WJ, Caldwell JH (1984) Mapping electric currents around skeletal muscle with a vibrating probe. *J Gen Physiol* **83**: 143–156.

Betz WJ, Caldwell JH, Harris GL et al (1986) A steady electric current at the rat neuromuscular synapse. *Prog Clin Biol Res* **210**: 205–212.

Black J (1987) *Electrical stimulation: Its role in growth, repair and remodelling of the musculoskeletal system*. New York, Praeger.

Borgens RB (1981) Injury, ionic currents and regeneration. In Becker RO (ed) *Mechanisms of Growth Control*. Springfield, IL, Charles C Thomas: 107–136.

Borgens RB (1982) What is the role of naturally produced electric current in vertebrate regeneration and healing? *Int Rev Cytol* **76**: 245–298.

Borgens RB (1984) Endogenous ionic currents traverse intact and damaged bone. *Science* **225**: 478–482.

Borgens RB, McCaig CD (1989) Endogenous currents in nerve repair, regeneration and development. In Borgens RB (ed) *Electric Fields in Vertebrate Repair*. New York, Alan R Liss Inc: 77–116.

Borgens RB, Robinson KR, Vanable JW et al (1989) *Electric Fields in Vertebrate Repair: Natural and Applied Voltages in Vertebrate Regeneration and Healing*. New York, Alan R Liss Inc.

Burr HS, Harvey SC, Taffel M (1938) Bio-electric correlates of wound healing. *Yale J Biol Med* **11**: 103–107.

Chakkalakal DA, Wilson RF, Connolly JF (1988b) Electrophysiologic basis for prognosis in fracture healing. *Med Inst* **22**(6): 312–322.

Chakkalakal DA, Wilson RF, Connolly J (1988a) Epidermal and endosteal sources of endogenous electricity in injured canine limbs. *IEEE Trans Biomed Eng* **35**: 19–29.

Chang KS, Snellen JW (1982) Bioelectric activity in the rabbit ear regeneration. *J Exp Zool* **221**: 193–203.

Chang K, Chang WH, Wu ML et al (2003) Effects of different intensities of extremely low frequency pulsed electromagnetic fields on formation of osteoclast-like cells. *Bioelectromagnetics* **24**(6): 431–439.

Charman RA (1990) Bioelectricity and electrotherapy: towards a new paradigm. Introduction. *Physiotherapy* **76**(9): 502–508.

Charman RA (2000) *Complementary therapies for physical therapists*. Oxford, Butterworth–Heinemann.

Charman RA (2002) Electrical properties of cells and tissues. In Kitchen S (ed) *Electrotherapy: Evidence Based Practice*. Chapter 2, pp 31–44. Oxford, Elsevier.

Ciombor DM, Aaron RK (2005) The role of electrical stimulation in bone repair. *Foot Ankle Clin* **10**(4): 579–593, vii.

Cleary SF (1987) Cellular effects of electromagnetic radiation. *IEEE Eng Med Biol* **6**(1): 26–30.

da Silva RV, Camilli JA (2006) Repair of bone defects treated with autogenous bone graft and low-power laser. *J Craniofaci Surg* **17**(2): 297–301.

De Pedro JA, Perez-Caballer AJ, Dominguez J et al (2005) Pulsed electromagnetic fields induce peripheral nerve regeneration and endplate enzymatic changes. *Bioelectromagnetics* **26**(1): 20–27.

Diniz P, Shomura K, Soejima K et al (2002) Effects of pulsed electromagnetic field (PEMF) stimulation on bone tissue like formation are dependent on the maturation stages of the osteoblasts. *Bioelectromagnetics* **23**(5): 398–405.

El-Husseini T, El-Kawy S, Shalaby H et al (2006) Microcurrent skin patches for postoperative pain control in total knee arthroplasty: a pilot study: a pilot study. *Int Orthop* **31**(2): 229–233.

Evans RD, Foltz D, Foltz K (2001) Electrical stimulation with bone and wound healing. *Clin Podiatr Med Surg* **18**(1): 79–95, vi.

Foulds IS, Barker AT (1983) Human skin battery potentials and their possible role in wound healing. *Br J Dermatol* **109**: 515–522.

Friedenberg Z, Brighton CT (1966) Bioelectric potentials in bone. *J Bone Joint Surg (A)* **48**: 915–923.

Friedenberg ZB, Brighton CT (1981) Bioelectricity and fracture healing. *Plast Reconstr Surg* **68**(3): 435–443.

Friedenberg Z, Harlow MC, Heppenstall RB et al (1973) The cellular origin of bioelectric potentials in bone. *Calc Tiss Res* **13**: 53–62.

Fukada E, Yasuda I (1957) On the piezoelectric effect of bone. *J Phys Soc Japan* **12**: 1158–1162.

Gapeyev AB, Chemeris NK (2000) Nonlinear processes of intracellular calcium signaling as a target for the influence of extremely low-frequency fields. *Electro Magnet Biol* **19**(1): 21–42.

Garavello-Freitas I, Baranauskas V, Joazeiro PP et al (2003) Low-power laser irradiation improves histomorphometrical parameters and bone matrix organization during tibia wound healing in rats. *J Photochem Photobiol B* **70**(2): 81–89.

Gebauer D, Mayr E, Orthner E et al (2005) Low-intensity pulsed ultrasound: effects on nonunions. *Ultrasound Med Biol* **31**(10): 1391–402.

Grodzinsky AJ (1983) Electromechanical and physiochemical properties of connective tissue. *CRC Crit Rev Biomed Eng* **9**(2): 133–199.

Guzelsu N, Walsh WR (1993) Piezoelectric and electrokinetic effects in bone tissue – review. *Electro Magnet Biol* **12**(1): 51–82.

Illingworth CM, Barker AT (1980) Measurement of electrical currents emerging during the regeneration of amputated finger tips in children. *Clin Phys Physiol Meas* **1**(1): 87–89.

Jaffe LF (1986) Ion currents in development: An overview. *Prog Clin Biol Res* **210**: 351–357.

Jaffe LF, Vanable JW (1984) Electric fields and wound healing. *Clin Dermatol* **2**(3): 34–44.

Juutilainen J (2005) Developmental effects of electromagnetic fields. *Bioelectromagnetics* **Suppl 7**: S107–S115.

Karu TI (1987) Photobiological fundamentals of low power laser therapy. *J Quant Elect QE* **23**(10): 1703–1717.

Kesani AK, Gandhi A, Lin SS (2006) Electrical bone stimulation devices in foot and ankle surgery: types of devices, scientific basis, and clinical indications for their use. *Foot Ankle Int* **27**(2): 148–156.

Kloth LC (2005) Electrical stimulation for wound healing: a review of evidence from in vitro studies, animal experiments, and clinical trials. *Int J Low Extrem Wounds* **4**(1): 23–44.

Kloth LC, McCulloch JM (1996) Promotion of wound healing with electrical stimulation. *Adv Wound Care* **9**(5): 42–45.

Lafargue AL, Cabrales LB, Larramendi RM (2002) Bioelectrical parameters of the whole human body obtained through bioelectrical impedance analysis. *Bioelectromagnetics* **23**(6): 450–4.

Lambert MI, Marcus P, Burgess T et al (2002) Electro-membrane microcurrent therapy reduces signs and symptoms of muscle damage. *Med Sci Sports Exerc* **34**(4): 602–7.

Legare A, Garon M, Guardo R et al (2002) Detection and analysis of cartilage degeneration by spatially resolved streaming potentials. *J Orthop Res* **20**: 819–826.

Loewenstein WR (1981) Junctional intercellular communication: The cell to cell membrane channel. *Physiol Rev* **61**(4): 829–913.

Lokietek W, Pawluk RJ, Bassett CAL (1974) Muscle injury potentials: a source of voltage in the undeformed rabbit tibia. *J Bone Joint Surg* **56B**(2): 361–369.

Luchian T, Bancia B, Pavel C et al (2002) Biomembrane excitability studied within a wide-band frequency of an interacting exogenous electric field. *Electromag Biol Med* **21**(3): 287–302.

Luger EJ, Rochkind S, Wollman Y et al (1998) Effect of low-power laser irradiation on the mechanical properties of bone fracture healing in rats. *Lasers Surg Med* **22**(2): 97–102.

MacDonald N, Watson J (1982) Measurement of skin potential patterns. *Trans Bioelect Repair Growth* **2**: 33.

Malizos KN, Hantes ME, Protopappas V et al (2006) Low-intensity pulsed ultrasound for bone healing: an overview. *Injury* **37 Suppl 1**: S56–S62.

Marino AA (1988) *Modern Bioelectricity.* New York, Marcel Dekker Inc.

Marino AA, Kolomytkin OV, Frilot C (2003) Extracellular currents alter gap junction intercellular communication in synovial fibroblasts. *Bioelectromagnetics* **24**(3): 199–205.

McMakin CR (2004) Microcurrent therapy: a novel treatment method for chronic low back myofascial pain. *J Bodywork Mov Ther* **8**: 143–153.

Mortimer AJ, Dyson M (1988) The effect of therapeutic ultrasound on calcium uptake in fibroblasts. *Ultrasound Med Biol* **14**(6): 499–506.

Nordenstrom BE (1983) *Biologically Closed Electric Circuits: Clinical, Experimental and Theoretical Evidence for an Additional Circulatory System.* Stockholm, Nordic Medical Publications.

Nordenstrom BE (1994) The paradigm of biologically closed electric circuits (BCEC) and the formation of an International Association (IABC) for BCEC systems. *Eur J Surg Suppl* **574**: 7–23.

Nuccitelli R (2003) A role for endogenous electric fields in wound healing. *Curr Top Dev Biol* **58**: 1–26.

O'Leary JL, Goldring S (1964) D-C potentials of the brain. *Physiol Rev* **44**: 91–125.

Ojingwa JC, Isseroff RR (2002) Electrical stimulation of wound healing. *Prog Dermatol* **36**(4): 1–12.

Oschman JL (2005) Energy and the healing response. *J Bodywork Mov Ther* **9**(1): 3–15.

Park SH, Silva M (2004) Neuromuscular electrical stimulation enhances fracture healing: results of an animal model. *J Orthop Res* **22**(2): 382–387.

Pokorny J (2001) Endogenous electromagnetic forces in living cells; implications for transfer of reaction components. *Electro Magnet Biol* **20**(1): 59–73.

Pollack SR, Salzstein R, Pienkowski D (1984) Streaming potentials in fluid filled bone. *Ferroelectrics* **60**: 297–309.

Rubinacci A, Brigatti L, Tessari L (1984) A reference curve for axial bioelectric potentials in rabbit tibia. *Bioelectromagnetics* **5**(2): 193–202.

Ryaby JT (1998) Clinical effects of electromagnetic and electric fields on fracture healing. *Clin Orthop* **355** (Suppl): S205–S215.

Saunders RD, McCaig CD (2005) Developmental effects of physiologically weak electric fields and heat: an overview. *Bioelectromagnetics* **Suppl 7**: S127–S132.

Sevitt S (1981) *Bone Repair and Fracture Healing in Man.* London, Churchill Livingstone.

Shibib K, Brock M, Buljat G et al (1988) Structural and regenerative changes in deafferented and deefferented ulnar nerves. *Surg Neurol* **29**: 282–292.

Singh S, Katz J (1989) Electromechanical properties of bone: a review. *J Bioelectricity* **7**(2): 219–238.

Smith RB (2002) Microcurrent therapies: emerging theories of physiological information processing. *NeuroRehabilitation* **17**(1): 3–7.

Sonnier H, Marino AA (2001) Sensory transduction as a proposed model for biological detection of electromagnetic fields. *Electro Magnet Biol* **20**(2): 153–175.

Trock DH (2000) Electromagnetic fields and magnets. Investigational treatment for musculoskeletal disorders. *Rheum Dis Clin North Am* **26**(1): 51–62, viii.

Vanable J (1989) Integumentary potentials and wound healing. In borgens R (ed) *Electric Fields in Vertebrate Repair.* New York, Alan Liss Inc: 171–224.

Wachtel H (1992) Bioelectric background fields and their implications for ELF dosimetry. *Bioelectromagnetics* **Suppl 1**: 139–145.

Walsh WR, Guzelsu N (1993) Ion concentration effects on bone streaming potentials and zeta potentials. *Biomaterials* **14**(5): 331–336.

Warden SJ, Fuchs RK, Kessler CK et al (2006) Ultrasound produced by a conventional therapeutic ultrasound unit accelerates fracture repair. *Phys Ther* **86**(8): 1118–1127.

Watson T (1995) *Bioelectric Correlates of Musculoskeletal Injury and Repair.* PhD Thesis, Department of Mechanical Engineering. University of Surrey, Guildford, Surrey.

Watson T (1996) Electrical stimulation for wound healing. *Phys Ther Rev* **1**(2): 89–103.

Watson T (2000) The role of electrotherapy in contemporary physiotherapy practice. *Man Ther* **5**(3): 132–141.

Watson T (2006) Electrotherapy and tissue repair. *Sportex Med* **29**: 7–13.

Weiss DS, Kirsner R, Eaglstein WH (1990) Electrical stimulation and wound healing. *Arch Dermatol* **126**: 222–225.

Wilber MC (1978) Surface direct current bioelectric potentials in the normal and injured human thigh. *Texas Rep Biol Med* **36**: 197–204.

Zhang Y, Ding J, Duan W et al (2005) Influence of pulsed electromagnetic field with different pulse duty cycles on neurite outgrowth in PC12 rat pheochromocytoma cells. *Bioelectromagnetics* **26**(5): 406–411.

Zhao M, Forrester JV, McCaig CD (1999) A small physiological electric field orients cell division. *Proc Natl Acad Sci USA* **96**: 4942–4946.

Chapter 4

Tissue repair

Sheila Kitchen and Stephen R. Young

INTRODUCTION

Physiotherapists and others treat acute and chronic inflammatory lesions, open and closed wounds. Use is made of a wide variety of electrophysical agents, discussed in later chapters, to initiate or enhance the repair process, including ultrasound, the diathermies, lasers, and low-frequency stimulating currents. To understand how electrophysical agents can affect the healing of tissues, and the rationale underlying their selection and application, it is essential that the processes underlying healing are understood.

Healing is a complex but essential process without which the body would be unlikely to survive. It involves the integrated actions of cells, matrix and chemical messengers and aims to restore the integrity of the tissue as rapidly as possible. It is a homoeostatic mechanism to restore physiological equilibrium, and can be initiated as a result of loss of communication between adjacent cells, between cells and their support, or by cell death. Healing can be described in terms of chemokinesis, cell multiplication and differentiation. A complex series of events occurs, involving the migration of cells of vascular and connective tissue origin to the site of injury. This process is governed by chemotactic substances liberated *in situ*. The healing process, which is common to all body tissue types, can be divided into three overlapping phases:

1. inflammation
2. proliferation
3. remodelling.

Healing of all tissue is based on these phases and normally results in the formation of scar tissue. Limited regeneration of certain tissues, such as the epidermis, skeletal muscle and adipose tissue, can also occur. The basic principles that underlie repair and which lead to scar formation will be described first; subsequently, a brief summary of the regenerative healing of specific tissues is provided; finally, a number of factors that might be detrimental to repair are addressed.

THE PRINCIPLES OF TISSUE HEALING

The duration of each phase varies slightly depending on the type of wound, tissue involved and any complicating factors. Table 4.1 provides a general guide.

INFLAMMATORY PHASE

Inflammation is the immediate response to injury. The cardinal signs of inflammation are redness, swelling, heat and pain. The acute, or early, phase inflammatory response lasts between 24 and 48 hours and is followed by a subacute, or late, phase, which lasts between 10 and 14 days. The subacute phase can be extended if there is a continuing source of trauma or if some form of irritation, such as a foreign body or infection, is present.

Tissue injury causes both cell death and blood vessel disruption. The primary purpose of the inflammatory phase of healing is to rid the area of debris and dead tissue and to destroy any invading infection prior to the repair. This phase can be described in terms of vascular and cellular changes, which are mediated through the actions of chemical agents. Figure 4.1 shows a typical wound after 3 days.

VASOREGULATION AND BLOOD CLOTTING

The initial vascular reaction involves haemorrhage and fluid loss due to destruction of vessels; this is followed by vasoconstriction, vessel plugging and blood coagulation, to prevent further blood loss. These processes lead to the activation of the repair process. Blood loss into the tissues initiates platelet activity and blood coagulation directly, both of which then result in the production of chemical factors which initiate and control the healing process. In addition, the blood clot provides a provisional matrix that facilitates the migration of cells into the wound (Clark 1991b, Singer & Clark 1999).

Primary vessel constriction occurs. This is due to the release of noradrenaline (norepinephrine); the reaction lasts for only a few seconds to a few minutes. During vasoconstriction the opposing cell walls are brought into contact, and adhesion between the surfaces results. Secondary vessel vasoconstriction might follow, due to the action of serotonin, adenosine diphosphate, calcium and thrombin.

Both lymphatics and blood vessels are plugged to limit fluid loss. Initial platelet adhesion and aggregation is stimulated by the presence of thrombin (Terkeltaub & Ginsberg 1988). The platelets adhere to one another, to the vessel walls and to the interstitial extracellular matrix, leading to the build-up

Table 4.1 Duration of and factors affecting repair phases

Phase of repair	Approximate duration	Factors affecting duration
Inflammation		
Acute phase	24–48 hours	• Tissue involved
Subacute phase	10–14 days	• Levels of nutrients, oxygen, cytokines, etc.
		• Mechanical tensions on tissues
Proliferation		
	Variable intermediate phase	As above
Remodelling		
	Begins at around 2 weeks; can last for a year or more	As above

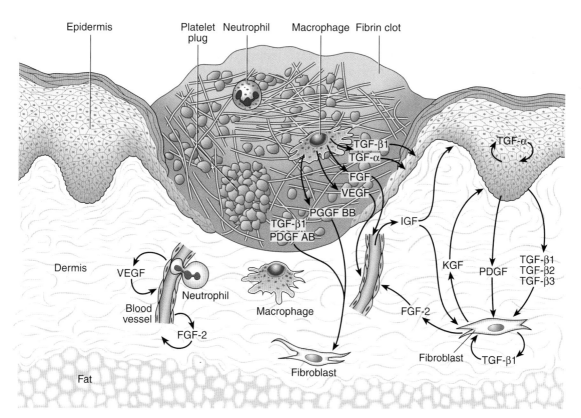

Figure 4.1 A cutaneous wound 3 days after injury. FGF, fibroblast growth factor; IGF, insulin-like growth factor; KGF, keratinocyte growth factor; PDGF, platelet-derived growth factor; TGF, transforming growth factor; VEGF, vascular endothelial growth factor (from Singer & Clark 1999).

of relatively unstable platelet plugs. The process is continued and consolidated by the release of adhesive proteins such as fibrinogen, fibronectin, thrombospondin and von Willebrand factor by the platelets (Ginsberg et al 1988). Coagulation of extravascular blood is thought to be due to the action of platelets and intrinsic and extrinsic clotting mechanisms. Prothrombin is converted to thrombin and thus fibrinogen to fibrin, providing an early wound matrix.

Blood coagulation not only aids haemostasis through clot formation but adds to the early wound matrix and results in the generation of chemical mediators such as bradykinin (Proud & Kaplan 1988). These substances affect the local circulation, stimulate the production of further chemical mediators and act as attractants to cells such as neutrophils and monocytes.

Following this period of vasoconstriction, secondary vasodilation and increased permeability of venules occur owing to the effects of histamine, prostaglandins and hydrogen peroxide production (Issekutz 1981, Williams 1988). Subsequently, both bradykinin and the anaphyllatoxins initiate mechanisms that increase the permeability of undamaged vessels, leading to the release of plasma proteins which contribute to the generation of the extravascular clot.

CELL MIGRATION AND ACTION

Neutrophils and monocytes are the earliest cells to reach the site of injury. They migrate in response to a wide variety of chemical and mechanical stimuli, including the products of the clotting mechanism, the presence of bacteria and cell-derived factors.

The primary action of neutrophils is phagocytosis; their task is to rid the site of bacteria and of dead and dying materials. Neutrophilic margination within the vascular structures leads to the passage of neutrophils through vessel walls by amoeboid action, enabling them to reach damaged extravascular tissues. Phagocytosis is achieved by neutrophilic lysis. This results in the release of protease and collagenase, which begin the lysis of necrotic protein and collagen respectively, as shown in Figure 4.2. Infiltration of the neutrophils into the extravascular tissue ends after a couple of days, marking the end of the early phase of inflammation.

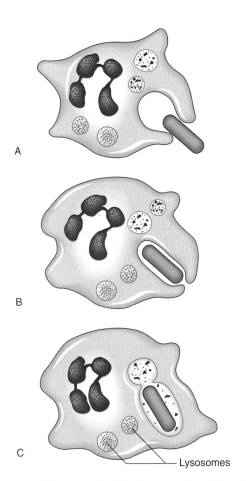

A

B

C

Lysosomes

Figure 4.2 Phagocytosis. A, in phagocytosis, cells such as neutrophils and macrophages ingest large solid particles such as bacteria and dead and dying material. B, folds of the plasma membrane surround the particle to be ingested, forming a small vacuole around it, which then pinches off inside the cell. C, lysosomes fuse with the vacuole and pour their digestive enzymes (such as protease and collagenase) on to the digested/ingested material.

Macrophages are essential to the healing process and can perform the normal function of neutrophils in addition to their other tasks. Monocytes migrate from the vasculature into the tissue space and rapidly differentiate into macrophages; the factors responsible for this change have not been fully identified, but may include the presence of insoluble fibronectin (Hosein et al 1985), low oxygen tension (Hunt 1987), chemotactic agents (Ho et al 1987) and bacterial lipopolysaccharides and interferons (Riches 1996). Macrophages phagocytose pathogenic organisms, tissue debris and dying cells (including neutrophils), and release collagenase and proteoglycans, both of which are degrading enzymes that lyse necrotic material (Leibovich & Ross 1975, Tsukamoto et al 1981).

CHEMICAL FACTORS

Many growth factors that influence and control the initial inflammatory process and trigger further developments in the proliferative phase are released by cells during the stage of inflammation; some key factors are shown in Table 4.2.

Macrophages release factors that attract fibroblasts to the area (Tsukamoto et al 1981) and enhance collagen deposition (Clark 1985, Weeks 1972). Platelets release growth factors that contribute to the control of fibrin deposition, fibroplasia and angiogenesis through their action on a variety of cells. Platelets also release fibronectin, fibrinogen, thrombospondin and von Willebrand factor (Ginsberg et al 1988); these are necessary for the aggregation of platelets and for their binding to tissue structure. In addition, serotonin, adenosine diphosphate, calcium and thromboxin are released; these are necessary for blood vessel constriction to prevent haemorrhage.

Dead and dying cells release substances that influence the development of the neomatrix; these include a variety of tissue factors, lactic acid, lactate dehydrogenase, calcium, lysosomal enzymes and fibroblast growth factor (Clark 1991a). In addition, prostaglandins (PG) are produced by almost all cells of the body following damage, due to alterations in the phospholipid content of the cell walls (Janssen et al 1991); some types of PG are proinflammatory, increasing vascular permeability, sensitising pain receptors and attracting leucocytes to

Table 4.2 Key cytokines affecting tissue repair (adapted from Singer & Clark 1999)

Cytokine groups	Arising from	Targets tissues and effects
Epidermal growth factors		
EGF	Platelets	Epidermal and mesenchymal structures:
TGF-α	Macrophages, epidermal cells	cell motility and proliferation
Heparin binding EGT	Macrophages	
Fibroblast growth factors	Macrophages, endothelial cells, fibroblasts	Wound vascularization, fibroblast proliferation, epidermal cell proliferation and motility
Transforming growth factor-β family	Platelets, macrophages	Fibrosis and increased tensile strength
Platelet-derived growth factor	Platelets, macrophages	Fibroblast proliferation and chemoattraction; macrophage chemoattraction and activation
Interleukin-1	Neutrophils	Production of growth factors
Insulin-like growth factor-1	Fibroblasts, epidermal cells	Granulation tissue formation; re-epithelialisation
Tumour necrosis factor	Neutrophils	Production of growth factors
Interferon-α/β	Lymphocytes, fibroblasts	Macrophage activation, inhibit fibroblast proliferation
Thromboxane A_2	Destroyed cells	Potent vasoconstrictor

EGF, epidermal growth factors; EGT, epidermal growth factor; TGF, transforming growth factor.

the area. Other classes of PG are anti-inflammatory. Both can be involved in early stages of repair.

PROLIFERATIVE PHASE

Granulation tissue is formed during the proliferative phase. This is a temporary structure that evolves after a period of a couple of days and comprises neomatrix, neovasculature, macrophages and fibroblasts. Granulation tissue precedes the development of mature scar tissue. 'Fibroplasia' is a term that encompasses the processes of fibroblast proliferation and migration, and the development of the collagenous and non-collagenous matrices.

Fibroplasia

Fibroblasts produce and organize the major extracellular components of the granulation tissue. They migrate into the wound in response to both chemical and physical attractants (Clark 1990, McCarthy et al 1996, Repesh et al 1982). The fibroblast is primarily responsible for the deposition of the new matrix. Once present within the wound, fibroblasts synthesize hyaluronic acid, fibronectin and types I and III collagen; these form

the early extracellular matrix. Changes take place as the matrix matures: the amount of hyaluronic acid and fibrinogen is gradually reduced, type I collagen becomes the predominant component, and proteoglycans are deposited.

Hyaluronic acid, present only in early wound healing, appears to facilitate cell motility and might be important in fibroblast proliferation (Lark et al 1985, Toole 1981). Fibronectin has many functions within a wound, including acting as a chemoattractant to cells such as fibroblasts and endothelial cells, augmenting the attachment of fibroblasts to fibrin, facilitating the migration of fibroblasts, and possibly providing a template for collagen deposition (Clark 1996). Proteoglycans contribute to tissue resilience and help to regulate cell motility and growth, and the deposition of collagen.

Collagen is a generic term covering a number of different types of glycoprotein found in the extracellular matrix. Collagen provides a rigid network, which facilitates further healing. The types of collagen within a wound, and their quantities, are gradually modified with time. Type III (embryonic collagen) is gradually absorbed and replaced by type I collagen, which is mature fibrillar collagen. Type IV collagen might be produced as a part of the basement membrane when skin damage occurs, and type V collagen is deposited around cells, forming a structural support.

Two primary factors affect collagen metabolism and, therefore, production. The first is the effect of the cytokines; Table 4.3 lists some of the cytokines believed to affect collagen metabolism. There appears to be a balance between the stimulatory and inhibitory effects of these substances, leading to optimal healing with neither over- nor underproduction of collagen.

The second factor influencing collagen metabolism is the nature of the extracellular matrix (Kulozik et al 1991, Mauch & Krieg 1990). The extracellular matrix provides both a structural scaffold for the tissue and signalling for the cells. Reduced collagen synthesis results from cell contact with mature, type I collagen, upon which the production of collagenase is activated.

ANGIOGENESIS

An extensive vascular system is required to provide for the needs of the proliferative phase. Angiogenesis is thought to be initiated by the presence of multiple stimuli. The process initially involves capillary budding, with the disruption of the basement membrane of the venule at a point adjacent to the angiogenic stimulus. Endothelial cells migrate towards the stimulus as a cord of cells

surrounded by a provisional matrix (Ausprunk et al 1981, Clark et al 1982). Individual sprouts link to form capillary loops, which might in turn develop further sprouts. Lumina appear within the arched cords and blood flow is gradually established, initially in immature, permeable vessels, and later in more mature capillary beds having developed basement membrane components (Ausprunk et al 1981, Hashimoto & Prewitt 1987).

The anastomosis of existing vessels and the coupling or recoupling of vessels within the wound space also occurs, leading to a well-developed blood supply within the granulation tissue. However, this state is not retained, as the granulation tissue is later remodelled into scar tissue. Capillary regression occurs, possibly in response to a loss of angiogenic stimuli, and is characterized by changes in the mitochondria of the endothelial cells, their gradual degeneration and necrosis, and final ingestion by macrophages.

Angiogenesis is stimulated and controlled through the action of many substances; these have been reviewed by Folkman & Klagsburn (1987), Madri & Pratt (1996) and Zetter (1988). Effects can be direct and indirect, and arise from stimuli generated both at the time of injury and during the early stages of repair.

WOUND CONTRACTION

Wound contraction begins soon after injury and peaks at around 2 weeks. It involves the complex interaction of cells, extracellular matrix and cytokines. There are still many gaps in our knowledge about wound contraction in humans; a helpful review of the various possibilities is provided by Nedelec et al (2000). What is presented here is a simplified over view of the most likely factors.

During the second week of repair, fibroblasts appear to develop into myofibroblasts – cells that have characteristics of both fibroblasts and smooth muscle cells. The contractile activity of these cells draws the edges of the wound together against the constant centrifugal tension of the surrounding tissues. More recently, a form of actin has been identified in myofibroblasts, and these microfilaments form cell-to-cell and cell-to-matrix linkages. They then retract, holding the collagen in place until it has stabilized its position. This process is probably

Table 4.3 Cytokines controlling collagen production

Cytokine	Action	Reference
TGF-β	Induces collagen synthesis	Ignotz & Massague 1986
IL-1	Induces collagen synthesis	Prostlethwaite et al 1988
TNF	Induces collagen synthesis	Duncan & Berman 1989
IFN	Decreases collagen synthesis	Czaja et al 1987
TNF-α	Decreases collagen synthesis	Scharffetter et al 1989
PGE2	Decreases collagen synthesis	Nicholas et al 1991

IFN, interferons; IL-1, interleukin-1; PGE_2, prostaglandin E_2; TGF, transforming growth factor; TNF, tumour necrosis factor.

initiated and controlled by growth factors such as transforming growth factor (TGF)- β1, TGF-β2 and platelet-derived growth factor (PDGF); cross-links between bundles of collagen have a direct affect on this process (Woodley et al 1991), as does the attachment of the fibroblasts to the collagen matrix (Schiro et al 1991).

REMODELLING

Remodelling of the immature tissue matrix commences at about the same time as new tissue formation, although for clarity it is normally regarded as comprising the third phase of healing. The matrix that is present at this stage is gradually replaced and remodelled over the subsequent months and years as the scar tissue matures.

Collagen is immature and gel-like in construction in the early stages of wound healing, and exhibits little tensile strength. Remodelling occurs over a period ranging from several months to years, with type III collagen (which has more cross-links) being partly replaced by type I. Fibres reorientate themselves along the lines of stress applied to the lesion, thus resulting in greater tensile strength of the tissue. Wound breaking strength increases with the deposition of collagen, reaching approximately 20% of the normal strength by day 21. The final strength attained will be in the region of 70–80% of the normal value.

REPAIR OF SPECIALISED TISSUES

The repair of certain specialised tissues can result in a number of modifications or additions to the normal healing process. A brief description of the processes that might occur when epidermal tissue, muscle, ligament/tendon, nerve and bone are damaged follows. A number of reviews and texts have addressed these areas in more detail (e.g. Carpenter & Karpati 1984, Heppenstall 1980, Singer & Clark 1999, Williams et al 1989).

EPIDERMAL TISSUE

Injuries to the skin can involve either the epidermis alone or both the epidermis and the dermis. When the skin is broken, rapid coverage of the surface is essential to reduce the hazards associated with environmental stress and contamination. While dermal healing is proceeding, as described above, re-epithelialization of the surface occurs to repair damage to the epidermis.

Re-epithelialization is initiated within 24 hours of injury. Epidermal basal cells undergo changes that allow them to migrate toward the site of the lesion; they loosen their intercellular attachments (desmosomes), lose their cellular rigidity and develop actinic pseudopodia – all of which facilitate cell mobility. In addition, the bond (hemidermasomal link) between the epidermal and dermal layers loosens, allowing lateral movement of the cells. Epidermal cells migrate rapidly towards the base of a wound, travelling across the remaining viable basal lamina or the fibrin scaffolding of the blood clot formed in deeper lesions. They separate the eschar ('scab') from the viable tissue. This process is controlled by a variety of factors; cells move across the wound surface in response to a number of substances in the wound matrix, including fibronectin, fibrin and collagen (type IV), which provide a structural network for migration (Hunt & Dunphy 1980). Separation of the epidermal from the dermal layers, and of the eschar from viable tissue, is controlled by factors, including chemotactic factors, structural macromolecules, degradative enzymes, tissue geometry (such as the free-edge effect), fibrin, collagen, fibronectin, thrombospondin and growth factors.

A few days after injury, epidermal cells at the edge of the wound begin to proliferate and spread across the wound. The absence of neighbouring cells, increased numbers of growth factors or increased numbers of growth factor receptors might all stimulate this process. Basement membrane proteins reappear and the hemidesmosomes re-form to link the basement membrane and the epidermal layer of cells. Normal keratinization follows, initially in the uppermost layers, followed by the development of a full stratum corneum.

MUSCLE TISSUE

The degree to which regeneration takes place in muscle appears to depend both on the degree to which the basement membranes of the original fibres have been retained and on the vascular and nerve supply to the area (Carlson & Faulkner 1983). Muscle repair involves the removal of damaged cell components, the proliferation of satellite cells to form new muscle fibre building materials and the fusion of satellite cells to form new myotubes and muscle fibres (Fig. 4.3).

In the early degenerative phase, myofibrils lose their regularity and disorganization of the Z disc occurs. Mitochondria become more rounded and lose their regular distribution within the cell. Actin and myosin filaments lose their regularity, glycogen particles disappear and tissue no longer stains positive for the enzymes, such as phosphorylase, that are used in glycogenolysis.

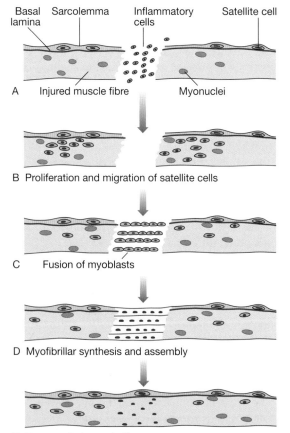

A Injured muscle fibre

B Proliferation and migration of satellite cells

C Fusion of myoblasts

D Myofibrillar synthesis and assembly

E Regenerated muscle fibre

Figure 4.3 Muscle repair. A, damaged cellular components are digested by cellular infiltration and inflammation. B, satellite cells proliferate and then, C, fuse into myotubules to form new myofibrils. D, myofibrillar proteins are synthesized to 'fill' the new fibre, resulting in, E, regenerated muscle fibre.

Proliferation of skeletal muscle satellite cells (or presumptive myoblasts) follows, and these provide a source of myonuclei for the regenerating muscle cells. Bischoff (1986, 1990) hoped to identify the factors that might initiate this process; he suggested that under normal conditions the sarcolemma exerted a negative control on satellite cells to prevent proliferation; this inhibition was removed after structural damage. Bischoff (1990) also suggested positive control through the action of mitogenic factors, although the nature of this is as yet unclear.

Regeneration subsequently follows the normal pattern of muscle development, with satellite cells aligning themselves along the basal lamina and fusing into myotubules. The presence of the basal lamina appears to influence this process, providing a substrate upon which alignment can occur and expressing a number of extracellular matrix components. It is not, however, essential to the process, as reduced levels of regeneration occur in the absence of an intact lamina.

As the myotubules mature and differentiate, they synthesise myofibrillar proteins; these are deposited in the outer subsarcolemmal region. During this process, the muscle nuclei are normally pushed to the periphery, although a few remain centrally as testimony to the repair process.

TENDON, LIGAMENT AND CARTILAGE REPAIR

Ligaments and tendons

Ligaments and tendons are less vascular than many other tissues, being largely made up of collagen with varying amounts of ground substance. Some repair relatively well, with little surgical or other intervention (e.g. the medial collateral ligament (MCL) of the knee) whereas others are more of a problem (e.g. the Achilles tendon).

The repair process fundamentally follows that described above. During the first 72 hours, a matrix consisting of randomly aligned collagen fibres and ground substance is developed. The process continues over a period of approximately 6 weeks. Type III collagen appears in higher levels than normal and is thought to be especially useful because it has the ability to form cross-links, which provide some stability to the repair. During this phase there is an increased level of organization within the tissue, although the collagen fibres continue to remain relatively disorganized; the remodelling phase is therefore important and takes a year or more. During this phase, the structure is relatively weak, although it improves as the fibres are reoriented along the lines of force. As noted with other tissues, growth factors are important in the repair of these tissues; these include insulin-like growth factor (IGF-1), PDGF, TGF-β and -α and EGF (Molloy et al, 2003; Woo et al, 2000). They bring repair cells to the wound and stimulate the production of collagen and ground substance materials; for example, TGF-β and PDGF have been shown to increase the rupture point of healing tendon, and TGF-β1 and EGF affect matrix synthesis by fibroblasts.

Management of these types of injury varies and includes surgical intervention, which is essential if the ends of the structures are no longer in contact, and possibly immobilization in a cast. However, not all ligament and tendon injuries require this and it has been shown that MCL healing is often good without either intervention. Studies of healing of tendons and ligaments has shown that some have a very poor capacity for repair; both poor morphological and biomechanical properties are often evident, making them susceptible to repeated injury. More recently, work has developed to investigate whether doses of growth factors can stimulate better repair, and there is some evidence of benefits.

Cartilage

In the adult cartilage has a very poor ability to repair itself following damage. One reason for this is its very low vascularity, another is that the collagen network in the cartilage does not repair effectively, with in-vivo studies suggesting that collagen production is very limited. Possible interventions to assist repair are currently very limited. Recently, however, there has been an increased amount of work examining the possibilities of tissue engineering with respect to cartilage. Some reports have looked at the role of growth factors and shown some promise in terms of the generation of new cartilage in vitro. In normal healthy tissue, cartilage undergoes a very slow but continual process of remodelling, with a balance between destruction and synthesis. This is under the control of a variety of growth factors. It is hoped that in time this knowledge will be of help in the in-vivo repair of damaged cartilage.

NERVOUS TISSUE

When a peripheral axon is damaged it is sometimes possible for it to undergo repair, which allows normal conduction to resume. In mammals, however, repair of central axons is generally not possible, possibly owing to the absence of definite endoneurial tubes and the proliferation of macroglia cells. Considerable research is currently being conducted in this area to clarify matters.

When an axon is subject to trauma, changes occur on both sides of the injury. Distally, the axon swells and then disintegrates, with total degeneration and removal of the cytoplasmic matter occurring within the membrane of the axon. A similar process occurs in the proximal direction, gradually progressing toward the cell body. This normally leads to effects in the cell body, such as changes in cytoplasmic RNA, dispersion of Nissl granules, production of protein-synthesizing organelles, and positional reorganization of both nucleoli and ribosomes (Fig. 4.4).

When regrowth of the axon is possible, as occurs in the peripheral nervous system when the cell body has not been destroyed, an intact endoneurial sheath at or near to the site of damage helps to establish satisfactory contact with the peripheral receptors and end organs. Following degeneration of the myelin sheath, the Schwann cells proliferate and occupy the endoneurial tube. In addition, they form a bridge across any gap in the continuity of the axon. The proximal part of the axon develops a swelling, which gives rise to a large number of axonal 'sprouts'. These spread out within the tissue surrounding the wound. Although many ultimately serve no useful purpose, one will enter the tube and grow distally, accompanied by the Schwann cells. When the axon finally makes successful contact with the end organs, the Schwann cells begin to synthesize a myelin sheath. Finally, the axonal diameter and the myelin-sheath thickness increase, leading to near-normal conduction behaviour.

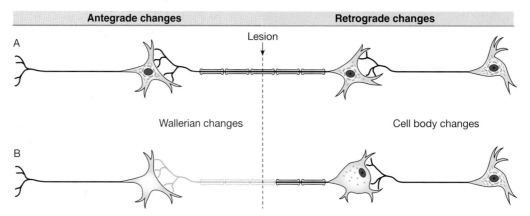

Figure 4.4 Repair of nervous tissue. A, both antegrade and retrograde changes occur following damage to a neuron. B, Wallerian changes, which include generation of the myelin sheath and axon, occur in the antegrade direction. Cell body changes include movement of the nucleus to the periphery, removal of the protein synthesis apparatus and dispersion of Nissl granules.

BONE TISSUE

The repair of bone tissue follows the same basic pattern as that described in the section on the principles of healing, with an added osteogenic component. Haemorrhage occurs immediately after injury. A clot forms and the acute inflammatory phase of repair is initiated. Mast cells, polymorphonuclear leucocytes and macrophages move into the area and appear to be responsible for the release of factors that stimulate tissue repair. Dead and dying tissues are removed by macrophages and osteoclasts and a gradual ingrowth of granulation tissue occurs to replace the clot. This is completed normally by about 4 days.

Osteoblasts, whether derived from osteocytes, fibroblasts or a number of other sources, become active. They are stimulated into activity by a number of factors, including mast cell factors, decreased oxygen levels and bone morphogenic substances. In addition, chondroblasts can become active under certain conditions, especially when oxygen levels are particularly poor. Small groups of cartilaginous cells appear within this early tissue, chiefly in the region of the periosteum. Osteoblasts deposit calcium both directly in the tissue matrix and in the islands of cartilage. The fracture is now united by a firm but pliable material known as *provisional* (or *soft*) *callus*.

Subsequently, both subperiosteal and endochondral ossification continues and, after about 2 months, the bone ends become united by primitive (or *woven*) bone, which is known as *hard callus*.

Finally, this woven bone is remodelled to form mature lamellar bone. Both osteoblasts and osteoclasts are involved in this process. The marrow cavity is restored, the contour of the bone smoothed, and the internal structure of the bone reorganized as the type of bone changes and the tissue responds to the normal external forces to which it is again submitted. Figure 4.5 illustrates the process of repair.

ABNORMAL TISSUE REPAIR

Wound healing is a complex and intricate process and for normal repair the processes need to be well orchestrated. The body generally manages this very efficiently, but a number of possible problems can occur and are discussed below.

EXCESSIVE SCARRING

This is characterized by excessive accumulations of collagen within a wound. It is most commonly associated with complex injuries, such as severe burns, but can be the result of repeated injuries and surgical interventions, or occasionally arise spontaneously. Abnormal cell migration and proliferation, abnormal synthesis and secretion of extracellular proteins and growth factors (cytokines) and abnormal remodelling of the wound have been identified

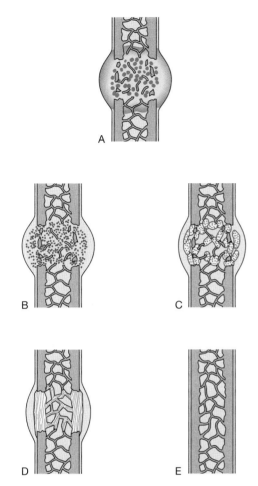

Figure 4.5 Repair of bone. A, fracture leads to bleeding and blood clot. B, granulation tissue forms. C, calcification gradually occurs, leading to D, new bone and E, remodelling (after Williams et al 1989).

as factors (Burd & Huang 2005, Tredget et al 1997). As noted above, myofibroblasts – with their actinic microfilaments – are active in the contraction phase of normal would repair. Under normal conditions, they cease their action when the wound is closed, most likely due to their death (Desmouliere 1995). However, it seems that in wounds where excessive scars appear they continue to be active.

Two main types of excess scarring are found: hypertrophic and keloid. Hypertrophic scars, which are most common and follow injury, follow the normal process of repair (see above) but the time course can be considerably protracted with increased repair matrix, increased morphology and abnormal biochemistry. They are restricted to the area of the original injury and are found to contain nodular structures containing myofibroblasts which produce actin (α-SM actin) and fine, randomly organized collagen fibres. Although these scars do regress, they affect both appearance and function by producing contractures.

Keloid scars are less common than hypertrophic ones and do not follow the normal pattern of repair. They can arise following injury, some time later or even spontaneously. They do not regress with time, extend into the adjacent tissue and contain thick collagen fibres, with very few cells and low vascularity. However, they do not produce contractures and so might affect function to a lesser extent.

The abnormal activity of the growth factors that are associated with control of collagen production would appear to be a major factor in the development of these problems; they can include TGF-β1, IGF-1 and interleukin (IL)-1. However, Desmouliere (1995) notes that many more might be implicated, and that additional factors such as the extracellular matrix, proteoglycans, and heparin could be factors.

SECONDARY HYPOXIC INJURY

It has recently been suggested that tissue can suffer from later-stage injury, which leads to further tissue death. This form of injury is termed 'hypoxic' and results from a disturbed oxygen supply to the tissue, poor tissue metabolism and a degraded repair process involving abnormal enzymatic activity. Additional damage to tissues adjacent to the original injury can therefore occur. It is most often seen following major insults, such as myocardial infarction and strokes. However, it might also arise in some wounds, especially if they are severe or chronic in nature.

Both intra- and extracellular effects occur. Within the cell, mitochondria appear to be most strongly affected and, as they are key to any repair process, this has a considerable impact. In addition, hypoxia, especially if associated with ischaemic conditions, triggers a general acute inflammatory response that increases cell injury and can lead to cell death.

Mitochondria are major sites of oxygen metabolism and also appear to act as the 'oxygen sensor' of the cell, giving rise to more general cell responses. The mitochondrial electron transport chain (ETC) enzyme complexes appear to be specifically targeted (Corbucci et al 2001, 2003). Cytochrome oxidase (COX) is part of the mitochondrial ETC and is reported to be crucial in determining the extent of damage due to lack of oxygen. The process involves an increase in nitric oxide generation; this diffuses into cells and binds with COX at the same site as oxygen, thus reducing the potential for oxygen uptake. The result is a rapid and detrimental effect on mitochondrial respiration. These changes affect other processes, including signal transduction pathways, and produce a response at the level of the cell nucleus; in turn, the cell membrane can be affected.

This process is reversible when nitric oxide levels are relatively low and with an increase in oxygen tension. Thus whereas low levels of nitric oxide are essential to healing, high levels are cytotoxic and therefore detrimental to the repair process.

CHRONIC WOUNDS AND DELAYED REPAIR

Most wounds heal very effectively; however, certain individuals, such as those with diabetes and spinal cord injuries, have more problems. Even minor wounds are slow to heal and can develop into large, non-healing areas. For good healing, a complex and interactive sequence of events must occur, orchestrated by a wide variety of factors both chemical and physical.

Scarring can lead to poor healing; the material is both largely vascular and has a distorting effect on adjacent tissue. Both affect the repair process, the later through its effects on biochemical factors. Mechanical factors, such as those arising from Dupuytren's contracture, can result in inhibition of collagenase and the proteases, and so affect healing. An adequate blood supply is essential to bring nutrients, chemical factor and cells to the area; its importance is highlighted by the levels of angiogenesis occurring in wound repair. An adequate lymphatic drainage system is required to remove detritus and excess fluid. Many common conditions can lead to impairment in the microvascular structure, with increased pressures and effects on flow.

Deficiencies in the oxygen tension of wounds have a major impact on repair, and a direct relationship between repair and oxygen tension has been demonstrated. For example, proliferation of both fibroblasts and epithelium is largely dependent on this factor, with cell division being severely affected at tension below 20 mmHg. Collagen cross-linking activity has been reported to be optimal between 20 and 60 mmHg, whereas the rate of collagen accumulation and the tensile strength of wounds is affected by oxygen concentrations. With severe depletion, cells can die (see 'Secondary hypoxic injuries' above).

Infections also affect wound repair and are particularly problematic in poorly perfused tissues, such as pressure sores, diabetic tissues and venous leg ulcers. Again, oxygen is essential to kill bacteria as the process is highly oxygen dependent, as are the nutrients and chemical messengers brought by the circulatory system.

Poor healing of wounds in the elderly has sometimes been considered to be age related. However, evidence suggests that delayed repair is more likely to be due to related conditions suffered by the elderly, rather than simply age. Age-related changes to the skin do occur, and can include those due to chronic exposure to the sun and certain life-style factors (smoking, stress, excess alcohol, etc.). A number of studies have looked at the tensile strength of wounds, wound-healing factors and the rate of wound closure and have found little relationship to age. However, related conditions such as diabetes, poor circulation and general debility can have a major impact and need to be considered when treating wounds in the elderly.

References

Ausprunk DH, Boudreau CL, Nelson DA (1981) Proteoglycans in the microvasculature II. Histochemical localization in proliferating capillaries in the rabbit cornea. *Am J Pathol* **103**: 367–375.

Bischoff R (1986) A satellite cell mitogen from crushed adult muscle. *Dev Biol* **115**: 140–147.

Bischoff R (1990) Interaction between satellite cells and skeletal muscle fibres. *Development* **109**: 943–952.

Burd A, Huang L (2005) Hypertrophic response and keloid diathesis: two very different forms of scar. *Plastic Recon Surg* **116**(7): 150e–157e.

Carlson BM, Faulkner JA (1983) The regeneration of skeletal muscle fibres following injury: a review. *Med Sci Sport Exercise* **15**: 187–198.

Carpenter S, Karpati G (1984) *Pathology of Skeletal Muscle.* New York, Churchill Livingstone.

Clark RAF (1985) Cutaneous tissue repair: basic biological considerations. *J Am Acad Dermatol* **13**: 701–725.

Clark RAF (1996) Overview and general considerations of wound repair. In Clark RAF, Henson PM (eds) *The Molecular and Cellular Biology of Wound Repair 2nd ed.* New York, Plenum Press, 3–33.

Clark RAF (1990) Fibronectin matrix deposition and fibronectin receptor expression in healing and normal skin. *J Invest Dermatol* **94**, 6(supplement): 128S–134S.

Clark RAF (1991a) Cutaneous wound repair. In Goldsmith LE (ed) *Biochemistry and Physiology of the Skin.* Oxford, Oxford University Press, 576–601.

Clark RAF (1991b) Cutaneous wound repair: a review with emphasis on integrin receptor expression. In Janssen H, Rooman R, Robertson JIS (eds) *Wound Healing.* Petersfield, UK, Wrightson Biomedical Publishing Ltd, 7–17.

Clark RAF, Della Pelle P, Manseau E et al (1982) Blood vessel fibronectin increases in conjunction with endothelial cell proliferation and capillary ingrowth during wound healing. *J Invest Dermatol* **79**: 269–276.

Corbucci CG, Ricchi A, Cardu G et al (2001) Biomolecular and biochemical response of myocardial cell to ischaemia and reperfusion in the course of heart surgery. *J Cardiovasc Surg (Torino)* **42**: 605–610.

Corbucci CG, Tupputi M, Marchi A et al (2003) Cardiac pre-conditioning and reperfusion stunning in human left ventricle. *Minerva Anesthesiol* **69**: 657–672.

Czaja MJ, Weiner FR, Eghbali M et al (1987) Differential effects of interferon-gamma on collagen and fibronectin gene expression. Journal of Biological Chemistry, 262, 13348–13351.

Desmouliere A (1995) factors influencing myofibroblast differentiation during wound healing and fibrosis. *Cell Biol Int* **19**(5): 471–476.

Duncan MR, Berman B (1989) Differential regulation of collagen, glycosaminoglycan, finronectin and collageninase activity production in cultured human adult fibroblasts by interleukin-1 alpha and beta and tumour necrosis factor alpha and beta. Journal of Investigative Dermatology, 92, 699–706.

Folkman J, Klagsburn M (1987) Angiogenic factors. *Science* **235**: 442–447.

Ginsberg MH, Loftus JC, Plow EF (1988) Cytoadhesions, integrins and platelets. *Thromb Haemost* **59**: 1–6.

Hashimoto H, Prewitt RL (1987) Microvascular changes during wound healing. *Int J Microcirc Clin Exp* **5**: 303–310.

Heppenstall RB (1980) Fracture healing. In Heppenstall RB (ed) *Fracture Treatment and Healing.* Philadelphia, PA, WB Saunders, 35–46.

Ho Y-S, Lee WMF, Snyderman R (1987) Chemoattractant induced activation of *c-fos* gene expression in human monocytes. *J Exp Med* **165**: 1524–1538.

Hosein B, Mosessen MW, Bianco C (1985) Monocyte receptors for fibronectin. In van Furth R (ed) *Mononuclear Phagocytes: Characteristics, Physiology and Function.* Dordrecht, Holland, Martinus Nijhoff, 72–99.

Hunt TK (1987) Prospective: a retrospective perspective on the nature of wounds. In Barbul A, Pines E, Caldwell M, Hunt TK (eds) *Growth Factors and Other Aspects of Wound Healing.* New York, Alan R Liss, Inc, xiii–xx.

Hunt TK, Dunphy JE (1980) *Fundamentals of Wound Healing and Wound Infection: Theory and Surgical Practice.* New York, Appleton-Century Crofts.

Ignotz RA, Massague J (1986) Transforming growth factor β stimulates the expression of fibronectin and collagen and their incorporation into the extracellular matrix. Journal of Biochemistry, 260, 4337–4342.

Issekutz AC (1981) Vascular responses during acute neutrophilic inflammation: their relationship to *in vivo* neutrophil emigration. *Lab Invest* **45**: 435–441.

Janssen H, Rooman R, Robertson JIS (1991) *Wound Healing.* Petersfield, UK, Wrightson Biomedical Publishing Ltd.

Kulozik M, Heckmann M, Mauch C et al (1991) Cytokine regulation of collagen metabolism during wound healing *in vitro* and *in vivo.* In Janssen H, Rooman R, Robertson JIS (eds) *Wound Healing.* Petersfield, UK, Wrightson Biomedical Publishing Ltd, 33–39.

Lark MW, Laterra J, Culp LA (1985) Close and focal contact adhesions of fibroblasts to a fibrinectin-containing matrix. *Fed Proc* **44**: 394–403.

Leibovich SJ, Ross R (1975) The role of macrophages in wound repair. *Am J Pathol* 78: 71.

Madri JA, Pratt BM (1996) Angiogenesis. In Clark RAF, Henson PM (eds) *The Molecular and Cellular Biology of Wound Repair 2nd ed.* New York, Plenum Press, 335–371.

Mauch C, Krieg Th (1990) Fibroblast-matrix interactions and their role in the pathogenesis of fibrosis. *Rheum Dis Clin North Am* **16**: 93–107.

McCarthy JB, Sas DF, Furcht LT (1996) Mechanism of parenchymal cell migration in wounds. In Clark RAF, Henson PM (eds) *The Molecular and Cellular Biology of Wound Repair 2nd ed.* New York, Plenum Press, 373–390.

Molloy T, Wang Y, Murrell G (2003) The role of growth factors in tendon and ligament repair. *Sports Med* **33**: 381–394.

Nedelec B, Ghahary A, Scott P, Tredget E (2000) Control of wound contraction. Basic and clinical features. *Hand Clin* **16**(2): 289–302.

Nicholas JF, Gaycherand M, Deplaporte E et al (1991) Wound healing: a result of co-ordinate kertinocyte-fibroblast interactions. In: Janssen H, Rooman R, Robertson JIS, Wound Healing. Wrightson Biomedical Publishing Limited, Petersfield. pp 71–80.

Proud D, Kaplan AP (1988) Kinin formation: mechanisms and roles in inflammatory disorders. *Ann Rev Immunol* **6**: 49–83.

Prostlethwaite AE, Raghow R, Stricklin GP et al (1988) Modulation of fibroblast function by interleukin-1 increased steady state accumulation of type 1 procollagen mRNA and stimulation of other functions but not chemotaxic by human recombinant interleukinin-1 α and β. Journal of Cell Biology, 106, 311–318.

Repesh LA, Fitzgerald TJ, Furcht LT (1982) Fibronectin involvement in granulation tissue and wound healing in rabbits. *J Histochem Cytochem* **30**: 351–358.

Riches DWH (1996) Macrophage involvement in wound repair, remodeling and fibrosis. In Clark RAF, Henson PM (eds) *The Molecular and Cellular Biology of Wound Repair 2nd ed*. New York, Plenum Press, 25–55.

Scharffetter K, Heckmann M, Hatamocji A et al (1989) Synesgistic effect of tumour necrosis factor-a and interferon gamma on collagen synthesisin human fibroblasts in vitro. Experimental Cell Research, 181, 409–419.

Schiro JA, Chan BMC, 95–141, Roswit WT et al (1991) Integrin α2β1 (VLA-2) mediates reorganization and contraction of collagen matrices by human cells. *Cell* **67**: 403–416.

Singer AJ, Clark RAF (1999) Cutaneous wound healing. *N Engl J Med* **341**(10): 738–746.

Terkeltaub RA, Ginsberg MH (1988) Platelets and response to injury. In Clark RAF, Henson PM (eds) *The Molecular and Cellular Biology of Wound Repair*. New York, Plenum Press, 25–55.

Toole BP (1981) Glycosaminoglycans in morphogenesis. In Hay ED (ed) *Cell Biology of the Extracellular Matrix*. New York, Plenum Press, 167–189.

Tredget EF, Nedelec B, Scott PG, Ghahary A (1997) Hypertrophic scars, keloids, and contractures: the cellular and molecular basis for therapy. *Surg Clin North Am* **77**: 701–730.

Tsukamoto Y, Helsel JE, Wahl SM (1981) Macrophage production of fibronectin, a chemoattractant for fibroblasts. *J Immunol* **127**: 673–678.

Woo S, Debski R, Zeminski J et al (2000) Injury and repair of ligaments and tendons. *Ann Rev Biomed Eng* **2**: 83–118.

Woodley DT, Yamauchi M, Wynn KC et al (1991) Collagen telopeptides (cross-linking sites) play a role in collagen gel lattice contraction. *J Invest Dermatol* **97**: 580–585.

Weeks JR (1972) Prostaglandins. *Ann Rev Pharmacol Toxicol* **12**: 317.

Williams PL, Warwick R, Dyson M, Bannister LH (eds) (1989) *Gray's Anatomy*. Edinburgh, Churchill Livingstone.

Williams TJ (1988) Factors that affect vessel reactivity and leucocyte emigration. In Clark RAF, Henson PM (eds) *The Molecular and Cellular Biology of Wound Repair*. New York, Plenum Press, 115–147.

Zetter BR (1988) Angiogenesis: state of the art. *Chest* **93**: 1595–1665.

Chapter 5

Sensory and motor nerve activation

Mary Cramp and Oona Scott

INTRODUCTION

Skeletal muscle is one of the most abundant and adaptable tissues in the human body. The heterogeneity and plasticity of mammalian muscle have become major topics of interest (Pette & Staoron 1997, Pette & Vrbová 1992). In the past two decades, the physiological mechanisms that influence the neural adaptations that accompany and contribute to these changes in skeletal muscles have been under increasing scrutiny (Gandevia 2001). They are gradually being recognized as playing a key role in evaluating the efficacy of therapeutic interventions (Enoka 1997, Pette & Vrbová 1999). This chapter outlines basic muscle and peripheral nerve physiology. Particular attention is paid to the propagation of nerve and muscle action potentials, to differing characteristics of motor units and to the concept of nerve–muscle interaction.

MOTOR NEURON TO MUSCLE ACTIVATION

NEURAL CONTROL OF MUSCLE

Smooth, coordinated movement is the output of a complex neuromuscular system. Skeletal muscle is capable of generating varying tensions and, at its very simplest, smooth, coordinated movement depends on the practical issue of contracting the required muscles in the right sequence at the right time. The control of coordinated movement is complex as different muscles combine in a variety of patterns. Appropriate combinations of excitation or inhibition of different motor neurons in dynamic series provide the required overall functional effect. Even now, there is much to understand about the way in which the neural system devises these patterns of excitation and inhibition, about the interrelationship of the afferent and efferent neural systems, and not least about how motor units are selected to achieve a particular movement and about how firing patterns are updated as the movement evolves.

The brain uses stereotypical electrical signals – nerve action potentials – to convey information received in the central nervous system (CNS) and to encode information at various levels. The signals consist of potential changes produced by electrical currents flowing across cell membranes, currents carried by ions such as those of sodium (Na^+), potassium (K^+) and chlorine (Cl^-) (see 'Electrophysiological properties of nerves and muscles', below). The coding of information depends principally on the frequency of impulses being transmitted along a nerve fibre, the number of fibres involved and on the synaptic connections made within the spinal cord and at higher levels of the CNS. Variability of response occurs at the level of neuronal synapses and the ability to modify processes of excitation and inhibition is thought to be critical to changes which occur in central control mechanisms.

THE MOTOR UNIT

The smallest unit of movement that the CNS can control is a *motor unit*. Defined by Sherrington in 1906, this unit consists of a motor neuron, together with its axon and dendrites, motor end plates and the muscle fibres it supplies. Motor neurons are the largest cells in the ventral horn of the spinal cord. The activity or firing frequency of these cells is dependent on their connections with afferent fibres from muscles, joints and skin, as well as their connections with other parts of the CNS.

Each motor neuron integrates excitatory (EPSP) and inhibitory (IPSP) postsynaptic potentials from thousands of synapses spread over the dendrites and cell body or soma, and these influence whether the motor neuron generates an action potential.

When an action potential is discharged down the axon, its amplitude remains constant. The action potential is an *all or nothing* impulse regenerated at regular intervals along the axon until it reaches the nerve–muscle synapse. There the action potential triggers transmitter release, which in turn causes a muscle action potential and contraction of all the muscle fibres that particular axon supplies. External electrical stimulation is used therapeutically to elicit skeletal muscle contraction supplementing or enhancing normal physiological processes. To understand such uses, it is important to understand the underlying electrophysiological processes.

ELECTROPHYSIOLOGICAL PROPERTIES OF NERVES AND MUSCLES

All nerve fibres have essentially the same structure and resemble a shielded electric cable. As described by Keynes & Aidley (2001), inside there is a central long conducting cylinder of cytoplasm or axoplasm surrounded by insulation: outside is another conducting layer, the electrically excitable *nerve membrane*. Similarly, skeletal muscle fibres are embedded in a basal lamina – a glycoprotein and collagen layer – and have an electrically excitable cell membrane (sarcolemma) that contains the intracellular fluid (sarcoplasm) and intracellular structures. Conduction of *action potentials* along

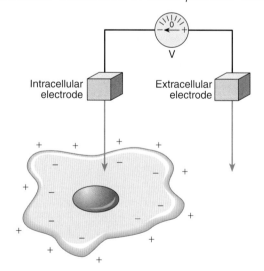

Figure 5.1 The potential difference across a cell membrane measured with an intracellular electrode and an extracellular electrode.

membranes of nerves and muscles occurs because there is a potential difference between the intracellular fluid and the extracellular fluid (Fig. 5.1). The *resting potential* is of the order of -90 mV for skeletal muscle, and -70 mV for lower motor neurons. The minus sign indicates that the inside of the cell has a negative potential relative to the exterior; this *potential difference* can be altered by passage of ions.

In the cell membranes of both nerves and muscles, protein molecules are embedded in a double layer of lipid molecules arranged with their hydrophilic heads facing outward and hydrophobic tails extending into the middle of the layer. Some protein molecules make contact with both the extracellular and the intracellular fluids; these exert control functions, with one region being a selectivity filter and another providing a gate that can be open or closed. The intracellular and extracellular fluids are in *osmotic equilibrium*, that is, the concentration of ions in the intracellular and extracellular fluids is similar. There is, however, a difference in the proportions of different ions in the two solutions: there is a higher concentration of K^+ ions in the intracellular fluid, and higher concentrations of both Na^+ and Cl^- ions in the extracellular fluid.

MOVEMENT OF IONS

Ions at high concentration tend to diffuse to areas of low concentration; their movement is also influenced by voltage gradients, with positive ions being attracted down the negative gradient, and vice versa. An outward movement of K^+ ions down their concentration gradient would be expected but, at the same time, the inner surface of the membrane is at a negative potential with respect to the outside and this tends to restrain the outward movement of positively charged ions.

The *equilibrium potential* of any ion is proportional to the difference between the logarithms of intracellular concentration and the extracellular concentration. It is defined by the *Nernst equation* as the electric potential necessary to balance a given ionic concentration across a membrane so that the overall passive movement of the ion is zero.

By 1955, Hodgkin and Keynes had established that cell membranes of both muscles and nerves were permeable to K^+ and Na^+ ions, and that these ions are in a continuous state of flux across the

membrane against both the concentration and the electrical gradients. Their findings supported the concept of an active transport system with voltage-sensitive mechanisms that uses energy supplied by the hydrolysis of adenosine triphosphate (ATP) to pump Na^+ ions out of the cell and to accumulate K^+ ions within the cell. Evidence suggests that the expulsion of Na^+ ions to the influx of K^+ ions is of the order of $3:2$.

GENERATION AND PROPAGATION OF ACTION POTENTIALS

The unequal distribution of ions across the cell membrane of both nerve and muscle cells forms the basis for generation and propagation of action potentials. Nerve and muscle cells are *excitable*, that is, they are able to produce an action potential after the application of a suitable stimulus (see 'Threshold', below). An *action potential* is a transient reversal of the membrane potential – a *depolarization*. This lasts for about 1 ms in nerve cells and up to 2 ms in some muscle fibres.

Threshold

An initial opening of a few of the voltage-activated sodium channels occurs, followed by a rapid transient increase in Na^+ permeability. This allows Na^+ ions to diffuse rapidly into the cell, causing a sudden accumulation of positive charge on the inside surface of the neural or muscle fibre membrane. The increased permeability to Na^+ ions is followed by repolarization via the opening of voltage-activated K^+ channels; there is some hyperpolarization beyond the resting potential.

The nature of the regenerating mechanism was demonstrated both in terms of the time course of the action potential and of ionic conductance by Hodgkin & Huxley (1952). Stimulus below the threshold required to produce an action potential reduces, but does not reverse, the membrane potential. As the stimulus is increased, the potential difference across the cell membrane is reduced until it reaches the critical threshold level. At this level, the stimulus will lead to the automatic generation of an action potential. The level of the threshold varies according to a number of factors, including how many action potentials the nerve fibre has recently conducted.

After an action potential, two changes occur that make it impossible for the nerve fibre to transmit a second action potential immediately. First, *inactivation* (the *absolute refractory period*) occurs during the falling phase of the action potential. During this period, no amount of externally applied depolarization can initiate a second regenerative response. After the absolute refractory period, there is a *relative refractory period* during which the residual inactivation of the Na^+ conductance and the relatively high K^+ conductance combine to produce an increase in the threshold for action potential initiation.

To stimulate a nerve, the stimulus has to be both of sufficient intensity and of sufficient duration to depolarize the nerve membrane. Action potentials can be initiated in peripheral nerves by the application of suitable electrical stimuli (pulses). The rate of change and frequency of stimuli are important.

STRENGTH–DURATION CURVES

The strength–duration relationship can be determined by applying single rectangular pulses of differing pulse widths to a peripheral nerve. The intensity of current required to produce a single muscle contraction (often called a twitch contraction) is recorded along with the time (pulse width) for which it is applied. Figure 5.2 illustrates the relationship between the duration of an electrical stimulus and the intensity of stimulation.

If the stimulus is applied very slowly, that is, its rise time is slow, then the rate of depolarization is very slow. There is a steady flow of ions in one direction and no action potential is generated. A slow, steady, unidirectional current and a slow fall is typical of currents used in 'galvanic' treatment or 'iontophoretic' treatments, and no stimulation of muscle or nerve occurs. If the stimulus is applied quickly and the duration of the stimulus is long enough, the nerve fibre is rapidly depolarized to the threshold and an action potential is generated. The slower the stimulus applied, the greater the magnitude of depolarization required to bring the fibre to threshold. This test has clinical applications and is used both to determine the state of innervation and to monitor re-innervation of skeletal muscle following trauma to peripheral nerves.

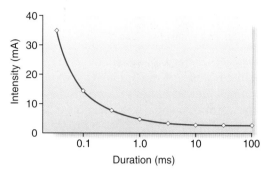

Figure 5.2 The relationship between strength and duration of a stimulus required to generate an action potential in a motor nerve fibre.

NEURONS AS CONDUCTORS OF ELECTRICITY

Although permeability properties of cell membranes result in regenerative electrical signals, there are other factors to be considered. Many peripheral motor and sensory nerves are myelinated. *Myelin* is an insulating material formed by Schwann cells and forms as many as 320 membranes in series between the plasma membrane of a nerve fibre and the extracellular fluid. This sheath of membranes is interrupted at regular intervals by the *nodes of Ranvier*, which are arranged such that the greater the diameter of the nerve fibre, the greater are the internodal distances. Because myelin is an insulator and ions cannot flow easily into and out of the sheathed internodal region, excitation skips from node to node (*saltatory conduction*), thereby greatly increasing the conduction velocity and, because ionic exchange is limited to the nodal regions, using less energy. While the excitation is progressing from one node to the next on the leading edge of the action potential, many nodes behind are still active. Myelinated nerve fibres can fire at higher frequencies and for more prolonged periods than other nerve fibres.

As a general rule, larger-diameter nerves (group Aα motor nerves) conduct impulses more rapidly and have a lower threshold of excitability than the much smaller Aδ pain fibres (Fig. 5.3). This means that threshold and motor nerve conduction velocities can be tested without exciting the pain fibres. On stimulation, larger nerve fibres

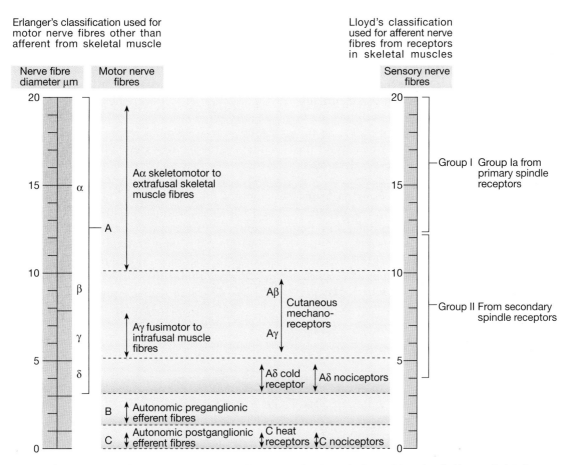

Figure 5.3 Classification of peripheral nerves according to conduction velocity and junction (with permission from Erlanger & Gasser 1970 *Human Neurophysiology*, 2nd edn, Chapman and Hall).

also produce larger signals, their excitatory response lasts for a shorter time and they have shorter refractory periods.

Within muscle, the axon of a motor neuron loses pits myelin sheet. It divides into a number of fine intramuscular branches to innervate muscle fibres that are scattered throughout the muscle and together make up the motor unit. The region of contact between the motor nerve and the muscle fibre is called the neuromuscular junction. Each muscle fibre has one neuromuscular junction, lying usually about midway along the fibre.

SYNAPTIC TRANSMISSION

Synapses are points of contact between nerve cells, or between nerves and effector cells such as muscle fibres. At electrical synapses, the current generated by an impulse in the presynaptic nerve terminal spreads into the next cell through low-resistance channels. More commonly, however, synapses are chemical in action: the gap between the presynaptic and postsynaptic membranes is filled with extracellular fluid, and the nerve terminal secretes a chemical, a *neurotransmitter*, which activates the postsynaptic membrane. The motor end plate is the specialized region on the muscle where the axon terminal comes into close contact with the muscle fibre that it innervates.

Acetylcholine release

When an action potential arrives at a neuromuscular junction, it causes voltage-dependent calcium ions channels in the axon terminal to open, and allows calcium ions (Ca^{2+}) to diffuse into the intracellular fluid. Increased intracellular Ca^{2+} concentration causes a cascade mechanism that results in synaptic vesicles binding to the membrane in close contact with the muscle fibres. Acetylcholine released from the synaptic vesicles in the nerve terminal diffuses across the synaptic cleft in multimolar packages (or quanta) to combine with the receptor sites on the motor end plate. This alters the end-plate membrane permeability to Na^+ and K^+ ions and immediately depolarizes the membrane. The end-plate potential (EPP) causes a local change in potential of the muscle membrane in close contact with it. This propagates a regenerative motor unit action potential (MUAP) in all directions along the adjacent muscle membrane using the mechanism already described for the propagation of action potentials along the axon membrane. The magnitude of a single MUAP is normally sufficient to cause contraction of a muscle fibre and all fibres within the motor unit will be activated simultaneously – following the *all-or-none principle*.

The action of acetylcholine at the neuromuscular junction is terminated by an enzyme, acetylcholinesterase. This enzyme, embedded in the basal lamina of the synaptic cleft of the motor end plate, hydrolyses acetylcholine and thereby prevents prolonged action of the transmitter. Along the length of the muscle fibre, the muscle cell membrane (the sarcolemma) has numerous infoldings forming a system of membranes called the transverse tubular system or T tubules. As the action potential progresses along the sarcolemma, it passes close to the myofibrils down the T tubules (Figs 5.4 and 5.5).

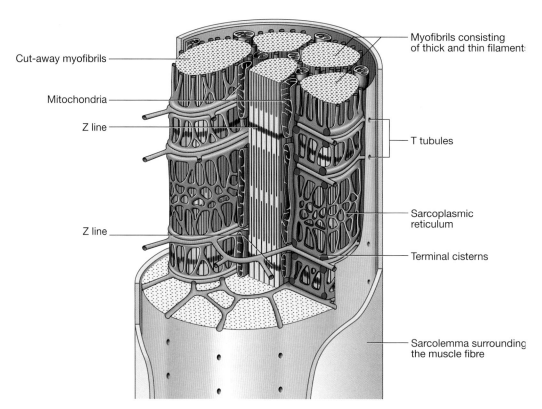

Cut-away myofibrils

Mitochondria

Z line

Z line

Myofibrils consisting of thick and thin filaments

T tubules

Sarcoplasmic reticulum

Terminal cisterns

Sarcolemma surrounding the muscle fibre

Figure 5.4 A section of mammalian skeletal muscle. A single muscle fibre has been cut away to show the individual myofibrils and the thick myosin and thin actin filaments within a sarcomere. The sarcoplasmic reticulum is seen surrounding each myofibril, together with the T system of tubules in which the Ca^{2+} ions are stored and released during muscle contraction.

Calcium release

Arrival of the action potential in the T tubules depolarizes the sarcoplasmic reticulum, another complex membrane system in close contact with the myofibrils. The main function of the sarcoplasmic reticulum is to release and take up Ca^{2+} during contraction and relaxation. Depolarization of the transverse tubular system signals the release of calcium ions from the sarcoplasmic reticulum into the sarcoplasm and allows the actin–myosin cross-bridges to bond (see 'The sliding-filament hypothesis', below). Calcium ions are then actively pumped back into the sarcoplasmic reticulum and contraction ceases (see Fig. 5.5).

MUSCLES: BASIC CHARACTERISTICS, CLASSIFICATION AND THE INFLUENCE OF THE MOTOR NEURON

GROSS STRUCTURE AND FUNCTION

Muscles vary in function as well as in shape, size and in method of attachment to bone or to cartilage. A muscle might fulfil more than one

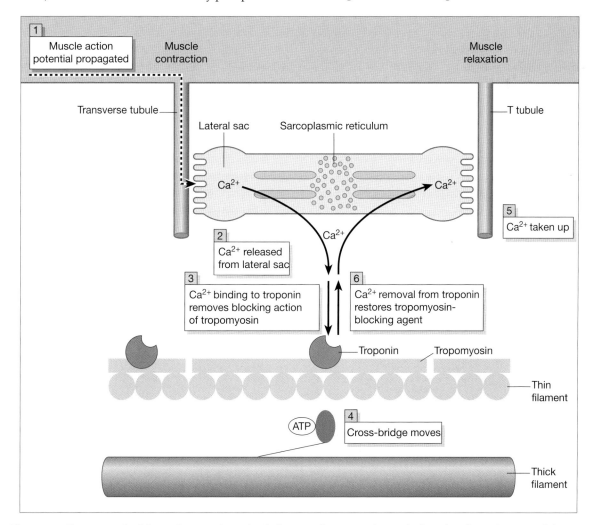

Figure 5.5 Sequence of calcium release and uptake during muscle contraction and relaxation. An action potential causes release of calcium ions (Ca^{2+}) from the sarcoplasmic reticulum into the sarcoplasm, which, in the presence of adenosine triphosphate (ATP), causes the interaction of the cross-bridges of the myosin filaments with the actin filaments and hence muscle contraction. When calcium is released from the sarcoplasmic reticulum, the myofibril contracts; when calcium is reabsorbed by the sarcoplasmic reticulum, the myofibril relaxes.

function: stabilizing, producing power and sustaining posture, as well as performing one or more specifically controlled movement during what is for the person a single sequence of movements.

Each muscle's composition and structure is often seen as a compromise between the different needs for speed of movement, force and economy of energy. There are, however, basic principles to the mechanical properties of muscle: the maximum force that can be produced by a muscle is generally proportional to its cross-sectional area and the maximum rate of contraction of a long muscle is greater than that of a short muscle.

As a rule, small muscles with precision tasks, such as those in the hand, are composed of motor units with few muscle fibres, whereas trunk and proximal limb muscles contain motor units with a large number of muscle fibres. At a simple level, two components are integrated in a single muscle: a contractile component, which is altered by stimulation and can develop an active tension, and an elastic component, connective tissue, through which the contractile component transmits the generated force to the muscle tendon.

When a single electrical stimulus of sufficient intensity is applied to a muscle, the muscle responds with a *twitch contraction* and then returns to its resting state (Fig. 5.6). If more than one impulse is given within an interval that is shorter than the contraction–relaxation cycle time of the motor unit, the muscle does not return to its resting state, and the forces produced by each impulse are said to *summate* or *fuse*.

At a sufficiently high frequency of stimulation, a fused, tetanic or smooth, contraction is produced as the force fluctuations of each impulse are indistinguishable in practical terms (Fig. 5.7). Because slow-contracting muscle fibres summate and produce a tetanic contraction at lower frequencies of nerve stimulation, investigators realized that slow muscles such as the soleus might be more suitable for sustained 'tonic' function at low levels of activation, whereas fast-contracting muscle fibres, which fuse at higher frequencies of stimulation, might be more appropriate for 'phasic' function, and for generating high forces for short periods of time.

MYOSIN AND ACTIN: CONTRACTILE PROTEINS

At the molecular level, the main elements visible under a light microscope are myofibrils, and these, arranged in parallel, make up a muscle fibre. Each myofibril has longitudinal myofilaments with the alternating light I (isotropic) and dark A (anisotropic) bands that give skeletal muscle its typical striated or striped appearance (Fig. 5.8).

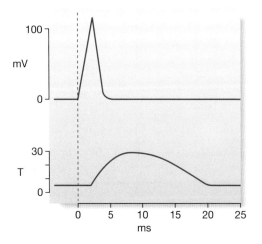

Figure 5.6 The electrical (mv, potential change) and mechanical (T, tension) response of a mammalian skeletal muscle fibre to a single action potential resulting in a twitch contraction.

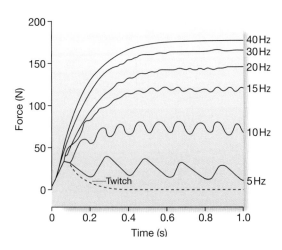

Figure 5.7 The response of human skeletal muscle to different rates of stimulation.

Under an electron microscope, it becomes apparent that each myofibril is composed of a series (end to end) of repeating units or *sarcomeres*, the functional unit of muscle contraction. Within each sarcomere are myofilaments composed mainly of either actin or myosin. Each sarcomere has two sets of thin actin filaments anchored at one end to a network of interconnecting proteins, called the Z line, and at the other end interdigitating with a set of thick myosin filaments. The myosin molecules, packed tail to tail, form the wide dark A band. The I band and the H zone are regions where there is no overlap between the actin and the myosin myofilaments: the I band has only the thin actin molecules and the H zone only the thick myosin myofilaments. Finally, in the centre of the

H zone is the M line, formed by proteins that bind all the myosin filaments together (Fig. 5.8).

Myosin molecules are relatively large proteins that consist of two globular heads attached to a long tail. Each molecule is made up of six polypeptide chains, two heavy myosin chain portions and four short light chains. The two heavy chains wind round each other forming a long double-helical 'tail' region also known as the light meromyosin (LMM) portion. Extending from the 'tail' by the hinge region, the heavy chain (HMM) portion consists of the flexible, so-called neck portion (the S_2 portion), and the two globular head portions (S_1 head portions), each with two associated light chains. The composition of these light chains differs in fast and slow muscles, but so far their role has not been established. Each globular portion contains the ATP-binding site and the actin-binding site (Fig. 5.9). Enlargement of the globular head shows the cleft, the opening and closing of which is regulated by the interaction of ATP. This determines the rate of cross-bridge reactions with the actin filaments and, in consequence, the speed of muscle contraction (McComas 1996).

Each actin protein molecule is relatively small and roughly spherical in shape. The thread-like actin filaments are made up of between 300 and 400 actin molecules polymerized (combined into a more complex molecule) to form two intertwined helical chains. Two regulatory proteins, troponin and tropomyosin, are located on the actin filament. The two chains of tropomyosin molecules, each about the length of seven actin molecules, fit end to end along the strands of the actin double helix into a groove along the filament length, and partially cover the myosin binding site (see Fig. 5.9).

THE SLIDING–FILAMENT HYPOTHESIS

The force-generating mechanism appears to be cyclical, and the formation of cross-bridges between actin and myosin in the presence of ATP plays an essential role. Both this concept of cross-bridge action, and the model of myosin with a head that rotates and stretches a compliant portion of the molecule, follow from theories advanced by AF Huxley in 1957 and extended by Huxley and Simmons in 1971. They observed no change in length of either the thick myosin or the thin actin

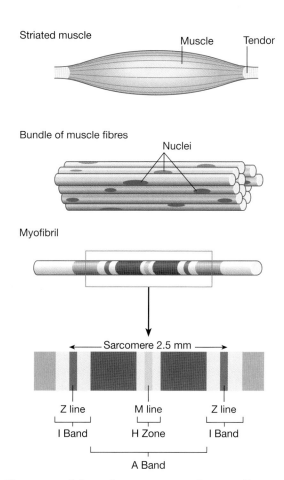

Figure 5.8   Schematic arrangements of contractile components.

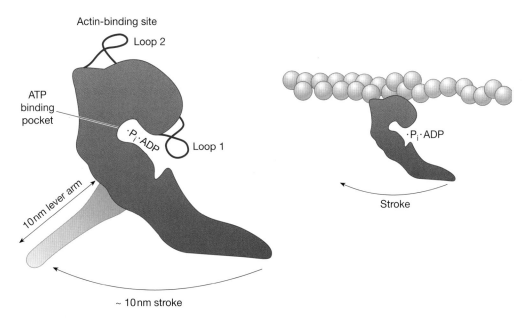

Figure 5.9 Myosin consists of two heads and a long α-helical tail. The figure shows a close-up of the S_1 (one of the two head portions) of the myosin molecule at the actin AM*•ADP · P_i state (see Fig. 5.10). The arrow shows the direction of the conformational movement. Loop 1 sets the rate constant for the adenosine diphosphate (ADP) release rate and loop 2 interacts with the amino terminal of the actin molecule (after Spudich 1994, with permission of *Nature* and Professor J.A. Spudich).

filaments and suggested that a sliding motion forces the thin actin filaments on either side of the sarcomere in the A band towards the M line, thereby shortening the sarcomere. Although the exact mechanism is still uncertain, recent work on molecular motors has provided considerable support for the mechanochemical actin-activated myosin-ATPase cycle (Spudich 1994). One form of this mechanism is illustrated in Figure 5.10 and discussed below.

In step 1, the adenosine diphosphate (ADP) and inorganic phosphate (P_i) are bound to the myosin head. The myosin heads are free to bind to the actin molecules and form an actin–myosin –ADP–P_i complex (step 2). This binding triggers the release of energy, the myosin head rotates, and force is exerted between the two filaments. Movement occurs between the filaments if they are free to move; if they are not, an 'isometric (static) contraction' occurs. The link between the myosin and the actin molecules must be broken to allow the myosin cross-bridge to reattach to a new actin molecule and repeat the cycle. Binding of a molecule of ATP breaks the link between actin and myosin (step 3).

The ATP that is bound to the myosin then splits (step 4), forming the energized state of myosin, which can now reattach to a new site on the actin filament.

ROLE OF CALCIUM IN CONTRACTION

At a critical Ca^{2+} concentration, Ca^{2+} binds to specific binding sites on troponin, one of the regulatory proteins. Troponin changes its conformation, moving the tropomyosin, and thereby exposing binding sites on the actin molecule (see Fig. 5.9). This enables the head of the myosin filament to interact with the binding sites on the actin molecule, forming cross-bridges cyclically and so developing force. Removal of Ca^{2+} reverses this process and tropomyosin moves back into its blocking position.

MATCHING MOTOR NEURONS TO THE MUSCLE FIBRES

Ranvier (1874) observed that the soleus muscle was a deeper red colour and contracted more

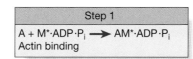

Step 1

$A + M^* \cdot ADP \cdot P_i \longrightarrow AM^* \cdot ADP \cdot P_i$
Actin binding

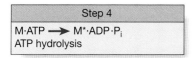

Step 4

$M \cdot ATP \longrightarrow M^* \cdot ADP \cdot P_i$
ATP hydrolysis

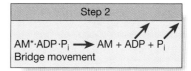

Step 2

$AM^* \cdot ADP \cdot P_i \longrightarrow AM + ADP + P_i$
Bridge movement

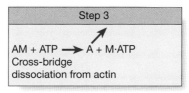

Step 3

$AM + ATP \longrightarrow A + M \cdot ATP$
Cross-bridge
dissociation from actin

Figure 5.10 Chemical and physical events occurring during first four steps of the cross-bridge cycle. M* indicates myosin in a high energy state. ⁄ indicates disassociation of reaction products.

slowly than other calf muscles. Eccles and his co-workers (1958) established that fast-firing, so-called 'phasic' motor neurons innervated muscle fibres with fast contraction times and that slow, 'tonic' motor neurons innervated muscle fibres with slow contraction times. Edström and Krugelberg (1968) confirmed the similarity of muscle fibres belonging to a single motor unit by a method of glycogen depletion of individual motor units in response to prolonged stimulation of single motor nerve fibres. Using their methodology of glycogen depletion, human muscle can be seen to be heterogeneous in that each muscle is composed of a wide variety of different muscle fibres. Fibres belonging to any one motor unit are spread over a large territory rather than being clustered together. Edström and Krugelberg's finding was later modified (Martin et al 1988) as more sophisticated techniques showed that subtle differences do exist within individual motor units.

SPEED OF CONTRACTION AND HISTOLOGICAL PROPERTIES

Burke and colleagues (1973), working on cat gastrocnemius muscle, showed a close association between physiological or mechanical properties and histochemical (*histo* = tissue, implying chemical reaction occurring in tissues themselves) properties of the muscle fibres in each motor unit. They identified three main types of motor unit based on their speed of contraction and resistance to fatigue,

and stated that each physiological category of muscle unit had a corresponding unique histochemical profile.

- 'FF' motor units: fast contracting with short contraction times, developing relatively high tension, fatiguing quickly, with high anaerobic glycolytic capacity and low oxidative capacity.

- 'FR' units: fast contracting, short twitch-contraction times, developing less tension than the 'FF' units, less fatigable, with high glycolytic capacity and moderate-to-high oxidative capacity.

- 'S' units: slow contracting with longer twitch–contraction times, developing least tension, with high oxidative and low glycolytic capacity.

This classification by Burke et al (1973) of motor units by their resistance to fatigue matches that based on enzyme histochemical characteristics of whole muscle fibre populations by Barnard et al (1971), which is described in further detail below.

MUSCLE FIBRE CLASSIFICATION

Muscle fibres are now currently classified using three different methods:

1. Histochemical staining for myosin ATPase.

2. Immunocytochemical investigations of myosin heavy chain isoforms.

3. Biochemical identification of metabolic enzymes to reflect adaptations in structural and functional aspects of muscle characteristics (Pette & Vrbová 1992, Pette & Staron 1997, Scott et al 2001).

The first two methods distinguish muscle fibres solely on the basis of differences with regard to the myosin molecule. The third is based primarily on histochemical differences using selected key enzymes of anaerobic–glycolytic and aerobic–oxidative metabolism (Pette & Vrbová 1992).

Myosin ATPase staining

Bárány (1967) was the first to demonstrate a close relationship between actomyosin adenosine triphosphatase (mATPase) activity and speed of muscle shortening. In human studies, the histological method frequently used to distinguish muscle fibre types is based on staining techniques for myofibrillar mATPase activity. The differences in mATPase activity relate to specific myosin heavy-chain complements and make it possible to distinguish between specific muscle fibre types, called type I and type II for those fibres staining light and dark, respectively. Based on differences in pH stability, type II fibres can be further subdivided into two major subgroups: IIA and IIB fibres (see Dubowitz

1995). More recently, further subgroups – IC, IIC, and IIAB, which have intermediate mATPase staining – have been identified (Table 5.1). It is now possible to distinguish, on a qualitative basis of intensity of staining, between seven specific muscle fibre types: types I, IC, IIC, IIAC, IIA, IIAB and IIB (from slowest to fastest contraction speeds).

Myosin heavy chain isoforms

More recently, the development of immunocytochemistry has made it possible both to identify and quantify the different molecular forms (isoforms) of myosin heavy chains using single-fibre electrophoretic separation (the SDS-PAGE technique). The link is between mATPase activity, speed of contraction and location of the mATPase binding site in the globular heads of the myosin molecule (Weiss et al 1999).

Initially, three different myosin isoforms – MHCI, MHCIIa and MHCIIb – were identified. These corresponded to those identified by ATPase staining, i.e. types IA, IIA and IIB. Table 5.1 shows that this classification follows a similar profile to that described for mATPase staining. More recently, an additional fast-fibre subtype, type IIx (also known as type IId) has been identified. Type IIx is intermediate to types IIa and IIb and is characterized as

Table 5.1 Comparison of 4 different human skeletal muscle classifications: Physiological properties; histochemical staining for myosin adrenosinetriphosphatase (mATPase), myosin heavy chain identification and biochemical identification of metabolic enzymes. In humans it is now established that MHCIIb are now more accurately referred to as MHCIIx/d. The dotted lines indicate that the correlation between the different classification schemes is weak.

Fibre type classification						
Physiological Biochemical		mATPase properties		Myosin heavy		chain
S	←——→	I	←——→	MHCI	←——→	SO
		IC				
		IIC				
		IIAC				
FR	←——→	IIA		MHCIIa	←----→	FOG
		IIAB				
FF	←——→	IIB		MHCIIx/d	←----→	FG

S, slow fatigue resistant; FR, fast fatigue resistant; FF, fast fatiguable; SO, slow oxidative; FOG, fast oxidative, glycolytic; FG, fast glycolytic. (Table adapted from Scott et al 2001.)

being more fatigue resistant than type IIb fibres. It is now confirmed that human muscles do not express the fastest myosin heavy chain isoform MHCIIb (Pette & Staron 1997, Scott et al 2001).

Each muscle fibre can contain more than one myosin heavy chain isoform, explaining both the molecular and functional diversity of muscle fibres as well as their adaptability, i.e. their change of phenotype or transition of genetic functional expression that can occur throughout life (see Pette & Staron 2001).

Biochemical identification of metabolic enzymes

This scheme is based on histochemically identified enzymes that reflect the metabolic pathways and are classified as either aerobic/oxidative or anaerobic/glycolytic. This classification leads to three fibre types: fast-twitch glycolytic (FG), fast-twitch oxidative (FOG), and slow-twitch oxidative (SO) (Barnard et al 1971). As already indicated (see above), Burke et al's (1973) classification of motor units by their resistance to fatigue matches that based on enzyme characteristics of whole muscle-fibre populations so that fast glycolytic (FG) fibres probably belong to the 'FF' (most fatiguable) motor units, the fast oxidative glycolytic (FOG) to the 'FR' (less fatiguable) units and the slow oxidative (SO) to the 'S' (fatigue resistant) units. Care is needed when combining information on muscle fibre myosin ATPase histochemistry and qualitative histochemistry for certain metabolic enzymes (Pette & Staron 1997).

RECRUITMENT OF MOTOR UNITS IN VOLUNTARY CONTRACTIONS

In 1929, Adrian and Bronk introduced the concentric-needle electrode and showed that by inserting this electrode directly into the muscle it was possible to record the electrical events that cause contraction of the muscle fibres. They showed that voluntary muscle force could be increased both by increasing the firing frequency of motor neurons and by recruiting additional motor units. In the same year, Denny Brown (1929) found that the smaller motor neurons that innervate slow-contracting muscle fibres were more readily activated than the larger phasic motor neurons, which innervate faster-contracting muscle fibres.

Denny Brown's finding supports the theory (see 'Gross structure and function', above) that slow muscle fibres are used for sustained activities whereas faster-contracting muscle fibres are used when short bursts of high levels of force are required. Henneman & Olson (1965) investigated the excitability of motor neurons and the order of their recruitment during movement. The size of the cell body of a motor neuron is related to the number of muscle fibres that it innervates. Large motor neurons have larger cell bodies, large-diameter axons (and high conductance velocities) and a lower input resistance to an applied input current than do small neurons. For a similar input current, small motor neurons reach their threshold for firing sooner than large motor neurons. Henneman & Olson (1965) showed that the excitability or firing pattern of a motor neuron was directly correlated with its size and that, in any given movement, motor neurons were recruited in an orderly manner according to their size. It is now thought that this hierarchy of motor unit recruitment might be responsible for the heterogeneity of muscle fibres within the same muscle (see Pette & Vrbová 1992, 1999).

In 1973, Milner-Brown and colleagues showed that slower-contracting motor units in humans were recruited first in both reflex and voluntary movements involving low tensions and that the larger, faster, motor units were activated 'only by rapid vigorous and briefly sustained contractions' with bursts of rapid firing. Patterns of firing and of recruitment of voluntary muscle force can be increased both by increasing the firing frequency of motor neurons and by recruiting additional motor units.

Only in very fast (ballistic) movements, where speed is of the essence, does the faster conduction speed of the large motor neurons play a part; the slow motor units, because of the slower conduction times of their axons, might fire after the faster motor units. Normal frequencies of firing of motor neurons in human muscles rarely exceed 40 Hz and are rarely less than 6–8 Hz. Under most conditions, motor units fire asynchronously; they fire synchronously only during powerful contractions and during fatigue.

INFLUENCE OF THE MOTOR NEURON

The change of muscle properties in response to a change of neural input was first demonstrated by Buller and colleagues in 1960 (Buller et al 1960a,b).

They sutured a nerve that normally supplied a slow-contracting muscle of a cat into the fast-contracting flexor digitorum longus (FDL). The soleus was innervated by suturing the nerve from FDL. This experiment showed not only that contractile properties of the two muscles exchanged but also that there were extensive sequential changes in their metabolic and histological properties.

The close association of the activity pattern of a motor neuron and the contractile properties of the motor unit was underlined when it was shown, using chronic stimulation at 10 Hz, that it was possible to preserve the contractile characteristics of the soleus muscle of the rabbit following tenotomy (Vrbová 1966). The slow soleus would normally have become fast-contracting following section of its tendon and the spinal cord. However, when the muscle was stimulated chronically at 5–10 Hz for 8 hours each day, its contractile properties remained slow. If higher frequencies of stimulation were used (i.e. 20–40 Hz), the silenced soleus muscle became fast contracting (Salmons & Vrbová 1969, Vrbová 1966). This matching of the pattern of activity of motor neurons to the properties of the muscle fibres is fundamental. It underlies the hypothesis that activity has an impact on the phenotype of skeletal muscle (Pette & Vrbová 1999) and provides an explanation for changes in skeletal muscle associated with clinical neurological situations (see Chapter 14).

AFFERENT INPUT TO THE CENTRAL NERVOUS SYSTEM

The ability to react to external stimuli is important for human function and many receptors in the human body are responsive to external stimuli. There are receptors that respond to light, to sound, to mechanical stimuli, or to heat and to cold; some stimuli are perceived as pain; some chemical influences are perceived as smells or as tastes. The nervous system receives information from a wide variety of receptors via sensory nerve fibres (also called *afferent* nerve fibres). Such neurons are sometimes called primary or first-order neurons because they are the first cells entering the CNS in the synaptically linked chains of neurons that handle the incoming information.

Afferent neurons differ from motor neurons in that they have no dendrites and only one process or axon. On leaving the cell body, the axon divides into two branches: one, the peripheral process, ends in a receptor and the other, the central process, enters the CNS and makes synaptic contact with its target neurons. A single afferent neuron might end in one receptor. More commonly, the afferent neuron divides into fine branches, each terminating in a receptor, all of which are preferentially sensitive to the same type of stimulus or input. A single afferent neuron and all its receptor endings make up a *sensory unit*, a concept similar to the motor unit described above.

SENSORY TRANSMISSION

Sensory receptors act as transducers and the input signal is transformed into an electrical signal. In response to an adequate stimulus, the receptor generates a receptor potential that reflects the intensity, duration and location of the stimulus. A stimulus that is too weak to initiate nerve impulses is said to be *subthreshold*. Adequate stimuli generate *receptor potentials*, which result in trains of action potentials that are propagated along afferent nerve fibres. These stimuli have the same all-or-none nature of action potentials that were described earlier for motor neurons. The greater the intensity of the stimulus, the higher the frequency of action potentials; the more widespread the stimulus, the greater the number of receptors that are stimulated.

ADAPTATION

A stimulus that is applied and maintained results in different patterns of impulses, depending on the particular receptor that is being stimulated. In some receptors, there is an initial burst of impulses on stimulation and then the discharge rate falls greatly or may cease altogether. This process is called *adaptation* and involves a decline in the intensity of response during stimulation that is sustained at constant intensity. Other receptors show no adaptation and the pattern of impulses accurately reflects the duration and intensity of the input stimulus. Adaptation of the subject to the sensory effects of electrical stimulation is important and is sometimes overlooked in evaluating tolerance to superimposed electrical stimulation (see Chapter 6 on Pain and Chapter 15 on TENS).

CLASSIFICATION OF AFFERENT NERVE FIBRES

Sensory nerves, like motor nerves, can be myelinated and have been classified according to their function and the receptors that they innervate. Two methods of classification have been used (see Fig. 5.3). Lloyd & Chang (1948) proposed a system of classification of grades, I–IV, for muscle afferents based on fibre diameter, which is related to conduction velocity. The largest and fastest-conducting sensory nerves are group Ia afferents (12–20 mm in diameter) and they have the lowest threshold of any sensory nerves to electrical stimulation. They correspond to motor neurons having conduction velocities that range from 50 to 70 m/s. Group Ib and group II afferents, are smaller and have slower conduction velocities. The other afferent nerves share Erlanger's A, B and C classification based on the conduction velocities for the motor nerves (see Fig. 5.3). The A group have a wide spectrum of fibre diameter (1–20 mm). Erlanger & Gasser (1937) were the first to realize that the compound action potential of a peripheral nerve in a frog shows several distinct peaks. For convenience, these were divided according to their conduction velocity; peak A is subdivided into α, β, γ and δ. Efferent nerve fibres supplying skeletal muscle are classified as Aα and γ peaks.

SENSORY RECEPTORS

Skin is equipped with three categories of cutaneous receptor: mechanoceptors or pressure receptors, thermoceptors for sensing hot and cold, and nociceptors signalling damage to the skin. Skeletal muscle contains the following sensory receptors: free nerve endings, Golgi tendon organs, pacinian corpuscles and muscle spindles. Both nociceptors and muscle receptors are of particular interest.

NOCICEPTIVE SYSTEMS AND PAIN

The pain receptors are free nerve endings without specialised accessory structures. Information about noxious or painful stimuli is passed to the spinal cord by two distinct sets of fibres. The myelinated Aδ axons (1–4 μm in diameter) conduct at 6–24 m/s. They are stimulated by sharp, pricking, well-localized pain, respond to noxious stimuli such as burning and cutting, and are mechano-thermal receptors. The non-myelinated C axons, at 0.1–1 μm in diameter, conduct more slowly (at 0.5–2 m/s) and provide the second wave of pain, which is associated with a burning or aching sensation and is poorly localized.

The signals are either carried in ascending pathways to the brainstem and thalamus, and then relayed to a specific area of cerebral cortex, or are relayed from the interneurons along non-specific ascending pathways into the brain reticular formation and regions of the thalamus and cortex. The subject of pain modulation has received considerable attention and is addressed in detail in Chapter 6. Many experiments have shown that no noxious stimulus can fail to activate other receptors responding to touch, pressure, displacement, stretch and cooling, and much interest in the treatment of pain by stimulation of the afferent system is based on these findings.

SENSORY RECEPTORS IN SKELETAL MUSCLE

Muscle receptors are sophisticated and their function is moderated by the CNS. Mathews, in his book published in 1972, and Jami (1992) provide comprehensive reviews of the function of muscle receptors.

Free nerve endings are found in association with every structure in muscle; they are the endings of all non-myelinated afferent fibres and the smallest myelinated nerve endings-type Aδ fibres. Types of stimuli that excite these endings are pressure, pain, increase in osmolarity, tetanus and infusion of potassium ions – all conditions that might be expected to exist in exercising or stimulated muscle.

Golgi tendon organs are mechanoreceptors found at the points of attachment of muscle fibres to tendinous tissue. They are encapsulated structures composed of collagen bundles innervated by large, myelinated (8–12 μm diameter) group Ib afferent fibres. Golgi tendon organs, originally believed to be high-threshold stretch receptors, actually have a low threshold and a dynamic sensitivity that signals small and rapid changes in contractile forces in the muscle. Their widespread distribution at the musculotendinous junction enables monitoring of contractions of every portion of muscle. In addition to ascending pathways, activation of Ib axons from the tendon organs produces inhibition of homonymous and synergic motor neurons and excitation of antagonist motor neurons.

Pacinian corpuscles are usually found in association with Golgi tendon organs and are supplied by group II (3 μm diameter) myelinated fibres. Their function is not yet fully understood.

Muscle spindles are highly complicated receptors. They are found in greatest number in skeletal muscles, which undergo small length variation requiring precision movement. Figure 5.11 shows a schematic diagram of a spindle. The spindles are structures of about 10 mm in length, which lie parallel to the extrafusal muscle fibres. They are attached at either end to extrafusal fibres or to tendinous insertions and consist of a bundle of specialized muscle fibres or intrafusal fibres. They have a rich nerve supply, the role of which, again, is not yet fully established. The central part of the spindle is contained within a thick connective tissue capsule. There are two types of intrafusal muscle fibre in the spindle: two- or three-bag fibres, and up to eight-chain fibres. Bag fibres can be further subdivided into bag_1 and bag_2 fibres.

The large, group Ia afferent fibres (12–20 μm diameter) have primary spiral endings on all of the muscle fibres in a spindle. These endings are on the most central region of each fibre. On either side of them, there might be up to five secondary spiral endings of the group II afferent neurons, lying mainly on the bag_2 and chain fibres. The primary and secondary afferent endings differ in their responses to stretch and to vibration. The primary endings are very sensitive to stretch, which is thought to be due to the mechanical response of bag_1 fibre. These endings respond with a rapid discharge during actual extension, have a slower rate of discharge during static stretch, and do not fire during the release of stretch. The secondary endings fire during static stretch. The primary endings are more highly sensitive to vibration than the secondary endings.

Unusually for a sensory receptor, the muscle spindles have a motor supply. The motor supply is provided mainly by small motor nerves fusimotor or γ fibres, (2–8 mm in diameter) which are found at the poles of the spindles within the capsule. The extrafusal muscle fibres are supplied by Aα fibres. There are two main classes of γ efferent motor fibres: one group, γ_δ innervates the dynamic bag fibres, whereas the other group γ_σ innervate ends on static bag_2 fibres and chain fibres. Stimulation of the fusimotor nerves elicits no increase in muscle tension but produces an increase in sensory discharge. More recently, it has been recognized that some of the

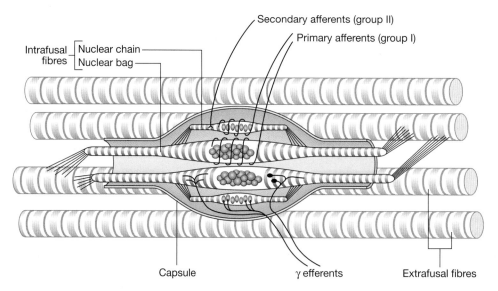

Figure 5.11 Diagrammatic representation of a muscle spindle. The two types of afferent sensory ending (group Ia and group II) are shown on the upper chain, and bag fibres and the efferent endings on the lower fibres.

motor supply to the spindles comes from branches of the motor neuron supplying extrafusal muscles.

All information coming into the CNS is subjected to control mechanisms at synaptic junctions either by other afferent neurons or by descending pathways from higher regions, such as the reticular formation and the cerebral cortex. These inhibitory controls are exerted at two main sites:

1. the axon terminals of the afferent nerves
2. the interneurons, which are activated directly by the afferent neurons.

Motor neurons that innervate a particular muscle form a *motor neuron pool*; α and γ motor neurons are mixed together in this pool, which is located in the ventral horn of one of several segments of the spinal cord. The motor neurons receive afferent input from all the muscle spindles in the innervated muscle. The group Ia and group II afferent fibres make mono- and polysynaptic excitatory connections to the motorneurons in the spinal cord. Thus receptor activation has a direct influence on the activity patterns of motor neurons.

References

Adrian ED, Bronk DW (1929) The discharge of impulses in motor nerve fibres II, the frequency of discharge in reflex and voluntary contractions. *J Physiol* **67**: 119–151.

Bárány M (1967) ATPase activity of myosin correlated with speed of muscle shortening. *J Genet Physiol* **50**: 197–218.

Barnard RJ, Edgerton VR, Furukawa T, Peter JB (1971) Histochemical, biochemical and contractile properties of red, white and intermediate fibres. *Am J Physiol* **220**: 410–414.

Buller AJ, Eccles JC, Eccles RW (1960a) Differentiation of fast and slow muscles in the cat hind limb. *J Physiol* **150**: 399–416.

Buller AJ, Eccles JC, Eccles RW (1960b) Interactions between motor neurones and muscles in respect of the characteristic speeds of their responses. *J Physiol* **150**: 417–439.

Burke RE, Levine DN, Tsiaris P, Zajac FE (1973) Physiological types and histochemical profiles in motor units of the cat gastrocnemius. *J Physiol* **234**: 723–748.

Denny Brown D (1929) The histological features of striped muscle in relation to its functional activity. *Proc Roy Soc (Series B)* **104**: 371–411.

Dubowitz V (1995) *Muscle Disorders in Childhood*. London, WB Saunders.

Eccles JC, Eccles RN, Lundberg A (1958) The action potentials of the alpha neurones supplying fast and slow muscles. *J Physiol* **142**: 275–291.

Edström L, Krugelberg E (1968) Histochemical composition, distribution of units and fatigability of single motor units. *J Neurol Neurosurg Psychiatry* **31**: 424–433.

Enoka RM (1997) Neural adaptations with chronic physical activity. *J Biomech* **30**: 447–455.

Erlanger J, Gasser HS (1937) *Electrical Signs of Nervous Activity*. Philadelphia, PA, University of Pennsylvania Press.

Erlanger J, Gasser HS (1970) *Human Neurophysiology*, 2nd edn. London, Chapman and Hall.

Gandevia SC (2001) Spinal and supraspinal factors in human muscle fatigue. *Physiol Rev* **81**: 1725–1789.

Henneman E, Olson C (1965) Relations between structure and function in the design of skeletal muscles. *J Neurophysiol* **28**: 581–598.

Hodgkin AL, Keynes RD (1955) Active transport of cations in giant axons from Sepia and Lologo. *J Physiol* **128**: 28–60.

Hodgkin AL, Huxley AF (1952) Currents carried by sodium and potassium ion through the membrane of the giant axon of Loligo. *J Physiol* **116**: 449–472.

Huxley AF (1957) Muscle structure and theories of contraction. *Prog Biophys* **7**: 255–318.

Huxley AF, Simmons RM (1971) Proposed mechanism of force generation in striated muscle. *Nature* **233**: 533–538.

Jami L (1992) Golgi tendon organs in mammalian skeletal muscle: functional properties and central actions. *Physiol Rev* **72**: 623–666.

Keynes RD, Aidley DJ (2001) *Muscle and Nerve*, 3rd edn. Cambridge, Cambridge University Press.

Lloyd DPC, Chang HT (1948) Afferent nerves in muscle nerves. *J Neurophysiol* **11**: 488–518.

Martin TP, Bodine-Fowler S, Roy RR et al (1988). Metabolic and fibre size properties of cat tibialis anterior motor units. *Am J Physiol* **255**: C43–C50.

Mathews PBC (1972) *Mammalian Muscle Receptors and their Central Actions*. London, Edward Arnold.

McComas AJ (1996) *Skeletal Muscle: Form and Function*. Champaign, IL, Human Kinetics.

Milner-Brown HS, Stein RB, Yemm R (1973) The orderly recruitment of human motor units under voluntary isometric contractions. *J Physiol* **230**: 371–390.

Pette D, Staron RS (1997) Mammalian skeletal muscle fiber type transitions. *Int Rev Cytol* **170**: 143–223.

Pette D, Staron RS (2001) Transitions of muscle fiber phenotypic profiles. *Histochem Cell Biol* **115**: 359–372.

Pette D, Vrbová G (1992) Adaptation of mammalian skeletal muscle fibres to chronic electrical stimulation. *Rev Physiol Biochem* **120**: 116–202.

Pette D, Vrbová G (1999) What does chronic electrical stimulation teach us about muscle plasticity? *Muscle Nerve* **22**: 666–677.

Ranvier L (1874) De quelques faits relatifs a l'histologie et la physiologie des muscles striès. *Arch Physiol Normal Pathol* 6: 1–15.

Salmons S, Vrbová V (1969) The influence of activity on some contractile characteristics of mammalian fast and slow muscles. *J Physiol* **201**: 535–549.

Scott W, Stevens J, Binder-Macleod SA (2001) Human skeletal muscle fiber type. *Phys Ther* **81**(11): 1810–1816.

Sherrington CS (1906) *The Integrative Action of the Nervous System* (reprinted 1961). New Haven, CT, Yale University Press.

Spudich JA (1994) How molecular motors work. *Nature* **372**: 515–518.

Vrbová G (1966) Factors determining the speed of contraction of striated muscle. *J Physiol* **185**: 17P–18P.

Weiss A, Schiaffino S, Leinwand LA (1999) comparative sequence analysis of complete human sarcomeric myosin heavy chain family: implications for functional diversity. *J Mol Biol* **290**: 61–75.

Chapter 6

Physiology of pain

Leslie Wood

INTRODUCTION

Ask any group of people to define what is meant by the word 'pain' and they will invariably each come up with a different set of words and terms to describe it. This reflects the general difficulty shared by scientists in trying to come up with a meaningful and accurate definition of what pain is and, perhaps more importantly, what it means in the context of the normal functioning of the human body. In addition, the relationship between the physiological events occurring in the body and the psychological state of the subject during the experience of pain is an important one.

As a starting point, therefore, it might be useful to provide a loose definition of pain as being the subjective sensations that accompany the activation of nociceptors (pain receptors) and which signal the location and strength of actual or potential tissue-damaging stimuli. As will be discussed later, this definition does not always apply in situations where pain might be experienced without apparent nociceptor activation.

Despite the difficulty in arriving at an acceptable definition of pain, most people would agree that it can be of a variable quality, ranging from mild irritation, through itching, burning and pricking sensations to more intense stabbing and throbbing sensations and finally to agonizing, intractable pain, which for some subjects can be beyond endurance. In most cases these sensations are associated with the activation of nociceptors and the sensation of pain, but the differences in the

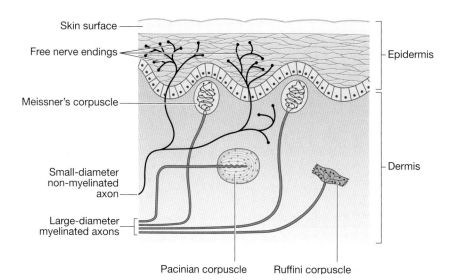

Skin surface

Free nerve endings

Epidermis

Meissner's corpuscle

Small-diameter non-myelinated axon

Dermis

Large-diameter myelinated axons

Pacinian corpuscle   Ruffini corpuscle

Figure 6.1 Types of sensory endings found in the skin. The endings giving rise to large-diameter afferents are those serving the sensations of touch, vibration, pressure and temperature. The non-myelinated afferents from the free nerve endings convey nociceptive information to the central nervous system.

subjective responses reflect both the strength and severity of the nociceptor activation and subjects' individual psychological and emotional responses to this information. As will be discussed later, these differences can be important in the modulation of pain in certain circumstances.

There are also circumstances, however, where subjective pain can be felt in the absence of any tissue damage or nociceptor activation. In these cases, the pain arises as a result of changes in the sensitivity of cells within the central nervous system (CNS; see later).

PERIPHERAL ASPECTS

Nociceptors are generally free nerve endings embedded throughout the tissues; there are variations in the density of these receptors in different tissues. The free nerve endings are no more than simple nerve endings without any of the associated accessory structures that can be found with other sensory nerve endings (Fig. 6.1). The free nerve endings have a relatively high threshold to activation and are sensitive to potentially tissue-damaging stimuli such as mechanical, thermal, electrical and chemical stimuli.

These free nerve endings give rise to small-diameter afferent nerve fibres, which convey action potentials to the spinal cord and higher centres in the CNS. These afferent fibres are classed as either myelinated Aδ fibres, with conduction velocities of between 5 and 30 m/s, or non-myelinated C fibres, which conduct action potentials at velocities between 0.5 and 2 m/s. (*Note*: Aδ fibres are sometimes referred to as group III fibres and C fibres as group IV fibres.) These two types of afferent fibre are responsible for what is termed 'fast' and 'slow' pain, the properties of which are outlined in Table 6.1.

These two pain modalities underlie the concepts of transient and prolonged pain sensations. Transient pain is the first sensation to accompany a noxious stimulus and usually involves only minimal tissue damage. It is of short duration and has no real long-term consequences for the subject. The Aδ afferent nerve fibres that are responsible for these sensations are also involved in the withdrawal reflex (see below). Prolonged pain is associated with activation of the group C afferent nerve fibres and usually accompanies a greater degree of tissue damage. This damage to the tissue cells results in the release of chemical mediators – such as bradykinin, substance P, histamine, 5-hydroxytryptamine (5-HT) and prostaglandins – from the damaged cells themselves and from activated nociceptor nerve endings. These chemical mediators can activate nociceptive nerve terminals directly and can also sensitize the response of the nociceptors to normal stimuli by altering the transduction properties of the free nerve endings.

Table 6.1 Properties of 'fast' and 'slow' pain fibres

Properties	Fast pain	Slow pain
Receptors	Free nerve endings	Free nerve endings
Afferents	Aδ (group III) fibres	C (group IV) fibres
Action potential conduction velocity	Relatively slow, 5–30 m/s	Very slow; 0.5–2 m/s
Subjective sensation	Sharp, pricking pain	Dull, burning, throbbing pain
Onset of sensation	Short latency, quick onset	Long latency, slow onset
Localization	Well localized, easily identified	Poorly localized, diffuse
Duration of sensation	Short lasting	Long lasting
Subjective response	Reflex withdrawal, less difficult to endure, possible emotional involvement	Emotional and automatic response

As well as activating group C nociceptive endings, these chemical mediators are also responsible for initiating the inflammatory responses in the damaged tissue. Figure 6.2 summarizes how tissue damage and the release of chemical mediators can activate nociceptors and transmit this information to the CNS.

The subjective involvement of both transient and prolonged pain can be best illustrated by referring to the pain sensations that accompany an injury such as stubbing a toe. Initially, there is a sharp pain associated with the physical contact of the toe with a hard object. This transient pain is followed by a duller, throbbing pain, which lasts for much longer. This is the prolonged pain caused by the ongoing release of chemical mediators from the damaged tissue in the toe. As part of this process, the injured area can become much more sensitive to what were previously innocuous stimuli but which now produce painful sensations. This sensitization can take place either at the free nerve endings themselves (peripheral sensitization; see above) or in the neurons of the dorsal horn of the spinal cord (central sensitization; see later). This increase in sensitivity is termed hyperalgesia and is also associated with allodynia (tenderness) attributed to the affected tissue.

CENTRAL ASPECTS

Information from the nociceptive afferent nerves is transmitted to the spinal cord, where it influences reflex activity, or is further transmitted via

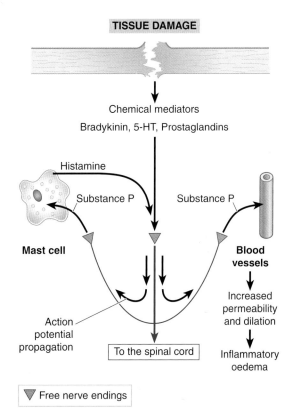

Figure 6.2 The role of chemical mediators in the activation of nociceptors and in the generation of inflammatory processes. Action potentials generated in the nociceptive afferents can travel along axonal branches to cause the release of the neurotransmitter substance P from other terminals. This, in turn, can influence mast cells, causing them to release histamine, which further activates the free nerve endings and also causing vasodilation and increased permeability of nearby blood vessels. 5-HT, 5-hydroxytryptamine.

specific pathways to higher brain centres. Nociceptive afferents enter the spinal cord via the dorsal root and make synaptic connections with other neurons located in the dorsal horn of the spinal cord grey matter. The dorsal horn is the site of convergence of several inputs relating to nociception, including the peripheral afferents described above, spinal interneurons and also descending neurons from higher centres in the brain.

The main reflexes involving nociceptive afferents are the flexor withdrawal and crossed extensor reflexes. These are polysynaptic reflexes and involve several muscle groups as well as operating over several spinal segmental levels. Nociceptive inputs make excitatory polysynaptic connections with motoneurons supplying flexor muscle groups and inhibitory polysynaptic connections with extensor motoneurons on the ipsilateral side. When these pathways are activated, they produce flexion in the limb where the original noxious stimulus arose while simultaneously switching off activity in the extensor muscles of this limb. These actions serve to move the limb away from the initial stimulus and, therefore, act in a protective fashion by removing the area from potential damage. At the same time, different polysynaptic connections from the same nociceptive afferents excite extensor motoneurons and inhibit flexor motoneurons in the contralateral limb. This action serves to stabilize the body during flexion of the ipsilateral limb. Figure 6.3 summarizes these connections.

The nociceptive afferents entering the spinal cord grey matter terminate in the dorsal horn, where they make synaptic connections either with interneurons serving the reflexes described above or with second-order neurons (so-called transmission cells, or T cells). These cross the midline of the spinal cord to transmit information to the higher centres via the lateral spinothalamic pathways on the contralateral side of the spinal cord (Fig. 6.4). The axons travelling in these pathways are therefore always second-order neurons, which have their cell bodies in the marginal zone or substantia gelatinosa (SG) of the spinal cord grey matter. Some of these second-order axons will ascend ipsilaterally for a few spinal segments before crossing the midline, whereas others will cross immediately. When these ascending neurons reach the ventrobasal nucleus of the thalamus, they terminate on third-order neurons, which

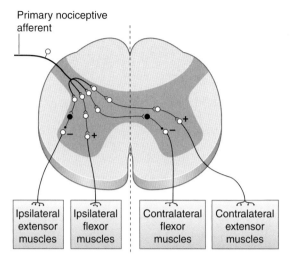

Primary nociceptive afferent

| Ipsilateral extensor muscles | Ipsilateral flexor muscles | Contralateral flexor muscles | Contralateral extensor muscles |

Figure 6.3 Spinal reflex pathways for the flexor withdrawal and crossed extensor reflexes. Excitatory interneurons are shown in white, and inhibitory interneurons in black.

then convey the information on the noxious stimulus to the cerebral cortex.

In addition, information is also passed to higher centres via the multisynaptic spinoreticular tract. This pathway sends projections from several brainstem terminations via the intralaminar nucleus of the thalamus to areas such as the hypothalamus, the frontal lobe and the limbic system of the brain. These areas coordinate the autonomic, psychological and emotional responses to pain.

MODULATION OF PAIN TRANSMISSION

It is in the spinal cord that the possibility for the modulation of transmission of nociceptive information to higher centres exists. To understand how this operates, it is useful to look in more detail at what happens in the dorsal horn of the spinal cord grey matter.

As we have already noted, primary nociceptive afferents terminate on second-order neurons, which then transmit the nociceptive information to higher centres. The excitability of this pathway can be altered by other interneurons present in the dorsal horn. Cells of the substantia gelatinosa (SG cells)

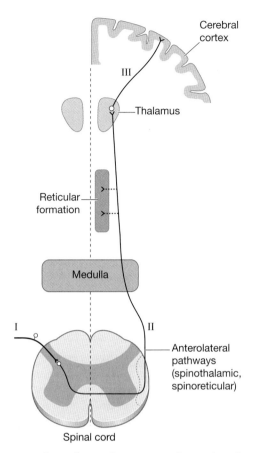

Figure 6.4 Ascending pathways conveying nociceptive information to higher centres. Primary nociceptive afferents (I) enter the dorsal horn where they synapse with second-order neurons, which cross the midline to ascend in the anterolateral pathways (II). Some axons terminate in the reticular formation of the pons and medulla (dashed lines) whereas other axons ascend to the thalamus where they synapse with third-order neurons (III), which ascend to the somatosensory cortex.

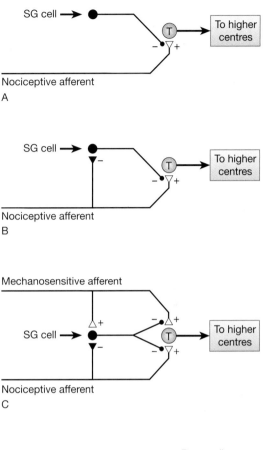

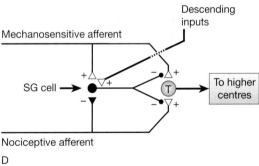

Figure 6.5 Neural circuits in the dorsal horn that influence pain transmission to higher centres. See text for detailed explanation. SG, substantia gelatinosa; T, transmission cell.

have an inhibitory influence on the transmission cells. This is achieved by presynaptic inhibition of the nociceptive afferent terminals at the point where they synapse with the transmission cells (Fig. 6.5A). However, the SG cells are inhibited when the nociceptive afferents are activated (Fig. 6.5B), reducing the presynaptic inhibition of the nociceptor afferent terminal and thereby allowing nociceptive information to be passed to higher centres.

The SG cells are influenced by other inputs, however. Activation of low-threshold, large-diameter, mechanosensitive afferents stimulates the SG cells via an excitatory synapse, and therefore increases the amount of presynaptic inhibition acting on the nociceptor afferent terminals and preventing the transmission of nociceptive information to higher centres (Fig. 6.5C). It should be noted here that the large-diameter afferents also have excitatory inputs onto the T cells, but that this is also inhibited by presynaptic inhibition of these terminals (Fig. 6.5C).

In addition to these inputs to SG cells from peripheral afferents, descending inputs from higher centres also have excitatory connections to the SG cells (Fig. 6.5D), thereby allowing descending control on the overall excitability of the T cells (see below). The important point to note is that activation of the SG cells will inhibit pain transmission to higher centres. The overall balance of excitation and inhibition impinging on the T cells is therefore of great importance in determining whether nociceptive information is relayed to the higher cognitive centres of the brain. By altering the balance in favour of inhibition via the SG inhibitory interneurons, transmission of nociceptive information to higher centres can be reduced or abolished (Fig. 6.6).

This modulation of pain transmission by altering the influences of the different inputs to the transmission cells is known as the gate control theory, which was established by Melzack and Wall in 1965. In its simplest form, this mechanism can be regarded as a system in which the 'gate' is either open, to allow nociceptive information to be passed on to higher centres, or closed, preventing this information from being transmitted. In terms of producing analgesia, it is the goal of the therapist to ensure that the balance of inputs is always in favour of closing the gate.

As the SG cells receive inputs both from large-diameter mechanosensitive afferents and from

descending inputs, activation of these inputs will provide a mechanism whereby pain transmission can be modulated. Large-diameter mechanosensitive afferents can be activated by a number of means, including direct, simple mechanical stimulation of receptors in the skin, muscles and joints, as well as being activated artificially by electrical stimulation. This has implications for the management of pain in physiotherapy. Any technique that activates these afferents has the potential to modulate pain transmission in the spinal cord. Techniques such as massage, joint manipulation, traction and compression, thermal stimulation and electrotherapy can all produce sensory inputs from low-threshold afferents, which can ultimately inhibit pain transmission in the spinal cord by 'closing the gate', i.e. inhibiting T-cell activity via the SG cells. Transcutaneous electrical nerve stimulation (TENS) can be used to stimulate the large-diameter afferents in the skin directly and, when administered in an appropriate area and at an appropriate voltage, can therefore influence pain transmission in the relevant spinal segments. In this way, both the therapist and the patient can have control over pain modulation and can adjust the levels of this at any time.

The descending influences on the T cells are also important. These inputs come principally from the periaqueductal grey matter (PAGM, the grey matter surrounding the cerebral aqueduct, located in the midbrain) and the raphe nucleus (located in the medulla). These both have excitatory effects on the inhibitory interneurons of the substantia gelatinosa in the dorsal horn of the spinal cord, and so have the ability to reduce pain transmission at the level of the spinal cord. These descending pathways are thought to exert their effects on the SG cells by releasing monoaminergic neurotransmitters such as norepinephrine and 5-HT. Under normal circumstances, though, these pathways are usually inactive due to further influence of inhibitory interneurons from other areas of the brain. These inputs therefore turn off or reduce the activity of the cells of the PAGM or raphe nucleus.

In certain situations, this inhibition of the PAGM and the raphe nucleus can be removed. This is achieved by the actions of neurons projecting from other areas of the CNS associated with pain modulation. These neurons arise from the limbic system – a term used collectively to describe

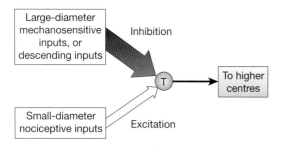

Figure 6.6 Inhibition of pain transmission is achieved by altering the balance of inputs to the transmission cells such that it favours those from large-diameter mechanosensitive afferents or from descending inputs. When this happens, the larger amount of inhibitory input (large arrow) overrides the excitatory input generated by the nociceptive afferents (small arrow). T, transmission cell.

structures such as the hypothalamus, the hippocampus and the amygdala – as well as from other areas within the PAGM itself. The limbic areas are involved in emotion and mood and can have wide-ranging influences on other aspects of nervous control, including the control of pain.

Activity in these areas stimulates the production of naturally occurring (endogenous) opioids (opiate-like chemicals). There are three families of endogenous opioids, the enkephalins, the endorphins and the dynorphins. Neurons containing and utilizing these opioids have clearly distinct distributions throughout the brain and spinal cord and have different roles to play in the modulation of pain transmission. The actions of the endogenous opioids on their target neurons are generally inhibitory. Therefore, these opioids allow excitation of the descending PAGM neurons by inhibiting the background inhibition of the PAGM cells, rather than by direct excitation (i.e. these opioids turn off, or block, the inhibition of the PAGM neurons). When this happens, these cells are now free to exert their own descending influences on the SG cells of the dorsal horn of the spinal cord grey matter, which, in turn, will inhibit transmission of nociceptive information via the T cells (Fig. 6.7).

In addition, these descending pathways might also activate spinal cord interneurons, which release enkephalins that subsequently inhibit the transmission cells both pre- and postsynaptically at the spinal level.

It is thought that these effects of the endogenous opioids are associated with producing analgesia related only to the prolonged aspects of pain, rather than the initial, faster pain responses produced when an injury first occurs, that is, the inhibitory effects of PAGM and raphe nucleus activation influence only the transmission of pain mediated by C fibres and not that by Aδ fibres.

However, there is an alternative theory for the role of the descending pathways in pain modulation. There is some evidence to suggest that the descending pathways are activated by nociceptive inputs and actually enhance pain transmission in the spinal cord. The effect of the release of endogenous opioids is therefore to suppress the activity in these descending pathways and thereby reduce the transmission of pain to higher centres. Research is ongoing to establish a clearer understanding of the nature of the descending modulation of pain transmission.

Whatever the mechanism of descending pain modulation, it is clear that higher cognitive centres in the brain can have some influence on these processes. Fear, stress, excitement and even pain itself can all reduce, or even abolish, the feelings of pain associated with injury. A well-known example of this is the so-called 'battlefield analgesia', where a soldier who has sustained a severe injury to part of the body is initially unaware of it until some time later, usually after reaching safety. Similar reduced responses to pain are observed in many sports, with players or athletes managing to continue despite having sustained what would otherwise be a debilitating injury. This higher suppression of pain sensation is probably mediated from the cerebral cortex via the limbic system to the descending pain control systems described above.

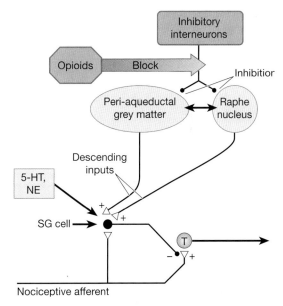

Figure 6.7 Descending influences on substantia gelatinosa (SG) cell activity. The periaqueductal grey matter (PAGM) and raphe nucleus inputs are normally held in check by the actions of inhibitory interneurons. Release of endogenous opioids blocks this inhibition, leading to activation of these descending pathways, which exert excitatory effects on the SG cells utilizing 5-hydroxytryptamine (5-HT) and norepinephrine (NA). T, transmission cell.

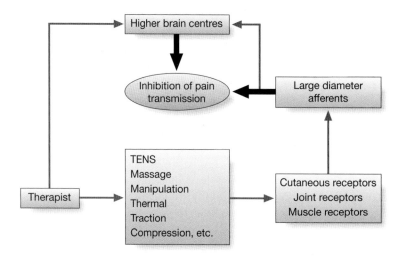

Figure 6.8 The role of the therapist in influencing the inhibition of pain transmission.

Such mechanisms can also be of importance for therapeutic interventions at a psychological, rather than a physiological, level. The fact that patients might simply be receiving attention from a therapist, regardless of the techniques being employed, could be sufficient to induce an emotional or psychological response that modulates the pain they are experiencing. Figure 6.8 summarizes the possible influences of the therapist on pain modulation.

SENSITIZATION

We have already noted the possibility of increased sensitivity of the free nerve endings due to the action of inflammatory chemical mediators (peripheral sensitization). We should also note that, following activation by group C afferents, the excitability of the dorsal horn transmission cells can remain elevated for several hours, via alterations in intracellular second messengers in these cells. This leads to changes in membrane channels and membrane receptors that, in turn, increase both the excitability of the neurons and their sensitivity to synaptic transmitters. This phenomenon is termed central sensitization (see below).

The altered sensitivity of the transmission cells means that they now respond abnormally to inputs from the large-diameter mechanosensitive group A afferents, which can now elicit flexor withdrawal reflexes as well as pain sensations. The consequences of these abnormal responses of the transmission cells to innocuous afferent input are that any clinical pain reduction treatment aimed at preventing or reducing nociceptive input to the spinal cord will not be sufficient to prevent pain sensations in the subject, as these can now be elicited by simple stimulation of the large-diameter mechanosensitive afferents. Such alterations to the sensitivity of the dorsal horn cells can last for several hours or longer. These mechanisms underlie the development of the phenomena of hyperalgesia and allodynia. In some cases, injury and the subsequent sensitizing effects on spinal cord neurons can produce longer-lasting changes in the expression of receptors, transmitters and ion channels in peripheral and central neurons and in modification of synaptic connections in the dorsal horn, resulting in reorganized neural circuitry in the pathways mediating pain transmission. In such cases the reorganization might be such that the sensitization of the pain transmission pathways becomes permanent and irreversible, leading to persistent abnormal responses to peripheral stimuli, which are subjectively interpreted as pain.

CHRONIC PAIN

Chronic pain is defined as pain that persists beyond the duration of the normal period for tissue healing and beyond the time when pain might normally be expected to occur after injury; this is nominally about 3 months postinjury. Chronic pain is also associated with prolonged structural and functional changes within the CNS. These features differentiate chronic pain from the shorter-lasting acute pain.

Central sensitization is a feature of chronic pain. There is a gradual increase in the sensitivity of T cells in the dorsal horn of the spinal cord to both noxious and non-noxious stimuli, resulting in a greater discharge response of these cells when they are stimulated. This phenomenon is termed 'wind-up'. Although associated with chronic pain, it should be noted that wind-up is also involved in acute pain responses.

The increase in sensitivity of dorsal horn cells is brought about by the repetitive firing of peripheral C fibres and is mediated in part by activation of the N-methyl-D-aspartate (NMDA) subtype of postsynaptic glutamate receptors on the dorsal horn cells. These receptors are normally blocked by the presence of a magnesium ion (Mg^{2+}) at the receptor site, but with sustained depolarization (see Chapter 4) of the dorsal horn cells this Mg^{2+} is removed and glutamate is then free to bind to the NMDA receptors, producing an increased sensitivity of these cells: wind-up. Subsequent to these changes, the NMDA receptors on the dorsal horn cells undergo longer-lasting modifications (e.g. phosphorylation of receptors), which cause further cellular changes that increase the sensitivity of the cells to previously subthreshold inputs: central sensitization. If wind-up and central sensitization persist, they eventually result in changes in gene expression together with plastic changes in the cells, resulting in a chronic pain state. These mechanisms are summarized in Figure 6.9.

COMPLEX REGIONAL PAIN SYNDROME

Complex regional pain syndrome (CRPS) is a collection of abnormal painful disorders that arise as a result of, in some cases, relatively minor trauma to tissues (e.g. bone fractures, surgery, sprains). The pain associated with CRPS is often out of proportion to the initial precipitating injury and there are additional accompanying autonomic responses. CRPS is most commonly observed in distal limb areas, with the upper limbs more susceptible than the lower.

Two types of CRPS exist: type I, which has no obvious involvement of damage to peripheral nerves; and type II, where nerve injury is present. Previous terminologies used to describe CRPS include reflex sympathetic dystrophy for type I, and causalgia for type II.

The diagnostic criteria set by the International Association for the Study of Pain for CRPS were modified in 1999 and include (Bruehl et al 1999):

- An initial noxious event.

- Continuing pain that is disproportionate to any initiating event (including allodynia and hyperalgesia).

- Hyperaesthesia.

- Temperature and skin colour asymmetry.

- Oedema and/or sweating changes and/or sweating asymmetry.

- Decreased range of movement and/or motor dysfunction (tremors, muscle weakness, hyperreflexia, dystonia).

The pain associated with type I CRPS is a diffuse, burning, spontaneous pain that is intractable and becomes worse and more widespread with time. In addition, allodynia and hyperalgesia might be present. Disordered sympathetic nervous system responses are also evident, affecting sweating patterns, skin temperature and colour (abnormal skin blood flow) and tissue swelling. The underlying cause of these effects has not been fully elucidated but might involve abnormalities in central autonomic (sympathetic) control, leading to dysregulation of blood vessel and sweat gland function. It has also been suggested that peripheral interaction between sympathetic neurons and nociceptive afferents in the skin, muscles and joints might promote spontaneous pain in these tissues (sympathetically maintained pain; SMP). This is possibly brought about by increased sympathetic activity stimulating the synthesis and release of inflammatory chemical mediators that affect the growth and excitability of nociceptive afferents. In addition, increased nociceptive input to the dorsal horn cells in the spinal cord might lead to central sensitization, as described in the section on chronic pain above.

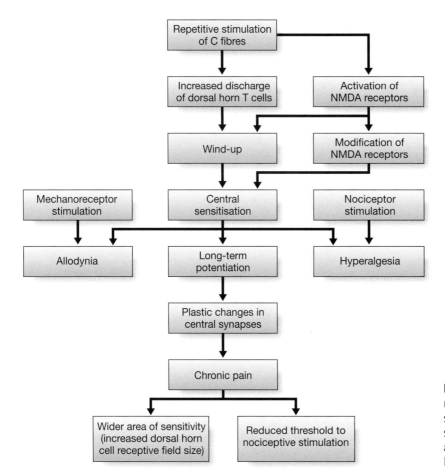

Figure 6.9 Summary of the mechanisms and interrelationships underpinning central sensitisation, chronic pain, allodynia and hyperalgesia. NMDA, *N*-methyl-D-aspartate.

PAIN STATES

It should be apparent by this stage that the delivery of nociceptive information to higher centres is highly dependent on the state of the nervous pathways serving the transmission processes. Put simply, these pathways can be in the normal state, the suppressed state or the enhanced, sensitized state. These three states therefore equate with the concepts of 'normoalgesia', 'hypoalgesia' and 'hyperalgesia'. In each of these three different possible states, the same stimulus intensity can produce different subjective sensations of pain depending on how the nociceptive information is delivered to, and processed by, the CNS. For example, a particular stimulus intensity might produce a painful sensation in the normoalgesic state, whereas the same stimulus intensity would not elicit any subjective pain in the suppressed, hypoalgesic state.

Similarly, an innocuous stimulus might not elicit pain in either the normoalgesic or hypoalgesic states but will produce subjective pain in the hyperalgesic state. The reasons for this are summarized diagrammatically in Figure 6.10.

In this figure we can see that the threshold for eliciting a subjective painful sensation is altered depending on how readily the nervous pathways respond to the incoming afferent information. In the suppressed, hypoalgesic state (Fig. 6.10B), the threshold is reached only at higher stimulus intensities, whereas it is reached at lower (often innocuous) intensities in the enhanced, hyperalgesic state (Fig. 6.10C).

For these reasons, it is important for therapists to be aware that stimuli applied to a patient as part of a therapeutic treatment programme might not, in fact, result in the desired outcome of pain relief and might instead exacerbate a painful condition.

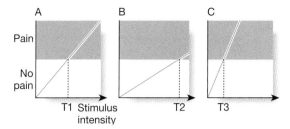

Figure 6.10 Generation of subjective pain sensations in three pain states: normoalgesia, hypoalgesia and hyperalgesia. A, normoalgesia – increasing stimulus intensity eventually reaches a threshold level (T1), which crosses the boundary between no pain sensation and pain. B, hypoalgesia – suppressed pain transmission (reduced slope) means that greater stimulus intensities are required to reach the threshold level (T2 higher than T1), i.e. it is more difficult to elicit pain sensations. C, hyperalgesia – sensitized pain transmission (increased slope) means that the threshold level is reached much sooner (T3 lower than T1), i.e. pain sensations are elicited with weaker stimuli.

Table 6.2 Sites of referred pain and their common sites of origin

Origin of pain	Site of referred pain and spinal segments involved
Heart (angina pectoris)	Chest, left shoulder, left arm (T1–T5)
Gall bladder and bile ducts	Right upper quadrant of abdomen, below right shoulder (T7, T8)
Diaphragm	Top of shoulder (C3–C5)
Stomach	Upper central region of abdomen (epigastrium) (T7, T8)
Duodenum (e.g. duodenal ulcer)	Anterior abdominal wall above umbilicus (T9, T10)
Kidneys and ureter	Loin and groin (L1, L2)
Appendix	Umbilicus initially, then to lower right quadrant of abdomen when peritoneum becomes inflamed (T10)

REFERRED PAIN

Pain that arises from deep structures in the body – visceral pain – is often felt by the subject in locations that are far removed from the site of origin. Such translocation of pain sensation is known as referred pain. An example of this is the pain associated with angina pectoris. Here, the organ that is affected is the heart but the pain is often described as arising in (or referred to) the upper chest, left shoulder and arm. Other sites of referred pain and their sites of origin are given in Table 6.2.

The explanation for the pattern of referred pain lies in the pattern of convergence of afferent nerve fibres in the dorsal horn of the spinal cord. Dorsal horn neurons, including those that act as transmission cells, receive inputs from a wide variety of sources that are innervated by the same spinal segments (T1–T4 in the case of the heart and left arm). These convergent inputs can include nociceptive inputs from both cutaneous areas and visceral areas (Fig. 6.11A). As described above, these transmission cells pass this nociceptive information to higher centres, where it is perceived and interpreted as pain sensation. However, the higher centres cannot distinguish the source of this information as

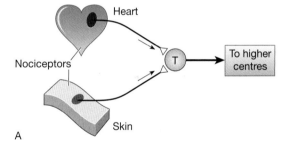

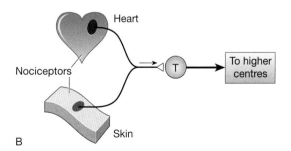

Figure 6.11 Mechanisms of referred pain. A, nociceptive afferents from two different locations (here the hart and the skin) converge on the same transmission cell in the dorsal horn of the spinal cord. B, the nociceptors from the two different areas share the same primary afferent axon entering the spinal cord.

being either cutaneous or visceral in origin because they receive inputs only from single transmission cells. Peripheral nociceptive input from cutaneous or skeletal muscle receptors normally predominates in normal, everyday circumstances (rather than nociceptive input from the heart) and so the higher centres incorrectly ascribe the information passed on by the transmission cells as coming from their usual source of the skin or muscles, rather than the deeper, visceral organ, the heart.

There is also some evidence that, in some cases, referred pain might arise owing to bifurcations in the peripheral neurons that converge on the transmission cells in the dorsal horn – that is, single peripheral afferents might split to supply both skin areas and deeper visceral areas (Fig. 6.11B).

It is important for the therapist to be aware of the possible patterns of referred pain (see Table 6.2) because the patient might describe pain as arising in a structure that has no underlying lesion, misleading the therapist as to the real source of the complaint.

PHANTOM LIMB PAIN

When a limb has been amputated or the sensory nerves from a limb have been destroyed, the sensation of the limb still being present can exist in some cases (phantom limb) and sometimes pain referred to the missing limb can be perceived. Pain associated with a missing limb is known as phantom limb pain. Phantom limb pain is often described as burning, electric or cramping sensations, and can persist for many years after the loss of the limb.

The source of this phantom limb pain might be the severed ends of the peripheral nerves that were cut during the amputation or injury. This could set up abnormal patterns of discharge in the peripheral nerve fibres, particularly nociceptive

afferents, which are then relayed to higher centres and perceived as pain sensations arising in the areas these nerves formerly supplied. Additionally there might be altered activity in the neurons of the dorsal horn associated with pain transmission (see Sensitization above). This altered activity might arise as a result of afferent degeneration inducing postsynaptic changes in the dorsal horn neurons.

Recent research (Hill 1999) has suggested a further cause of phantom limb pain. This proposes that phantom limbs and the sensations associated with them are a consequence of activity in neural networks in higher centres of the brain. These neural networks form a so-called neuromatrix, the structure and functioning of which might be genetically determined, and which is susceptible to inputs from peripheral structures. This neuromatrix is not localized but widespread throughout the brain. It provides a neural framework that underpins subjects' experience of their own body as a physical entity that 'belongs' to them. Sensory inputs from all areas of the body can manipulate and modify the activity of the neuromatrix. It has been suggested that phantom limb pain arises as a result of abnormal or absent modulating input to this neuromatrix and missing channels of output from the neuromatrix to the muscles. Interestingly, more recent research has proposed a novel method of relieving phantom limb pain in some patients. This effectively involves fooling the patients' CNS by allowing the patient to 'see' the phantom limb using a mirror reflection of their intact opposite limb. When this is done, manipulation or movement of the intact limb is viewed in the mirror and is transposed by the brain on to the phantom limb. In certain circumstances, this simple technique can be used to remove painful sensations arising from the phantom limb.

References

Bruehl S, Harden RN, Galer BS et al (1999) External validation of IASP diagnostic criteria for complex regional pain dyndrome and proposed research diagnostic criteria. *Pain* **81**: 147–154.

Hill A (1999) Phantom limb pain: a review of the literature on attributes and potential mechanisms. *J Pain Symptom Manage* **17**(2): 125–142.

Melzack R, Wall PD (1965) Pain mechanisms – a new theory. *Science* **150**: 971–979.

Bibliography

Costigan M, Woolf CJ (2000) Pain: molecular mechanisms. *J Pain* **1**: 35–44.

Herrero JF, Laird JMA, Lopez-Garcia JA (2000) Wind-up of spinal neurones and pain sensitisation: much ado about something? *Prog Neurobiol* **61**: 169–203.

Janig W, Baron R (2003) Complex regional pain syndrome: mystery explained. *Lancet Neurol* **2**: 687–697.

Kandel ER, Schwartz JH, Jessell TM (2000) *Principles of Neural Science*, 4th edn. New York, McGraw-Hill.

McBride A, Atkins R (2005) Complex regional pain syndrome. *Curr Orthop* **19**: 155–165.

Melzack R (1990) Phantom limbs and the concept of a neuromatrix. *Trends Neurosci* **13**: 88–92.

Melzack R, Wall PD (1996) *The Challenge of Pain*, 2nd edn (updated). London, Penguin.

Priest TD, Hoggart B (2002) Chronic pain: mechanisms and treatment. *Curr Opin Pharmacol* **2**: 310–315.

Ramachandran VS, Blakeslee S (1998) *Phantoms in the Brain*. London, Fourth Estate.

Ru-rong J, Woolf CJ (2001) Neuronal plasticity and signal transduction in nociceptive neurons: Implications for the initiation and maintenance of pathological pain. *Neurobiol Dis* **8**: 1–10.

Shipton EA (1999) *Pain – Acute and Chronic*. London, Edward Arnold.

Wall PD, Melzack R (eds) (1994) *Textbook of Pain*, 3rd edn. New York, Churchill Livingstone.

Woolf CJ, Costigan M (1999) Transcriptional and posttranslational plasticity and the generation of inflammatory pain. *Proc Natl Acad Sci* USA **96**: 7723–7730.

Chapter 7

Thermal effects

Sheila Kitchen

INTRODUCTION

Chapter 2 presented the basic scientific principles underpinning the way in which changes in temperature affect materials. This chapter examines in more detail the effects that are produced in biological materials, particularly when these are part of a functioning body.

THERMAL HOMOEOSTASIS

In health, humans preserve a constant body temperature by means of a highly efficient thermoregulatory system. This process involves close temperature regulation of the deep body (or core) temperature, with more varied but managed temperature regulation of the peripheral layers.

BODY TEMPERATURE

The body is usually considered to consist of two thermal compartments: the core or central compartment, and the shell or superficial layer (Fig. 7.1).

CORE TEMPERATURE

Core temperature is approximately 37°C; arbitrary variations of ± 2°C define hyper- and hypothermia, despite much larger variations in the ambient temperature in which the person is functioning (International Union of Physiological Sciences 1987).

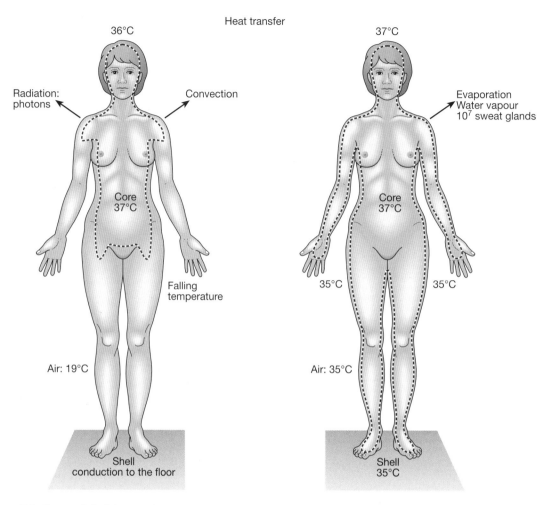

Figure 7.1 Core and shell temperatures.

Hyperthermia can therefore be regarded as a core temperature in excess of 39°C and hypothermia a temperature below 35°C. At rest, and in a neutral environment, core temperature can be kept within a narrow band of control (±0.3°C). However, although the core temperature tends to be kept within this narrow range around 37°C, it is not a fixed entity and there are significant temperature gradients within the anatomical core. Organs such as the liver and active skeletal muscles, for example, have a higher rate of metabolic heat production than other tissues and therefore maintain a higher temperature. Similarly, there are temperature gradients within the vascular compartment perfusing both the core and the shell. In addition, core temperature varies with the body's intrinsic diurnal temperature rhythm.

SHELL TEMPERATURE

Whereas the core temperature is relatively stable, the shell – at the interface between the body and the environment – is subject to much greater variations in temperature. Across approximately 1 cm of the body shell, from the skin surface to the superficial layer of muscle, the temperature gradient varies according to the temperature of the core and the external environment (demonstrated for the forearm in Fig. 7.2). The gradient is not uniform and changes with the thermal conductivity of the tissue layers and the rate of blood flow in the different regions. Skin temperatures differ widely over the body surface, especially in hot or cold conditions. When an individual is in a comfortable environment of, say, 24°C, the skin of the

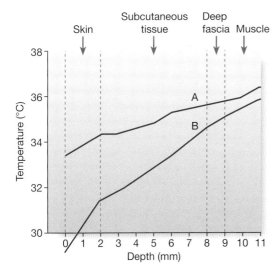

Figure 7.2 Temperature gradients in the forearm between the skin surface and deep tissues in A, comfortably warm conditions and B, cold conditions.

toes might be 27°C, that of the upper arms and legs 31°C and the forehead 34°C; the core is maintained at 37°C.

DIURNAL (CIRCADIAN) CORE TEMPERATURE RHYTHM

The diurnal (circadian) core temperature rhythm is one of the most stable of biological rhythms, with a well-marked intrinsic component (Fig. 7.3). Body temperature is lowest in the early morning and highest in the evening, although in a small minority of people this phase is reversed. The diurnal range of variation is usually about 0.5–1.5°C in adults, depending on other external factors, such as the effects of meals, activity, sleep and ambient temperature. Different intrinsic biological rhythms are often in phase with each other and there is evidence that when they are not, synchronization function is compromised. For example, desynchronization of the sleep–wake cycle and the core temperature cycle by continuous light exposure can bring about impairment of thermoregulatory function (Moore-Ede & Sulzman 1981). Other rhythms, which are not daily (e.g. the female menstrual cycle) also affect core temperature.

BODY TEMPERATURE MEASUREMENT

Core temperature is measured conventionally by a mercury-in-glass or electrical thermometer placed in the mouth; both are quick and accurate. Errors occur with mouth breathing or talking during measurement, following hot or cold drinks, or if the tissues of the mouth are otherwise affected by the external environment. Alternatives are rectal or urinary measurement of core temperature (more reliable but generally less practical), which give results that are on average about 0.5°C higher than mouth temperatures. For accurate and fast recording, measurement can be made in the ear canal (near to but not touching the tympanic membrane) by thermistor or thermocouple. The reliability of measurement at all sites can be affected by a variety of conditions, which need to be controlled, especially when accuracy – as required in research conditions – is essential.

THERMAL BALANCE

For the core temperature to remain constant there needs to be a balance (equilibrium) between internal heat production, heat gain from the environment and external heat loss. This is shown pictorially in Figure 7.4 and expressed in the form of a *heat balance equation* (Box 7.1).

Metabolic heat production (M) is the heat produced during the work of metabolism. It can be calculated from the measurement of total body oxygen consumption. Basal metabolic rate, which occurs during complete physical and mental rest,

---

Box 7.1 Heat balance equation

$$M \pm w = \pm K \pm C \pm R - E \pm S$$

where:
- M is the rate of metabolic heat production
- w is the external work performed by or on the body
- K, C and R are the loss or gain of heat by conduction, convection and radiation, respectively
- E is the evaporative heat loss from the skin and respiratory tract
- S is the rate of change of body heat storage (resultant = 0 at thermal equilibrium).

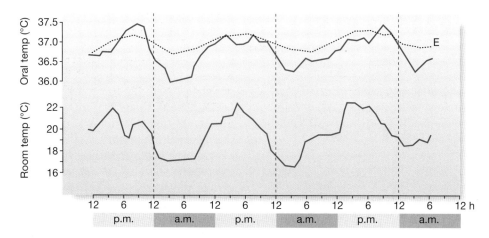

Figure 7.3 Diurnal variation in body temperature showing the influence of ambient (room) temperature on the oral temperature when meals and physical activity are kept constant. E, intrinsic temperature rhythm.

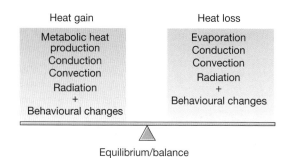

Figure 7.4 Heat balance.

is about $45\,W/m^2$ (i.e. watts per square metre of body surface) for an adult male of 30 years and $41\,W/m^2$ for a female of the same age. These values can be almost doubled during severe physical work and might be as high as $900\,W/m^2$ for brief periods. A small increase in M follows the eating of a meal; M is also increased by shivering.

Heat loss or gain by conduction (K) depends on the temperature difference between the body and the surrounding medium, on thermal conductivity between the two and on the area of contact. Little heat is normally lost by conduction to the air because air is a poor heat conductor, but immersion in cold water, as in a winter sea or during a long swim, can lead to rapid cooling. Subcutaneous fat is important in determining the level of cooling because this provides tissue insulation; applying

grease to the body before a marathon swim aims to reduce heat loss by conduction.

Convective heat exchange (C) depends on the fluid (most commonly air) surrounding the body, and its flow patterns. Normally, an individual's surface temperature is higher than the temperature of the surrounding air, so that heated air close to the body moves upwards by natural convection and colder air takes its place, thus cooling the body.

Radiant heat transfer (R) depends on the nature of the surfaces involved, their temperature and the geometrical relationship between them. Extending the arms and legs effectively increases the surface area over which convective and radiant heat exchange can take place.

Evaporative heat loss (E): at rest in a comfortable ambient temperature, an individual loses water by evaporation through the skin and from the respiratory tract. This is described as insensible water loss. It occurs at a rate of about $30\,g$ per hour and produces a heat loss of about $10\,W/m^2$. Sweating (sensible water loss) contributes a much greater potential heat loss (E). Complete evaporation of 1 litre of sweat from the body surface in 1 hour will dissipate about $400\,W/m^2$.

Rate of heat storage (S): the specific heat of the human body is $3.5\,kJ/kg$. If a person of $65\,kg$ increases mean core temperature by $1°C$ over a period of 1 hour, S becomes $230\,kJ/h$, or $64\,W$. S can be positive or negative.

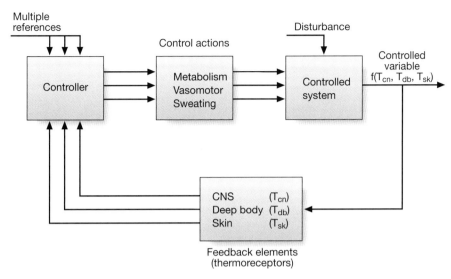

Figure 7.5 The human thermoregulatory system.

CONTROL OF BODY TEMPERATURE

The above factors contribute to changes in body temperature, and control of these processes (thermoregulation) is essential for survival. Good health requires that very limited variation occurs, despite people working and playing in environments of very different temperatures.

Thermoregulation is integrated by a controlling mechanism in the central nervous system (CNS) that responds to the heat of the tissues, which is detected by thermoreceptors. These receptors are sensitive to heat and cold information arising in the skin, the deep tissues and the CNS itself. They provide feedback signals to CNS structures, which are situated mainly in the hypothalamus of the brain, via a servo- or loop system (Fig. 7.5). The temperature of the blood perfusing the hypothalamus is also a major physiological drive to thermoregulation. The hypothalamus monitors ambient temperature in relation to the heat balance discussed above, and initiates appropriate physiological responses (vasodilatation and sweating in hot conditions, or vasoconstriction and shivering in cold) that counteract any deviation in the core temperature (Fig. 7.6). Apart from these involuntary responses, thermal information is transmitted by afferent nerves to regions of the brain that control

endocrine functions and to the cerebral cortex, which makes individuals aware of their thermal sensations by inducing behavioural changes such as moving away from/toward heat sources, donning/removing clothing or opening/closing windows.

An essential role in processing thermal signals is ascribed to the preoptic region of the anterior hypothalamus and to a region in the posterior hypothalamus, described respectively as the 'heat loss' and 'heat gain' centres because they are considered to exert the primary control on vasodilatation/sweating in the heat and on vasoconstriction/shivering in a cold environment. The integration of incoming and outgoing information, and the 'set-point' from which the hypothalamic centres operate, is the basis on which present views of thermoregulatory control are constructed (Collins 1992, Hensel 1981).

PHYSIOLOGICAL EFFECTS OF THERMAL CHANGES

The general physiological effects of heating and cooling of tissue are described in some detail here; the individual sections and chapters following highlight issues related to individual agents.

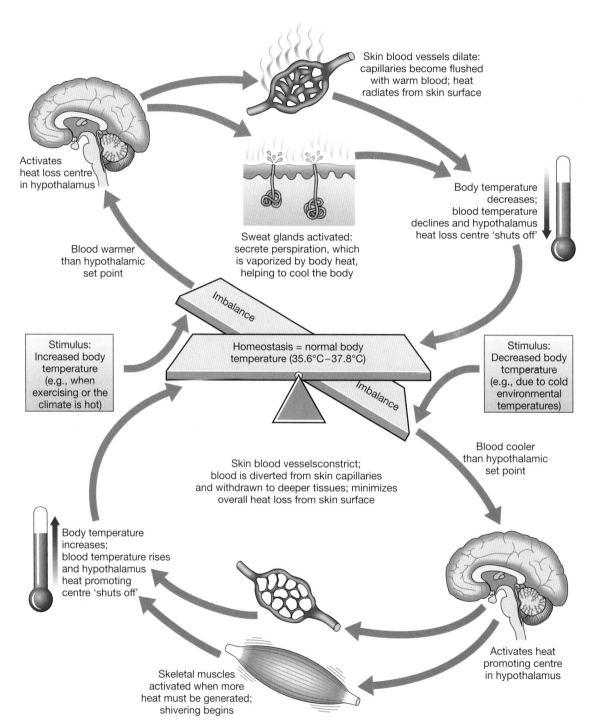

Skin blood vessels dilate: capillaries become flushed with warm blood; heat radiates from skin surface

Activates heat loss centre in hypothalamus

Body temperature decreases; blood temperature declines and hypothalamus heat loss centre 'shuts off'

Blood warmer than hypothalamic set point

Sweat glands activated: secrete perspiration, which is vaporized by body heat, helping to cool the body

Imbalance

Stimulus: Increased body temperature (e.g., when exercising or the climate is hot)

Homeostasis = normal body temperature (35.6°C–37.8°C)

Imbalance

Stimulus: Decreased body temperature (e.g., due to cold environmental temperatures)

Blood cooler than hypothalamic set point

Skin blood vesselsconstrict; blood is diverted from skin capillaries and withdrawn to deeper tissues; minimizes overall heat loss from skin surface

Body temperature increases; blood temperature rises and hypothalamus heat promoting centre 'shuts off'

Skeletal muscles activated when more heat must be generated; shivering begins

Activates heat promoting centre in hypothalamus

Figure 7.6 The role of the hypothalamus in thermoregulation (from Marieb 2002, with permission of Benjamin Cummings).

PHYSIOLOGICAL EFFECTS OF COLD

This overview is necessarily somewhat simplistic, and readers are referred to the literature for further detail. For example, the effects on cells and, particularly, enzymes are temperature dependent and therefore variable. In addition, there are still considerable gaps in knowledge, which must be borne in mind.

Local effects

Once cooling has occurred, how this was brought about is immaterial. Therefore the issues discussed here are dependent on the actual temperature rather than the process of cooling. The varied effects of cooling are the consequence of factors such as the:

- volume of tissue
- composition of the tissue
- capacity of tissue to moderate the effects of cooling: largely a factor of blood supply
- rate of temperature fall
- temperature to which the tissue is lowered.

Cell activity

It is generally, but not universally, true that chemical and biological processes slow down with decreasing temperature. As most enzyme systems operate at an optimal temperature, lowering the temperature results in a slowing of activity. Cell viability is critically dependent on membrane transport systems involving active biochemical pumps and passive leaks in membranes, which maintain intracellular ionic composition. The failure of pumps at low temperatures relative to the leaks brings about a gain in Na^+ and Ca^{2+}, and a loss of K^+ from cells: that is, membranes lose their selective permeability in cold conditions.

Freezing damage to cells occurs when the local temperature drops to zero. Viscosity increases, ice crystals form and the remaining solution in the cells is reduced in volume as water leaks into the interstitial space. A characteristic feature of cold injury is the vascular damage that occurs with intravascular aggregation of platelets and red blood cells to form blockages in vessels.

Blood flow

Cooling skin causes immediate vasoconstriction, which diminishes body heat loss. Thermoreceptors

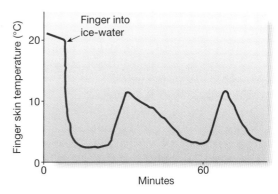

Figure 7.7 Cold vasodilatation in the finger immersed in ice-water, measured by skin temperature changes.

in the skin are stimulated and produce vasoconstriction over the body surface through an autonomic reflex. In addition, there is a direct constrictor effect of cold on the smooth muscle of arterioles and venules. Countercurrent heat exchange between blood vessels helps to reduce heat loss. This is most effective in the limbs because of the relatively long parallel pathways between the deep arteries and veins. In these ways, body core temperature is prevented from falling rapidly. Arteriovenous anastomoses that open to allow more blood flow to the skin in hot conditions are constricted in the cold.

A further effect is seen, for example, in the hand. Immersion of the hands in water at 0–12°C at first causes the expected vasoconstriction, this is followed after a delay of 5 minutes or more by a marked vasodilatation. This is then interrupted by another burst of vasoconstriction and subsequent waves of increased and decreased local blood flow. This phenomenon is known as cold-induced vasodilatation (CIVD) and demonstrates a hunting reaction of the vessels, which can be measured simply by thermocouple readings on the cooled skin (Fig. 7.7). CIVD is most likely to be due to the direct effect of low temperature causing paralysis of smooth muscle contraction in the blood vessels (Keatinge 1978). The reaction – which does not only occur in the hand – might provide protection to tissues from damage caused by prolonged cooling and relative ischaemia. There is a marked difference in the appearance of the skin erythema due to CIVD compared to that produced by skin heating. In CIVD, the skin has a brighter red colour owing to the presence of more oxyhaemo-globin and less reduced haemoglobin in blood. The reason for this is that at low temperatures there is a shift in the oxygen dissociation curve so that the blood tends to hold on to its oxygen, with oxyhaemoglobin dissociating less readily.

Muscle blood flow is not much influenced by thermal reflexes but is determined largely by local muscle metabolic rate. A striking feature of attempts at muscle cooling is the prolonged period taken to reduce intramuscular temperatures: muscles are insulated from temperature changes at the skin surface by a layer of subcutaneous tissue (Jutte et al 2001, Otte et al 2002).

Collagen

Although most studies examining stretch in collagen focus on the effects of higher temperatures (e.g. Rigby et al 1959, 1964, Warren et al 1971) with little below 25°C, it is reasonable to expect that collagen tends to become stiffer when cooled. The degree to which this happens, and at what temperatures, is not clear. Experience tells us that very cold hands can feel 'stiff' and individuals with rheumatoid arthritis often complain of an increase in stiffness as temperatures are reduced. However, whether this effect is purely the result of changes in collagen requires much more work.

Pain relief

Cold applied to the skin initially stimulates both cold and pain sensations. If the cold is sufficiently intense, both sensations are suppressed because of inhibition of nerve conduction. The reduction in pain that accompanies cooling can be due to either direct or indirect factors.

Cold can be used as a counterirritant, and it has been suggested that such responses might be explained on the basis of the pain gate theory (see Chapter 6). Effects can also be mediated through the effects of the morphine receptors in the CNS, and the role of the enkephalins and endorphins (Doubell et al 1999, Fields & Basbaum 1999). It has been demonstrated that peripheral nerve conduction is slowed by cold (Lee et al 1978), finally ceasing altogether. Fibres vary in their sensitivity according to their diameter and whether they are myelinated, and animal studies have demonstrated that the small-diameter myelinated fibres (i.e. Aδ fibres), which conduct pain, are most responsive to cold. Although it would be unwise to extrapolate all these findings wholly to humans, this combined evidence suggests that effects on nerve fibres and free nerve endings lead to a reduction in pain.

Pain can sometimes be due to particular tissue irritants. For example, a number of studies have suggested that patients with arthritis experience pain relief as a result of the adverse effects of cooling on the activity of destructive enzymes within the joints (Harris & McCroskery 1974, Pegg et al 1969).

Muscle performance

The effect of temperature on muscle performance is complex, involving the effects of cold on the contractile process, neuromuscular transmission and circulatory oxygen. Some muscle properties have a large thermal dependence (e.g. power, velocity, maximal isometric force by stimulation at high frequencies) whereas others are barely influenced by temperatures between 25 and 37°C (e.g. maximal isometric force by stimulation at low frequencies; Jones et al 2004). The time to peak and time to half relaxation of an isometric twitch increases with cooling, suggesting a slowing of contraction and relaxation. Maximum tetanic tension is relatively stable between temperatures of 25 and 35°C, which is within the normal physiological range; greater effects can be seen below 25°C. With cooling, therefore, muscle contractions tend to slow but attain a reasonably normal level of force, provided the cooling is within reasonable limits. The ability to sustain a maximal muscle contraction is also temperature dependent and is optimum at 27°C. Temperatures below this might reduce muscle performance. Factors affecting this are most likely to result from failure of the electrical properties of the muscle, although increased fluid viscosity and reduced metabolism can compound the problem.

Again, it is worth noting that the actual temperature achieved in the muscle will vary enormously according to its size, the thickness of subcutaneous insulation layers (Otte et al 2002) and external temperatures. Not all studies measure muscle temperature directly and therefore results need to be interpreted with caution.

Exercise–induced muscle damage

It has been suggested that the symptoms of muscle damage, particularly from strenuous or eccentric exercise, might be affected by cooling. However, evidence to support this is very limited. Easton and Peters (1999) examined the effect of cooling following maximal reciprocal contractions of the elbow flexors in a randomized controlled trial. Immersion at a temperature of 15°C immediately after activity and at 12-hour intervals for 3 days demonstrated that there was no difference in perception of tenderness and strength loss in the treated group, although the authors suggest that there was some indication of reduced muscle stiffness and damage.

Muscle tone

Although the underlying physiology is not totally understood, cold can reduce muscle tone. The neural effects might be due to changes in the activity of muscle spindles, Ia and secondary afferents, α motor neurons, γ fibres, neuromuscular junctions or the muscle itself (when increased twitch-contraction and half-time relaxation might result). Muscle spindles respond more rapidly than other neural and muscular structures as the reduction in temperatures required for activation are not so great. With reduced temperatures, muscle spindle sensitivity drops in proportion to the degree of cooling, possibly as a result of a direct effect on the sensory terminal, or as the firing rate of Ia afferents is decreased, or both (Eldred et al 1960, Ottoson 1965). Many muscles are well insulated, and thorough cooling appears necessary to achieve a muscle spindle response, presumably to ensure cooling of the spindles, which are embedded in the muscle structure. Miglietta (1973) and Trnavsky (1983) showed that prolonged cooling was needed to reduce clonus. This was confirmed by Price et al (1993), who demonstrated a significant reduction in spasticity at the ankle (secondary to head injury) following the application of liquid ice in a bag to the gastrocnemius muscle after thorough cooling for 20 minutes. Again, the work of Jutte et al (2001) demonstrates that it might take quite a long time (up to an hour) to produce cooling of 7°C in muscle beneath a skin-fold thickness of 30–40 mm.

The authors discussed above suggest that the effect seen is most likely to be due to effects on muscle spindles. However, it is also possible that greater degrees of cooling can affect other tissues. Effects might be the result of a slowing of conduction in both the muscle and motor nerves, a reduction in the sensitivity of the muscle spindle or impaired conduction in the γ or α efferents. However, because rapid responses are also seen on skin cooling (30 s after the application of ice) other explanations have also been sought. It is postulated that reflexes from the cold skin might inhibit the dominant excitatory stimuli that operate in the region of the anterior horn neurons of the spinal cord, causing spasticity and spasm (Lehmann & De Lateur 1990b). In addition, following an acute injury, a reduction in muscle spasm could in part be attributed to the reduction of pain.

Despite all these inhibitory effects, it is important to note that cooling can result in an immediate increase in tone for a short period. In line with other researchers, Price et al (1993) note that two patients treated with cold to reduce tone exhibited an aggravated response, and attributed this to the effects of tactile stimulation; Chiara et al (1998) reported an increase in spasticity in patients with multiple sclerosis. Lehmann and de Lateur (1999) suggest that evidence points to an initial increase in excitability of α motor neurons. An increase in tone has also been demonstrated with the use of ice massage.

Thus it is important to use an appropriate method of cooling to produce either excitation (e.g. a brief stimulus such as ice massage) or inhibition (more prolonged cooling such as with an ice pack). The response to cold might be rapid, occurring in a matter of seconds, but to obtain muscle cooling treatments must be at appropriate temperatures and adequate times (30 minutes or more).

Tissue repair

The fundamental process of tissue repair is discussed in Chapter 4. Cooling has both negative and positive effects on repair, and the key issue in clinical practice is what specific effect is required at any particular stage of healing; the practitioner must consider what physiological effects are to be obtained and how they relate to the whole process of tissue repair. Reduced blood supply, cellular and chemical activity can have detrimental effects if prolonged. Other, broader, changes are beneficial and might, however, outweigh possible negative effects. These include a reduction in bleeding, swelling and local muscle spasm, and pain relief. These indirect effects are largely addressed above under circulatory and neurological changes. Reduced swelling is attributed to the immediate, albeit short-lived, vasoconstriction of the arterioles and venules, which reduces the circulation to the area and therefore reduces the extravasation of fluid into the interstitium. This effect is enhanced by a reduction in cell metabolism and the activity of vasoactive substances, such as histamine, and a number of clinical studies support the empirical evidence for the use of ice to reduce swelling (e.g. Basur et al 1976, Hecht et al 1983). Cooling in clinical practice is often accompanied by compression, which means that it is difficult to ascribe the benefits to cooling alone.

Recent work has suggested that cold might also be beneficial during a 'secondary injury' phase when – in some more serious injuries – secondary hypoxia and enzymatic activity might cause additional damage to tissues adjacent to the original injury. Cooling slows down cellular and chemical activity, reduces oxygen release and reduced blood flow. It might be that, through these mechanisms, cooling is able to reduce destructive enzyme activity and the metabolic rate of the damaged tissue, thereby helping to preserve their integrity during this phase. Most work in this area relates to cardiac damage after infarctions, although one study by Merrick et al (1999) suggests that in an animal model using prolonged cooling (far beyond that normal in cryotherapy) there is a reduction in mitochondrial damage in muscle tissue. Further work in this area is under way.

Systemic effects

These are summarized in Box 7.2.

Generalized vasoconstriction develops over the skin surface when a cold stimulus is applied, and can produce large changes in heat transfer (e.g. 60W/m^2 transferred across the shell of the body with peripheral vasodilation; 10W/m^2 with

---

> **Box 7.2 Systemic effects of cooling**
>
> - Generalized vasoconstriction
> - Increased blood viscosity
> - Increased arterial blood pressure
> - Shivering, including preshivering
> - Voluntary activity
> - Altered (contracted) posture
> - Behavioural changes
> - Tissue injury, nerve paralysis and 'hypothermia'

---

vasoconstriction). Skin vasoconstriction and increased blood viscosity raise peripheral resistance and produce an increase in arterial blood pressure. As the skin temperature decreases, the drive to internal heat production grows. This is brought about by an involuntary increase in muscle tone (preshivering tone) that eventually develops into shivering. Voluntary movement and muscular exercise tend to inhibit shivering, mostly by helping to raise the body temperature, and reduce the central nervous drive. Behavioural responses such as adopting a contracted posture with arms and legs drawn up to the body can reduce the surface area exposed for heat loss by up to 50%.

Severe local cooling of the limbs can induce non-freezing cold injury in the extremities, and cooling for short periods below 12°C might cause sensory and motor paralysis of local nerves. Hypothermia is a condition of low core temperature, defined as a deep body temperature below 35°C (Collins 1983). It is potentially life threatening and often develops insidiously without the subject being aware of the threat. As the body temperature falls below 35°C there are increasing disturbances of brain and cardiac function. Consciousness is lost at a body temperature between 33 and 26°C, with considerable variability between individuals.

PHYSIOLOGICAL EFFECTS OF HEAT

Local effects

Once energy is absorbed, it is immaterial as to how the heat was delivered. There are no *different* heats, only different means of generating the same heat.

The different effects of heating are the consequence of such factors as the:

- volume of tissue absorbing the energy
- composition of the absorbing tissue
- capacity of the tissue to dissipate heat, which is largely a factor of blood supply
- rate of temperature rise
- temperature to which the tissue is raised.

Cell activity

Chemical reactions involved in metabolic activity are increased by a rise in temperature (Van't Hoff's law). Metabolic rate increases by about 13% for each 1°C rise in tissue temperature, with a corresponding increase in tissue demands for oxygen and nutrients and an enhanced output of metabolic waste products.

An increase in temperature can produce useful effects, as it speeds up or increases most cell activity. However, this is not always the case, as there comes a point when the increase is too great. For example, enzyme systems are heat sensitive and increasingly destroyed by raising the temperature beyond a threshold value. Rising tissue temperature first produces an increase in enzyme activity to a peak value, followed by a decline, and then finally abolition of activity. As an example, an increase in temperature to 36°C brings about an increase in the destructive enzyme collagenase (active in rheumatoid arthritis) when compared with that at 30°C in tissue experiments (Harris & McCroskery 1974). Clinically, it has been demonstrated that normal knee joints have a temperature of 30.5–33°C, whereas joints with active synovitis have temperatures between 34 and 37.6°C. Raising the joint temperature to, say, 40–45°C, might inactive the destructive collagenase; the problem is, of course, that in vivo other enzyme systems with similar or lower thresholds may also be destroyed. Similarly, heat might increase problems associated with secondary hypoxic damage to tissue surrounding wounds as it increased cell metabolism and enzyme activity.

It has been found that 'heat-shock proteins' accumulate in cells and tissues exposed to high temperatures, the function of which is thought to be to confer a degree of protection to cells upon subsequent heat exposure. Infrared radiation has been shown to cause an alteration in the amino acid composition of proteins which develop thermal tolerance (Westerhof et al 1987). This effect is overcome by allowing between 36 and 72 hours to elapse between applications.

At temperatures of about 45°C, so much protein damage occurs that there is destruction of cells and tissues. At this temperature, skin burns also occur if contact is maintained for long enough. Cell membranes are particularly sensitive: the lipoprotein structure of membranes may become more fluid with increasing temperature and cause a breakdown in permeability (Bowler 1987). Whereas normal cells are unaffected by mild heating, the effects of temperatures of around 40°C on cancer cells can include the inhibition of the synthesis of ribonucleic acid (RNA), deoxyribonucleic acid (DNA) and proteins (Westerhof et al 1987). This can cause irreversible structural damage to cell membranes and the disruption of organelles.

Blood flow

Heat can induce changes both in the superficial and deep tissues. When the skin is heated, the surface reddens (erythema) and blood vessels become vasodilated leading to increased blood flow. Vasodilatation may be due to: (1) a direct effect on the smooth muscle of arterioles and venules; (2) a local axon reflex; and (3) increased levels of certain metabolites in the blood. If local tissue damage occurs, further dilatation may be produced by histamine-like mediators, such as bradykinin. Increased skin blood flow occurs in areas remote from the heated tissue owing to long spinal nervous reflexes (Kerslake & Cooper 1950). There is a complex response in deeper tissues, involving a balance between vasodilatation due directly to heating and increased blood flow due to increased metabolic activity (e.g. in skeletal muscle) on the one hand and a reduced blood flow because of a relative vasoconstriction brought about by thermoregulation as blood is directed towards the surface to enable heat loss, on the other. In addition, heat exchange occurs between arterial and venous vessels, with heat flow from the arterial to the cooler venous blood. Vasodilation of the large superficial veins can have considerable effects of heat loss, as can the opening of the arteriovenous anastomoses deep below the skin capillaries.

Slight differences in circulatory changes occur with superficial (e.g. infrared irradiation or contact methods) and deep methods of heating (e.g. short-wave diathermy), although only due to depth of penetration. Infrared radiation has been shown to cause an increase in blood flow in the cutaneous circulation (Crockford & Hellon 1959, Millard 1961, Wyper & McNiven 1976), whereas microwave and short-wave diathermy (Chapter 10) penetrate further and affect deeper structures. Local heat in the early stages of injury should be avoided. Some increased blood flow and the presence of chemical mediators such as bradykinin and histamine, which are associated with heating, can affect capillary and postcapillary venule permeability. This, together with the increase in capillary hydrostatic pressure, may result in oedema. Clinical and laboratory research has demonstrated an increase in oedema together with a prolonged healing time in acute injuries treated with heat (e.g. Feibel & Fast 1976, Wallace et al 1979).

Collagen

The properties of collagen change with heat. Thus the properties of tendon, ligaments and, to some degree, muscle can be altered. Early work examined the behaviour of animal collagen tissue under passive stretch with and without heat. Gersten (1955) initially showed an increase in the extensibility of frog Achilles' tendons following heating with ultrasound. In a series of key studies, Rigby and colleagues (1959, 1964) showed that the viscoelastic properties of tendon are temperature dependent between 37 and 40°C, with an increase in the stress–relaxation relationship. Changes were reversible with loads of less than 4% and at temperatures below 40°C, and it was shown that repeated stress could be applied at temperatures of below 37°C with no change in stress–strain curves. Lehmann et al (1970) and Warren et al (1971, 1976), using rat-tail collagen heated in a water bath to temperatures between 41 and 45°C, showed reduced tensile strength, residual elongation followed the application of force at temperatures of 45°C, and the need for lower forces to produce rupture (30–50% of normal). A temperature of 39°C relates to the transition phase of collagen. All this suggests that normal body temperatures could allow collagen to perform optimally, although when permanent elongation is required, such as to mobilize a stiff joint, a raised temperature of over 39°C is needed.

Owing to the large number of confounding factors that can affect results, few studies have examined the effect of heat on stretch of collagenous tissues such as ligaments and tendons in people/patients. Recent work by Draper and colleagues has examined the effect of heating collagenous tissue to a known temperature of around 40°C prior to specific stretch. Using normal college students (aged between 30 and 43 years) over three studies and applying deep heat with shortwave diathermy, they obtained conflicting results (Draper et al 2002, 2004a, Evans et al 2002). Small numbers and differing protocols may have contributed to the variability; however, there is some indication that adequate heating does facilitate stretch. This view is supported by a number of case studies with patients, heating with both diathermy and ultrasound, which obtained good results (Draper et al 2004b, Oates & Draper 2006). These studies need to be replicated with larger numbers, in clinical settings, and by other researchers.

Muscle tone

It is evident from practice that increased muscle tone can sometimes be relieved by heat, and some research supports this view. Lehmann and de Lateur (1990a), for example, describe work that shows that heating to temperatures of between 40 and 45°C results in a reduction of spasm. Although the physiological basis for this is still unclear, a number of possibilities have been investigated.

The responses of muscle spindles, secondary afferents and Golgi tendon organs to heating have all been investigated. The Ia afferents of muscle spindles have been shown to increase their firing rate with a moderate rise in temperature (Mense 1978), whereas most (although not quite all) secondary afferents demonstrate decreased firing with temperature increases (Lehmann & de Lateur 1999). In addition, there is increased firing from Golgi tendon organs, resulting in increased inhibition. These factors are likely to reduce tone, assuming that secondary muscle spasm is largely a tonic phenomenon. There is also some evidence that heating of the skin results in reduced tension, probably due to γ fibre activity affecting the muscle spindles (Fischer & Solomon 1965). Thus superficial heating, such as hot packs and infrared, can reduce tone as well as the deeper-penetrating modalities.

Increased tone associated with upper motor neuron lesions can be reduced to some degree by heating. These effects tend to be short term, however, and the use of cold may be a more effective method of treatment as the temperature of muscle returns to normal less rapidly following cooling than following heating.

Pain relief

Heat is often used to relieve pain. Various mechanisms may be responsible. Pain may be relieved by reducing secondary muscle spasm (see above) and increasing circulation to ischaemic muscle. Heat has also been claimed to act as a 'counterirritant'. Changes in nerve conduction velocity may also be a factor. Kramer (1984) used infrared as a control when evaluating the heating effect of ultrasound in nerve conduction tests on normal subjects. Both were applied separately to the ulnar nerve in dosages that increased temperature by 0.8°C; an increase in ulnar nerve conduction velocity was found in both cases. Studies by Halle et al (1981) and Currier and Kramer (1982), again on human subjects, supported this work, suggesting possible implications with respect to motor and sensory conduction.

Muscle performance

Few studies have looked at the effect of an increase in temperature on muscle in situ beyond that in normal physiological ranges, and certainly not much beyond 40°C, as above this tissue damage occurs rapidly. The principles governing temperature changes are discussed in previous sections relative to the effects of cold. However, a number of studies have indicated some points for consideration. Strength and endurance might be affected by an increase in temperature. Following immersion of the lower limbs in a water bath at 44°C for 45 minutes (actual temperature of muscle not known), Edwards et al (1970) demonstrated a reduction in the ability of subjects to sustain an isometric contraction. Similarly, an immediate reduction in the strength of the quadriceps muscle following the application of heat through the use of shortwave diathermy has also been demonstrated (Chastain 1978). In this study, a temperature of 42.4°C at a depth of 3.22 cm was reported. However, Chastain (1978) also noted that over the ensuing 2 hours the muscle strength increased and remained above pretreatment levels. These findings are important for clinical practice and should be considered both when making objective measurements of muscle strength in order to evaluate treatment efficacy and when implementing exercise programmes.

Tissue healing

Although it is important to remember that heating can be detrimental to tissue repair in the early stages because it can increase bleeding, oedema, chemical activity and associated pain, in mild doses it has a number of beneficial effects in the later stages, possibly being of greatest use for chronic injuries with delayed repair.

Positive changes can arise from an increase in the chemical reaction rates. An increase in oxygen uptake is associated with a muscle temperature of about 38.6°C (Abramson et al 1958). The right-sided shift of the oxygen dissociation curve that occurs with an increase in temperature means that oxygen is more readily available for tissue repair. Haemoglobin releases twice as much oxygen at 41°C than at 36°C, and releases it twice as quickly (Barcroft & King 1909). An increase in blood flow means that there are likely to be a greater number of white cells and more nutrients available for the healing process. Heat has secondary pain-relieving effects as the vasodilation accelerates the removal of pain-inducing metabolites or inflammatory products and so reduces congestion. There is conflicting evidence arising from animal studies regarding the efficacy of heating in the management of haematomas. Fenn (1969) and Lehmann et al (1983) in controlled studies showed a greater resolution of artificially induced haematomas in rabbits (shortwave diathermy) and pigs (915 MHz microwaves) with heating. In contrast, a randomized, controlled study by Brown and Baker (1987) treated experimental haematomas in rabbits with pulsed shortwave diathermy (PSWD) and found no difference.

Systemic effects

These are summarized in Box 7.3.

Local heating causes a rise in temperature of tissues and reflex vasodilatation in remote areas of the body and, if heating is extensive and prolonged, a general rise in core temperature can ensue. The immediate systemic response is a generalized skin vasodilatation, which serves to transport heat by conduction and convection from the core to the shell. There is a concomitant reduction in splanchnic blood flow resulting in reduced hepatic clearance rate and reduction in urine flow.

Box 7.3 Systemic effects of heat

- Reflex vasodilation remote to site of heating
- Increase in core temperature
- Reduced renal function
- Sweating
- Heat illness:
  - swelling of feet and ankles
  - prickly heat
  - water deficiency
  - salt loss: below 25°C greater effects can be seen
- Heat stroke and death

If the heat stress is great, the skin temperature rises and approaches 35°C over the whole of the body. At or near this point, the body temperature becomes stabilized by the stimulation of sweat glands, which secrete hypotonic sweat on to the body surface so that increased evaporative cooling can take place. High radiant temperatures can be tolerated for many minutes if the environment is dry (as in a sauna). An increase in ambient humidity makes these conditions immediately unbearable as it reduces the possibility of evaporation of sweat (which simply runs off the body).

Heat illness may occur with sudden increases in heat stress, most readily in those who are not adapted (acclimatized) to heat. Generalized skin vasodilatation may cause swelling of the feet and ankles (heat oedema) or syncope during postural change or prolonged standing. Prickly heat, a papulovesicular rash accompanied by a dermal prickling sensation when sweating is provoked, occurs in some people when areas of the skin are continuously wetted by sweat. More serious heat illnesses, such as heat exhaustion from water deficiency or salt deficiency, are due to imbalance of body water and salt, respectively, with excessive sweating, and lead to collapse. Left untreated, they may result in potentially fatal heat stroke when the core temperature reaches high levels of 41°C and above and the central heat-regulatory mechanisms fail (Khogali & Hales 1983).

References

Abramson DI, Kahn A, Tuck S et al (1958) Relationship between a range of tissue temperature and local oxygen uptake in the human forearm. I: changes observed under resting conditions. *J Clin Invest* **37**: 1031–1038.

Barcroft J, King W (1909) The effect of temperature on the dissociation curve of blood. *J Physiol* **39**: 374–384.

Basur R, Shephard E, Mouzos G (1976) A cooling method in the treatment of ankle sprains. *Practitioner* **216**: 708.

Bowler K (1987) Cellular heat injury: are membranes involved? In Bowler K, Fuller BJ (eds) *Temperature and Animal Cells*. Cambridge, Company of Biologists: 157–185.

Brown M, Baker RD (1987) Effects of pulsed shortwave diathermy on skeletal muscle injury in rabbits. *Phys Ther* **67**: 208–214.

Chastain PB (1978) The effect of deep heat on isometric strength. *Phys Ther* **58**: 543.

Chiara T, Carlos J, Martin D et al (1998) Cold effect of oxygen uptake, perceived exertion and spasticity in patients with MS. *Arch Phys Med Rehab* **79**: 523–528.

Collins KJ (1983) *Hypothermia the Facts*. Oxford, Oxford University Press.

Collins KJ (1992) Regulation of body temperature. In Tinker J, Zapol WM (eds) *Care of the Critically Ill Patient*, 2nd edn. London, Springer-Verlag: 155–173.

Crockford GW, Hellon RF (1959) Vascular responses of human skin to infra-red radiation. *J Physiol* **149**: 424–432.

Currier DP, Kramer JF (1982) Sensory nerve conduction: heating effects of ultrasound and infrared. *Physiothe–Canada* **34**: 241–246.

Doubell P, Mannon J, Woolf CJ (1999) The dorsal horn: state dependent sensory processing, plasticity and the generation of pain. In Wall PD, Melzack R (eds) *Textbook of Pain*, 4th edn. New York, Churchill Livingstone: 165–182.

Draper DO, Miner L, Knight KL, Ricard MD (2002) The carry over effect of diathermy and stretching in developing hamstring flexibility. *J Athletic Training* **37**: 37–42.

Draper DO, Castro JL, Feland B et al (2004a) Shortwave diathermy and prolonged stretching increase hamstring flexibility more than prolonged stretching alone. *J Orthop Sports Phys Ther* **34**: 13–20.

Draper DO, Castel JC, Castel D (2004b) Low watt pulsed shortwave diathermy and metal plate fixation of the elbow. *Athletic Ther Today* **September**: 28–32.

Easton R, Peters D (1999) Effect of cold water immersion on the symptoms of exercise induced muscle damage. *J Sports Sci* **17**: 231–238.

Edwards R, Harris R, Hultman E et al (1970) Energy metabolism during isometric exercise at different temperatures of m. quadriceps femoris in man. *Acta Physiol Scand* **80**: 17–18.

Eldred E, Lindsey DF, Buchwald JS (1960) The effects of cooling on the mammalian muscle spindle. *Exp Neurol* **2**: 144–157.

Evans RK, Knight KL, Draper DO et al (2002) Effects of warm-up before eccentric exercise on indirect markers of muscle damage. *Med Sci Sport Exer*, http://www.acsm-msse.org.

Feibel H, Fast H (1976) Deep heating of joints: A reconsideration. *Arch Phys Med Rehab* **57**: 513–514.

Fenn JE (1969) Effect of pulsed electromagnetic energy (Diapulse) on experimental haematomas. *Can Med Assoc J* **100**: 251.

Fields HL, Basbaum AI (1999) Central nervous system mechanisms of pain. In Wall PD, Melzack R (eds) *Textbook of Pain*, 4th edn. New York, Churchill Livingstone: 309–330.

Fischer E, Solomon S (1965) Physiological responses to heat and cold. In Licht S (ed) *Therapeutic Heat and Cold*, 2nd edn. New Haven, CT, E Licht: 126–169.

Gersten JW (1955) Effect of ultrasound on tendon extensibility. *Am J Phys Med* **34**: 362–369.

Halle JS, Scoville CR, Greathouse DG (1981) Ultrasound's effect on the conduction latency of the superficial radial nerve in man. *Phys Ther* **61**: 345–350.

Harris ED Jr, McCroskery PA (1974) The influence of temperature and fibril stability on degradation of cartilage collagen by rheumatoid synovial collagenase. *N Engl J Med* **290**: 1–6.

Hecht PJ, Backmann S, Booth RE, Rothman RH (1983) Effects of thermal therapy on rehabilitation after total knee arthroplasty: a prospective randomized study. *Clin Orthop Rel Res* **178**: 198–201.

Hensel H (1981) *Thermoreception and Temperature Regulation*. Monographs of the Physiological Society no. 38. London, Academic Press.

International Union of Physiological Sciences (1987) Commission for Thermal Physiology. A glossary of terms for thermal physiology. *Pflugers Arch* **410**: 567–587.

Jones D, Round, J, de Haan A (2004) *Skeletal Muscle from Molecules to Movement*. London, Churchill Livingstone.

Jutte LS, Merrick MA, Ingersoll CD, Edwards JE (2001) The relationship between intramuscular temperature, skin temperature and adipose thickness during cryotherapy and rewarming. *Arch Phys Med Rehab* **82**: 845–850.

Keatinge WR (1978) *Survival in Cold Water*. Oxford, Blackwell: 39–50.

Keatinge WR, Sloane REG (1975) Deep body temperatures from aural canal with servo-controlled heating to outer ear. *J Appl Physiol* **38**: 919–921.

Kerslake D McK, Cooper KE (1950) Vasodilatation in the hand in response to heating the skin elsewhere. *Clin Sci* **9**: 31–47.

Khogali M, Hales JRS (1983) *Heat Stroke and Temperature Regulation*. London, Academic Press.

Kramer JF (1984) Ultrasound: evaluation of its mechanical and thermal effects. *Arch Phys Med Rehab* **65**: 223–227.

Lee JM, Warren MP, Mason SM (1978) The effects of ice on nerve conduction velocity. *Physiotherapy* **64**: 2–6.

Lehmann JF, De Lateur BJ (1990a) Therapeutic heat. In Lehmann, JF (ed) *Therapeutic Heat and Cold*, 4th edn. Baltimore, MD, Williams & Wilkins: 444.

Lehmann JF, De Lateur BJ (1990b) Cryotherapy. In Lehmann, JF (ed) *Therapeutic Heat and Cold*, 4th edn. Baltimore, MD, Williams & Wilkins: 590–632.

Lehmann JF, de Lateur B (1999) Ultrasound, shortwave, microwave, laser, superficial heat and cold in the treatment of pain. In Wall PD, Melzack R (eds) *Textbook of Pain*, 4th edn. New York, Churchill Livingstone: 1383–1397.

Lehmann JF, Masock AJ, Warren CG, Koblanski JN (1970) Effects of therapeutic temperatures on tendon extensibility. *Arch Phys Med Rehab* **51**: 481–487.

Lehmann JF, Dundore DE, Esselman PC et al (1983) Microwave diathermy: effects on experimental muscle haematoma resolution. *Arch Phys Med Rehab* **64**: 127–129.

Marieb EN (2002) *Essentials of Human Anatomy & Physiology*, 7th edn. Reading, Benjamin Cummings.

Mense S (1978) Effects of temperature on the discharges of motor spindles and tendon organs. *Pflugers Arch* **374**: 159–166.

Merrick M, Rankin J, Andres F, Hinman C (1999) A preliminary examination of cryotherapy and secondary injury in skeletal muscle. *Med Sci Sports Exerc* **31**: 1516–1521.

Miglietta O (1973) Action of cold on spasticity. *Am J Phys Med* **52**: 198–205.

Millard JB (1961) Effects of high frequency currents and infrared rays on the circulation of the lower limb in man. *Ann Phys Med* **6**: 45–65.

Moore-Ede MC, Sulzman FM (1981) Internal temporal order. In Aschoff, J (ed) *Handbook of Behavior Neurobiology*. New York, Plenum Press: 215–241.

Oates D, Draper DO (2006) Restoring wrist range of motion using ultrasound and mobilization: a case study. *Athletic Ther Now* **January**: 57–59.

Otte JW, Merrick MA, Ingersoll CD, Cordova ML (2002) Subcutaneous adipose tissue thickness alters cooling time during cryotherapy. *Arch Phys Med Rehab* **83**: 1501–1505.

Ottoson D (1965) The effects of temperature on the isolated muscle spindle. *J Physiol* **180**: 636–648.

Pegg SMH, Littler TR, Littler EN (1969) A trial of ice therapy and exercise in chronic arthritis. *Physiotherapy* **55**: 51–56.

Price R, Lehmann JF, Boswell-Bessette S et al (1993) Influence of cryotherapy on spasticity at the human ankle. *Arch Phys Med Rehab* **74**: 300–304.

Rigby BJ (1964) The effect of mechanical extension upon the thermal stability of collagen. *Biochem Biophys Acta* **79**: 634–636.

Rigby BJ, Hirai N and Spikes JD (1959) The mechanical behaviour of rat tail tendon. *J Gen Physiol* **43**: 265–283.

Trnavsky G (1983) Die Beeinflussing des Hoffman-Reflexes durch Kryoangzeittherapie. *Wiener Medizinische Wochenschrift* **11**: 287–289.

Wallace L, Knortz K, Esterton P (1979) Immediate care of ankle injuries. *J Orthop Sports Phys Ther* **1**: 46.

Warren CG, Lehmann JF, Koblanski JN (1971) Elongation of rat tail tendon: effect of load and temperature. *Arch Phys Med Rehab* **52**: 465–475.

Warren CG, Lehmann JF, Koblanski JN (1976) Heat and stretch procedures: an evaluation using rat tail tendon. *Arch Phys Med Rehab* **57**: 122–126.

Westerhof W, Siddiqui AH, Cormane RH, Scholten A (1987) Infrared hyperthermia and psoriasis. *Arch Dermatol Res* **279**: 209–210.

Wyper DJ, McNiven DR (1976) Effects of some physiotherapeutic agents on skeletal muscle blood flow. *Physiotherapy* **62**: 83–85.

Chapter 8

Low-energy treatments: non-thermal or microthermal?

Sheila Kitchen and Mary Dyson

INTRODUCTION

The body is a complex mechanism, and the ways in which the various electrophysical agents discussed in this book interact with it are still being investigated. In particular, the relationship between the thermal and so-called 'non-thermal' effects that can arise is still a matter of debate.

The thermal changes that can occur following the use of hot packs, infrared irradiation, ultrasound and shortwave diathermy and other agents are outlined in Chapter 7. Although these effects are significant, heating is not the only way in which physiological changes can be brought about in body tissues by electrophysical agents. Other effects include the use of low-frequency currents to produce stimulation of muscle or nervous tissue, whereas wound repair can be stimulated by electromagnetic fields and currents. Finally, certain high-frequency agents, such as ultrasound, pulsed shortwave diathermy and light, are used by practitioners in very low and/or pulsed doses to facilitate tissue repair and reduce pain.

The term 'non-thermal' is frequently used in clinical practice to mean a treatment that does not result in the patient being conscious of any warming. It must be remembered, however, that all forms of energy can degrade ultimately into heat energy, although the level may be extremely low. Although there is clear evidence of the non-thermal effects of agents such as ultraviolet irradiation, visible light, X-rays and gamma rays, there is currently much controversy surrounding the possible existence of such effects from the use of low-intensity, non-ionizing radiations and mechanical waves in physiotherapy practice and further a field. The press and academic literature continues to report research about the possible effects on people of many devices that we encounter regularly, such as power cables, mobile telephones (e.g. effects on brain tissue; Ferrerri et al 2006), transmission masts and televisions.

Arguments for and against the existence of these effects arose early in clinical practice (e.g. with ultrasound and pulsed shortwave diathermy) and controversies have continued. For example, in 1990 Frizzell and Dunn believed there to be no evidence of biological effects arising with the use of low-energy ultrasound. By contrast, Mortimer and Dyson (1988) reported changes in the permeability of the cell membrane to calcium ions, while Dyson et al (1974) noted the temporary banding at half wavelength intervals of blood cells and endothelial cell damage within blood vessels exposed to ultrasound in a stationary wave field in vivo.

Similarly, Barker and Freestone (1985) and Barker (1993) had reservations with respect to pulsed shortwave diathermy, and many people have doubted the benefits of therapeutic laser. Although for many years the American Food and Drug Administration (FDA) was unconvinced of the clinical efficacy of low-level laser therapy (LLLT), this has now changed due to an increase in scientifically valid clinical trials. In 2002 the FDA granted approval for some LLLT devices to be marketed for specific indications, such as 'adjunctive use in providing temporary relief of minor chronic neck and shoulder pain of musculoskeletal origin' and for 'adjuncted use in the temporary relief of hand and wrist pain associated with carpal tunnel syndrome' (Swedish Laser Medical Society 2004).

A variety of suggestions has been made about the underlying ways in which predominantly non-thermal effects may occur. Many of those postulated are based on the suggestion that electrophysical agents can influence the mechanisms that lead to cell communication. Tsong (1989) suggested that cells communicate both *directly* through chemical means and *indirectly* through the influence of electrical, physical and acoustic signals, and it seems that electrophysical agents may produce physiological changes through these mechanisms.

Work in this area has gained momentum recently, particularly as knowledge of growth factors and their role in tissue repair and function increases, as research workers have examined the possible effects derived from using electromagnetic fields to stimulate cell activity. Recent work, using a variety of field parameters, has examined changes in growth-factor production, signalling pathways (e.g. Ca^{2+} mediated), cell growth and survival, cell cycle distribution, cyclic AMP content and gap-junction-mediated communication between cells (e.g. George et al 2002, Schimmelpfeng et al 2005, Takashima et al 2006).

For any agent to be effective it must be active through one of more sites, or components, of tissues. It is generally considered that these sites are intracellular, although energy transduction within extracellular molecules such as collagen might also be involved and lead to the activation of these intracellular sites, here termed interactive targets.

INTERACTIVE TARGETS

'Interactive targets' are cellular components that may be receptive to interventions. These interactive targets include the plasma membrane of the cell, also termed the cell membrane, and intracellular structures such as the intracellular membranes, microtubules, mitochondria, chromophores, cell-associated ions and the nucleus.

PLASMA MEMBRANE

The cell was described in terms of its electrical structure and function in Chapter 3, and it will be recalled that the plasma membrane consists of a bilayered, phospholipid structure which surrounds the cell and is studded with transmembranous proteins (Alberts et al 1994). These proteins have a number of functions: they strengthen the membrane; they transport substances such as proteins, sugars, fats and ions across the membrane; and they form specialist receptor sites for hormones, neurotransmitters and enzymes. In addition, the plasma membrane is electrically charged, possessing a negative charge on its internal surface and a positive charge on its external surface. The resulting potential difference of approximately 70 mV is maintained through the passive and active movement of ions across the cell membrane.

A number of electrophysical agents are thought to effect changes at the level of the plasma membrane. For example, Adey (1988) postulated the transduction of a pulsed magnetic field (PMF) signal across the cell membrane and regarded this structure as the primary site of interaction between the oscillating electrical field and the cellular components of the tissue. Adey suggested that a large amplification of an initial weak trigger can occur as the result of the binding of hormones, antibodies and neurotransmitters to their specific binding sites on the cell membrane owing to the effects of magnetic fields.

Other workers, such as Tsong (1989), Westerhoff et al (1986) and Astumian et al (1987), have postulated that proteins can undergo conformational changes as a result of interaction with an oscillating electrical field. For this to occur with any degree of efficiency, the frequency of the field must match the kinetic characteristics of the reaction and be at an optimum field strength (Tsong 1989). This reaction can result in pumping effects, with substances being actively transported across the cell membrane, leading to subsequent ATP synthesis. Although none of these researchers has specifically examined the effects of agents used in clinical practice, it might be that pulsed shortwave diathermy acts upon cells in one or more of these ways.

Mechanical energy might also effect changes in cell membrane behaviour; such changes have been shown to occur when therapeutic levels of ultrasound are applied to cells in vitro. Hill and ter Haar (1989) state that acoustic cavitation results in sound energy being converted into other forms of energy, including shear energy. The sound energy induces the oscillation of minute bubbles within the tissues, which in turn induce microstreaming of liquids both around the bubbles themselves and around the cell walls (further details are provided in Chapter 12). Some writers, such as Repacholi (1970) and Repacholi et al (1971), suggest that microstreaming may alter membrane permeability and secondary messenger activity and be responsible for changes in the surface charge of cells, resulting in the transduction of signals. This view has been reinforced by

both Dyson (1985) and Young (1988), who have suggested that microstreaming (at therapeutic doses) may influence cell function by reversibly affecting the permeability of the plasma membrane and modifying the local environment through mechanisms such as altered cell metabolite gradients. Mortimer and Dyson (1988) have demonstrated that therapeutic levels of ultrasound can induce permeability changes to calcium ions, and that this is associated with cavitation.

Finally, writers such as Smith (1991a, b) have suggested that infrared, low-level laser radiation may initiate reactions at the cell membrane level, possibly through photophysical effects on Ca^{2+} channels. This suggestion has been supported by the work of other groups. In 1997, Lubart et al reported changes in calcium transport in plasma membranes caused by 780 nm irradiation. In 2004, Kujawa et al (2004) reported that low-intensity (3.75–25 J/cm^2) near-infrared (810 nm) laser irradiation of erythrocytes induces long-term conformational plasma membrane transitions related to changes in the structural states of both membrane proteins and the lipid membrane; these resulted in changes in the activity of membrane ion pumps and, therefore, in plasma membrane permeability to ions. It has been proposed that optimization of the structure and function of the erythrocyte plasma membrane may be the basis for improvement of cardiac function in patients undergoing laser therapy (Kujawa et al 2004). Some of the cellular effects of LLLT can be mediated by nitric oxide (NO; Karu et al 2005); in erythrocytes this may be released by LLLT from NO-haemoglobin (Vladimirov et al 2000).

INTRACELLULAR MEMBRANES

Intracellular membranes surround the internal organelles of the cell and exhibit similar electrical characteristics to cell membranes. One of their functions is to exercise control over the movement of substances into and out of these structures (Alberts et al 1994, Frohlich 1988) and thereby control the behaviour and actions of the organelles and ultimately of the entire cell. Similar effects to those induced at the cell surface may occur across these membranes, resulting in changes in activity of the organelles.

MICROTUBULES

Microtubules are elongated cylinders made of protein that are present within cells. Electrically, they consist of dimers, which are charged dipole units, their internal ends being negatively charged relative to the periphery. This arrangement results in the cell having similar electrical properties to electrets, which are insulators carrying a permanent charge analogous to permanent magnets. These properties include the ability to exhibit piezoelectric and electropiezo effects and, in addition, such dipole units rotate under the influence of oscillating fields. However, they do not respond equally to all frequencies of energy, but instead have preferred resonant frequencies, which are governed by their moment of rotation (Frohlich 1988).

Such dipole units may respond to the alternating magnetic and electrical fields produced by shortwave diathermy equipment. In general, it seems likely that such motion will give rise to *microthermal* changes, and Muller (1983) has suggested that an oscillation in temperature might allow a biological system to absorb free energy. Westerhoff et al (1986) note that an electrical field is a 'thermodynamic quantity' and suggest that it may be the oscillation in this parameter that results in changes in the cyclical enzymatic activity of cells.

MITOCHONDRIA

It has been suggested that mitochondria may be stimulated directly by the application of electrophysical energy, and a number of researchers have suggested that laser radiation at certain wavelengths may initiate changes at this site in the cell. Karu (1988) has postulated the following sequence of events: certain wavelengths of red light, when absorbed by components of the respiratory chain within the mitochondria, cause a brief activation of that chain; oxidation of the nicotinamide adenine dinucleotide (NAD) pool occurs, leading to changes in the redox status of the mitochondria and cytoplasm; these changes lead to altered membrane permeability, and consequently to changes in the transport of ions across the cell wall. For example, changes in the $Na^+:H^+$ ratio across the membrane occur, and there are subsequent increases in Na^+/K^+-ATPase activity. The

calcium flux is consequently altered, resulting in modulation of DNA and RNA synthesis and changes in cell growth and proliferation. Smith (1991) has suggested that other wavelengths (e.g. infrared radiation) not absorbed by mitochondrial cytochromes may be absorbed by cytochromic components of the cell membrane, producing direct changes in calcium flux at this site. More recently Kujawa et al (2004) have shown that in human red blood cells, which do not contain mitochondria, and in isolated cell membranes, near-infrared (810 nm) LLLT induced structural changes in the membranes.

IONS

Ions are electrically charged particles that are present in both intracellular and extracellular fluids. Being electrically charged, they respond to oscillating electrical fields and ionic vibration is likely to occur (Frohlich 1988). Such movement again may lead to changes in ionic distribution within the cells, affecting the cells' activity.

NUCLEUS

The interaction of electromagnetic fields with the nucleus of the cell has been reviewed by Nicolini (1985) and Frohlich (1988), who note that relatively little is known about these effects. Hiskenkamp et al (1978) and Takahashi et al (1986) are among those who believe that direct effects on the nucleus may occur, and they have suggested that pulsed magnetic fields may influence DNA synthesis and transcription. Adey (1988), however, postulates that any changes that have been noted are more likely to be the result of the presence of secondary messengers such as cAMP and calcium ions, which may exert such an influence at the membrane level.

CHROMOPHORES

Chromophores are molecules that absorb specific wavelengths of electromagnetic radiation. They include melanin, nucleic acids and proteins, and are therefore distributed widely in the tissues and cells of the body. Ultraviolet radiation, visible light and infrared radiation may all be absorbed by these structures. When energy is absorbed by chromophores, an atom of the molecule affected becomes temporarily excited, resulting in the movement of an electron to a higher energy level. It subsequently degrades, releasing energy which may be passed on to other molecules, be used to effect a variety of biochemical changes or degrade into heat.

CELLS

If free to move and subjected to ultrasonically induced standing waves, entire cells can be transported in a predominantly non-thermal fashion to pressure nodes spaced at half-wavelength intervals (Dyson et al 1974). Although this is generally a reversible phenomenon, it can be irreversibly damaging to the endothelial cells lining blood vessels in which the blood corpuscles have been caused to band and should therefore be avoided, for example, by moving the transducer slowly during treatment so that the position of the pressure nodes and energy peaks change.

THE EFFECT OF DOSAGE

Although it has been suggested that many forms of energy (including electrical, mechanical and chemical) may initiate changes in cell behaviour, it is becoming increasingly clear that the dosage parameters of the energy imparted to the cell are likely to affect the end result. For example, Frohlich (1988) has suggested that ion oscillation and dipole rotation are dependent upon the frequency and amplitude of the electrical field in question. In addition, enzyme activity depends on the availability of specific charge sites on membrane surfaces, which, Frohlich (1988) suggests, may be unlocked by the application of electrical signals of an 'appropriate type'. Tsong (1989) states that 'in principle, each class of protein is adapted to respond to an oscillating force field (electrical, sonic or chemical potential) of a defined frequency and strength'. Smith (1991a, b) has suggested that laser radiations of different wavelengths may affect different structures; he postulates that radiation at 633 nm may initiate activity at the mitochondrial level, as suggested by Karu (1987), whereas at 904 nm it may initiate reactions at the cell membrane

level, possibly through photophysical effects on calcium channels. In addition, it is known that ultraviolet irradiation at certain frequencies is more likely to produce erythematous changes ('sunburn') and carcinogenic changes than others. Recently, Takashima et al (2006) demonstrated the importance of dosage. They exposed cells to radiofrequency electromagnetic fields (2.45 GHz) ranging from 0.05 to 1500 W/kg. Results varied from suppression of activity (continuous, 200 W/kg), no effect (continuous application, 0.05–100 W/kg; intermittent application, 300, 900, 1500 W/kg_{pk} (100 W/kg_{mean}) and an effect (continuous application, 50 W/kg for 2 hours). This final effect appeared to occur as a result of thermal changes. George et al (2002) specify that they selected their intervention based on 'the mitogenic (i.e. cell-cycle-stimulating) properties of a specific spatial–temporal conformation of low level, confined, high-frequency electromagnetic filed'. Li et al (1999) highlight the dose- and time-dependent nature of the effects seen in fibroblasts with the application of electromagnetic energy.

There is still relatively little information about the precise dosage parameters of many of these agents which are most likely to achieve therapeutic effects in clinical practice. The Arndt–Schultz law applies with ultrasound and light, too little energy having no measurable effect, too much being damaging, while energy levels between these extremes can be therapeutic. Although there is some evidence that low intensities are adequate to stimulate cell activity in vitro, more work is needed to establish the most effective wave bands and pulsing frequencies and to confirm this in clinical practice. It should, however, be noted that many therapeutic forms of energy act as stimuli at the cellular level, whether in vitro or in vivo. The cells transduce these stimuli and amplify them, so the energetic output of the cells far exceeds the energetic input, an extremely efficient mode of activity which would not occur should the changes be of a purely thermal nature.

CONCLUSION

This overview has highlighted the many theories that are currently being explored with respect to the ways in which the electrotherapy agents used by physiotherapists may effect therapeutically significant changes in cell behaviour. As this discussion has shown, it is possible that a number of similarities exist between the mechanisms whereby physiological changes are induced by the use of agents such as low-level ultrasound, pulsed non-thermal levels of shortwave diathermy and low-level laser radiation. However, concrete evidence both of the mechanisms of interaction and of the physiological effects that occur in living, injured tissue is limited, a fact that should be borne in mind as the various agents are studied and used in clinical practice.

Later chapters in this book examine in further detail the effects and efficacy of a number of agents used by physiotherapists at predominantly non-thermal intensities to treat soft tissue lesions and reduce pain.

References

Adey WR (1988) Physiological signalling across cell membranes and co-operative influences of extremely low frequency electromagnetic fields. In Frohlich H (ed) *Biological Coherence and Response to External Stimuli*. Heidelberg, Springer-Verlag.

Alberts B, Bray D, Lewis J et al (1994) *Molecular Biology of the Cell*, 2nd edn. New York, Garland Publishing.

Astumian RD, Chock PB, Tsong TY et al (1987) Can free energy be transduced from electrical noise? *Proc Natl Acad Sci USA* **84**: 434–438.

Barker AT (1993) Electricity magnetism and the body. *IEE Science, Education and Technology Division* **December**: 249–256.

Barker AT, Freestone, IL (1985) Medical applications of electric and magnetic fields. *IEE Electronics and Power* **October**: 757–760.

Dyson M (1985) Therapeutic applications of ultrasound. In Nyborg WL, Ziskin MC (eds) *Biological Effects of Ultrasound (Clinics in Diagnostic Ultrasound)*. New York, Churchill Livingstone.

Dyson M, Pond J, Woodward B et al (1974) The production of blood cell stasis and endothelial damage in the blood vessels of chick embryos treated with ultrasound in a stationary wave field. *Ultrasound in Medicine and Biology* **1**: 133–148.

Ferreri F, Curci G, Pasqualetti P et al (2006) Mobile phone emissions and human brain excitability. *Ann Neurol* **60(2)**: 188–196. Online 26 June 2006.

Frizzell LA, Dunn F (1990) Biophysics of ultrasound. In Lehmann JF (ed) *Therapeutic Heat and Cold*, 4th edn. Baltimore, MD, Williams and Wilkins: 362–397.

Frohlich H (1988) *Biological Coherence and Response to External Stimuli*. Heidelberg, Springer-Verlag.

George FR, Lukas RJ, Moffett J, Ritz MC (2002) *In vitro* mechanisms of cell proliferation induction: a novel bioactive treatment for accelerating wound healing. *Wounds* **14**: 107–115.

Hill CR, ter Haar G (1982) Ultrasound. In Suess MJ, Benwell-Morison DA (eds) *Nonionizing Radiation Protection* Series no. 10 199–228, 2nd edn. Geneva, World Health Organization.

Hiskenkamp M, Chiabrera A, Pilla AA, Bassett CAL (1978) Cell behaviour and DNA modification in pulsing electromagnetic fields. *Acta Orthop Belg* **44**: 636–650.

Karu TI (1987) Photobiological fundamentals of low power laser therapy. *IEEE Quant Elect* **23**: 1703–1717.

Karu TI (1988) Molecular mechanism of the therapeutic effects of low intensity laser radiation. *Lasers Life Scie* **2**: 53–74.

Karu TI, Pyatbrat LV, Afanasyeva NI (2005) Cellular effects of low power laser therapy can be mediated by nitric oxide. *Lasers Surg Med* **36**: 307–314.

Kujawa J, Zavodnik L, Zavodnik I et al (2004) Effect of low-intensity (3.75–27 J/cm^2) near-infrared (810 nm) laser radiation on red blood cell ATPase activities and membrane structure. *J Clin Laser Med Surg* **22**: 111–117.

Li R, Ritz MC, Lukas RJ et al (1999) Cell proliferation induction (CPI); dose- and time-dependent effects on fibroblast proliferation in vitro. *FASEB J* **13**: 351.

Lubart R, Friedmann H, Sinyakov M et al (1997). Changes in calcium transport in mammalian sperm mitochondria and plasma membranes caused by 780 nm irradiation. *Lasers Surg Med* **21**: 493–499.

Mortimer AJ, Dyson M (1988) The effect of therapeutic ultrasound on calcium uptake in fibroblasts. *Ultrasound Med Biol* **14**: 499–506.

Muller AWJ (1983) Thermoelectric energy conversion could be an energy source of living organisms. *Phys Lett A* **96**: 319–321.

Nicolini C (1985) Cell nucleus and EM fields. In Chiabrera A, Nicolini C, Schwan HP (eds) *Interactions between Electromagnetic Fields and Cells*. London, Plenum Press.

Repacholi MH (1970) Electrophoretic mobility of tumour cells exposed to ultrasound and ionising radiation. *Nature* **227**: 166–167.

Repacholi MH, Woodcock JP, Newman DL, Taylor KJW (1971) Interaction of low intensity ultrasound and ionising radiation with the tumour cell surface. *Phys Med Biol* **16**: 221–227.

Schimmelpfeng J, Stein J-C, Dertinger H (2005) Action of 50 Hz magnetic fields on cyclic AMP and intercellular communication in monolayers and spheroids of mammalian cells. *Bioelectromagnetics* **16**: 381–386.

Smith KC (1991) The photobiological basis of low level laser radiation therapy. *Laser Ther* **3**: 19–24.

Swedish Laser Medical Society (2004) Online. Available: http://www.laser.nu/lllt/fda.htm

Takahashi K, Kaneko I, Date M, Fukada E (1986) Effects of pulsing electromagnetic fields on DNA synthesis in mammalian cells in culture. *Experientia* **42**: 185–186.

Takashima Y, Hirose H, Koyama S et al (2006) Effects of continuous and intermittent exposure to RF fields with a wide range of SARs on cell growth, survival and cell cycle distribution. *Bioelectromagnetics* **27**: 392–400.

Tsong TY (1989) Deciphering the language of cells. *TIBS* **14**: 89–92.

Vladomirov Y, Borisenko G, Boriskina N et al (2000) NO-haemoglobin may be light-sensitive source of nitric oxide both in solution and in red blood cells. *J Photochem Photobiol B: Biol* **59**: 115–122.

Westerhoff HV, Tsong TY, Chock PB et al (1986) How enzymes can capture and transmit free energy from an oscillating electrical field. *Proc Natl Acad Sci USA* **83**: 4734–4738.

Young SR (1988) *The Effect of Therapeutic Ultrasound on the Biological Mechanisms Involved in Dermal Repair*. PhD Thesis, London University.

SECTION 2

Thermal and non-thermal modalities

SECTION CONTENTS

Chapter 9

Heat and cold application

Sheila Kitchen

INTRODUCTION

Both cold and heat can be effective forms of treatment, for example to manage pain, stiffness, oedema and spasticity. Chapter 7 describes in some detail the physical and physiological changes that can arise in the human body due to thermal variation. This chapter discusses the use of agents that effect temperature changes through direct physical contact with tissue and through radiation.

COLD OR HEAT?

Many, although not all, of the clinical benefits produced by heat and cold are similar. Selection is therefore sometimes based on a number of factors that might, on occasion, be empirical but are nevertheless important.

- **Stage of inflammation.** Generally, cold is preferable during the acute stage of inflammation to relieve pain, reduce the level of bleeding and swelling (these benefits are especially effective if applied early and, in practice, often combined with compression) and possibly retard secondary injury following trauma (see Chapter 4). Heat, in contrast, can exacerbate the early inflammatory process.

- **Oedema (swelling).** Heat tends to increase oedema whereas cold can help to limit it in recent injuries (see above).

- **Collagen extensibility.** A rise in temperature increases collagen extensibility, whereas it becomes stiffer with cold.

- **Pain.** Both heat and cold can be used to relieve pain. The effect of cold may be more prolonged but in certain situations can cause/increase pain.

- **Spasm.** Both heat and cold can decrease muscle spasm associated with musculoskeletal injuries and nerve root irritation. Similarly, both will reduce spasticity due to upper motor neuron dysfunction, though heat will do so for only a short period of time; cold is generally more effective under these circumstances as the return to normal temperatures takes longer.

- **Muscle contraction.** There appears to be a slight increase in the power of contraction with a rise in temperature within normal temperature ranges (approximately 25–37°C), especially in type 1 muscles, whereas cooling below this leads to a decrease.

- **Area to be treated.** In some subjects (e.g. those with Raynaud's disease) the application of cold to the hands and feet leads to severe pain, and this may therefore be an indication for heat therapy.

- **Ease of use.** This can be especially important when considering home therapy administered by the patient.

- **Patient preference.** Some subjects find cold intolerable; the use of heat to relieve both pain and muscle spasm may be more acceptable.

- **Specific contraindications** to either heat or cold.

WET OR DRY?

A second important factor to be considered when selecting thermal treatments is that of choosing between wet and dry contact techniques. Little is known about the relative efficacy of one compared with the other; however, Abramson (1967) has suggested that dry heat can elevate surface temperature to a slightly greater degree, whereas wet heat can lead to rises in temperature at slightly deeper levels. Thus either can be used for closed injuries, with choice largely dependent on pragmatic considerations. Wet techniques have the potential to introduce infection into an open wound and to waterlog tissue. Drying, for example with infrared heating, can be detrimental to wound repair but

has been demonstrated to be effective in the management of some skin conditions.

COLD *AND* HEAT

The effects of cold, contact heating methods and infrared irradiation are described separately in the following sections. However, occasionally cold and heat can be used alternately, most commonly in contrast baths. These comprise two water baths at different temperatures: a hotter bath at 40–42°C (immersion for 3–4 minutes) and a colder one at 15–20°C (immersion for about 1 minute). The body part is placed in each bath alternately, and it is normal practice to begin and end with the hotter bath. Lehmann and de Lateur (1990) have suggested that a 10-minute immersion in the warmer bath prior to the use of the colder contrasting temperature may be useful in producing an initial hyperaemia.

Few studies have examined the efficacy of this treatment but it is suggested that hyperaemia, reduced oedema due to vasodilation (Woodmansey et al 1938) and pain relief – possibly through the pain gate mechanism – may be implicated (Lehmann & de Lateur 1999). Myrer et al (1994) demonstrated that contrast baths are unlikely to result in an increase in intramuscular temperature.

CRYOTHERAPY (THERAPEUTIC COLD)

Tissues can be cooled for therapeutic reasons. The changes in temperature that can be achieved have been reported in many studies and vary enormously. This variation can be attributed to:

- different methods of application
- the length of time over which cooling has been applied
- the initial temperature of the technique used, e.g. water temperature.

THE EFFECTS ON TISSUES

Skin temperature

The greatest changes in temperature reported in a variety of studies for the different methods of application are as follows:

- Immersion in water: a drop of 29.5°C at a water temperature of 4°C after 193 minutes.

- Ice massage: a drop of 26.6°C at an ice temperature of 2°C after 10 minutes' application.

- Evaporation sprays: a drop to between 15–20°C with spraying for 3 seconds at 15 cm (using dimethyl ether).

- Ice packs: a drop of 20.3°C at a contact temperature of 0–3°C after 10 minutes.

- Ice towels: a drop of 13°C after a 7-minute period (with repeated application of towels).

Intramuscular temperature

The associated drop in temperature depends on the duration of the treatment, the depth of the muscle from the surface, the thickness of adipose tissue that insulates the underlying muscle and the initial temperature of the treatment agent; cooling persists for several hours (Meussen & Lievens 1986). Using a crushed ice bag, Otte et al (2002) reported drops in temperature of around 7°C at a depth of 1 cm in muscle in a patient with a skin fold of 20 mm in approximately 25 minutes; however, it took around 40 minutes to achieve this drop when the skin fold was between 21 and 30 mm.

Joint temperature

This appears to remain low after the application of cold, although some investigators have reported an initial brief rise in temperature (Kern et al 1984). Given the above report of limited cooling of muscle when insulated by adipose tissue, it is important to note that joint cooling will be very limited in most, especially deeper, joints.

PHYSIOLOGICAL EFFECTS

These are described in detail in Chapter 7 and include effects on cell function in general, circulation (reduced blood flow, oedema, haemorrhaging), collagen, neurological tissue (pain, spasm), muscle (contraction rates and power) and tissue repair. It is important to remember that contact methods of cooling produce only relatively superficial changes, so effects will be very limited in the deeper tissues of the body.

CLINICAL EFFICACY

Studies examining clinical efficacy support the empirical evidence for the use of ice for a number of symptoms. Cooling can reduce swelling following injury (e.g. Basur et al 1976), and Hecht et al (1983) demonstrated that 10 treatments can reduce swelling in patients with osteoarthritis (OA) of the knee. However, in clinical practice, cooling is often accompanied by compression or other treatments, which means that it is often difficult to ascribe the benefits to cooling alone.

Pain is normally reduced by cooling, mediated by the neurological effects described in Chapter 6. Examples include patients with OA of the knee (Clarke 1974) and following arthroscopy (Lessard et al 1997), and (Curkovic et al 1993) demonstrated an elevation of the pain threshold in patients with rheumatoid arthritis immediately after treatment; this declined within 30 minutes. Pain may be due to tissue irritants; a number of studies have suggested that patients with arthritis may experience pain relief owing to the adverse effects of cooling on the activity of destructive enzymes within the joints (Harris & McCroskery 1974, Pegg et al 1969).

The report by Lessard et al (1997) demonstrates a significant difference between the postarthroscopy groups (exercise regimen plus cold, or exercise regimen only) in terms of increased compliance and weight bearing. Effects on muscle performance are described in Chapter 7 and clinical studies lend some support to these findings (e.g. Oliver et al 1979): there is some evidence that it improves above pretreatment levels during the hours following cooling. Yurtkkurtan and Kocagil (1999) demonstrated increased quadriceps strength, range of movement of the knee and timed walking in patients with OA.

Finally, cooling recently injured tissues may confer some protection against secondary damage of adjacent cells due to hypoxia and enzyme activity by lowering the metabolic demands of the cells (see Chapter 7 for further discussion). Although this indicates good effects from cooling, it is important to note that clinical scenarios are complex and attributing effects exclusive to cooling can be difficult.

METHODS OF APPLICATION

Cold can be applied in a number of ways. These include the more common contact methods employing conduction (see Chapter 2 for details), such as wet and dry packs, and baths. In addition, evaporating sprays, relying on evaporation for their effect, may be used. During the application of cold therapy the subject will experience a number of sensations; these may include:

- intense cold
- a 'burning' sensation
- aching
- analgesia.

Before any application, the body part should be inspected for any contraindications and an explanation and safety warnings given (see the next section).

Cold packs

Cold packs can be either 'homemade' by the clinician or purchased. Satisfactory packs can be made by wrapping flaked ice in damp terry towels. These can be applied to the body part to be treated for anything up to 20 minutes. The rate of initial cooling is rapid but decreases as a film of water forms between the pack and the skin; this means that the temperature of the skin is usually above that of the melting ice and is generally in the region of 5–10°C.

Cold packs produced commercially are of two types. First, bags that contain a mixture of water and an antifreeze substance are available, and are cooled in a freezer. Care should be taken on initial application as the temperature of the pack can be below 0°C and can therefore cause very rapid cooling of the surface tissue and possible injury. A damp towel placed between the skin and the pack can ensure that the contact temperature remains a little above 0°C. Second, packs that rely on a chemical reaction for their cooling properties are available. Such packs may be used only once. Although both types of pack are effective in reducing tissue temperatures, McMaster et al (1978) demonstrated that chemical packs are more effective in lowering subcutaneous temperatures. However, as suggested earlier in this section, the final temperature developed depends on a variety of factors.

Very superficial cooling may be achieved through the use of ice towels and gels. Towelling may be placed in a mush of flaked ice and water, wrung out and applied to the part. Large areas may be covered, but the towel will need to be replaced frequently as it warms up rapidly. Treatment may be given for up to 20 minutes.

Application Some form of barrier is normally placed between the skin and cooling medium to prevent damage; this may be a damp towel which ensures the temperature is above 0°C or a barrier cream to prevent adhesion between the skin and agent; neither is needed with gels or sprays. The part should be observed regularly during treatment to avoid cold burns.

Cold baths

One of the simplest methods of cooling tissue is to place the body part in cold water or a mixture of ice and water. The temperature can be controlled by varying the ratio of ice to water. Lee et al (1978) suggest that a temperature of 16–18°C may be tolerated for 15–20 minutes. Lower temperatures may be used but will require intermittent immersion of the part. Clinical and experimental studies have used a wide variety of temperatures depending on the aim of the work.

Vaporizing sprays

Chapter 2 discusses the role of evaporation in producing cooling of the skin. Techniques that use this method of reducing skin temperature result in effective but short-lived tissue cooling. As yet unpublished work suggests that rewarming begins at about 15–20 seconds after the preceding application, and that statistically significant decreases in temperature to around 15–20°C can be produced with repeated applications (Cocker 2004, Collier 2004, Griffin 1997).

Application A volatile liquid (e.g. dimethyl ether) is sprayed directly on to the area to be treated. For safety reasons, it is important that the spray is both non-flammable and non-toxic. It should be applied over the area in a number of short bursts (of approximately 3–5 seconds each). Generally, three to five bursts are adequate.

Ice massage

Ice massage can be used to produce analgesia. The technique, which uses ice 'lollipops' or blocks, is normally performed over a small area such as a muscle belly or trigger point, and may be used prior to other techniques such as deep massage. Waylonis (1967) discusses the physiological effects of ice massage and suggests that an area of up to $10-15\,cm^2$ may be treated for up to 10 minutes or until analgesia occurs. A slow, circular motion over a small area is used. Temperatures do not drop to levels below 15°C with this method. Ice massage may also be used to facilitate muscle activity. In this case, ice is applied briskly and briefly over the skin dermatome of the same nerve root as the muscle in question. A number of studies have looked again at this area. Melzack et al (1980) reported that ice massage and transcutaneous electrical stimulation reduced pain to a similar degree; Roberts et al (1992) that it was more effective than both heat and cold packs; Yurtkurtan & Kocagil (1999), in a randomized controlled trial, showed improvements in a variety of outcomes in subjects with OA (see above). All suggest that ice massage has an effect on pain.

HAZARDS AND DETRIMENTAL EFFECTS

Not all the effects of cooling are beneficial. Damage due to the therapeutic use of cold therapy is, however, relatively rare in clinical practice, and the following precautions and contraindications contribute to this record (Box 9.1).

Ice burns can occur if cold is excessive or the pathology of the patient is such as to predispose to damage at temperatures that are normally acceptable. Damage appears a few hours after the application of cold and takes the form of erythema and tenderness and possibly blistering. More severe damage leads to fatty necrosis and the appearance of bruising; ultimately, severe cooling can lead to frostbite. Cuthill and Cuthill (2005) reported a case of self-administered cooling leading to superficial and partial-thickness burns and a survey of 80 practitioners, half of whom reported having seen one or more instances of frostbite injuries of limited severity. They note that many reported instances were associated with the self-administration of cold, often with the apparent assumption that 'more is better'; this suggests that education of the public is of considerable importance.

Care should be taken when cooling areas where nervous tissue is superficial. A number of authors have reported neural damage, including confirmed axonotmesis, following cooling of the peroneal nerve, the lateral cutaneous femoral nerve and the cutaneous femoral nerve (Covington & Bassett 1993, Green et al 1989, Parker et al 1983).

Other detrimental effects can occur. The immediate increase in peripheral vascular resistance associated with vasoconstriction on cooling causes an increase in blood pressure. This may preclude the use of cooling in patients with a history of severe hypertension. Ice should not be applied to areas affected by peripheral vascular disease as vasoconstriction will further impair the blood supply to an area that is already compromised. The shift to the left of the oxygen-dissociation curve with cooling means that oxygen is not readily available to the tissues and may retard repair, although this is unlikely to have significant therapeutic effects with intermittent use. The effects of temperature on collagen are discussed in Chapter 7; a reduction in temperature causes an increase in the mechanical stiffness of collagenous tissue and is therefore likely to increase joint stiffness, especially in superficial joints such as those of the hand (e.g. Hunter et al 1952). Use when attempting mobilization of joints may therefore be inappropriate. Finally, it should be noted that certain therapeutic effects may not occur in patients with sympathetic dysfunction, as some circulatory responses are mediated by the sympathetic nervous system.

CONTRAINDICATIONS

The following conditions generally contraindicate the use of cryotherapy:

- Acute febrile illness.

- Vasospasm, e.g. conditions such as Raynaud's disease, which is associated with excessive vasospasm leading to white/blue digits.

- Cryoglobinaemia: abnormal blood proteins can precipitate at low temperatures and this can lead to vessel blockage; the condition may be associated with rheumatoid arthritis and systemic lupus erythematosus.

- Cold urticaria: histamine, released by mast cells, leads to local weal formation, itching and the development of an erythema; changes in blood pressure (lowered) and pulse rate (raised) occur occasionally.

PRECAUTIONS, TESTS AND WARNINGS

Caution should also be exercised when treating patients with the following problems:

- Open wounds, infected or damaged tissue (e.g. skin conditions, allergies, etc.).

- Cardiac disease and high/low blood pressure may be important if a large area is cooled.

- Defective skin sensation: loss of sensory awareness may indicate other neuromuscular and autonomic problems, which may make the skin susceptible to damage if cold is used.

- Skin hypersensitivity.

- Adverse psychological factors: some subjects have a strong dislike of cold and it should therefore not be used in these cases.

- Very large areas (e.g. bilateral lower limbs) should not be subject to very low temperatures.

- The treatment can give rise to initial pain.

- The treatment can result in cold burns.

HEAT (CONTACT AND RADIANT)

Heat, like cold, has probably been used to manage pain for as long as man has had access to specific usable sources such as hot springs and pools, hot rocks, or simply wrapping parts in blankets. More recently, much work has been undertaken to examine what happens to tissues when they are heated.

PHYSIOLOGICAL EFFECTS

The physiological effects of heat are described in detail in Chapter 7 and relate to both contact and radiant heating. It is generally assumed by most specialists that infrared photons do not give rise to significant photochemical effects and so both methods have similar effects. These include effects on cell function, circulation (rate of blood flow, increased oedema and haemorrhaging, especially at the early stages of injury), collagen, neurological tissue (pain, spasm), muscle (contraction rates and power) and tissue repair. It is important to remember that both heating methods produce only relatively superficial thermal changes and that effects will be limited in the deeper tissues of the body.

CLINICAL EFFICACY

The physiological changes noted are thought to affect more functional aspects (which have more overt importance to most of us), such as range of movement, muscle function, walking distances and quality of life, parameters that are examined in a number of clinical trials. Much of the core work to examine the clinical efficacy of heat described in Chapter 7 has been conducted using contact methods such as water baths and so is not repeated here. The principles derived from this research can be largely applied to heating through radiation. Lehmann and de Lateur (1990) and Chapman (1991) review this literature in some detail, and a number of recent Cochrane reports shed some light on the current levels of knowledge; these form the basis of the discussion in Chapter 7. Some additional evidence for specific studies examining the efficacy of radiant therapy is noted below.

METHODS OF APPLICATION: CONTACT TECHNIQUES

Contact methods of heating, by definition, require physical contact between the therapeutic agent and the tissues. Changes in temperature are the result of heat transfer through conduction (see Chapter 2 for details) and are relatively superficial. Some heating of deeper tissues occurs and is due to conduction within the tissues, as well as convection through fluids (e.g. blood and lymph) and their circulation.

When superficial contact heat is applied, the surface tissue temperature change will depend on:

- the intensity of the heat (watts/cm^2)
- the length of exposure to the heat (minutes)
- size of area exposed (cm^2)
- the thermal medium: this is a product of the thermal conductivity, density and specific heat characteristics of the tissue (Hendler et al 1958).

To achieve therapeutic effects, the temperature obtained in the tissues should be between 40 and 45°C (Lehman & de Lateur 1990). Burning and destruction of proteins is likely to occur above this level and below 40°C the effects of heating are considered too mild to be of therapeutic use. Maximal elevation of the temperature of the skin and very superficial tissue will occur within 6–8 minutes. The underlying muscle will respond to a lesser extent and more slowly, and, at tolerable temperatures, muscle temperature can be expected to be raised by about 1°C at a depth of 3 cm. However, where subcutaneous fat is present, heating of deeper tissues is reduced because of insulation. Although no specific work has been identified in relation to tissue heating replicating that of Otte et al (2002) and Jutte et al (2001) with cold, it is very likely that the insulating effects of adipose tissue will have similar effects. Where a greater depth of penetration is required, deep-heat modalities such as shortwave diathermy should be considered.

Surface heat can be applied in a number of ways. All raise superficial tissue temperatures, but some may be more suitable in given situations owing to the material used (e.g. wet or dry heat) and practicalities. The most common are considered here.

Before any application, the body part should be inspected for any contraindications and washed; an explanation and safety warnings should be given (see the next section).

Wax

Paraffin wax, with a melting point of approximately 54°C, is combined with a mineral oil such as liquid paraffin to produce a temperature-controlled bath at a temperature between 42°C and 50°C. These temperatures are slightly higher than would be tolerated if the body part were placed in hot water. This is because the specific heat of paraffin wax is less than that of water (2.72 kJ/kg per degree centigrade for wax and 4.2 kJ/kg per degree centigrade for water). Wax therefore releases less energy than water when cooling. Selkins and Emery (1990) note that the amount of heat imparted to the tissue due the solidification of the wax – the latent heat of fusion – is small. At the same time, heat loss is prevented owing to the insulating nature of the material. The net result is a well-insulated, low-temperature method of heating tissue. Slightly higher temperatures may be used for the upper extremities than for the lower extremities and newly healed tissue (Burns & Conin 1987, Head & Helms 1977).

Application In the *dip and wrap* method, the part is first immersed in the warm wax, then withdrawn and the wax allowed to set. The procedure is repeated, normally 6 to 12 times, to develop a 'wax glove'. The whole is then wrapped in plastic or waxed paper and an insulating layer of material such as towelling. Alternatively, the part may be retained in the bath following the development of the wax glove – the *dip and reimmerse* method. This technique results in a greater increase in temperature (Abramson et al 1964, 1965).

Heated pads and packs

A variety of heated pads/packs may be used to provide heat to small areas:

● Dry pads/packs: these are most common, vary greatly, and include many that can be bought over the counter or are home made. They include those that contain heat-retentive gels, hot water (hot-water bottles), grains such as wheat, electrical elements or heat-producing chemicals, and can be heated in microwave ovens, by electrical means or through mixing chemical components within a sachet (often by simply crushing). The temperature of the final pack should be around 40–42°C. Gradual cooling will occur.

● Moist pads/packs: these are immersed in hot water (at approximately 36–41°C) and perform a similar function to those above but tend to cool more quickly as it is not usually practical to provide an insulation layer. Such pads need to be replaced after approximately 5 minutes.

Application The type of pack is selected based on the comments above. Replacement of the packs during treatment can result in prolonged heating, although no significant differences in subcutaneous temperatures result (Lehmann et al 1966).

Hydrotherapy

The use of hot water to heat tissue is an effective way of increasing temperature and both still and – less often – whirlpool baths may be used for local treatment. Temperatures are usually between 36 and 41°C (lower than wax temperatures for the reasons discussed above). Borell et al (1980) confirmed that treatment at these temperatures results in an increase in subcutaneous temperature. The motion of the water in whirlpool baths may, in addition, stimulate receptors in the skin surface, giving rise to pain relief through the pain gate mechanism.

Application This treatment should only be used when wet application is appropriate; see above. Movement of the part can occur during heating.

METHODS OF APPLICATION: RADIANT TECHNIQUES (INFRARED RADIATION)

Infrared radiation (IR) is a superficial thermal agent used therapeutically for the relief of pain and stiffness, to increase joint motion and to enhance the healing of soft tissue lesions and skin conditions (Kitchen & Partridge 1991, Lehmann & de Lateur 1999, Michlovitz 1986).

All hot bodies emit IR to varying degrees and sources can be either natural (e.g. the sun) or artificial. Artificial IR is generally produced by passing an electrical current through a coiled resistance wire, and therapeutically both luminous generators (radiant heaters) and non-luminous generators are available. Their characteristics are shown in Table 9.1.

Physical characteristics

IRs lie in that part of the electromagnetic spectrum that gives rise to heating when absorbed by matter (see Fig. 2.20), between microwaves and visible light. Many sources that emit visible light or ultraviolet (UV) radiation also emit IR. The International Commission on Illumination (CIE) describes IR in terms of three biologically significant bands, which differ in the degree to which they are absorbed by biological tissues and therefore in their effect upon those tissues. The wavelengths mainly used in clinical practice are between 0.7 mm (700 nm) and 1.5 mm (1500 nm), and are concentrated in the IRA band.

IR is produced as a result of molecular motion. An increase in temperature above absolute zero results in the vibration or rotation of molecules within matter, which leads to the emission of IR. The temperature of the body affects the wavelength of the radiation emitted, with the mean frequency of emitted radiation rising with an increase in temperature. Thus, the higher the temperature of the body the higher the mean frequency output and, consequently, the shorter the wavelength. However, most bodies do not emit IR of a single waveband – a number of different wavelengths may be emitted owing to interplay between the emission and absorption of radiations affecting the behaviour of molecules.

Physical behaviour of infrared irradiation

IR can be reflected, absorbed, transmitted, refracted and diffracted by matter (see Chapter 2), the reflection and absorption being of most biological and clinical significance. These effects moderate the penetration of energy into the tissues and thus the biological changes which take place.

Absorption, penetration and reflection

Skin is a complex material, so its reflective and absorptive characteristics are not uniform (Moss et al 1989). Radiation must be absorbed to facilitate

Table 9.1 Characteristics of luminous and non-luminous generators

Generator	Peak wavelength emitted	Power levels emitted	Comments
Luminous	1 mm IR and visible radiations emitted	250 and 1500 W	Red filters used; minimal warm-up period required (few minutes)
Non-luminous (resistance wire embedded in insulating material)	4 mm IR radiation emitted; wider spectrum of emission	250 and 1000 W	No filter; warm-up period required (approximately 15 minutes)

changes within the body tissues, and absorption depends on the structure and type of tissue, vascularity and pigmentation. Penetration of energy into a medium is dependent upon the:

- intensity of the source of infrared
- wavelength (and consequent frequency of the radiation)
- angle at which the radiation hits the surface
- coefficient of absorption of the material.

Maximum penetration occurs with wavelengths of 1.2 mm, whereas the skin is virtually opaque to wavelengths of 2 mm and more (Moss et al 1989). Hardy (1956) showed that at least 50% of radiations of 1.2 mm penetrated to a depth of 0.8 mm, allowing interaction with capillaries and nerve endings. Selkins and Emery (1990) demonstrated that almost all energy is absorbed at a depth of 2.5 mm, and Harlen (1980) noted penetration depths of 0.1 mm for long IR wavelengths and up to 3 mm for the shorter wavelengths. In addition, because energy penetration decreases exponentially with depth, the greatest heating will occur most superficially. Some heating occurs at greater depths owing to the transfer of heat from the superficial tissue by conduction between layers of tissue, convection through the local circulation and increased blood flow. Infrared should, however, be regarded as a surface heating modality (for further details of conduction/convection see Chapter 2).

Evidence for clinical efficacy

There is limited evidence of efficacy directly related to the use of IR as few studies have been undertaken; nevertheless, evidence from other studies of heating that give rise to superficial thermal changes only (e.g. conduction heating as above) is applicable. Specific studies relating to the use of IR are noted here.

Pain

Lehmann et al (1958) demonstrated that when IR was applied to the region of the ulnar nerve at the elbow, an analgesic effect was noted distal to the point of application. Kramer (1984) utilized IR as a control when evaluating the heating effect of ultrasound in nerve conduction tests of the ulnar nerve

on normal subjects and reported an increase in the post-treatment ulnar nerve conduction velocity in both cases with an increase in tissue temperature of 0.8°C. The studies by Halle et al (1981) and Currier and Kramer (1982) also indicate that IR can cause an increase in nerve conduction velocity in normal humans.

Joint stiffness

Joint stiffness is due to a number of factors, including ligaments, joint capsule and periarticular structures, and fluid pressure. Wright and Johns (1961) applied IR to a normal hand joint in vivo, producing a surface temperature of 45°C. They measured a 20% drop in joint stiffness at 45°C compared to the stiffness at a temperature of 33°C. However, this work was performed with two subjects only, and no replication studies have been identified using IR. More recent work using other agents is reported in Chapter 7 but its applicability is unclear, as IR is such a superficial form of heating; it might be effective for small joints such as those of the hand.

Skin lesions

Some skin lesions may benefit from a drying heat. Psoriasis and fungal infections, such as paronychia, may be managed with IR treatment. Westerhof et al (1987) exposed patients with psoriasis to IR for 1 month, with skin temperatures of 42°C. Eighty per cent of subjects experienced remission, with 30% experiencing a dramatic improvement. Orenberg et al (1986) confirmed these results. Infrared irradiation should not be used to treat open wounds, however, as evidence indicates that its tendency to dehydrate the tissue causes further damage and inhibits healing.

Application

Before treatment, the body part should be inspected for any contraindications and an explanation and safety warnings given (see the following section). The following procedure should be used when giving infrared therapy:

1. Select and warm up equipment.

2. Patient: a comfortable, supported position is required to allow the subject to remain still.

The skin should be uncovered, clean and dry, all liniments and creams having been removed.

3. Lamp position: at a right-angle to the skin to facilitate maximum absorption of energy but not directly above a part to avoid burns should it fall. Distance: between 50 and 75 cm.

4. Dosage: this is determined in clinical practice by the response of the subject. It is essential, therefore, that the patient is advised of the appropriate level of heating and understands the importance of reporting any changes from this.

Dosage

The amount of energy received by the patient will be governed by the:

- intensity of the output of the lamp (in watts)
- distance of the lamp from the patient
- duration of the treatment.

For therapeutic effects to occur, it has been suggested there is need for a temperature of between 40 and 45°C to be maintained for at least 5 minutes (Lehmann & de Lateur 1990). Crockford and Hellon (1959) demonstrated a gradual rise in temperature during the first 10 minutes of irradiation, with the return to normal taking an average of 35 minutes. The intensity is altered either by changing the distance of the lamp from the body part or by altering the output of the generator. By the end of a treatment, a mild dose should generate skin temperatures in the region of 36–38°C, and a moderate dose should produce temperatures of between 38 and 40°C. Infrared treatment is normally continued for a period of between 10 and 20 minutes, depending on the size and vascularity of the body part, and the type and chronicity of the lesion. Small avascular parts and acute/subacute conditions tend to be treated for shorter periods.

HAZARDS AND DETRIMENTAL EFFECTS

The hazards associated with heating by any of the above methods are similar. Differences are largely due to the size of the area heated, wet/dry application or the nature of the areas treated. They include:

- Burns (normally superficial, involving only the skin): can occur if there is inadequate testing of materials and equipment, the tissue is devitalized or the patient has severely impaired skin sensation and is unable to note overheating. Burns normally occur at exposure to temperatures of 46–47°C and above. Pain, however, occurs at 44.5 ± 1.3°C and should, therefore, provide protection by evoking a withdrawal response (Hardy 1951, Stevens 1983). Electrical burns (which can be deeper) can occur if equipment is faulty.

- Chronic damage to tissue: this may follow prolonged exposure to IR at higher, tolerable temperatures (Kligman 1982); epidermal hyperplasia and a large increase in ground substance occurred in guinea pigs. Permanent pigmentation may occur with prolonged use of IR.

- Foreign material/infection: may be introduced into open wounds by contact methods.

- Open wounds: tissues exposed to IR during surgical procedures show an increased tendency to develop adhesions, suggesting that open wounds should not be exposed to dry heating.

- Testicles: there is a temporary lowering of sperm count following heating.

- Apnoea: infants exposed to radiant warmers may be subject to periods of apnoea.

- Optical damage: corneal burns, retinal and lenticular injury may occur if drying of the eyes occurs (Moss et al 1989)

- Susceptible subjects, e.g. elderly people may suffer dehydration and temporary lowering of the blood pressure, or symptoms including dizziness and headaches following treatment, especially to large areas such as the back or neck/shoulders.

CONTRAINDICATIONS

Although not all factors listed have been substantiated fully through research, the following contraindications have resulted in minimal reporting of injury to patients:

- lack of local thermal sensitivity on the part of the patient
- local areas of recent bleeding (haemorrhaging)
- devitalized skin, e.g. after deep X-ray treatment
- certain skin conditions, e.g. skin carcinomas, acute dermatitis (especially with wax).

Caution should also be exercised when treating patients with the following problems:

- impaired local circulation
- damaged or infected tissues: moist heat may encourage breakdown.

PRECAUTIONS, TESTS AND WARNINGS

- A thermal skin test should be carried out to determine the ability of the patient to differentiate between hot and cold.

- The treatment can give rise to burns.

The electrical safety of the equipment should be checked regularly (Chartered Society of Physiotherapy 2006). The output of the lamp should be checked, and the mechanical stability, alignment and security of all parts of the lamp should be examined.

References

Abramson DI (1967) Comparison of wet and dry heat in raising temperature of tissue. *Arch Phys Med Rehab* **48**: 654.

Abramson DI, Tuck S, Chu L et al (1964) Effect of paraffin bath and hot fomentations on local tissue temperature. *Arch Phy Med Rehab* **45**: 87–94.

Abramson DI, Chu LSW, Tuck S (1965) Indirect vasodilation in thermotherapy. *Arch Phys Med Rehab* **46**: 412.

Basur R, Shephard E, Mouzos G (1976) A cooling method in the treatment of ankle sprains. *Practitioner* **216**: 708.

Borell PM, Parker R, Henley EJ et al (1980) Comparison of *in vivo* temperatures produced by hydrotherapy, paraffin wax treatment and fluidotherapy. *Phys Ther* **60**: 1273–1276.

Burns SP, Conin TA (1987) The use of paraffin wax in the treatment of burns. *Physiother Canada* **39**: 258.

Chapman CE (1991) Can the use of physical modalities for pain control be rationalized by the research evidence? *Can J Physiol Pharmacol* **69**: 704–712.

Chartered Society of Physiotherapy (CSP) (2006) *Guidance for the Clinical Use of Electrophysical Agents*. London, CSP.

Clarke GR, Willis LA, Stenner L, Nichiols PJR (1974) Evaluation of physiotherapy in the treatment of osteoarthrosis of the knee. *Rheumatol Rehab* **13**: 190–197.

Cocker A (2004) *The Skin Temperature Achieved with a Commercially Available Cooling Spray Applied to Areas of Different Vascular Perfusion*. MSc thesis. King's College London.

Collier C (2004) *The Skin Temperature Achieved with a Commercially Available Cooling Spray Applied to Areas of Different Vascular Perfusion*. MSc thesis. King's College London.

Covington DB, Bassett FH (1993) When cryotherapy injures. *Phys Sports Med* **21**(3): 78–93.

Crockford GW, Hellon RF (1959) Vascular responses of human skin to Infrared Radiation. *J Physiol* **149**: 424–432.

Curkovic B, Vitulic V, Babic-Naglic D, Durrigl T (1993) The influence of heat and cold on the pain threshold in rheumatoid arthritis. *Zeitschr Rheumatol* **52**: 289–291.

Currier DP, Kramer JF (1982) Sensory nerve conduction: heating effects of ultrasound and infrared. *Physiother Canada* **34**: 241–246.

Cuthill JA, Cuthill SC (2005) Partial thickness burn to the leg following application of a cold pack: case report and results of a questionnaire survey of Scottish physiotherapists in private practice. *Physiotherapy* **92**: 61–65.

Green GA, Zachazewski JE, Jordan SE (1989) Peroneal nerve palsy induced by cryotherapy. *Phys Sports Med* **17**(9): 63–70.

Griffin S (1997) *Study to Examine the Change in Skin Temperature Produced by the Application of Ice Spray on the Ankle*. BSc dissertation. King's College London.

Halle JS, Scoville CR, Greathouse DG (1981) Ultrasound's effect on the conduction latency of the superficial radial nerve in man. *Phys Ther* **61**: 345–350.

Hardy JD (1951) Influence of skin temperature upon pain threshold as evoked by thermal irradiation. *Science* **114**: 149–150.

Hardy JD (1956) Spectral transmittance and reflectance of excised human skin. *J Appl Physiol* **9**: 257–264.

Harlen F (1980) Infrared irradiation. In Docker MF (ed) *Physics in Physiotherapy, Conference Report Series-35*. London, Hospital Physicists Association: 180.

Harris ED, McCroskery PA (1974) The influence of temperature and fibril stability on degradation of cartilage collagen by rheumatoid synovial collegenase. *N Engl J Med* **290**: 1–6.

Head MD, Helms PS (1977) Paraffin and sustained stretching in the treatment of burns contracture. *Burns* **4**: 136.

Hecht PJ, Backmann S, Booth RE, Rothman RH (1983) Effects of thermal therapy on rehabilitation after total knee arthroplasty: a prospective randomized study. *Clin Orthop Rel Res* **178**: 198–201.

Hendler E, Crosby R, Hardy JD (1958) Measurement of heating of the skin during exposure to infrared radiation. *J Appl Physiol* **12**: 177.

Hunter J, Kerr EH, Whillans MG (1952) The relation between joint stiffness upon exposure to cold and the characteristics of synovial fluid. *Can J Med Sci* **30**: 367–377.

Jutte LS, Merrick MA, Ingersoll CD, Edwards JE (2001) The relationship between intramuscular temperature, skin temperature and adipose thickness during cryotherapy and rewarming. *Arch Phys Med Rehab* **82**: 845–850.

Kern H, Fessl L, Trnavsky G, Hertz H (1984) Das Verhalten der Gelenkstemperatur unter Eisapplikation-Grundlage für die praktische Anwendung. *Wiener Klini Wschr* **96**: 832–837.

Kitchen SS, Partridge CJ (1991) Infrared therapy. *Physiotherapy* **77**(4): 249–254.

Kligman LH (1982) Intensification of ultraviolet-induced dermal damage by infrared radiation. *Arch Dermatol Res* **272**: 229–238.

Kramer JF (1984) Ultrasound: evaluation of its mechanical and thermal effects. *Arch Phys Med Rehab* **65**: 223–227.

Lee JM, Warren MP, Mason SM (1978) Effects of ice on nerve conduction velocity. *Physiotherapy* **64**: 2–6.

Lehmann JF, de Lateur JB (1990) Therapeutic heat. In Lehman JF (ed) *Therapeutic Heat and Cold*, 4th edn. Baltimore, MD, Williams & Wilkins: 417–581.

Lehmann JF, de Lateur JB (1999) Ultrasound, shortwave, microwave, laser, superficial heat and cold in the treatment of pain. In Wall PD, Melzack R (eds) *Textbook of Pain*, 4th edn. New York, Churchill Livingstone: 1383–1397.

Lehmann JF, Brunner GD, Stow RW (1958) Pain threshold measurements after therapeutic application of ultrasound, microwaves and infrared. *Arch Phys Med Rehab* **39**: 560–565.

Lehmann JF, Silvermann DR, Baum B et al (1966) Temperature distribution in the human thigh produced by infrared, hot pack and microwave applications. *Arch Phy Med Rehab* **47**: 291–299.

Lessard LA, Scudds RA, Amendola A, Vaz MD (1997) The effect of cryotherapy following arthroscopic knee surgery. *J Orthop Sports Phys Ther* **26**(1): 14–22.

McMaster WC, Liddle S, Waugh TR (1978) Laboratory evaluation of various cold therapy modalities. *Am J Sports Med* **6**(5): 291–294.

Melzac R, Jeans ME, Stratfrod JG, Monks RC (1980) Ice massage and transcutaneous electrical stimulation: comparison of treatment for low back pain. *Pain*, **9**: 209–217.

Meussen R, Lievens P (1986) The use of cryotherapy in sports injuries. *Sports Med* **3**: 398–414.

Michlovitz SL (1986) *Thermal Agents in Rehabilitation, Contemporary Perspectives in Rehabilitation*, Vol. 1. Philadelphia, FA Davies.

Moss C, Ellis R, Murray W, Parr W (1989) *Infrared Radiation, Nonionising Radiation Protection*, 2nd edn. Copenhagen, WHO Regional Publications, European Series, no. 25.

Myrer JW, Draper DO, Durrant E (1994) Contrast therapy and intramuscular temperature in the human leg. *J Athletic Training* **29**(4): 318–322.

Oliver RA, Johnson DJ, Wheelhouse WW et al (1979) Isometric muscle contraction response during recovery from reduced intramuscular temperature. *Arch Phys Med Rehab* **60**: 126.

Orenberg EK, Noodleman FR, Koperski JA et al (1986) Comparison of heat delivery systems for hyperthermia treatment of psoriasis. *Int J Hypertherm* **2**(3): 231–241.

Otte JW, Merrick MA, Ingersoll CD, Cordova ML (2002) Subcutaneous adipose tissue thickness alters cooling time during cryotherapy. *Arch Phys Med Rehab* **83**: 1501–1505.

Parker JT, Small NC, Davis DG (1983) Cold induced nerve palsy. *Athletic Training* **18**: 76.

Pegg SMH, Littler TR, Littler EN (1969) A trial of ice therapy and exercise in chronic arthritis. *Physiotherapy* **55**: 51–56.

Roberts D, Wallis C, Carlile J et al (1992) Relief of chronic low back pain: heat versus cold. In Aronoff GM (ed) *Evaluation and Treatment of Chronic Pain*, 2nd edn. Baltimore, MD, Urban and Schwarzenberg: 263–266.

Selkins KM, Emery AF (1990) Thermal science for physical medicine. In Lehmann JF (ed) *Therapeutic Heat and Cold*, 4th edn. Baltimore, MD, Williams and Wilkins: 62–112.

Stevens J (1983) Thermal sensation: infrared and microwaves. In Adair, E (ed) *Microwaves and Thermal Regulation*. London, Academic Press: 134–176.

Waylonis GW (1967) The physiological effect of ice massage. *Arch Phys Med Rehab* **48**: 37–41.

Westerhof W, Siddiqui AH, Cormane RH, Scholten A (1987) Infrared hyperthermia and psoriasis. *Arch Dermatol Res* **279**: 209–210.

Woodmansey A, Collins DH, Ernst MM (1938) Vascular reactions to the contrast bath in health and in rheumatoid arthritis. *Lancet* **2**: 1350–1353.

Wright V, Johns RJ (1961) Quantitative and qualitative analysis of joint stiffness in normal subjects and in patients with connective tissue disease. *Ann Rheumatol Dis* **20**: 26–36.

Yurtkurtan M, Kocagil T (1999) Electroacupuncture and ice massage: a comparison of treatment for osteoarthritis of the knee. *Am J Acupuncture* **27**: 133–140.

Chapter 10

Pulsed and continuous shortwave therapy

Maryam M. Al-Mandeel and Tim Watson

INTRODUCTION

Shortwave therapy (SWT) involves the coupling of high-frequency electromagnetic (EM) energy to the tissues to treat a wide range of musculoskeletal or neurological conditions. Shortwave generators utilize the non-ionizing radiation of the electromagnetic (EM) spectrum. The frequency range of 10–100 MHz of EM constitutes the radiofrequency (RF) band that contains short, medium and long radio waves (see Fig. 2.20). The shortwave range of this band has been employed medically in the production of the physiotherapy-modality shortwave in its two forms: pulsed shortwave therapy (PSWT) and continuous shortwave therapy (CSWT). This chapter considers both modes of delivery and, where appropriate, differentiation between continuous and pulsed modes will be made. The term 'diathermy', although historically popular, will be largely omitted and the term 'shortwave therapy (SWT)' used in preference.

DEVELOPMENT OF SHORTWAVE THERAPY

Early experiences with high-frequency current started in the 1880s, when the French physiologist d'Arsonval passed a current of 1 ampere through his body and the body of his assistant. Despite the belief that a current of such strength would be deadly, they experienced only gentle warmth (Scott 2002). Based on this early work, experiments in the 1930s by the American physicist Arthur Milinowski and his colleague Dr Ginsberg focused on eliminating the heating effects and reducing the adverse outcomes associated with the application of CSWT (Lightwood 1989, Low & Reed 2000). Milinowski and Ginsberg introduced pauses in the electromagnetic field (EMF) output of the CSWT, which was thought at the time to allow for dissipation of heat and the prevention of thermal build-up (Arghiropol et al 1992). Their attempts culminated in 1936 in the production of an ultra-shortwave apparatus. They followed their efforts by experimenting on animals, but their task was terminated by the Second World War. In 1953, experiments were resumed and the first Diapulse apparatus (PSWT) was produced and marketed.

The revolution of Diapulse was followed by the production of Curapuls in 1970 and Megapulse in 1981, both of which were capable of producing continuous and pulsed output (Hayne 1984). Since then, the two modes of SWT have undergone fashionable shifts in utilization and, with the increasing move towards applying lower levels of energy (Watson 2000) and the belief that athermal modes of treatment could achieve therapeutic effects with minimal side effects, PSWT has become a more popular modality than CSWT (Al-Mandeel & Watson 2006, Shields 2003, Kerem & Yigiter 2002). Its increasing clinical use, however, has not been accompanied by an equivalent expansion of the supporting evidence. SWT remains an underexplored modality (Pope et al 1995) and relatively little is known of its bioeffects and its mechanism of action (Shields et al 2004), all of which warrant further research.

SHORTWAVE THERAPY GENERATORS

Therapeutic shortwave equipment is one of the many medical devices that utilizes high-frequency EMF. In an attempt to regulate the use of high-frequency currents in different disciplines, in 1947 the Federal Communication Commission assigned three frequencies at the short end of the RF band for the medical use of shortwave (Foley-Nolan 1990). These are: the frequency 40.68 MHz (± 20 KHz) and a wavelength of 7.5 m; the frequency of 13.56 MHz (± 6.25 KHz) and a wavelength of 22 m and the frequency of 27.12 MHz (± 160 KHz) and a wavelength of 11 m (Prentice & Draper 2001). The majority of the research reported in this chapter relates to the use of the 27.12 MHz frequency, which is the most widely employed in current clinical practice. The frequencies employed relate to international regulation rather than known optimal efficacy.

SWT generators produce high-frequency EMF by incorporating two electrical circuits: the machine and the patient circuits. The machine (or oscillator) circuit is composed of a high-frequency generator, amplifier (to raise the output to therapeutic levels), and a power supply (Fig. 10.1). The second circuit is the patient (or resonator) circuit, which is composed of a variable capacitor (to account for the changing capacity of the resonator circuit due to the type of tissue treated) and a method of transferring energy to the tissues; this is achieved by either capacitive or inductive electrodes.

The output of a SWT device can be delivered to the tissues in either a continuous or a pulsed mode. The difference between the two is that with CSWT the energy is delivered to the patient for the whole time of the treatment and, as such, it is primarily associated with thermal effects. With PSWT, the output is delivered to the tissues in a train of pulses of varying durations and repetition rate, as such allowing a high amplitude of energy to be delivered to the tissues with either thermal or non-thermal effects (Wadsworth & Chanmugam 1983, Watson 2006). Depending on the features of the machine being used, the main variables that can be controlled by the operator are pulse repetition rate (PRR), pulse duration (PD), pulse peak power (PP) and mean power (MP). In most machines MP can be controlled by changing PRR, PD and PP according to equation 10.1 (and illustrated

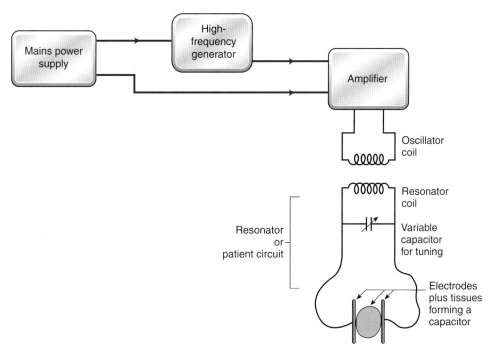

Figure 10.1 Electrical circuits with SWT generators (from Low & Reed 2000).

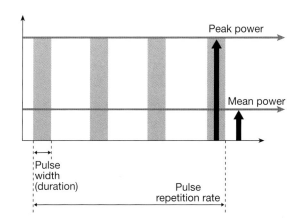

Figure 10.2 The essential relationship between pulse repetition rate, pulse duration, peak and mean power.

Table 10.1 Typical ranges of pulse parameters in modern pulsed shortwave therapy devices

Pulse parameter	Units	Typical range
Pulse repetition rate (frequency)	Pulses per second (pps) or Hz	26–800
Pulse duration	Microseconds (µs)	20–400
Pulse peak power	Watts	150–200
Applied mean power	Watts	0.1–30+

in Fig. 10.2). Table 10.1 illustrates the typical ranges of pulse parameters available on modern pulsed shortwave therapy devices.

Mean power (MP) = Pulse duration (PD)
            × Pulse repetition rate
            (PRR) × Peak pulse
            power (PP)   (10.1)

For example, using a machine with a mean power of 200 W, a pulse repetition rate of 400 pulses per second (pps) and a pulse duration of 200 µs, the mean power applied to the patient would be 16 W, whereas using the same machine (peak power 200 W) with a low pulse repetition rate (35 pps) and a short duration pulse (65 µs), the mean power would be 0.46 W. A modern PSWT device would typically be capable of delivering mean powers in the range of 0.3–30+ W.

PHYSICAL CHARACTERISTICS

Shortwave EM energy has two basic fields: the electric and magnetic fields, which are created in the tissues. It is the application of these fields and the subsequent currents that arise in the tissues that are responsible for the physiological effects, such as the rise in tissue temperature or the non-thermal changes in cellular activity.

An electric (E) field is set up whenever an electrical charges moves; this field is characterized by both its direction and its magnitude. An electrically charged particle, such as an electron or proton, placed within this field will experience a force (F). E and F are related according to equation 10.2:

$$F = qE \tag{10.2}$$

where q is the strength of the charge placed in the field and E is the charge. In electrically conductive materials, such as living tissues, these forces will result in the production of electrical currents.

A magnetic (H) field is set up in the tissue as a response to moving charges. This field is perpendicular in direction to the electric field. Magnetic fields are specified by both the magnetic flux density (B) and magnetic field strength (H), which are measured in units of tesla (T) and amperes per metre (A/m), respectively.

The interaction between the field and the tissues is affected by a macroscopic property of the tissue called the 'complex permittivity'; this is related to the dielectric constant (Delpizzo & Joyner 1987). The dielectric constant represents the depolarization characteristics of a tissue and is primarily dependent upon the water content. Complex permittivity is also a function of the field frequency and, therefore, the propagation and attenuation of the electromagnetic waves are dependent upon frequency.

Although SWT units produce both an E and an H field in the tissue, their ratio will differ according to the mode of application, the type of electrode in use, the carrying frequency and manufacturing characteristics. Differences in the base (carrying) frequency of operation can also result in variance of the ratio of H and E fields (Hand 1990, Markov & Colbert 2000).

METHODS OF COUPLING SHORTWAVE THERAPY TO THE TISSUES

There are two methods of transferring energy to the tissues when using SWT: the capacitance and the inductance methods. Each application affects different target structures and each has its own mechanism of producing heat in the tissues.

CAPACITIVE METHOD

Capacitor electrodes produce a higher proportion of E than H field in the tissues, with the field being stronger in the centre of the treated area (Prentice & Draper 2001). The strength of the field is governed by the electrode placement in relation to the tissue (there is a stronger field with the electrodes situated closer to the skin), the size of the electrodes (small electrodes have less penetration than medium and large electrodes) and spacing (uniform field in the tissues is achieved by using electrodes slightly larger than the treated area) (Hand 1990). The heat produced using capacitive method is the result of the movement of three components: charged molecules, dipolar molecules and non-polar molecules, and is governed by the strength of the E field and the conductivity of the tissues (more heat is produced in tissues with high conductivity), although capacitive application is actually expected to concentrate the field in the superficial tissues such as the skin and fat layers rather than the deep tissues such as muscles (Van der Esch & Hoogland 1991, Ward 1980). This is mainly caused by the reduction of field intensity as it propagates in the tissues. The refraction of the lines of force as they cross the muscle fat layer causes the loss of part of the applied field strength and termination of some field lines (Ward 1980). As the heating pattern with these electrode is mostly in the skin and subcutaneous fat layer, this method is possibly best suited for treating ribs, spine and areas of low subcutaneous fat such as hands and feet (Prentice & Draper 2001), and the use of capacitive delivery of SWT has diminished in recent years.

Two types of electrode are used with the capacitive method: air space plates and pad electrodes (Wadsworth & Chanmugam 1983).

1. Air space plates Air space plates are composed of two metal plates (ranging in diameter from 7.5 to 17.5 cm) enclosed in a plastic or glass guard (Fig. 10.3). Two electrodes are needed for this application and the patient is part of the electrical circuit acting as a dielectric. The distance between the skin and the electrodes can be adjusted by changing either the skin/electrode distance or by adjusting the metal plate position within the electrode housing. No consensus exists in the literature on the ideal skin electrode distance, with some suggesting 2.5 cm (Wadsworth & Chanmugam 1983) and others recommending 2–4 cm (Low & Reed 2000, Scott 2002). However, no justification was given for the choice of these values.

2. Pad (rubber) electrodes These electrodes are composed of a metal plate encased in rubber (Fig. 10.4). They are placed on the treated part with the electrode in a more uniform and even contact with the tissues. Two electrodes are used and the area treated is part of the circuit. Spacing between the skin and the electrodes is ensured by layers of towelling or felt spacers. The amount of heating generated in the tissue is dependent on the spacing between skin and electrodes (more distance

between the pads is thought to provide deeper penetration) (Prentice & Draper 2001). The use of one air spaced and one pad electrode is possible and at times provides an advantageous arrangement.

Electrode arrangement

With conductive techniques, electrodes can be positioned in a contraplanar, coplanar, longitudinal or crossfire arrangement. In contraplanar, the electrodes are placed opposite to each other on either side of the treated area. The distance between the skin and the electrodes can be symmetrical if an even field is desirable, or the electrodes can be positioned with uneven distances if the aim is to concentrate the field on one side of the treated area (Scott 2002, Wadsworth & Chanmugam 1983). To achieve heterogenous heating, it is considered important that the centre of the electrodes is centred with the centre of the treated area (Garret 2000, He et al 2005). Figure 10.5 illustrates a contraplanar air-spaced electrode arrangement at the knee.

Electrodes can also be positioned in a coplanar arrangement (Fig. 10.6), where both electrodes are placed on the same aspect of the treated area. For safety reasons, the distance between the two electrodes needs to be more than the sum of skin electrode distance in order to result in better field distribution. Although this technique produces a more superficial field, the depth of the field can be increased by increasing the distance between the two electrodes (Martin et al 1991).

Other electrode arrangements include the longitudinal application, when the electrodes are

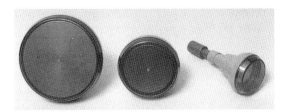

Figure 10.3 Air spaced electrodes of different sizes in clinical use.

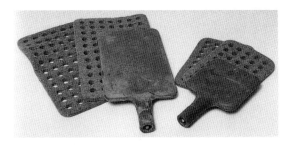

Figure 10.4 Flexible (rubber encased metal) electrodes and felt spacers.

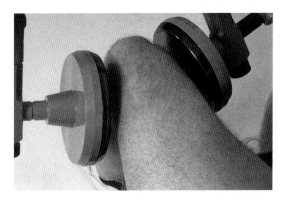

Figure 10.5 Contraplanar application using air-spaced electrodes.

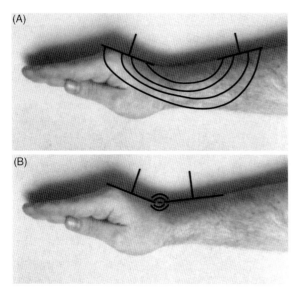

Figure 10.6 Coplanar electrode placement illustrating correct (A) and incorrect (B) electrode spacing.

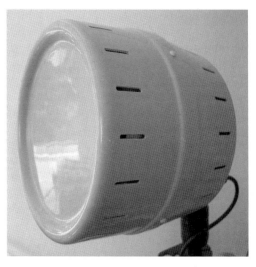

Figure 10.7 Monode (drum) type applicator for use with continuous or pulsed shortwave modes.

placed at either end of a limb parallel to the alignment of the tissues and the crossfire technique, when the electrodes are placed diagonally over the treated tissue for half the time and are then changed to the other diagonal for the rest of the time. Historically, this latter technique was used to treat cavities containing air, such as sinuses and the uterus (Forster & Palastanga 1985).

Electrode size

The size of the applicators is considered an important factor in determining the strength of the field in the tissues. The use of two electrodes of similar size results in uniform distribution of the field in the tissues. Using electrodes of different sizes, however, leads to the accumulation of the field on the side of the smaller electrode (Tzima & Martin 1994). Hand (1990) notes that applicators act as antennae for coupling the power to the tissues. When small applicators are used (small in relation to the other electrode or in relation to the size of the treated area) they act as poor radiators, decreasing the intensity of the field as the distance increases. This is believed to cause excessive heating at the superficial layers and reduction in the depth of penetration (Hand 1990).

INDUCTIVE METHOD

Inductive SWT can be applied to the tissues by means of either a drum or a cable electrode (Prentice & Draper 2001, Watson 2006). The inductive method produces predominantly an H field via a cable that is either wrapped around the extremity or coiled inside an electrode housing. The use of the monode or drum applicator has become the clinical norm in current practice, and the cable application is rarely employed. Unlike the conductive technique, the patient is not part of the circuit and the electrodes are placed perpendicular to the part to be treated (monode, circuplode) or wrapped around it (cable) (Hand 1990). A modern monode applicator is illustrated in Figure 10.7. Generation of the alternating high-frequency current in the cable produces an H field in the tissues, which is set up at right-angles to the direction of current flow (Scott 2002). The amount of E field emission from the monode-type electrodes is usually limited by using a Faradic screen. The strength of the H field is determined by the rate at which the current alternates and by the number of coils of the conducting wire contained within a conductor (Hand 1990).

The generated H field induces a secondary current in the tissues known as an eddy current (which consists of small circular E fields). Heat is generated as a result of the friction between eddy currents and intermolecular vibration of the tissue. It is believed that the effect of the H field produced by the inductive technique acts as a carrier for the eddy current, which acts as the main element responsible for the physiological effect gained during the application (Scott 2002). This form of heating is not associated with strong sensory stimulation as there is less superficial (skin and fat) heating and, as such, the heat may not be as obvious to the patient as in the capacitive application (Prentice & Draper 2001).

The inductive application is believed to result in selective energy absorption and heating. Tissues with a high electrolyte content and low impedance, such as muscle and blood, will be heated to a greater extent with the superficial layers such as skin and fat being minimally affected (Lehmann & DeLateur 1990, Watson 2006). Ward (1980) argues that with an inductive application there will be both superficial and deep heating. Structures such as blood and muscles will be heated as they have high dielectric content; however, the superficial fat layer will also be heated because fat is an inhomogeneous structure and usually incorporates areas of high conductivity found in the small blood and lymphatic vessels. These tissues lack an efficient way of dissipating heat and, as such, tend to absorb heat and concentrate it in the small blood vessels. Hand (1990) also argues that when the separation between the electrode and tissue is less than 3 cm, high intensities of the power are absorbed by the fat layer. However, by increasing this distance the field is expected to penetrate up to a depth of 4 cm. Although this study is one of the few that discussed the exact distance between inductive electrode and the tissues, it does not clearly state whether these findings were based on experimentation or on a theoretical model. Draper et al (1999) were able to demonstrate an increase in intramuscular temperature of up to 4°C using inductive electrodes. The inductive application (drum or cable method) can be employed with continuous or pulsed shortwave modes, although the most common combination in current practice is to use the drum applicator with shortwave in pulsed mode.

Drum electrode

The drum is composed of one or more monoplanar coils (sometimes referred to as a 'pancake'

arrangement) encased inside a plastic housing (see Fig. 10.7). The applicator has the advantage of being very straightforward to set up, although the disadvantage with this technique is that the drum electrode is less compliant with the skin contour. Maximum penetration with this technique is believed to be 3 cm, given that the subcutaneous fat layer does not exceed 2 cm. This is believed to be caused by the distortion of the field when it passes the fat layer and crosses the fat–muscle interface, which is expected to lead to unwanted increase in temperature in the fat layer (Prentice & Draper 2001, Low & Reed 2000, Ward 1980). Examining seven types of applicators, Lehmann et al (1983) demonstrated (using human tissue substitute substances) that the specific absorption rate (SAR) ratio of muscle to fat heating with inductive electrodes could vary between 0.4 and 2.7 : 1.

Cable electrode

The cable is a thick, insulated wire with plugs on either end. It can be wrapped in a pancake arrangement and placed over the treated area or it can be wrapped around the extremity. It has the advantage of fitting the contour of the body, unlike air-space or drum electrodes. A distance of at least 1 cm should be kept between the skin and the electrode, and a distance of about 5 cm should be kept between the turns of the cable to prevent overheating (Prentice & Draper 2001). The cable application method is rarely employed in current clinical practice, the drum or monode applicator being considered more efficient to set up and thus more effective.

It is of interest to know that most of the theories explaining the field distribution under the various types of electrode, their depth of penetration, and the possible approaches for arrangements remain theoretical, with little supportive researched evidence. Although these beliefs are widely accepted, further research is warranted, especially with regards the actual penetration depths achieved with these various fields and applicators.

HEAT PRODUCTION WITH SHORTWAVE THERAPY

Shortwave therapy can be employed in either thermal or 'non-thermal' modes: the use of continuous

SWT is always considered to be thermal, whereas pulsed SWT can bring about thermal or non-thermal effects. The rise in tissue temperature during the application of SWT depends on the SAR, which is the rate at which energy is absorbed by a known mass of tissue and is calculated in units of watts per kilogram (W/kg). SAR is a function of tissue conductivity and the electrical field magnitude. Tissue conductivity reflects the ease with which an electric field can be set up in the tissue. The SAR, and therefore the heating produced by SWT, is dependent upon the electrical properties of tissue within the electromagnetic field (Kloth & Ziskin 1996).

Electric field energy will concentrate in tissues with the greatest conductivity. It is accepted that tissues with high dielectric content, such as muscle and blood, are also good conductors of the current as they have the ability to absorb more energy and dissipate the resulting heat more efficiently (Scott 2002). Fatty tissues, on the other hand, have low dielectric constant and low conductivity (Ward 1980) and also tend to heat up, albeit for different reasons. Some have explained this by poor vascularity and the lack of thermoregulatory mechanism in the fatty layer (Wadsworth & Chanmugam 1983), whereas others suggest that it is the small blood vessels spread throughout the fatty layer that are responsible for retaining heat and the build-up of temperatures (Ward 1980). These views remain largely theoretical, with little directly supportive evidence.

It is accepted that CSWT application is always associated with heat production in the tissues unless applied at exceptionally low power levels. Pulsed-mode shortwave can be employed in a 'thermal' or 'non-thermal' fashion with the applied mean power (MP) being the main determinant. The thermal mode of PSWT can be achieved by using longer PD and high PRR. The non-thermal mode is achieved when short pulses are interposed by long interpulse periods. This is not strictly a 'non-thermal' mode, but that there is no net increase in temperature (ΔT) as the heat gained during the 'on phase' is dissipated by the circulating blood during the interpulse period (Scott 2002, Watson 2006). When long-duration treatments are applied with these parameters, it is possible that an accumulative heating effect may still be achieved. The differences between thermal and non-thermal effects of therapy are further considered in Chapter 8.

Heat generated in the tissues is the product of tissue resistance and current density as explained in equation 10.3 (Prentice & Draper 2001):

$$\text{Heating} = \text{Current density}^2 \times \text{Resistance} \quad (10.3)$$

Human tissues contain ions, polar molecules and non-charged molecules. Heat can be produced as a result of the oscillation of charged molecules such as protein and ions about a mean position along the lines of the E forces that are created by the EMF. The oscillation and friction converts the molecule kinetic energy to heat.

The second type of molecule, e.g. water, some proteins and hormones, possesses permanent electric dipoles. Normally, these dipoles are randomly arranged. Under the influence of an E field, these dipolar molecules undergo polarization and align themselves to the opposite charged pole of the E field. The alternating nature of the field causes the dipoles to rotate and collide, and the friction between these dipoles generates heat. The extent of this alignment is determined by the strength of the field (Hand 1990). Additionally, each of these polar molecules possesses a weak field of its own, extending from the positive to the negative pole and, when the substance is under the influence of the E field, the net result of these fields governs the electric properties of the matter. Dipolar molecules produce a mixture of real and displacement currents. Real current refers to the current that develops in the tissues and determines the electrical properties and heat production in a matter (Ward 1980) as opposed to the displacement current, which does not play a great role in the electrical properties of a matter (Scott 2002).

The third type of molecule is the non-charged molecule. The E field affects non-charged molecules by polarizing and distorting their electron cloud fields. Movement of the non-charged molecules in response to the E field results in displacement currents and as such contributes the least to heat production in the tissues, unlike the movement of charged molecules, which could result in real current. This is because the induced dipoles are not as strong as natural dipoles and tend to lose their properties as soon as the E field is removed (Delpizzo & Joyner 1987, Durney & Christensen 2000, Ward 1980).

Adey (1988) argues that EM energy absorbed by the tissues will always result in internal thermal energy regardless of the mode of application. The energy delivered to the tissues increases the kinetic energy of the molecules, resulting in random ionic movement. Atoms become excited and move into higher levels of energy, releasing photons of EMF, which may be transferred to other atoms or changed into heat (Low & Reed 2000, Scott 2002). Although no ΔT is detected externally on the skin, non-uniform heating occurs and microthermal effects are still occurring at the cellular level. However, these effects are believed to be caused by E rather than H fields (Durney & Christensen 2000).

Some argue that tissues could be irradiated with PSWT and that collision and friction of molecules could still be occurring; however, the proportion of E current converted into heat would be very slight and no real current is initiated in the tissues (Ward 1980), resulting in thermal agitation (Foster 1997), which lasts for the time of the 'pulse on' period (Michaelson & Elson 1996, Tenforde 1996). It could be added that even with tissues containing high dielectric molecules, under the influence of the E field it is the extent of dipolar alignment to the E field that determines the amount of heat produced, and this is dependent on the strength of the applied current and the amount of E field absorbed by these molecules (Hand 1990), which is governed by the proportion of displacement to real current that determines whether a given application is thermal or not. Longer treatment durations are expected to result in more energy delivered to the tissues, higher current densities, and a possibility of heat build-up compared to applications with short durations. It has not been customary so far to describe PSWT treatment doses in terms of power concentration (W/cm^2), although it has been suggested (as with ultrasound) that this may in fact be the most appropriate term.

The changes in the field distribution in response to implanted metal in the tissues has been considered in detail by Virtanen et al (2006) and the clinical use of PSWT with metal implants is discussed by Seiger and Draper (2006).

MECHANISMS OF ACTION

It is believed that the response of biological systems to EM energy could be the result of either thermal or 'athermal' effects. The heat developing in the tissues after 20 minutes of application of SWT was found to peak at 15 minutes, after which it levelled off for 5 minutes and then started to decline slowly at a rate of around 1° per 5 minutes (Draper et al 1999, Valtonen et al 1973). Therapeutically, a temperature increase of more than 1°C is useful for mild inflammation and an increase between 2 and 3°C is helpful in reducing pain and muscle spasm, whereas an increase of 3–4°C is necessary to cause changes in tissue extensibility (Lehmann 1990, Prentice & Draper 2001). The demonstrated changes in cell behaviour were found to be reversible immediately on termination of application if the increase in temperature was less than 1°C (Michaelson & Elson 1996, Tenforde 1996).

The mechanism of response to EM energy is thought to occur at several sites within the cell. One of the main sites for interaction between the applied energy and biological tissues is thought to be the cell membrane. It is suggested that EM energy changes the rate of opening and the formation of ion channels across the protein bilayer found in the cell membrane (Cleary 1997). This changes the charged ion build-up at the surface and the way new molecules are bound to the surface (Polk & Postow 1996). Cations such as Na^+ and K^+ leak from inside the cell to the extracellular fluid under the influence of the energy (Cleary 1997), altering the intracellular and extracellular environments (Adey 1988). It is also expected that these changes might restore ion, oxygen and nutrient concentrations to a more balanced state (Markov & Colbert 2000). It is believed that the E field could change membrane selectivity to ions hence altering ion transport across the membrane (Hand 1990).

Whereas the response of the nucleus to exogenous EM energy is governed by the presence of ions such as Ca^{2+} (Low & Reed 2000), the mitochondria are thought to change cell function by altering the rate of cell metabolism (Cleary 1997). Pope et al (1989) demonstrated that the interior of the cell reacts to the applied current by reducing mitochondrion size, increasing endoplasmic reticulum size, decreasing the cell lipid size, migration of lipid to cell poles and an increase in activity of ATPase. The size of the response was seen to correlate with the amount of energy delivered to the cell. For example, the reaction was higher with PD 400 μs, PRR 400 pps, intensity 1, for 10 minutes than with PD 400 μs, PRR 80 pps, intensity 4, duration 10 minutes.

Microtubules are dipoles and are expected to respond to the alternating E field by rotating and colliding, thereby producing heat (Charman 1990).

All the above changes are expected to revert the electrical potential of the diseased cell, correct the endogenous abnormalities and restore normal cell function (Chapter 3; Nordenstorm 1983). SWT coupling to endogenous fields is believed to alter physiological processes (Ward 1980).

It is thought that the vasodilatation observed with SWT occurs as a result of the accumulation of waste products or the direct stimulation of smooth muscles of the vessels in response to heat (Ward 1980). Blood vessels are also thought to dilate in response to the stimulation of sensory nerve endings at the skin surface as a result of heat production, initiating an axon reflex (Kitchen 2002). With vasodilatation, there may be a decrease in blood viscosity to ease the flow of blood.

Increase in blood flow is proportional to the gradual increase of energy, as demonstrated by Erdmann (1960), who examined the effect of radiating the epigastrium on the blood flow in the feet of 20 adults. Erdmann recorded a noticeable increase in blood flow, which started to increase in the first 8 minutes and reached a plateau within 35 minutes of application. Blood flow readings returned to baseline by 30 minutes post treatment. The increase in temperature was 2°C in the foot and ranged between 0.5 and 1.5°C under the treatment head. However, this increase was not associated with change in core temperature. These results were further supported by Morrissey (1966).

The increased amount of circulating blood and the accompanying thermal changes in and around the cell was found to be effective in speeding the recovery of open wounds, increasing tissue extensibility, decreasing oedema and haematoma, and relieving inflammation, joint stiffness and pain.

THERAPEUTIC EFFECTS OF SHORTWAVE THERAPIES

A reasonable amount of research has been published relating to the use of both continuous and pulsed SWT in various clinical areas. It is interesting to note that very little was published during the 1990s but the publication rate appears to have increased in more recent years (Shields et al 2001). There is a degree of ambiguity in the literature concerning the differences between pulsed electromagnetic fields (PEMFs) and pulsed shortwave therapy (PSWT), and the extensive literature concerning PEMFs is not reviewed here. It remains to be seen whether there is, or is not, a direct correlation between these two different forms of intervention. Treatment investigations involving SWT is divided up into several clinical topic areas in this section.

PAIN

Shortwave therapy can be used to relieve pain and although the evidence is largely poor in quality, reducing pain has been accepted widely to be one of the most widely employed clinical effects of SWT (Al Mandeel & Watson 2006). Reduction of pain could occur as a result of the inhibition of sensory impulse transmission, which may lead to a sedative effect in the treated area. Inflammatory pain is expected to reduce as a result of the vasodilatation and absorption of the exudates accumulating in the tissues (Ward 1980). The pain resulting from muscle spasm could decrease as a consequence of vasodilatation and the removal of excess lactic acid and other metabolic products in the muscle that cause muscle soreness (Kitchen 2002).

Several studies have investigated the therapeutic effects of SWT on pain. Studies have looked at pelvic pain, temporomandibular pain, back pain and pain at trigger points. Some studies were in favour of PSWT (Cheing et al 2005, Foley-Nolan et al 1992, Jorgensen et al 1994, McCray & Patton 1984, Varcaccio-Garofalo et al 1995), others were in favour of CSWT (Gibson et al 1985, Jan et al 2006, Nwuga 1982), others have found PSWT to be better than CSWT (Watgstaff et al 1986), and still others have found no significant difference between PSWT and laser or CSWT, although findings were better than for placebo (Gray et al 1994, Reed et al 1987).

FRACTURE

Using PSWT intensity 3, PRR 35 pps, 300 maximum pulse power, for 30 minutes on fracture of the neck of humerus, Livesley et al (1992) showed no significant difference between active and placebo groups.

A substantial volume of work relates to the application of pulsed EM fields to stimulate or accelerate fracture repair but a considerable proportion of this research does not utilize SWT applications and is beyond the primary remit of this chapter. Those with an interest in this field should consult Benazzo et al 1995, Hinsenkamp et al 1985, Livesley et al 1992, Thawer 1999 and Xu et al 1999. Further evidence regarding the specific use of SWT (in continuous or pulsed mode) is clearly needed.

PERIPHERAL NERVE REPAIR

The effect of SWT on nerves is an under-researched area, and whereas the increase in the rate of nerve regeneration has been demonstrated in animal studies, human studies are lacking. Wilson and Jagadeesh (1976) demonstrated that SWT was shown to aid the regeneration of nerves. In a rat nerve injury model, nerve conduction returned after 30 days of treatment compared to controls, which showed only a flicker of response after 60 days. Histological examination showed less fibrosis and scarring in the treated group. Additionally, large-diameter fibres were slower than small fibres in sprouting. Similar results were obtained by Raji and Bowden (1983), Raji (1984) and Zienowicz et al (1991). SWT was also shown to increase nerve conduction velocity in ulnar and median nerves (Abramson et al 1966, Currier & Nelson 1969). These outcomes, although promising, identify the need for quality investigations in human subjects prior to clinical acceptance of the technique.

RHEUMATOLOGY

In general, the findings of the studies are in favour of positive outcome, with the majority reporting improvement in function and reduction in pain (Ganguly et al 1996. Jan & Lai 1991, Klaber-Moffett et al 1996, Laufer et al 2005, Leclaire & Bourgouin 1991, Quirk et al 1985). In studies where PSWT was compared to other interventions, it was found to be more effective than placebo (Klaber-Moffett

et al 1996, Quirk et al 1985) and no better than interferential or ultrasound (US), exercise and stretching (Ganguly et al 1996, Jan & Lai 1991, Leclaire & Bourgouin 1991, Quirk et al 1985, Svarcova et al 1988) and less effective than manual mobilization (Guler & Kozanoglu 2004).

The thermal mode of SWT was found to reduce the viscosity of the synovial fluid (Jan et al 2006) and hence to decrease joint stiffness (Scott 2002, Yung et al 1986) and improve function. Unusually, the study by Jan et al (2006) evaluated the effectiveness of CSWT using a cable induction method in patients with osteoarthritis (OA) of the knee. Using a control group design, both the thickness of the knee synovium and pain were found to be significantly reduced following a programme of 10 SWT treatment sessions. The study by Callaghan et al (2005) compared the effectiveness of low dose (10 W), high dose (20 W) or placebo PSWT in a group of patients with OA of the knee. The outcome measures were related primarily to the inflammatory state of the tissue, and there was no significant beneficial outcome in any of the groups. It was concluded that PSWD used in this context did not have an 'anti-inflammatory' effect.

The pulsed mode of SWT can also be used to decrease inflammation associated with the flare-up stage of disease. PSWT is believed to aid the resolution of inflammation by increasing phagocytosis (Cameron et al 1999), increasing the number of white blood cells and antibodies that help reinforce body defence mechanisms, remove noxious toxins and improve oxygenation (Goldin et al 1981, Wadsworth & Chanmugam 1983). Evidence to support these claims was provided by Hill et al (2001), who demonstrated that there was a significant increase in fibroblast number after 10 minutes, PSWT with MP of 48 W applied twice daily. Cell proliferation has also been found to be time and energy dependent. This means that research findings on certain parameters cannot simply be extrapolated to other settings. Research results in this area are of mixed outcome. Laufer et al (2005) concluded that PSWT (comparing high, thermal dose, low, athermal dose and placebo) was of no therapeutic value in that pain scores improved in all groups and there were no significant differences across a range of other outcome measures. A recent review by Marks and van

Nguyen (2005) concluded from the RCT evidence considered that the continuing use of pulsed electromagnetic field applications for patients with OA of the knee was justified even though further research was needed to clarify dose and other treatment parameters.

MUSCULOSKELETAL

SWT was found to be effective in speeding the recovery of soft tissue injuries by increasing the activity of fibroblasts and the stimulation of ATP and protein synthesis (Cameron et al 1999), which may increase in the rate of collagen deposition (Low & Reed 2000).

SWT can increase tendon extensibility and improve muscle performance when used in the thermal mode as it can lead to elongation of collagenous structures and mobilization of scars, which will eventually improve flexibility, isometric strength and increase range of motion if the application is accompanied by stretching (Draper et al 2002, 2004, Evans et al 2002, Mucha 2005, Peres et al 2002). Robertson et al (2005) demonstrated the beneficial effects of a deep-heating-type treatment (using CSWT, capacitive method) on tissue extensibility in the calf and ankle, with the benefits being greater than those achieved with a superficial heat (hot pack) or no intervention, whereas Draper et al (2004) demonstrated significant benefit when using PSWT (monode applicator) to heat the hamstrings.

Dziedzic et al (2005) compared pulsed mode shortwave, manual therapy and advice with exercise in a patient group presenting with non-specific neck disorders. All patients received advice and exercise. In addition, one group was treated with manual therapy and one with PSWT. Although patients in all groups improved significantly, there were no significant differences for any of the outcome measures between groups, and the authors conclude that the addition of PSWT or manual therapy for this patient group is not justified.

The use of SWT in the pulsed mode can aid the resolution of haematomas and oedema by increasing the rate of interstitial fluid drainage (Goat 1989) and increasing venous return (Golden et al 1981, Wadsworth & Chanmugam 1983). Buzzard et al (2003) compared PSWT (26 Hz, 200 μs, twice daily for 15 minutes) and ice therapy (Cryocuff adjusted to 30 mmHg six times a day for 20 minutes) on oedema following calcaneal fractures. Although no control group was used and no reliability measurements were mentioned, the authors reported both modalities to be effective, with neither modality demonstrating significant superiority.

Subdeltoid bursitis

Early reports on the use of PSWT for soft tissue injury were published by Ginsberg (1961). The outcome of conditions treated over a period of 15 years were collated and analysed. Ninety-four subjects were treated with PRR 600 Hz, intensity 6 for 10 minutes at the affected site and another 10 minutes at PRR 400 Hz intensity 4 directed at the liver and the adrenals. Findings were encouraging, in that 86 of those subjects had partial to complete recovery with X-ray signs of Ca^{2+} reabsorption.

Ankle sprain

Pulsed SWT was found to be effective for ankle sprain (Barclay et al 1983, Barker et al 1985, McGill 1988, Pennington et al 1993, Santiesteban & Grant 1985, Wilson 1972, 1974), and better than CSWT (Wilson et al 1972). However, studies providing evidence on PSWT effectiveness are old and need to be replicated with better methodology.

Hand injuries

Barclay et al (1983) conducted a study on 230 patients complaining of hand and thumb injury. PSWT was delivered using a monode applicator with PP 975 W for 2½ hours daily. Patients in both the control and the active group received conventional treatment, which was not fully described. Findings were in favour of PSWT as the results have shown it to relieve pain, reduce swelling, and improve function in patients who have sustained a hand injury in the last 36 hours.

WOUND HEALING

Most of the studies identified examined the effect of PSWT, as opposed to CSWT, on wound healing. Evidence on the interaction between experimental wound healing and SWT in animals has shown conflicting results. Brown and Baker (1987), Constable et al (1971) and Krag et al (1979) found PSWT to be ineffective; Basal et al (1990) and Vanharanta et al (1982) have shown CSWT to be effective by histochemical and histoenzymic findings and the time to reach complete wound healing. PSWT was shown to be useful by Pope et al (1989), Ragi and Bowden (1983) and Fenn (1969).

Cell-based laboratory studies provide useful evidence regarding PSWT effectiveness. Badea et al (1993) investigated the effect of PSWT irradiation on the rate of microbial growth in a sample of cells prepared in the laboratory. The experiment was conducted over several stages and showed that PSWT interaction with the cell culture was most intensive at a narrow window of between 60 and 90 minutes, but not at 30 minutes. It was also reported that the application of PSWT at maximum setting for 30 minutes did not result in adverse reactions. A time/intensity window of effectiveness (see Chapter 1) was also demonstrated by Hill et al (2001), who compared different MPs (1, 3, 4, 8, 12, 48 W) and found that the best results were obtained with MP 12 W, and that when the MP delivered was kept constant (6 W) and other parameters were changed (100 μs/400 Hz; 200 μs/ 200 Hz; 400 μs/100 Hz) with four exposure times (5, 10, 15, and 20 minutes), it was found that cell proliferation varied considerably with different exposure times. The highest level of proliferation was seen with 5 minutes, application compared to longer treatments.

Skin graft

Goldin et al (1981) compared the effect of PSWT (Diapulse, 30 minutes, 400 pps, 65 μs, PP 975 W) on the rate of skin graft healing in a placebo group. Although the rationale for using the above-mentioned parameters was not reported, and despite the limited statistical analysis of the findings, the study demonstrated that PSWT does have a potential role in aiding the healing of wounds.

Skin ulcers and pressure sores

A limited number of research papers were located discussing the interaction between PSWT and pressure sores. PSWT was effective in reducing skin ulcer size (Itoh et al 1991), although the improvement was governed by the method of application (Salzberg et al 1995) and active treatment was found to be better than placebo (Comorosan et al 1993).

Itoh et al (1991) reported PSWT (600 Hz, power 6, for 30 minutes twice daily with approximately 8 hours in between applications) to increase the rate of healing of stage II and stage III ulcers. However, the number of subjects in each group was small and there was no control group, which makes it difficult to rule out the effect of natural recovery on the improvement levels obtained.

In a double-blind study, Todd et al (1991) investigated the effects of PSWT on 19 patients with resistant varicose ulcers. Although the reporting of the treatment dose was incomplete, the results were in favour of the active group. There was no significant difference between active and placebo PSWT in girth measurement, pain level and the presence of infection. However, it could be argued that the difference in mean ulcer size between groups at baseline (the treatment group had significantly larger ulcers at T = 0) might have been responsible for the statistically non-significant results.

In later research by Comorosan et al (1993), patients were randomly assigned into control, placebo and treatment groups (Diapulse, local application on site of ulcer: 600 pps, 30 minutes, intensity 6 twice a day; hepatic application: 400 pps, intensity 4, 20 minutes, 1/day). The PSWT group showed good to excellent results with complete healing achieved between 1 and 4 weeks for stage II and between 2 and 8 weeks for stage III ulcers in all patients. These results were accompanied by the disappearance of wound exudate after 48–72 hours. Although the authors have reported the intensity they used with their patients (4 and 6) the numbers are meaningless unless other parameters such as the brand of the PSWT machine, PP and MP are reported.

Salzberg et al (1995) provided data in broad agreement with these results when they examined the effect of PSWT on 30 spinal-cord-injured patients with skin ulcers. Patients were stratified according to the stage of the ulcer. The active group of stage II ulcer demonstrated better results than placebo (recovery of active group 84%, recovery of placebo group 40%), with a shorter duration needed to achieve recovery. However, patients with stage II ulcers were not compatible at baseline as most patients with large ulcers were in the active group and only one large ulcer was in the placebo group. In both groups, the site of the ulcer was not mentioned and the treatment parameters were not fully reported.

There were only 10 patients in the grade III sample, which was further divided into placebo and active groups.

Seaborne et al (1996) examined the effects of non-thermal application of PSWT on pressure sores (Curapuls 419 with PD fixed at 400 μs, and PP 700 W). Two groups were given PRR 20 pps, MP 5.6 W using either capacitive or inductive electrodes; the same was done with the remaining two groups but the treatment combinations were changed to PRR 110 pps, MP 30.8 W. The E field was delivered via a coplanar technique using air space electrodes, whereas H-field treatment was delivered using a circuplode. Routine dressing care was maintained throughout the study. All treatments were for 20 minutes twice a day for 2 weeks. All four protocols showed reduction in the size of the ulcer, with significant difference between the groups showing in weeks 4 and 5. Findings were better with H field 5.6 W, then by E field 5.6 W, then H field 30.8 W; least effective was E 30.8 W. It is difficult to conclude, however, that the improvement was related only to the PSWT treatment.

It has been proposed that SWT may assist healing by bringing about changes in the local nervous system rather than by cell activity alone. It is plausible that changes in nerve supply to the vessels in the damaged area have a direct effect on the redistribution of blood to the tissues. Moreover, SWT is believed to activate the sodium pump, resulting in the repolarizing of the depolarized cells in the injured area, which might restore the ionic level of the cell membrane to the preinjured state (Scott 2002). These proposed mechanisms need to be validated before being accepted as a confirmed mechanism in this context. On balance, and given the shortcomings of the research, the literature is in favour of using PSWT on pressure sores, with the studies generally demonstrating positive outcomes.

Postoperative wound healing

Several research papers have examined the effect of SWT on postoperative wound healing. All studies reported reduction in pain, swelling, oedema and an enhanced rate of healing. Aronofsky (1971) examined the effect of PSWT on dental wounds. The treatment was delivered in two parts using a Diapulse (15 minutes, 600 pps, intensity 6), administered 24 hours prior to surgery and for another 15 minutes immediately before surgery. The operated site was then irradiated with PSWT for 10 minutes postsurgery on the same dose and then again, at 24, 48, and 72 hours postsurgery; substantial improvements were reported.

A double-blind trial by Bentall and Eckstein (1975) examined the efficacy of PSWT in relation to children undergoing orchidopexy. Subjects underwent either active or sham PSWT treatment. PSWT was applied using Diapulse locally (550 pps, intensity 5, 20 minutes), followed by epigastric application (500 pps, intensity 4, 10 minutes). Findings revealed that both direct measurement of circumference and other subjective readings demonstrated increase in the speed of healing along with a quick return to normal appearance. However, no control group was used and it would be interesting to gauge the level of recovery to the natural process of recovery.

The effect of active and placebo PSWT on wound healing was investigated by Santiesteban and Grant in 1985. PSWT was delivered twice (immediately after surgery, and 4 hours post first application) for 30 minutes, 95 μs, power 12 (120 PP), 700 pps. The PSWT group consumed fewer drugs and their length of hospital stay was shorter than for the placebo group. Even with the use of a placebo group, it is difficult to confirm the effects being solely attributed to the PSWT intervention as both groups were exposed to continuing 'traditional' treatment.

Grant et al (1989) investigated the effect of PSWT on soft-tissue injury by comparing the rate of recovery of perineal trauma after childbirth using PSWT (100 pps, 65 μs for 10 minutes), ultrasound or a sham intervention. Therapy was started 12 hours after delivery and continued for up to 3 days. There was no significant difference between the groups immediately, at 10 days, or at 3 months post treatment, although it has been argued that the outcome measures employed were subjective and may not be sensitive in detecting real clinical change.

Arghiropol et al (1992) used a local PSWT (Diapulse) application for a period of 15 minutes on 400 pps, intensity 4 followed by hepatic application (600 pps, intensity 6, 30 minutes) to aid wound healing. Increase in fibronectin concentration was observed as an indication of the increase in the rate of wound healing.

OTHER CLINICAL PROBLEMS

Lightwood (1989) reported positive outcomes of PSWT with post operative soft tissue conditions, rheumatoid arthritis (RA), OA, pain, back pain, delayed bone healing and even spina bifida and stroke. The application was unusual in that rather than the more usual treatment time (of up to 30 minutes), treatments lasted for a minimum of 1 hour and were usually repeated several times a day. A lack of reported treatment parameters makes it difficult to evaluate these findings fully, but they may be consistent with a proposition by Low (1995) that the duration of the treatment directly affects the delivered energy and thus may in fact constitute a critical parameter.

Barker et al (1985) demonstrated the possibility of using PSWT (12 W) post abdominal surgery to stimulate peristalsis and aid the return of normal bowel sounds. Although the outcome was positive, the authors reported using an athermal mode of PSWT and thus the long duration of application might have been responsible for developing heat in the tissues, which may have been responsible for lack of significant results.

Keick et al (1994) compared the effect of laser and SWT on dry eye syndrome and reported increased tear flow with both modalities despite SWT being superior.

CLINICAL DECISION MAKING WITH SHORTWAVE THERAPY

When considering the available literature, an area that continues to generate considerable debate is the unresolved issue about SWT dosage. Considerable confusion exists between clinicians with respect to the application of SWT owing to the wide range and the variety of methods available for setting the treatment parameters.

There is a growing emphasis on basing clinical decisions on the best available evidence. Randomized clinical trials (RCTs) have been viewed as the highest level of evidence in terms of their ability to answer clinical questions (Gray 1997). However, while acknowledging the insights into electrotherapy practice offered by the available studies, the available literature contributes very little to resolve this dispute, with the majority of studies being not controlled or lacking important reporting such as the mode of application (whether PSWT or CSWT) or treatment protocols, absence of dose reporting and power setting (Table 10.2).

The choice of dose when applying CSWT and PSWT tends to follow the general principle of using a lower dose for more acute conditions and a higher dose for chronic conditions (van der Esch & Hoogland 1991, Watson 2006). To give a patient a low dose of PSWT, the pulse repetition rate, the pulse duration and the peak pulse power should be in the lower part of the available range. If the intention is to apply a high dose of PSWT, the above variables should be in the upper range or at their maximum. However, the same mean power of PSWT can be delivered by using different combinations of the above variables combining low and high variables.

Some of the newer SWT machines are fitted with preset programmes that can be used as guidelines during practice. Although these programmes and automated clinical recommendations are potentially of value, they do not always directly relate to the published evidence, and some caution needs to be employed in their use without critical evaluation.

THE USE OF THERMAL SENSATION FOR ASSESSING SHORTWAVE THERAPY DOSE

Skin testing has historically been a prerequisite prior to the application of any thermal modality,

Table 10.2 Example of studies conducted to study the effect of SWT on pain

Study	PSWT make	PP (Watts)	MP (Watts)	PD (μs)	PF (pps)	Intensity	Time (min)	Type of electrode
McCray and Patton, 1984	Magnotherm							Inductor coil
Wagstaff et al, 1986	Curapuls	700 300	23.2 23.4		82 200		15	Circuplode
Aronofsky, 1971	Diapulse	975	65		600	6	15	
Gray et al, 1994	Megapulse			60	100		20	
Jorgensen et al, 1994							15–30	
Varcaccio-Garofalo et al, 1995	Thelft							

The shaded area represents unreported treatment parameters.
MP, mean power; PD, pulse duration; PF, pulse frequency; PP, peak power.

including shortwave therapies. A standard method of determining dose is to ask the patient to report thermal sensation in response to a locally applied hot and cold source (commonly test tubes filled with water). However, it is questionable whether the skin is a reliable source for monitoring changes in temperature (Elder et al 1989). Patient statements of thermal sensation are reports of temperature in the skin and not in deeper tissues. Odia and Aigbogun (1988) extended the argument that certain areas of the body were more sensitive to changes in temperature than others because individuals were more accurate in reporting increases in the temperature of the facial skin than in the skin of the lower limb. Animal studies have shown that cells can be damaged if the tissue temperature exceeded 42°C (Elder et al 1989), which was below the threshold of thermally induced pain (45°C) in humans. Thus, when a patient is asked to report thermal sensation there is a possibility of high levels of heat and cell damage occurring in body areas with relatively low numbers of thermal receptors present in deeper tissue (Delpizzo & Joyner 1987). Extra care should be taken when the thermal sensory discrimination of the patient is less than optimum owing to pathology or to anatomical site.

This is particularly relevant where the energy absorbed in the superficial tissue may be lower than that absorbed in deep tissue as in inductive application (see the section above). The use of doses above this level of 'mild sensation' may have potentially detrimental effects. At the present time, and until more accurate methods of assessing treatment dose are established, therapists should be aware of the potential risk of causing thermal tissue damage and ensure that the maximum dose that a patient receives causes only a mild sensation of warmth.

Bricknell and Watson (1995) have demonstrated a definite heat perception with PSWT that was felt after 7 minutes of exposure with MP of 10.8 W. Murray and Kitchen (2000) have shown that definite thermal sensation can be experienced if the MP is 21.19 ± 8.27 W. Two other unpublished studies have examined the relationship between detectable and definite thermal sensation (see: http://www.electrotherapy.org). McMahon and Watson examined the effect of applying 400 μs, 400 pps, MP of 10.82 W on the time it takes subjects to report thermal sensation. It was reported that subjects took 104 ± 65 seconds to reach possible thermal sensation and 179 ± 107 seconds to reach definite perception. The other study (by Watson & Evans), examined the time it took for 20 non-injured subjects to report possible and definite thermal sensation using two different pulse parameter combinations providing the same MP. The doses used were 400 µs, 800 pps, MP 12 W, and 100 µs, 800 pps, MP 12 W. Only eight out of 20 subjects reported any heat sensation at either dose. Morrissey (1966) has demonstrated that, with an MP of 40 W, there was no statistical significant increase in measured skin temperature. Wadsworth and Chanmugam (1983) suggest the thermal effects could occur when the mean power is greater than 25 W. The work by Al-Mandeel (2004) has shown that with MP of 24 W only 11 subjects reported thermal sensation out of 31 healthy subjects despite the increase in skin temperature that ranged between 1.9 and 1.1°C. There is no doubt, therefore, that the application of PSWT can result in a real and measurable increase in tissue temperature. These results indicate that the relationship between applied energy and both subjective and objective thermal changes are complex, and cannot be resolved by demonstrating a simple linear relationship.

From the available literature, no measured thermal effect has been demonstrated with an applied MP of below 5 W and at the present time, therefore, this is considered to be the effective thermal threshold (Chartered Society of Physiotherapists (CSP) 2006). If a thermal effect is the intended outcome of the treatment, it will be necessary to deliver a dose with an MP in excess of this level. The higher the applied MP, the greater the tissue heating effect that will be achieved. If the intention of treatment is to avoid thermal effects in the tissues (e.g. because they are contraindicated), the treatment dose should not be raised above this level. Interestingly, Seiger and Draper (2006) have recently reported that apparently safe and effective delivery of much higher PSWT MP levels than identified in these guidelines.

The power meter incorporated in the SWT machine (if present) is a measure of the power emitted by the generator and as such provides no indication of the energy absorbed by the tissues nor of the magnitude of any temperature increase in the tissues (Depizzo & Joyer 1987, Wadsworth & Chanmugam 1983). Currently, the only method available for therapists is to monitor sensation via the patient's verbal response. As such, it is considered advisable to increase the machine intensity slowly and allow the temperature to stabilize, increasing the intensity further when a thermal effect is the intended outcome of treatment. Reliability of the patient's capacity to report thermal changes is clearly a necessary prerequisite for safe treatment. Further work to identify the key parameters that are responsible for thermal and non-thermal effects of PSWT is clearly needed.

SAFETY WITH SHORTWAVE THERAPY

ELECTROMAGNETIC RADIATION AROUND SHORTWAVE THERAPY MACHINES: ADVERSE EFFECTS AND OPERATOR SAFETY

Therapeutic SW machines can be a source of occupational hazard. These observations were underpinned by the fact that EM waves emitted from SW machines can propagate freely in air (Scott 2002) without the need for a medium, making it difficult to concentrate the energy in the area treated (Docker et al 1994, Martin et al 1991). This risk of 'electropollution' is increased by the small treatment cubicles and the cramped conditions in some hospitals (Coppell 1988), which could subject other patients in the vicinity of operating equipment to an increased risk of unintentional EM strays.

The majority of studies have considered associations between SW exposure and adverse effects such as heart pain among male physiotherapists (Hamburger et al 1983), fetal malformation (Hamburger et al 1983, Kallen et al 1992, Larsen et al 1991, Ouellet-Hellstrom & Stewart 1993, Stellman & Stellman 1980), abortion if physiotherapist exposure exceeds 10 hours/week (Lerman et al 2001) and abortion if exposure exceeds 5 hours/week and the therapist is beyond 10 weeks, gestation period (Taskinen et al 1990). Others have found no difference between therapists exposed to SW and those who were not in terms of congenital malformation (Guberan et al 1994, Larsen et al 1991).

No causal relationship (Shields 2003) can be established between the nature and methodology of these studies, due to the absence of quantitative measurements of EMF, and failure to take account of other confounding factors for abortions, such as heavy lifting or bad posture (Hollis 1992, West & Gardner 2001). However, despite the absence of   strong evidence, care should be taken to ensure operator safety when using SW. Studies on the strength of EMF around SW machines found differences according to the SWT make, mode of application (continuous or pulsed) and treatment setting (Coppell 1988, Shields 2003, Shields et al 2003, Skotte 1986).

The type of electrode used could affect the stray irradiation around SWT units. Capacitive electrodes recorded a higher E field than drum electrodes and inductive coils (Lau & Dunscombe 1984, Skotte 1986). Air-space electrodes were associated with 10 times higher values of stray emission than pad electrodes and 100 times higher radiation levels than inductive electrodes (Coppell 1988, Martin et al 1991). Tzima and Martin (1994) have evaluated the stray of E and H fields of several SW machines in pulsed and continuous mode and with different electrode configurations. Air-spaced electrodes were found to emit more EMR when used in continuous mode compared to pulsed, with field exceeding National Radiation Protection Board (NRPB) (1993) levels to 0.8–1.1 m in continuous and 0.4–0.8 m in pulsed modes. The strength of the field was also found to decrease with increasing distance from the unit. The E field was found to be higher near the electrodes while the H field was highest near the cables (Martin et al 1991, Shields 2003).

Li and Feng (1999) measured EMR intensities and the strength of both E and H fields from a distance of 30, 100, 150 cm from a SW machine at the level of the knee, waist and hand of the operator and reported the operator exposure to be below the recommended levels; the strength of the measured field was found to be variable in different directions around SW machines. The highest recorded value was in front of the diathermy at a distance of 30 cm at the level of the knee.

The size and placement of the electrodes on the body also plays a role in the strength of the field distribution. Field strength was found to be proportional to the size of the electrode. A 20–30% increase in field strength was demonstrated when the electrode diameter was increased from 6 to 14 cm (Tzima & Martin 1994).

The arrangement of the electrodes is another factor that could affect the strength of the field around SW machines. A coplanar arrangement was found to emit a lesser stray field than a contraplanar arrangement (Tzima & Martin 1994).

The distance between the electrodes and the area treated seems to play a role in the size of EMR emitted. The extent of the field was found to be proportional to the distance between the treated area and the electrodes, with less stray emission using closer applications (Lau & Dunscombe 1984, Tofani & Agnesod 1984). Changing the distance from 10 to 30 mm will result in uneven heating and concentration of the EMF field under the treatment head (Martin et al 1991).

However, these findings are not definitive because field strength could be altered in the clinical setting owing to the use or the presence of metallic furniture around the treatment area, another SW machine operating within a distance of 2 m, and the therapist standing in close proximity to SW cables (Coppell 1988, Delpizzo & Joyner 1987). Each of these factors could play a role in creating alternative conduction path, distorting the EMF (Docker et al 1994).

Studies have shown that therapists' average exposure time during a treatment is around 3 minutes (Stuchly et al 1982) and such short exposures are unlikely to exceed the levels recommended by NRPB (which state that, over a 6-minute period, maximum E field exposure should not exceed 61 V/m and maximum H field exposure should not exceed 0.16 V/m, SAR of 10 W/cm^2).

Despite all the above, following general practice recommendations, which state that, standing at the end of a diathermy console opposite the applicator instead of in front of the unit (Li & Feng 1999, Skotte 1986), and once the machine has been turned on, the therapist should maintain a distance of at least 1 m from the machine, cables and electrodes throughout the treatment period. It has been suggested that 0.5 m is a safe working distance with PSWT, but although this might be safe, it is generally held that a 1-m separation is preferred to reduce unwanted EMR exposure.

CONTRAINDICATIONS AND PRECAUTIONS

The contraindications that are applicable to the use of both continuous and pulsed SWT are detailed in Chapter 21, and only limited additional comments will be made here.

PACEMAKERS AND OTHER 'ACTIVE' IMPLANTS

It is strongly suggested that patients with pacemakers or other active implanted devices are not exposed to SWT as a therapy and that, furthermore, they should remain at a safe distance from an operating machine, as some implanted devices are susceptible to the 'stray' EM fields emitted from machines. There is currently a lack of definitive evidence concerning the absolute safe distance between a working SWT machine and a patient (or therapist) with an active implanted device, and the current recommendation is 3 m. Some pacemakers are much less susceptible to EM fields and it is likely that this separation is somewhat conservative, but unless the therapist is aware of the detailed information concerning which pacemaker has been used and the relative immunity of that pacemaker type to these interference fields, it is probably safest to adopt the 3-m separation. Further detailed evaluation is clearly needed in this area.

PREGNANCY

It is recommended that patients who are pregnant are not treated with SWT (continuous or pulsed) and remain at a safe (at least 1 m) distance from a working machine (CSP 1997). It is recommended that therapists who are pregnant do not operate SWT devices and maintain a safe working distance from operating machines (CSP 1997; see the previous section for a more detailed discussion).

METAL IN THE TISSUES

It is considered inappropriate to treat body segments that include (passive) metallic implants when using continuous SWT due to the higher heat capacity of metal compared with tissue and the potential for 'deep' tissue burns. It is currently suggested (CSP 2006) that metal in the tissues is not a contraindication with SWT in pulsed mode when applied with a mean power of less than 5 W. Given that mean power levels in excess of 5 W are considered to have a thermal capability, metal in the tissues *is* considered to be a contraindication when mean power over 5 W is applied. Interestingly, Seiger & Draper (2006) employed PSWT at much high mean power than this in patients with metal implants with no apparent adverse effect.

SKIN SENSATION TEST

It is considered necessary to perform a routine skin sensation test (see previous section) prior to a SWT application in continuous mode or in pulsed mode when a thermal effect is anticipated (i.e. a mean power in excess of 5 W). Although therapists may wish to use a thermal skin sensation test at mean power levels below 5 W, it is not considered to be an essential requirement.

Further details and referenced material relating to dangers, precautions and contraindications for continuous and pulsed shortwave are included in Chapter 21.

CONCLUSION

The use of SWT in continuous mode appears to have declined in the last 10 years, whereas in pulsed mode it has retained a significant degree of use (Al Mandeel & Watson 2006). It is known to be an effective heating modality (in continuous and pulsed modes) (e.g. Draper et al 1999, 2002) and this appears to be especially effective when the monode type applicator is employed. In its 'non-thermal' (pulsed) mode, it has similar effects to other modalities (ultrasound, laser therapy) but these effects are primarily achieved in the ionic tissues of low impedance, whereas ultrasound, for example, is most effective in tissues with a high collagen content (ter Haar 1999, Watson 2006).

Shortwave therapy has a useful effective penetration depth (several centimetres at least) and can be applied without the therapist needing to be in constant attendance. Although there is a strong need for additional research, especially in the clinical environment, the established benefits of the modality make it a useful adjunct to other forms of intervention and its potential use in the areas of fracture healing and open wound management are currently under-utilized in practice.

Additionally, unlike most other electrotherapy applications, SWT has been shown to have remote effects: that is, by applying it to the abdomen a desirable change in the circulatory system can be observed at the extremities and, as such, it can be used in cases where direct application of an electrotherapy modality to an area is not possible (Erdmann 1960, Morrissey 1966, Wessman & Kottke 1967). The concerns expressed with regard to therapist safety when using this modality are largely unfounded provided the practitioner complies with the essential safety guideline and remains at least 1 m from an operating machine.

Further work is continuing in this field of therapy, and it is anticipated that with an increasing number of laboratory and clinical trials being published, some of the current ambiguities will be resolved. It will be of significant interest to see whether the strongly beneficial effects of PEMFs (wound healing, fracture healing) are equivalent to the effects achieved by PSWT. They are not the same in terms of the mode of delivery, energy or the machine parameters available for manipulation, but their essential energy form is very similar and, thus, it is reasonable that their mode of action and range of clinical effects might overlap to a greater extent than is currently recognized. Demonstration of the similarity or difference between these modes is an important issue in the next generation of research in this field.

References

Abramson D, Chu L, Tuck S et al (1966) Effect of tissue temperature and blood flow on motor nerve conduction velocity. *J Am Med Assoc* **198**(10): 1082–1088.

Adey W (1988). Physiological signalling across cell membrane and co-operative influences of extremely low frequency EMF. In Frohlich H (ed) *Biological Coherence and Response to External Stimuli* pages 148–170. Heidelberg, Springer Verlag.

Al-Mandeel M (2004) *Pulsed Shortwave Therapy. Its Use and Physiological Effects with Healthy and Osteoarthritic Patients.* PhD thesis, University of Hertfordshire, UK.

Al Mandeel M, Watson T (2006) An evaluative audit of patients records in electrotherapy with specific reference to pulsed shortwave therapy. *Int J Ther Rehab* **13**(9): 414–419.

Arghiropol M, Jieanu V, Paslaru L et al (1992) The stimulation of fibronectin synthesis by high peak power electromagnetic energy (Diapulse). *Rev Roumaine Physique* **29**(3–4): 77–81.

Aronofky D (1971) Reduction of dental postsurgical symptoms using non thermal pulsed high peak power electromagnetic energy. *Oral Surg* **32**(5): 688–696.

Badea M, Vasilco R, Sandru D (1993) The effects of pulsed electromagnetic field (Diapulse) on cellular systems. *Rom J Physiol* **30**(1–2): 65–71.

Bansal PS, Sobti VK, Roy KS (1990) Histomorphochemical effects of shortwave diathermy on healing of experimental muscular injury in dogs. *Indian J Exp Biol* **28**(8): 766–770.

Barclay V, Collier R, Jones A (1983) Treatment of various hand injuries by pulsed electromagnetic energy (Diapulse). *Physiotherapy* **69**(6): 186–188.

Barker A, Barlow P, Porter J et al (1985) A double blind clinical trial of low power pulsed shortwave therapy in the treatment of a soft tissue injury. *Physiotherapy* **71**(12): 500–504.

Benazzo F, Mosconi M, Beccarisi G et al (1995) Use of capacitive coupled electric fields in stress fractures in athletes. *Clin Orthop* **310**: 145–149.

Bentall R, Eckstein H (1975) Trial involving the use of pulsed electromagnetic therapy on children undergoing orchidopexy. *Kinderchirugie* **17**(4): 380–389.

Bricknell R, Watson T (1995) The thermal effects of pulsed shortwave therapy. *Br J Ther Rehab* **2**(8): 430–434.

Brown M, Baker R (1987) Effects of pulsed shortwave diathermy on skeletal muscle injury in rabbits. *Phys Ther* **67**(2): 208–214.

Buzzard B, Pratt R, Briggs P et al (2003) Is pulsed shortwave diathermy better than ice therapy for reduction of oedema following calcaneal fractures? *Physiotherapy* **89**(12): 734–742.

Callaghan MJ, Whittaker PE, Grimes S et al (2005) An evaluation of pulsed shortwave on knee osteoarthritis using radioleucoscintigraphy: a randomised, double blind, controlled trial. *Joint Bone Spine* **72**(2): 150–155.

Cameron M, Perez D, Otano-Lata S (1999) Electromagnetic radiation. In Cameron M (ed) *Physical Agent in Rehabilitation from Research to Practice* chapter 10, pages 304–306. Philadelphia, WB Saunders.

Charman R (1990) Bioelectricity and electrotherapy towards a new paradigm, Part 2, Cellular reception. *Physiotherapy* **76**(9): 509–516.

Chartered Society of Physiotherapy (CSP) (1997) *Safe Practice with Electrotherapy (Shortwave Therapies)*. London, CSP.

Chartered Society of Physiotherapy (CSP) (2006) *2006 Guidance for the Clinical use of Electrophysical Agents*. London, CSP.

Cheing GL, Wan JW, Kai Lo S (2005) Ice and pulsed electromagnetic field to reduce pain and swelling after distal radius fractures. *J Rehab Med* **37**(6): 372–377.

Cleary S. (1997) In vitro studies of the effects of non-thermal radiofrequency and microwave radiation. In Bernhardt J, Mattes R, Repacholi M (eds) *Proceedings, International Seminar on Biological effects of Non Thermal Pulsed and Amplitude Modulated RF Electromagnetic Fields and Related Health Risks.* Munich Nov. 1996. Published by International Commission on Non-Ionizing Radiation Protection (ICNIRP) 1997, pages 119–130.

Comorosan S, Vasilco R, Archiropol M et al (1993) The effects of Diapulse therapy on the healing of decubitus ulcer. *Rom J Physiol* **30**(1–2): 41–45.

Constable J, Scapicchio A, Opitz B (1971) Studies of the effects of diapulse treatment on various aspects of wound healing in experimental animals. *J Surg Res* **11**: 254–257.

Coppell R (1988) Survey of stray electromagnetic emissions from microwave and shortwave diathermy equipment. *NZ J Physiother* **16**(3), 9–14.

Currier D, Nelson R (1969) Changes in motor conduction velocity induced by exercise and diathermy. *Phys Ther* **49**(2): 146–152.

Delpizzo V, Joyner K (1987) On the safe use of microwave and shortwave diathermy units. *Aust J Physiother* **33**(3): 152–162.

Docker M, Bazin S, Dyson M et al (1994) Guidelines for the safe use of the pulsed shortwave therapy equipment. *Physiotherapy* **80**(4), 233–235.

Draper D, Knight K, Fujiwara T (1999) Temperature change in human muscle during and after pulsed shortwave diathermy…including commentary with authors response. *J Orthop Sport Phys Ther* **29**(1): 13–22.

Draper D, Miner L, Knight K et al (2002) The carry over effects of diathermy and stretching in developing hamstring flexibility. *J Athletic Training* **37**(1): 37–42.

Draper D, Castro JL, Feland B et al (2004) Shortwave diathermy and prolonged stretching increase hamstring flexibility more than prolonged stretching alone. *J Orthop Sports Phys Ther* **34**(1): 13–20.

Durney C, Christensen D (2000). *Basic Introduction to Electromagnetics.* Boca Raton, FL, CRC Press.

Dziedzic K, Hill J, Lewis M, et al (2005) Effectiveness of manual therapy or pulsed shortwave diathermy in addition to advice and exercise for neck disorders: a pragmatic randomized controlled trial in physical therapy clinics. *Arthritis Rheum* **53**(2): 214–222.

Elder J, Czerski P, Stuchly M et al (1989) Radio-frequency radiation. In Suess M, Benwell-Morison D (eds) *Nonionizing Radiation Protection*, 2nd edn. Ottawa, WHO Regional Publications, European Series, no 25.

Erdman, W (1960) Peripheral blood flow measurements during application of pulsed high frequency currents. *Am J Orthop* **8**: 196–197.

Evans RK, Knight KL, Draper D et al (2002) Effects of warm-up before eccentric exercise on indirect markers of muscle damage. *Med Sci Sports Exerc* **34**(12): 1892–1899.

Fenn J (1969) Effect of electromagnetic energy (Diapulse) on experimental haematomas. *Can Med Assoc J* **100**: 251–253.

Foley-Nolan D (1990) Pulsed low energy high frequency fields: current status and future trends. *Compl Med Res* **4**(3), 41–45.

Foley-Nolan D, Moore K, Codd M et al (1992) Low energy high frequency pulsed electromagnetic therapy for acute whiplash injuries. *Scand J Rehab Med* **24**: 51–59.

Forster A, Palastanga N (1985). *Clayton's Electrotherapy Theory and Practice*, 9th edn. London, Baillière Tindall.

Foster K (1997) Interaction of radiofrequency fields with biological systems as related to modulation. In Bernhardt J, Mattes R, Repacholi M (eds) *Proceedings, International Seminar on Biological Effects of Non Thermal Pulsed and Amplitude Modulated RF Electromagnetic Fields and Related Health Risks*. Munich Nov. 1996. Published by ICNIRP 1997, pages 47–63.

Ganguly K, Sarkar A, Datta A et al (1996) A study of the effects of pulsed electromagnetic field therapy with respect to serological grouping in rheumatoid arthritis. *J Med Assoc* **96**(9): 272–275.

Garret C, Draper D, Knight K (2000) Heat distribution in the lower leg from pulsed shortwave diathermy and ultrasound treatment. *J Athletic Training* **35**(1): 50–55.

Gibson T, Grahame R, Harkeness J et al (1985) Controlled comparison of shortwave diathermy treatment with osteopathic treatment in non specific low back pain. *Lancet* **1**(1): 1258–1261.

Ginsberg A (1961) Pulsed shortwave in the treatment of bursitis with calcification. *Int Rec Med* **174**(2): 71–75.

Goat C (1989) Pulsed electromagnetic (shortwave) energy therapy. *Br J Sport Med* **23**(4): 213–216.

Goldin J, Broadbent N, Nancarrow J et al (1981) The effect of Diapulse on the healing of wounds: a double blind randomised controlled trial in man. *Br J Plastic Surg* **34**: 267–270.

Grant A, Sleep J, McIntosh J et al (1989) Ultrasound and pulsed electromagnetic energy treatment for perineal trauma. A randomised placebo controlled trial. *Br J Obs Gynaecol* **96**: 434–439.

Gray J (1997). *Evidence-based Healthcare: How to Make Health Policy and Management Decisions*. New York, Churchill Livingstone.

Gray R, Quayle A, Hall C et al (1994) Physiotherapy in the treatment of temporomandibular joint disorder: a comparative study of four treatment methods. *Br Dental J* **176**(7): 257–261.

Guberan E, Campana A, Faval P et al (1994) Gender ratio of offspring and exposure to shortwave radiation among female physiotherapists. *Scand J Work Environ Health* **20**(5): 345–348.

Guler-Uysal F, Kozanoglu E (2004) Comparison of the early response to two methods of rehabilitation in adhesive capsulities. *Swiss Med Weekly* **134**: 353–358.

Hamburger S, Logue J, Silverman P (1983) Occupational exposure to non ionising radiation and an association with heart disease: an exploratory study. *J Chronol Dis* **36**: 791–802.

Hand J (1990) Biophysics and technology of electromagnetic hyperthermia. In Gautherine M (ed) *Methods of External Hyperthermic Heating*. Berlin, Springer.

Hayne C (1984) Pulsed frequency energy, its place in physiotherapy. *Physiotherapy* **70**: 259–266.

He X, Weng X, Ye Y et al (2005) Study on thermal map distribution in phantom by shortwave capacitance coupled heating. *Chin J Biomed Eng* **24**(5): 560–565.

Hill J, Lewis M, Mills P et al (2001) Pulsed shortwave diathermy effects on human fibroblast proliferation. *Arch Phys Ther Rehab* **83**: 832–836.

Hinsenkamp M, Ryaby J, Burny F (1985) Treatment of non-union by pulsing electromagnetic field: European multicenter study of 308 cases. *Reconstr Surg Traumatol* **19**: 147–151.

Hollis M (1992) Back injuries: a review of liability reports in healthcare environments. *Occup Health* **44**(10): 296–299.

Itoh M, Montemayor J, Matsumoto E et al (1991) Accelerated wound healing of pressure ulcer by pulsed high peak power electromagnetic energy (Diapulse). *Decubitus* **4**(1): 24–34.

Jan M, Lai J (1991) The effects of physiotherapy on osteoarthritic knees of female. *J Formosan Med Assoc* **90**(10): 1008–1013.

Jan M, Ming H, Chung L et al (2006) Effects of repetitive shortwave diathermy for reducing synovitis in patients with knee osteoarthritis: an ultrasonographic study. *Phys Ther* **86**: 236–244.

Jorgensen W, Frome B, Wallach C (1994) Electrochemical therapy of pelvic pain: effects of pulsed electromagnetic fields (PEMF) on tissue trauma. *Eur J Surg* **574**: 83–86.

Kallen B, Malmquist G, Moritz U (1992) Delivery outcomes among physiotherapists in Sweden: is non-ionising radiation a fatal hazard? *Physiotherapy* **78**(1): 15–18.

Kecik T, Switka-Wieclawska I, Portacha L et al (1994) The efficacy of shortwave diathermy and laser stimulation of the lacrimal glands in the treatment of dry eye syndrome. *Adv Exp Med Bull* **350**: 601–604.

Kerem M, Yigiter K (2002) Effects of continuous and pulsed shortwave diathermy in low back pain. *Pain Clin* **14**(1): 55–59.

Kitchen S (2002) Thermal effects. In: Kitchen S (ed) *Electrotherapy: Evidence-Based Practice* chapter 6, pages 89–106. Edinburgh, Churchill Livingstone.

Klaber-Moffett J, Richardson P, Frost H et al (1996) A placebo controlled double blind trial to evaluate the effectiveness of pulsed shortwave therapy for osteoarthritic hip and knee pain. *Pain* **67**: 121–127.

Kloth L, Ziskin M (1996). Diathermy and pulsed radiofrequency radiation. In Michlovitz S (ed) *Thermal Agents in Rehabilitation*, 3rd edn. Philadelphia, FA Davis.

Krag C, Taudorf U, Siim E et al (1979) The effect of pulsed electromagnetic energy (Diapulse) on the survival of experimental skin flaps. A study on rats. *Scand J Plastic Reconstr Surg* **13**: 377–380.

Larsen A, Olsen J, Svane O (1991) Gender-specific reproductive outcomes and exposure to high frequency electromagnetic radiation among physiotherapists. *Scand J Work Environ Health* **17**: 324–329.

Lau R, Dunscombe P (1984) Some observation on stray magnetic fields and power outputs from shortwave diathermy. *Health Phys* **46**(4): 939–943.

Laufer Y, Ziberman R, Porat R et al (2005) Effect of pulsed shortwave diathermy on pain and function of subjects with osteoarthritis of knee: a placebo controlled double blind clinical trial. *Clin Rehab* **19**(3): 255–263.

Leclaire R, Bourgouin J (1991) Electromagnetic treatment of shoulder periarthritis: a randomised controlled trial of efficiency and tolerance of magnetotherapy. *Arch Phys Med Rehab* **72**: 248–287.

Lehmann J, DeLateur B (1990) Therapeutic heat. In Lehmann J (ed) *Therapeutic Heat and Cold* pages 470–474, 4th edn. Baltimore, MD, Williams & Wilkins.

Lehmann J, McDougall J, Guy A et al (1983) Heating patterns produced by shortwave diathermy applicators in tissue substitute models. *Arch Phys Med Rehab* **64**(12): 575–577.

Lerman Y, Jacubovich R, Green M (2001) Pregnancy outcome following exposure to shortwave among female physiotherapists in Israel. *Am J Industr Med* **39**: 499–504.

Li C, Feng C (1999) An evaluation of rdiofrequency exposure from therapeutic diathermy equipment. *Ind Health* **37**: 465–468.

Lightwood R (1989) The remedial electromagnetic field. *J Biomed Eng* **11**: 429–436.

Livesley P, Mugglestone A, Whitton J (1992) Electrotherapy and management of minimally displaced fracture of the neck of the humerus. *Injury* **23**(5): 323–327.

Low J (1995) Dosage of some pulsed shortwave clinical trials. *Physiotherapy* **81**(10): 611–616.

Low J, Reed A (2000) *Electrotherapy Explained: Principles and Practice*, 3rd edn. Oxford, Butterworth–Heinemann.

Markov M, Colbert A (2000) Magnetic and electromagnetic field therapy. *J Back Musculoskel Rehab* **15**(1): 17–29.

Marks R, van Nguyen J (2005) Pulsed electromagnetic field therapy and osteoarthritis of the knee: synthesis of the literature. *Int J Ther Rehab* **12**(8): 347–354.

Martin C, McCallum H, Strelley S et al (1991) Electromagnetic fields from therapeutic diathermy equipment: a review of hazards and precautions. *Physiotherapy* **77**(1): 3–7.

McCray R, Patton N (1984) Pain relief at trigger points: a comparison of moist heat and shortwave diathermy. *J Orthop Sport Phys Ther* **5**(4): 175–179.

McGill S (1988) The effect of pulsed shortwave therapy on lateral ligament sprain of the ankle. *NZ J Physiother* **16**: 21–24.

Michaelson S, Elson E (1996). Interaction of non modulated and pulse modulated radiofrequency fields with living matter: experimental results. In Polk C, Postow E (eds) *Handbook of Biological Effects of Electromagnetic Fields*. Boca Raton, FL, CRC Press.

Morrissey L (1966) Effects of shortwave diathermy upon volume blood flow through the calf of the leg. *J Am Phys Ther Assoc* **46**(9): 946–952.

Mucha C (2005) The Achilles reflex time after high and low frequency application. *Rehabiliticia* **42**(4): 244–249.

Murray C, Kitchen S (2000) Effects of pulse repetition rate on the perception of thermal sensation with pulsed shortwave diathermy. *Physiother Res Int* **5**(2): 73–85.

National Radiological Protection Board (NRPB) (1993) *Board Statement on Restrictions on Human Exposure to Static and Time Varying Electromagnetic Fields and Radiation*. NRPB vol 4, no. 5. HMSO, London.

Nordenstorm B (1983). *Biologically Closed Electric Circuits. Clinical Experiment and Theoretical Evidence for an Additional Circulatory System*. Stockholm, Nordic Medical Publications.

Nwuga V (1982) Relative therapeutic efficacy of vertebral manipulation and conventional treatment in back pain management. *Am J Phys Med* **61**(6): 273–278.

Odia G, Aibogun O (1988) Thermal sensation and the skin sensation test: regional differences and their effects on the issue of reliability of temperature ranges. *Aust J Physiother* **34**(2): 89–93.

Ouellet-Hellstrom R, Stewart W (1993) Miscarriage among female physical therapists who report using radio-and microwave electromagnetic radiation. *Am J Epidemiol* **138**(10): 775–786.

Pennington G, Danley D, Sumko M et al (1993) Pulsed, non-thermal, high frequency electromagnetic energy (Diapulse) in the treatment of grade I and grade II ankle sprains. *Military Med* **158**: 101–104.

Peres S, Draper D, Knight K et al (2002) Pulsed shortwave diathermy and prolonged long duration stretching increase dorsiflexion range of motion more than identical stretching without diathermy. *J Athletic Training* **37**(1): 43–50.

Polk C, Postow E (1996) *Handbook of Biological Effects of Electromagnetic Fields*, 2nd edn. Boca Raton, FL, CRC Press.

Pope G, Mocket S, Wright J (1995) A survey of electrotherapeutic modalities: ownership and use in the NHS in England. *Physiotherapy* **81**(2): 82–91.

Pope L, Muresan M, Comorosan S et al (1989) The effects of pulsed high frequency radio waves on rat liver (ultrastructural and biomedical observations). *Physiol Chem Phys Med NMR*, **21**(1): 45–55.

Prentice W, Draper D (2001) *Short and Microwave Diathermy*. In Prentice W (ed) *Therapeutic Modalities for Physical Therapists*, 2nd edn. New York, McGraw-Hill.

Quirk A, Newman R, Newman K (1985) An evaluation of interferential therapy, shortwave diathermy and exercise in the treatment of osteoarthrosis of the knee. *Physiotherapy* **71**(2): 55–57.

Raji A (1984) An experimental study of the effects of pulsed electromagnetic field (Diapulse) on nerve repair. *J Hand Surg* **9**(2): 105–112.

Raji A, Bowden R (1983) Effects of high peak pulsed electromagnetic field on the degeneration and regeneration of the common peroneal nerve in rats. *J Bone Joint Surg* **65**(4): 478–492.

Reed M, Bickerstaff D, Hayne C et al (1987) Pain relief after inguinal herniorrhaphy, ineffectiveness of pulsed electromagnetic energy. *Br J Clin Pract* **41**(6): 782–784.

Robertson VJ, Ward AR, Jung P (2005) The effect of heat on tissue extensibility: a comparison of deep and superficial heating. *Arch Phys Med Rehab* **86**(4): 819–825.

Salzberg C, Cooper-Vastola S, Perez F et al (1995) The effects of non thermal pulsed electromagnetic energy on wound healing of pressure ulcers in spinal cord injured patients: a randomised double blind study. *Osteot Wound Management* **41**(3): 42–51.

Santiesteban A, Grant C (1985) Post surgical effect of pulsed shortwave therapy. *J Am Podiatr Assoc* **75**(6): 306–309.

Scott S (2002) Diathermy. In Kitchen S (ed) *Electrotherapy Evidence-Based Practice* chapter 11, pages 145–165. Edinburgh, Churchill Livingstone.

Seaborne D, Quirion-Degirardi C, Rousseseau M et al (1996) The treatment of pressure sores using pulsed electromagnetic energy (PEME). *Physiother Canada* **48**(2): 131–137.

Seiger C, Draper D (2006) Use of pulsed shortwave diathermy and mobilization to increase ankle range of motion in the presence of surgical implanted metal: a case series. *J Orthop Sport Phys Med* **36**(9): 669–677.

Shields N (2003) *Operational, Quality Control and Safety Issues in Shortwave Diathermy*. PhD thesis. University of Dublin, Trinity College.

Shields N, Gormley J, O'Hare N (2001) Shortwave diathermy: a review of existing clinical trials. *Phys Ther Rev* **6**(2): 101–118.

Shields N, O'Hare N, Gormley J (2003) Shortwave diathermy and pregnancy: what is the evidence? *Adv Physiother* **5**(1): 2–14.

Shields N, O'Hare N, Gormley J (2004) Contra-indications to shortwave diathermy: survey of Irish physiotherapists. *Physiotherapy* **90**: 42–53.

Skotte J (1986) Reduction of radiofrequency exposure to the operator during shortwave diathermy treatments. *J Med Eng Technol* **10**(1): 7–10.

Stellman J, Stellman S (1980) Health effects of radiofrequency radiation in a cohort of physical therapists. *Am J Epidemiol* **112**: 442–443.

Stuchly M, Repacholi M, Leuyer D et al (1982) Exposure to the operator and the patient during shortwave diathermy treatments. *Health Phys* **42**: 341–366.

Svarcova J, Trnavsky K, Zvarova R (1988) The influence of ultrasound, galvanic currents and shortwave diathermy on pain in patients with osteoarthritis. *Scand J Rheumatol* **67**: 83–85.

Taskinen H, Kyyronen P, Hemminki K (1990) Effects of ultrasound, shortwaves, and physical exertions on pregnancy outcomes in physiotherapists. *J Epidemiol Commun Health* **44**: 196–201.

Tenforde T (1996) Interaction of ELF magnetic fields with living systems. In Polk C, Postow E (eds) *Handbook of Biological Effects of Electromagnetic Fields*. Boca Raton, FL, CRC Press.

ter Haar G (1999) Therapeutic ultrasound. *Eur J Ultrasound* **9**: 3–9.

Thawer HA (1999) Pulsed electromagnetic fields for osteogenesis and repair. *Phys Ther Rev* **4**(3): 203–213.

Todd D, Heylings R, McMillin W (1991) Treatment of chronic varicose ulcer with pulsed electromagnetic fields: a controlled pilot study. *Irish Med J* **84**(2): 54–55.

Tofani S, Agnesod G (1984) The assessment of unwanted radiation around diathermy RF capacitive application. *Health Phys* **47**(2): 235–241.

Tzima E, Martin C (1994) An evaluation of safe practice to restrict exposure to electric and magnetic fields from therapeutic and surgical diathermy equipment. *Physiol Meas* **15**: 201–216.

Valtonen E, Lilius H, Svinhufvud U (1973) Effects of three modes of application of shortwave diathermy on the cutaneuous temperature of the leg. *Eur Medicophys* **9**: 49–52.

Van der Esch M, Hoogland R (1991) *Pulsed shortwave therapy with Curapuls 403*. Delft, Enraf Nonius.

Vanharanta H, Eronen I, Videman T (1982) Shortwave diathermy effects on 35S-sulfate uptake and glycosaminoglycan concentration in rabbit knee tissue. *Arch Phys Med Rehab* **63**(1): 25–28.

Varcaccio-Garofalo G, Carriero C, Loizzo M et al (1995) Analgesic properties of electromagnetic field therapy in patients with chronic pelvic pain. *Clin Exp Obstet Gynaecol* **22**(4): 350–354.

Virtanen H, Keshvari J, Lappalainen R (2006) Interaction of radio frequency electromagnetic fields and passive metallic implants – a brief review. *Bioelectromagnetics* **27**(6): 431–439.

Wadsworth H, Chanmugam P (1983) *Electrophysical Agents in Physiotherapy*, 2nd edn. Marrickville New South Wales, Science Press.

Wagstaff P, Wagstaff S, Downey M (1986) A pilot study to compare the efficacy of continuous and pulsed magnetic energy (shortwave diathermy) on the relief of low back pain. *Physiotherapy* **72**(11): 563–566.

Ward A (1980) *Electricity, Fields and Waves in Therapy*. Marrickville New South Wales, Science Press.

Watson T (2000) The role of electrotherapy in contemporary physiotherapy practice. *Manual Ther* **5**(3): 132–141.

Watson T (2006) Electrotherapy and tissue repair. *Sport Ex Med* **29**: 7–13.

Wessman H, Kottke F (1967) The effects of indirect heating on peripheral blood flow, pulse rate, blood pressure and temperature. *Arch Phys Ther Rehab* **11**: 567–576.

West D, Gardner D (2001) Occupational injuries of physiotherapists in North and Central Queensland. *Aust J Physiother* **47**(3): 179–186.

Wilson D (1972) Treatment of soft tissue injuries by pulsed electrical energy. *Br Med J* **2**: 269–270.

Wilson D (1974) Comparison of shortwave diathermy and pulsed electromagnetic energy in the treatment of soft tissue injuries. *Physiotherapy* **60**(10): 309–310.

Wilson D, Jagadeesh P (1976) Experimental regeneration in peripheral nerves and the spinal cord in laboratory animals exposed to a pulsed electromagnetic field. *Paraplegia* **14**: 12–20.

Xu H, Feng L, Zeng Z et al (1999) Experimental study on ultrashortwave therapy on the healing of fracture. *Hunan Yi Ke Da Xue Xue Bao* **24**(2): 125–127.

Yung P, Unsworthy A, Haslock I (1986) Measurement of stiffness in the metacarpophalangeal joint: the effects of physiotherapy. *Clin Phys Physiol Meas* **7**(2): 147–156.

Zienowicz R, Thomas B, Hurtz W (1991) A multivariate approach to the treatment of peripheral nerve transection injury: the role of electromagnetic field therapy. *Plastic Reconstr Surg* **87**(1): 122–129.

Chapter 11

Low-intensity laser therapy

G. David Baxter

BRIEF HISTORY

The term 'laser' is an acronym for Light Amplification by Stimulated Emission of Radiation. Although Albert Einstein originally outlined the principles underlying the generation of such light in the early 1900s, it was not until 1960 that Theodore Maiman produced the first burst of ruby laser light at Hughes Laboratories in the USA. In the intervening decades, various laser devices based on Maiman's original prototype have found applications ranging from laser pointers and bar-code readers, to military range-finders and target acquisition systems.

Lasers have found a range of applications in medicine and particularly in surgery: ophthalmic surgeons were the first to use the pulsed ruby laser successfully for the treatment of detached retina in humans. In general, most medical applications to date have relied upon the photothermal (heating) and photoablative ('explosive') interactions of laser with tissue; thus lasers are routinely used to cut, weld and even destroy tissue. The widespread use of lasers as alternatives to metal scalpels, as well as for tumour ablation and tattoo removal, are all based upon these tissue reactions. In parallel with such developments, early interest also focused on the potential clinical applications of the non-thermal interactions of laser light with tissue, principally based upon initial work carried out by Professor Endre Mester's group in Budapest during the late 1960s and early 1970s. Results of this work indicated the potential of relatively low-intensity laser irradiation applied directly to tissue to modulate certain biological processes – in particular to *photobiostimulate* wound-healing processes (Mester et al 1985). Based on Mester's work in animals, and subsequently in patients, the ensuing decade saw the promotion of irradiation using the He-Ne laser (a laser device based upon a mixture of helium and neon gases as the lasing medium) as the treatment of choice for a variety of conditions throughout the countries of the former Soviet Union and in Asia, particularly China. However, it was not until the introduction of small, compact, laser-emitting photodiodes that the use of this therapy, known as low-level or low-intensity laser therapy (LILT), started to gain popularity in the West. The modality has found application by physiotherapists (for human and animal use), dentists, acupuncturists, podiatrists and some physicians, for a range of conditions including the treatment of open wounds, soft-tissue injuries, arthritic conditions and pain associated with various aetiologies (Baxter et al 1991). More recently, a series of approvals by the Food and Drug Administration (FDA) has led to increasing usage in the USA.

DEFINITIONS AND NOMENCLATURE

'Low-intensity laser therapy' (Baxter 1994) and 'low (reactive)-level laser therapy' (Ohshiro & Calderhead 1988), are generic terms that define the therapeutic application of relatively low-output (typically <500 mW for a single source) lasers and monochromatic superluminous diodes at dosages generally considered to be too low to effect any detectable heating of the irradiated tissues (usually <35 Jcm^{-2}). LILT is thus an athermal treatment modality. For this reason, this modality has also sometimes (inappropriately) been termed 'soft' or 'cold' laser therapy to distinguish the devices (and the resulting applications) from high-power sources of the type used in surgery and in other medical and dental applications; however, such terms are misleading and inappropriate, and are therefore best avoided.

This modality is also frequently referred to as laser (photo)biostimulation, particularly in the USA, where the term is sometimes abbreviated to 'biostim'. The use of such terminology derives from the early observations of Mester's group and others,

which suggested the potential of such devices to accelerate various wound-healing processes and cellular functions. However, the term is inappropriate to define the modality for two reasons. In the first instance, the applications of the modality exceed merely the treatment of wounds (e.g. laser therapy is also used to treat pain). Furthermore, and more importantly, lasers also have the potential, even at therapeutic intensities, to inhibit certain cellular processes (i.e. laser *photobioinhibition*; see the section on the Arndt–Schultz law, below); thus a more accurate generic term for the biological effects of low intensity laser irradiation is laser photobiomodulation.

PHYSICAL PRINCIPLES

Fuller accounts of the biophysical principles underpinning the therapeutic applications of lasers in LILT are available elsewhere (Nussbaum et al 2003a).

LIGHT EMISSION, ABSORPTION AND THE PRODUCTION OF LASER RADIATION

The basis of production of stimulated emission is illustrated in Figure 11.1. In non-laser sources, light is typically produced by *spontaneous emission of radiation* (Fig. 11.1A). In such circumstances and devices, the atoms and molecules comprising the central emitter (e.g. the element/filament in a typical household light bulb) are stimulated with (electrical) energy so that the electrons shift to higher energy orbits. Once in such orbits, the electrons are inherently unstable and fall spontaneously within a short period of time to lower energy levels. In so doing they release their extra energy as photons of light. The properties of the emitted photons are determined by the difference in energy levels (or valence bands) through which an excited electron 'dropped', as the difference in energy will be exactly the same as the quantal energy of the photon produced. As, for a given photon of light, the quantal energy (specified in electron-volts) is inversely related to the wavelength (in nm), the wavelength is effectively determined by the difference in valence bands; and in turn, molecules produce typical ranges of wavelengths or emission spectra when appropriately stimulated.

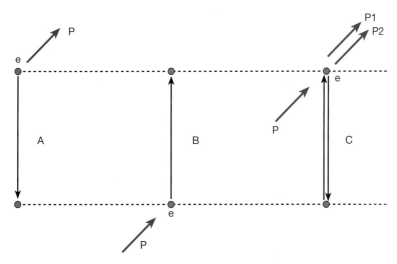

Figure 11.1 Spontaneous emission, absorption and stimulated emission of light. A, spontaneous emission: excited electron (e) drops to lower (resting) level, emitting a single photon (P). B, absorption: incident photon is absorbed by resting electron, which moves to higher level. C, stimulated emission: incident photon interacts with already excited electron to produce two identical photons (P1, P2).

ABSORPTION OF RADIATION

Absorption occurs when a photon of light interacts with an atom or molecule in which the difference in energy of the valence bands exactly equals the energy carried by the photon (Fig. 11.1B). This has two consequences: for a photon of a given quantal energy (and thus wavelength) only certain molecules will be capable of absorbing the light radiation; conversely, for a given molecule, only certain quantal energies (and thus wavelengths) can be absorbed (this is termed the *absorption spectrum* for the molecule). Thus absorption is said to be *wavelength specific*. This is an important concept in LILT applications, as this wavelength specificity of absorption effectively determines which types of tissue will preferentially absorb incident radiation, and (in turn) the depth of penetration of a particular treatment unit.

STIMULATED EMISSION OF RADIATION

Stimulated emission is a unique event that occurs when an incident photon interacts with an atom that is already excited (i.e. where the electron(s) are already in a higher energy orbit); additionally, the quantal energy of the incident photon must exactly equal the difference in energy levels between the electron's excited and resting states (Fig. 11.1C). Under these exceptional circumstances, the electron, in returning to its original orbit, gives off its excess energy as a photon of light with exactly the same properties as the incident photon, and completely in phase. In laser devices, the unique circumstances that give rise to stimulated emission of radiation are produced through the selection of an appropriate material or substance (the lasing medium), which, when electrically stimulated, will produce large numbers of identical photons through the rapid excitation of the medium. In order to produce such stimulated emission of radiation, laser treatment devices rely upon three essential components: the lasing medium, the resonating cavity and the power source.

Lasing medium

A lasing medium is capable of being 'pumped' with energy to produce stimulated emission; for therapeutic systems, the energy source is invariably electrical and the energy is delivered to the medium typically from the mains or (less commonly) from a battery (see below). The two media most commonly used in LILT applications are the gaseous mixture of helium and neon (He-Ne) operating at a wavelength of 632.8 nm (i.e. red light) and gallium arsenide (Ga-As), or gallium–aluminium–arsenide (GaAIAs) semiconductors, which typically produce radiation at 630–950 nm (i.e. visible red to the near infrared). Although He-Ne laser systems were the first to be used for LILT applications (i.e. they represented the 'first generation' of such systems), and a significant percentage of the papers published within this area are based upon such devices, these find few applications in routine physiotherapeutic practice. This is due to the relative expense of such units, and the comparatively low power output associated with He-Ne systems. In addition, the relatively greater collimation (see below) of these units when applied without fibre-optic applicators poses a significant hazard to the unprotected eye compared with the average semi-conductor-diode-based treatment unit.

Resonating cavity

A resonating cavity or chamber consists of a structure to contain the lasing medium and incorporates a pair of parallel reflecting surfaces or mirrors. Within this chamber, photons of light produced by the medium are reflected back and forth between the 'mirrors' to ultimately produce an intense photon resonance. As one of the reflecting surfaces (also termed the output coupler) is not a 'pure' mirror and so does not reflect 100% of the light striking its surface, some of the radiation is allowed to pass through as the output of the device. The resonating cavity for diode-based units is essentially the lasing medium itself (i.e. the semiconductor diode), the ends of which are carefully polished to form reflecting surfaces. This has important implications for the routine use of these units in clinical practice, as the treatment 'head' or 'probe' is usually not much larger than the size of a pen; this represents another reason why diode-based units (which may be regarded as 'second-generation' laser therapy systems), are so popular with clinicians (Fig. 11.2). Furthermore, most manufacturers now offer multi-source 'cluster' arrays, incorporating a number of diodes (up to 180) to allow simultaneous treatment of larger lesions and (in some cases) to allow several wavelengths of radiation to be used simultaneously (Fig. 11.2B). Such multisource cluster units may be

regarded as the 'third generation' of development for therapeutic lasers. More recently, several manufacturers have introduced 'fourth-generation' flexible multisource arrays to allow more efficient delivery of light to tissue surfaces with 'hands-free' application.

Power source

A power source is required to 'pump' the lasing medium to produce stimulated emission. In most cases, therapeutic devices tend to be mains supplied and incorporate a base unit to contain the transformer and control unit. Alternatively, some devices incorporate rechargeable and battery-powered units to enhance their portability (e.g. for sports injury applications).

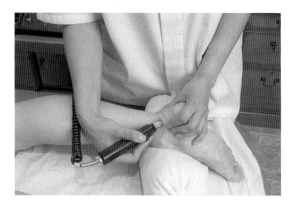

A

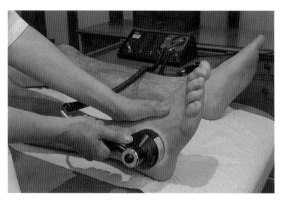

B

Figure 11.2 Modern laser treatment units. A, single diode treatment pen and B, multisource cluster array. (Photographs courtesy of Thor Laser Systems).

CHARACTERISTICS OF LASER RADIATION

The radiation generated by therapeutic laser devices differs from that produced by other similar sources (e.g. infrared heat lamps) in the following three respects:

1. **Monochromaticity**: the light produced by a laser is 'single coloured', the majority of the radiation emitted by the treatment device being clustered around a single wavelength with a very narrow band width. In contrast, light generated by other sources comprises a wide variety of wavelengths, sometimes ranging from the ultraviolet to the infrared, which result in the sensation of the colour white when the light strikes the retina of a human observer. Wavelength is a critical factor in determining the biological effects produced by laser treatments, as this parameter determines which biomolecules will absorb the incident radiation, and thus the basic photobiological interaction underlying any given treatment effect.

2. **Collimation**: in laser light, the rays of light or photons produced by the laser device are for all practical purposes parallel, with almost no divergence of the emitted radiation over distance; this property keeps the optical power of the device 'bundled' on to a relatively small area over considerable distances. However, highly collimated courses are also inherently more dangerous to the unprotected eye.

3. **Coherence**: the light emitted by laser devices is also in phase, so in conjunction with the two unique properties already outlined above, the troughs and peaks of the emitted light waves match perfectly in time (temporal coherence) and in space (spatial coherence). The biological and clinical relevance of this property is still debated (see Karu 1998, Tuner & Hode 1999), not least because of the widespread use of so-called 'superluminous diodes', which possess all the qualities of a 'true' laser diode, less the coherence, but which are a fraction of the cost of the latter. Multisource third- and fourth-generation cluster treatment units incorporating some 30 or 40 diodes would be prohibitively expensive for routine clinical use if they comprised nothing other than true laser diodes; thus these units typically incorporate no more than several laser diodes, the remainder being super-luminous diodes.

LASER–TISSUE INTERACTION

As already indicated above, laser–tissue interaction in medical applications has typically been associated with the potentially destructive effects of irradiation at relatively high power and energy levels; in these circumstances, high densities of laser light from highly collimated or focused sources with output in the watt range can easily produce photo-thermal reactions in tissues, including ablative or explosive effects. However, in LILT, the emphasis is by definition upon the non-thermal (or *athermal*) reactions of light with tissue. Light from a laser or monochromatic light therapy treatment device can interact with irradiated tissue in two ways:

1. **Scattering of incident light**: this is essentially a change in the direction of propagation of the light as it passes through the tissues, and is due to the variability in the refractive indices of tissue components relative to water. Such scattering will cause a 'widening' of the beam as it passes through irradiated tissue, and result in the rapid loss of coherence.

2. **Absorption of incident light by a chromophore**: a chromophore is a biomolecule that is capable, through its electronic or atomic configuration, of absorbing the incident photon(s). Light at the wavelengths typically employed in LILT are readily absorbed by a variety of biomolecules, including melanin and haemoglobin; as a consequence, the penetration depth associated with treatment devices is usually considered to be no more than several millimetres. It should be noted that, as the absorption is dependent upon the wavelength of incident light, the depth of penetration is similarly wavelength dependent.

Of these two modes of interaction, absorption may be regarded as the most important in terms of the photobiological basis of laser therapy, as without absorption, no photobiological (and thus clinical) effects would be possible.

CONCEPTUAL BASIS OF LASER PHOTOBIOMODULATION: THE ARNDT–SCHULTZ LAW

The photobiological effects of laser or monochromatic light upon tissue are many and complex, and to a large degree still poorly understood, particularly in terms of the variable stimulative/inhibitory reactions that can be effected by such irradiation. In providing a theoretical basis for the observed biological and clinical effects of this modality, the Arndt–Schultz law has been proposed as a suitable model; the main tenets of this law are illustrated in Figure 11.3. It should be stressed, however, that although this model can account for such phenomena as the 'inverse' dosage dependency reported in some papers (e.g. Lowe et al 1994), it essentially applies to radiant exposure (or energy density – see below); the putative relevance of manipulation of other irradiation parameters such as pulse repetition rate or power output remains, at least for the time being, a matter of debate (Nussbaum et al 2003b).

BIOLOGICAL AND PHYSIOLOGICAL EFFECTS

Investigations of the biological and physiological effects of low-intensity laser radiation can usefully be considered under three main areas: cellular studies involving the use of well-established cell lines and explanted cells, studies in various species of animals (in vivo and in vitro) and finally research in healthy human volunteers.

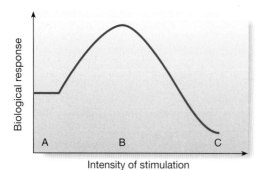

Figure 11.3 The Arndt–Schultz law. A, prethreshold: no biological activation (resting). B, biostimulation: activation of biological processes. C, bioinhibition: inhibition of biological processes.

Although the following provides an overview of the findings to date in these areas, a full and comprehensive review of the literature on the biological and physiological effects of low-intensity laser radiation is beyond the scope of this chapter; for further detail the reader is directed to the reviews of Basford (1995), Baxter (1994), Karu (1998), Schindl et al (2000), Shields and O'Kane (1994) and Tuner and Hode (1999).

CELLULAR RESEARCH

A large number of studies have examined the biological basis of low-intensity laser irradiation using a variety of bacteria, as well as cell lines and explanted cells, especially fibroblasts and macrophages (e.g. Pogrel et al 1997). In these studies, a number of possible indicators have been used to assess the photobiomodulatory effects of laser irradiation, including cell proliferation (Bolton et al 1995, Hawkins & Abrahamse 2006, Stein et al 2005), collagen production (Medrado et al 2003) and gene expression (Byrnes et al 2005). However, it should be stressed that although results from such studies are generally positive, findings in some areas are equivocal (Basford 1995, Posten et al 2005).

Cellular studies are important in two respects. In the first instance they provide a scientific basis for the clinical application of low-intensity lasers for the management of wounds, through demonstration of the photobiological mechanisms underlying such treatments (Karu 1998, Posten et al 2005). Second, by using such well-controlled laboratory research techniques, systematic investigations by some groups have demonstrated the importance of laser irradiation parameters such as wavelength, dosage and pulse repetition rate to the observed effects (O'Kane et al 1994, Rajaratnam et al 1994).

This notwithstanding, the precise relevance of the reported observations to clinical treatments is not always entirely clear. For example, where photobiostimulatory effects might be reported at a radiant exposure of $1.5\,\mathrm{Jcm^{-2}}$ in a laboratory study involving the direct irradiation of artificially maintained murine macrophage-like cell lines, what direct relevance has this for dosage selection in the laser treatment of a venous ulcer in a 67-year-old patient? Given such problems, e.g. the differences between the cell lines and the highly complex microenvironment of the clinical wound, a number of groups have employed animal studies and experimental studies on healthy human volunteers to further assess the biological and physiological effects of this modality in the laboratory.

ANIMAL STUDIES

To date, animal studies have concentrated on two main areas of research: the photobiostimulatory effects of laser irradiation on wound healing in experimentally induced lesions, and the neurophysiological and antinociceptive ('pain-blocking') effects of such irradiation. For the former studies, small, loose-skinned animals such as rats and mice have been traditionally, and most commonly, used (e.g. Mester et al 1985, Rabelo et al 2006). A range of experimental wounds have been employed in these species, including bone defects (Khadra et al 2004), burns (Bayat et al 2006), tendon and ligamentous injuries (Bayat et al 2005) and open skin wounds based upon models of compromised wound healing (Mester et al 1985, Rabelo et al 2006, Walker et al 2000). Although such studies have typically reported positive effects of laser irradiation (in terms of increased rates of healing, wound closure, enhanced granulation tissue formation, etc; see Woodruff et al 2004), the quality of much of the literature to date has been criticized (Lucas et al 2002) and the experimental lesions in these animals have long been considered to represent a poor model for wounds in humans, because of the species differences in tegument compared with humans (King 1990).

Perhaps the most interesting aspect of this type of animal work has been reports of the potential of laser irradiation to accelerate regeneration of damaged nerves, together with associated electrophysiological and functional recovery, after various types of experimental lesions (Anders et al 2004). If such effects are also possible in humans, the implications for future applications of this modality would be enormous (Gigo-Benato et al 2005).

The effects of laser irradiation have been studied in various animal models of pain, to investigate its mechanism of action, and dependence upon irradiation parameters (Ferreira et al 2005, Ponnudurai et al 1987, Wedlock & Shephard 1996, Wedlock

et al 1996). These studies have generally demonstrated a significant hypoalgesic effect of laser irradiation, which seems to be dependent upon the irradiation parameters used (pulse repetition rate: Ponnudurai et al 1987; dosage: Wedlock et al 1996). Furthermore, the observed hypoalgesia has been found to be naloxone reversible in some studies (Wedlock & Shephard 1996), but not in others (Ponnudurai et al 1987), suggesting that the pain relief obtained with laser irradiation may be underpinned by a variety of different mechanisms, and in some circumstances may be opiate mediated.

Notwithstanding the utility of such animal work, some of the problems in extrapolating the findings to humans remain. As a consequence, several groups have used controlled studies in healthy human volunteers as a useful means of investigation without recourse to patients and the problems inherent in undertaking controlled clinical research.

CONTROLLED STUDIES IN HUMANS

Whereas studies in this area have focused principally on the physiological and hypoalgesic effects of laser radiation, controlled studies on experimental lesions have also been completed and have shown benefits of laser irradiation (Hopkins et al 2004). Nerve conduction studies have long been used to study the effects of laser on peripheral nerves; such studies have typically demonstrated significant effects on peripheral nerve conduction in peripheral nerves, which would appear to depend upon the dosage and pulse repetition rate of the laser source (Basford et al 1993, Baxter et al 1994, Lowe et al 1994, Safavi-Farokhi & Bakhtiary 2005). However, the precise relevance of such observations to the clinical applications of this modality is debatable. Of more direct relevance to clinical practice, a number of studies have assessed the effects of laser upon various types of experimentally induced pain in humans; however these have produced variable findings (Brockhaus & Elger 1990, Douris et al 2006, Lowe et al 1997, Vinck et al 2006).

CLINICAL STUDIES

Although a large number of clinical studies have been completed and published in this area, generally with positive results, reviewers have consistently noted the following problems with the literature (Beckerman et al 1992):

- Most studies have been published in foreign-language journals, often without English abstracts, making the work inaccessible to anglophone researchers and clinicians.

- The studies reported in the literature (regardless of language) are often poorly controlled with only very limited blinding; indeed, a significant proportion of the studies is merely anecdotal in nature.

- The irradiation parameters and treatment protocols used are frequently inadequately specified, thus limiting comparison of results and rendering replication and application in the clinical setting impossible. Even where irradiation parameters are specified, the bewildering number of possible permutations and combinations of wavelength, irradiance, pulse repetition rate, etc. will often mean that precise replication is problematic.

This notwithstanding, it is important to stress that the published database of clinical studies on LILT represents a significant body of evidence in favour of the modality; although the constraints of this text preclude an exhaustive review of this literature, the following provides an overview of some of the most relevant recent reviews in the area.

WOUND HEALING

The popularity of laser therapy among physiotherapists for the treatment of various types of wound is evidenced by the results of the only large-scale survey of current clinical practice in this field (Baxter et al 1991). Treatment of various types of chronic ulceration was the first application for low-intensity laser to be trialled in humans during the late 1960s and early 1970s (Mester & Mester 1989), using He-Ne sources and dosages of up to $4\,Jcm^{-2}$. Based upon the reported success of these early studies, in terms of enhanced rates of wound healing and pain reduction, the modality quickly achieved popularity in this application. In the intervening decades, laser therapy has been assessed in the treatment of a variety of wounds and ulcerated lesions with positive results, especially when applied in more chronic,

intractable cases (Lagan et al 1998, Robinson and Walters 1991, Schindl et al 1999). However, and despite widespread and continuing clinical applications in wound treatment, research findings for laser therapy are not exclusively positive (Kopera et al 2005) and many of the reports published to date are of low quality and based upon relatively small numbers (Posten et al 2005). This notwithstanding, one comprehensive recent review in this area has reported clear evidence of the benefit of laser therapy for the promotion of wound healing, based upon animal experiments as well as clinical studies in humans (Woodruff et al 2004).

ARTHRITIC CONDITIONS

The role of laser therapy in the management of arthritic conditions such as rheumatoid arthritis, osteoarthritis and arthrogenic pain has been extensively investigated for almost three decades. The reviews of clinical trials in these conditions have produced mixed conclusions, and have been criticised as suffering from systematic biases (Bjordal et al 2005). The most recent systematic reviews in this area have provided some support for the effectiveness of laser therapy in rheumatoid arthritis (Brosseau et al 2005, Ottawa Panel 2004), particularly for relief of pain and early morning stiffness in the short term; in contrast, the evidence for its effectiveness in the treatment of osteoarthritis is more equivocal (Brosseau et al 2004). Although the precise reasons for contradictory research findings are not entirely clear, they may be due in part to the confusion surrounding the selection of laser parameters in these studies, including the use of relatively low output powers in some of the earlier studies (Basford et al 1987). Current opinion and evidence favours the use of infrared wavelengths (>700 nm), along with relatively higher power (>30 mW) and dosage (>2–3 J per point) levels for the effective treatment of arthritic conditions.

MUSCULOSKELETAL DISORDERS

Treatment of musculoskeletal disorders (including pain and soft-tissue injuries) represents the most common application of laser therapy in routine physiotherapy practice, and the area that has been studied most extensively. As for other areas of application, confusion over the clinical relevance of irradiation parameters and appropriate application techniques has confounded a systematic approach to research in musculoskeletal disorders (e.g. low-output powers: Waylonis et al 1988; use of non-contact treatment technique: Siebert et al 1987). Results from recent systematic reviews in this area have included inconclusive findings for the treatment of lateral epicondylitis ('tennis elbow'; Stasinopoulos & Johnson 2005), although this review has been criticized for including trials of laser acupuncture alongside 'regular' laser therapy treatments (Chow 2006). In tendinopathies, a systematic review by Bjordal and colleagues has provided evidence of effectiveness and also the potential relevance of dose to clinical effects for different types of tendinopathy (Bjordal et al 2001). Apart from reductions in pain associated with treatment effects in the musculoskeletal conditions already indicated, laser therapy has also been reported as effective in the treatment of various types of pain, including neuropathic and neurogenic pain syndromes. However, and despite positive reports, the treatment of pain has long been one of the most contentious areas of laser application, based in part upon what is regarded as the lack of an obvious mechanism of action (Devor 1990). This notwithstanding, the modality has been a popular treatment method with physiotherapists for the relief of pain, and is highly rated against alternative electrotherapeutic modalities (Baxter et al 1991). Furthermore, findings from a recent review in this area have provided some evidence for the effectiveness of laser therapy for the treatment of neck pain, although the authors again highlighted the problems associated with the lack of high-quality research within the field (Chow & Barnsley 2005).

PRINCIPLES OF CLINICAL APPLICATION

INDICATIONS

Laser therapy finds a variety of applications in clinical practice; these can be usefully summarized under the following headings:

- Wound management: stimulation of wound healing processes in various types of open wounds, and particularly chronic ulcers.

- Treatment of soft-tissue injuries.
- Treatment of arthritis: treatment of various arthritic conditions.
- Pain relief: relief of pain of various aetiologies.

These are considered in outline below, after an overview of the principles underlying effective laser treatment. As a basis for subsequent sections and to aid the reader in more critical review of the work published in this area, the method of calculating dosage and the importance of other irradiation parameters are presented below.

DOSAGE AND IRRADIATION PARAMETERS

Apart from wavelength, which is determined by the lasing medium used in the device, the other irradiation parameters that are important to consider in laser treatments are as follows.

Power output

The power output of a unit is usually expressed in milliwatts (mW), or thousandths of a watt. This is usually fixed and invariable. However, some machines allow operator selection of the percentage of the total power output (e.g. 10%, 25%); in addition, where pulsing of the output is provided as an option to be set by the operator, this can affect the power output of the unit in some devices. Over the last two decades, relatively higher-power output devices (30–200 mW per source), have replaced the once-popular 1–10 mW devices for routine clinical use, not least because higher-output units can deliver a specified treatment in a much shorter period of time.

Irradiance (power density)

The power per unit area (mW/cm^2) is an important irradiation parameter. It is usually kept as high as possible for a given unit by use of the so-called 'in-contact' treatment technique and by applying a firm pressure through the treatment head during treatment. It should be noted that, even with the small degrees of divergence associated with laser treatment devices, treatment out of contact with the target tissue will significantly reduce the effectiveness of treatment as the irradiance falls owing to the inverse square law (see Chapter 2) and because of increased reflection from the skin or tissue interface. For in-contact treatments for single point/probe devices, the irradiance is simply calculated by dividing the power output (or average power output for a pulsed unit) by the spot size of the treatment head; typical values for the latter are 0.1–0.125 cm^2.

Energy

This is given in joules (J) and is usually specified per point irradiated, or sometimes for the 'total' treatment where a number of points are treated. It is calculated by multiplying the power output in watts by the time of irradiation or application in seconds. Thus a 30 mW (i.e. 0.03 W) device applied for 1 minute (i.e. 60 seconds) will deliver 1.8 J of energy. For routine clinical practice, dosage is recorded in joules per point: thus, for treatment of a tendon using a 100 mW laser for 30 seconds per point, dose could be recorded as 3 J per point.

Radiant exposure (energy density)

This is generally considered to be the best means of specifying dosage, at least for research papers, and is given in joules per unit area (i.e. Jcm^{-2}); typical values for routine treatments may range from 1 to 30 Jcm^{-2}. Energy density is usually calculated by dividing the energy delivered (in joules) by the spot size of the treatment unit (in cm^2). It should be noted that this can lead to some variance in calculated dosage where manufacturers provide different estimates of spot size for their units (e.g. consider the same dose of 1 J delivered over spot sizes of 0.01 or 0.1 cm^2). Energy density can be a useful measure of dosage for treatment of wounds, especially where using 'cluster' units, where the total energy (in J) is divided by the wound area (in cm^2, established as part of wound assessment). Thus the treatment of a pressure sore (decubitus ulcer) using a multisource array with a total output of 500 mW for a total of 2 minutes (120 seconds) over a wound of 12 cm^2 would result in an average energy density of 5 Jcm^{-2}.

Pulse repetition rate

Although a percentage of the laser units routinely used in clinical practice are continuous wave (CW) output (i.e. the output power is essentially invariable over time), most units currently available allow for some form of pulsing of their output. For pulsed units, the pulse repetition rate is expressed in hertz (Hz, pulses per second). Typical values for pulse repetition rate can vary from 2 to tens of thousands of Hz (or kHz). Although the potential biological and clinical relevance of pulse repetition rate is still far from being universally accepted, cellular research would suggest that this parameter is critical to at least some of the biological effects of this modality (Nussbaum et al 2002, Rajaratnam et al 1994).

IMPORTANCE OF THE USE OF CONTACT TECHNIQUE

Although the method of application may vary depending on the presenting condition, wherever possible the treatment head or probe should be applied with a firm pressure to the area of tissue to be treated (Fig. 11.4). In the first instance, this makes the laser treatment inherently safer by reducing the potential for accidental intrabeam viewing (and thus the risk of eye injury). However, the primary reason for using so-called contact technique is to maximize the irradiance or power density on the tissue surface, and hence the light flux within the target tissue, which are important in ensuring the effectiveness of laser treatment. Where the treatment head is used out of contact, the light flux within the tissue is reduced owing to several factors; most importantly, the inverse square law applies to such non-contact applications, leading to reduced incident irradiance on surface of the irradiated tissue.

Apart from producing the highest levels of light flux within the tissue, application of the contact technique will also allow the operator to press the treatment probe into the tissues to treat deeper-seated lesions more effectively. As well as compensating for the relatively limited penetration of therapeutic laser devices by approximating the treatment probe with the target tissue, the deep pressure will drive red blood cells from the area of tissue directly under the probe head and thus reduce the attenuation of light due to absorption by such cells.

Application of the laser treatment probe also affords the opportunity of applying pressure treatments to key points (e.g. trigger or acupoints) and thus effectively combines laser with acupressure-type treatments; indeed, 'laser acupuncture' has long been proposed as a viable alternative (and

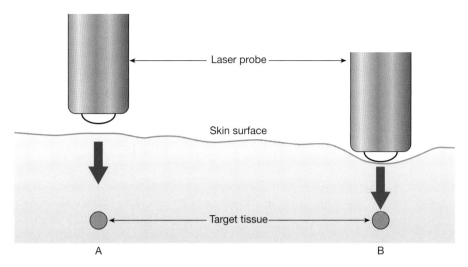

Figure 11.4 Contact versus non-contact technique. A, non-contact technique; B, contact technique.

non-invasive) means of stimulating acupuncture points (Baxter 1989).

Despite the above, there are situations in which laser treatment cannot be applied using contact technique, principally when such application would be too painful or when an aseptic technique is required (e.g. in cases of open wounds). Less commonly, the contours of the tissue to be treated may not allow use of a so-called 'cluster' head in full contact, and so non-contact technique must be used. Where this is the case, the treatment head should not be held more than 0.5–1 cm from the surface of the target tissue.

TREATMENT OF OPEN WOUNDS AND ULCERS

The treatment of open wounds and ulcers represents the cardinal application for low-intensity laser devices and combined phototherapy/LILT units (Fig. 11.5). For comprehensive treatment of such lesions, irradiation is applied in two stages: the first using standard contact technique around the edges of the wound; the second, during which the wound bed is treated, using non-contact technique.

Treatment of wound margins

For this, a single-diode probe is the ideal unit to apply treatment around the circumference of wound at approximately 1–2 cm from its edges. Points of application should be no more than 2–3 cm apart,

and the treatment unit should be applied with a firm pressure to the intact skin, within the patient's tolerances.

For such treatments of the wound margins, dosages should be initiated at 1 J per point (approximately $10 \, \mathrm{J/cm^2}$ assuming a $0.1 \, \mathrm{cm^2}$ spot size).

Treatment of the wound bed

As already indicated above, treatment of the wound bed will invariably be completed using non-contact technique. As the wound lacks the usual protective layer of dermis, the dosages applied during treatment will be much lower than during application over intact skin; typically cited radiant exposures are somewhere in the range of $1–10 \, \mathrm{J cm^{-2}}$, with $4 \, \mathrm{J cm^{-2}}$ being most commonly recommended as the so-called 'Mester protocol' (i.e. based upon the early work of Professor Endre Mester's group).

However, the problem of applying such a dosage in a standardized fashion across the surface of an open wound is obvious and has led to several means of application being recommended in these conditions. At the simplest level, where only a single probe or fibreoptic applicator is available, the wound may be 'mapped' with a hypothetical grid of equal-sized squares (typically $1–2 \, \mathrm{cm^2}$), each of which may be regarded as an individual area of target tissue and treated accordingly at the recommended dosage. Apart from such gridding, some therapists have also employed some variant of scanning technique to treat the wound bed where

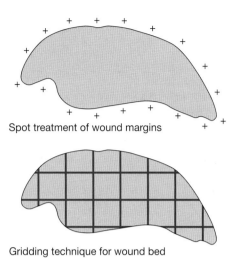

Spot treatment of wound margins

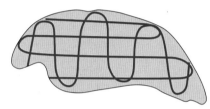

Gridding technique for wound bed

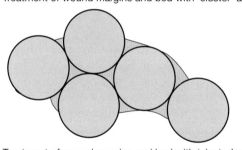

Treatment of wound margins and bed with 'cluster' array

Treatment of wound margins and bed with 'cluster' array

Figure 11.5 Laser treatment of wounds. Wound margin is treated with single probe using contact technique (1 cm from wound; 2-cm intervals); wound bed is treated using non-contact technique using either gridding or scanning technique (single-diode probe) or multidiode 'cluster' unit.

single-diode or fibreoptic applicators are used. In these cases, the probe is moved slowly over the area of the lesion using a non-contact technique and taking care to deliver a standardized radiant exposure to all areas, while maintaining the head at a distance of no more than 1 cm from the wound bed.

Special devices for treatment of wounds

A number of special devices have been produced and marketed to simplify and improve the efficiency and effectiveness of wound treatments. In the first instance, several manufacturers have produced scanning devices which mechanically direct the output of the device over an area defined by the operator by means of controls on the scanning unit. While such devices have been popular in some circles in offering a 'hands-off' approach to providing standardized treatment across the whole wound area, particularly in cases of more extensive wounds (e.g. burns), the relatively high cost and potentially greater hazards associated with these units have prevented them becoming popular.

As an alternative to scanners, most manufacturers now provide the option of so-called 'cluster' units, typically incorporating an array of diodes in a single hand-held unit. The number of diodes typically provided in these clusters varies between 3 and 200, but it is generally true that the larger units incorporate a mixture of superluminous (monochromatic) diodes as well as (true) laser sources in their arrays, owing to the prohibitive cost of the latter. Such cluster units allow simultaneous treatment of an area of tissue, the extent of which is decided by the number and configuration of the diodes included in the array. Furthermore, several manufacturers have incorporated diodes operating at a variety of wavelengths (i.e. multisource/multi-wavelength arrays) in their cluster units, claiming enhanced clinical effects through parallel (and possibly synergistic) wavelength-specific effects. In routine clinical practice, the relative difficulty in treating extensive ulceration with single-diode units has led to the use of cluster units being commonly cited by therapists (Baxter et al 1991). In treating wound beds, cluster units can be used in isolation or in conjunction with single probes to access deeper or recessed areas, and in either case provide a more time efficient means of treatment than single probes units used in isolation.

TREATMENT OF OTHER CONDITIONS

As already indicated, when treatment is applied to intact skin, contact technique is the application of choice. For such treatment of general musculoskeletal conditions, laser therapy can usefully be applied in a number of ways.

Direct treatment of the lesion

In such cases, the laser probe is applied directly to the lesion (area of bruising, site of pain, etc.) using a firm pressure within the patient's tolerance. Where extensive bruising/haematoma is present, an 'in contact' version of wound treatment (as above) is applied; for these cases, dosages applied are correspondingly higher than those used for the treatment of open wounds, given the presence of the skin as a barrier to laser irradiation.

Treatment of acupuncture and trigger points

In China and Japan, the main method of laser application is as an alternative to needles for acupuncture. Although the comparative effectiveness of such application with respect to needles or other non-invasive alternatives (e.g. TENS, acupressure) is still unclear, there are a number of positive reports in the literature of successful application of laser acupuncture for pain relief (Gur et al 2004, Hakguder et al 2003). Taut muscles with associated, well-localized areas of pain upon palpation (i.e. trigger points; Baldry 1993) may also be treated with laser irradiation; although no definitive recommendations can be made on dosage for such trigger-point therapy, to date the best results are achieved when an adequately high-power unit (i.e. >10 mW) is employed to deliver initial dosages of 1–3 J per point (i.e. in line with general recommendations for routine musculoskeletal treatments; World Association for Laser Therapy (WALT) 2005).

Irradiation over nerve roots, trunks, etc.

In the laser treatment of pain syndromes, or in cases where pain represents a major feature of the clinical presentation of the condition to be treated, irradiation may usefully be applied to the skin overlying the appropriate nerve root, plexus or trunk. For example, in treating upper limb pain, laser therapy might be applied over the relevant cervical nerve roots or the brachial plexus by irradiation over Erb's point, as well as to points where the nerves in the arm are relatively superficial, such as the radial, median or ulnar nerves at the elbow or wrist.

KEY POINTS ON LASER TREATMENT OF SOME SELECTED CONDITIONS

SOFT-TISSUE INJURIES

In such conditions, treatment should be initiated as early as is practically possible within the acute stage, using relatively low dosages in the region of 1 J per point or 10 Jcm^{-2} applied directly to the site of injury and any areas of palpable pain. Within the first 72–96 hours after injury, such treatment may be applied up to three times daily with no risk of overtreatment, provided that dosages are kept low. It is important to reiterate that low-intensity laser treatment is by definition athermal, and thus eminently suitable for treatment in these situations. As the condition resolves, the frequency of laser treatment may be reduced and dosage correspondingly increased, up to a maximum of 3–4 J per point, or 30–40 Jcm^{-2}. Where pulsed systems are available, early treatments should be initiated with relatively low pulse repetition rates (100 Hz) and increased into the kilohertz range as treatment progresses. Where haematoma or bruising is present, it should be treated using the general principles already outlined for the treatment of open wounds, although in this case a firm contact technique should be used within the patient's tolerance, particularly where the lesion is relatively deep.

In the treatment of muscle tears and injuries, laser therapy can be effective in accelerating the repair process and thus the return to normal function. This, coupled with its ability to be applied early in the acute stage – in some cases immediately after injury – makes it a popular modality in the treatment of sports injuries.

Neuropathic and neurogenic pain

Where the patient presents with chronic neurogenic pain, laser irradiation is typically applied in a systematic fashion to all relevant nerve roots, plexus and trunks, using a middle-range dosage of 1–2 J per point (10–20 Jcm^{-2}) to initiate treatment. Where trigger or tender points are identified, these are also treated, using the same dose level, which is increased to achieve desensitization of the point upon repalpation (i.e. as is normal practice with treatment of trigger points with other modalities). Irradiation is also applied directly to any areas of referred pain, and to the affected dermatome, etc.

Arthrogenic pain and arthritis

Arthritis and arthralgia of various aetiologies can be managed effectively with laser treatment when it is applied in a comprehensive manner to the affected joints at the appropriate dosages (2–10 J per point; WALT 2005). Care is needed (especially with regard to patient positioning) to ensure that all aspects of the joint are systematically treated.

HAZARDS

CLASSIFICATION OF LASERS AND OCULAR HAZARD

Under an internationally agreed classification system (revised in 2002), laser devices are classed on a scale from 1 to 4 according to the associated dangers to the unprotected skin and eye: 1, 1M, 2, 2M, 3R, 3B, 4. The units typically used in LILT are designated as class 3R or 3B lasers, although much lower output class 1 and 2 devices have also been used. This essentially means, for the majority of systems used in physiotherapy applications (i.e. class 3R and 3B units), that although the laser's output may be considered harmless when directed on to the unprotected skin, it poses a *potential* hazard to the eye if viewed along the axis of the beam (i.e. intrabeam viewing) owing to the high degree of collimation of the laser light. For this reason, the use of protective goggles, which must be appropriate for the wavelength(s) used, is recommended for operator and patient. Care is also recommended in ensuring that the beam is never directed towards the unprotected eye; the patient should be specifically warned about the ocular hazard associated with the device and asked not to stare directly at the treatment site during application. Furthermore, the laser treatment unit should ideally be used only in an area specifically designated for this purpose; outside this area, the appropriate laser warning symbols should be clearly displayed. Having outlined these fundamental safety rules, it is important to stress that the ocular hazard associated with therapeutic

units is (for all practical purposes) negligible, especially where the treatment head or probe is used with the recommended 'in-contact' technique (see the section Principles of clinical application, above). In addition, the output of the treatment unit should be regularly tested to ensure the optimal operation (and thus effectiveness) of the device; this is particularly important as it has been reported that a large proportion of laser units in routine use may not be providing adequate power output to be effective (Nussbaum et al 1999).

CONTRAINDICATIONS

Further information is available in Bazin et al (2006), Chartered Society of Physiotherapy (CPS) (1991) and Navratil and Kymplova (2002).

Apart from direct treatment of the eye (for whatever reason), the use of LILT is also contraindicated in the following cases.

- **In patients with active or suspected carcinoma** (with the exception of the treatment of wounds in people in hospice care, where the ethical considerations are different): studies at the cellular level testify to the potential photobiostimulatory effects of laser radiation; given this, it is possible that therapeutic laser application could accelerate carcinogenesis in patients where carcinoma is present. Despite this potential danger, it should be stressed that laboratory studies in normal cells have consistently failed to demonstrate any carcinogenic effects of laser radiation; indeed, results from controlled experiments in cells have found no evidence of either cytotoxic nor genotoxic effects (Logan et al 1995).

- **Direct irradiation over the pregnant uterus**: in the absence of hard evidence to show no associated hazard to fetus or mother, avoiding treatment directly over the pregnant uterus represents a prudent and standard precaution that applies to all forms of electrotherapy.

- **Irradiation of the testes**: it has also recently been recommended that laser therapy should be contraindicated for treatment of the testes (Bazin et al 2006; although hot packs, infrared and wax are *not* considered to be contraindicated in this area!).

- **Areas of haemorrhage**: this represents an absolute contraindication to laser treatment owing to the possibility of laser-induced vasodilatation, which would exacerbate the condition.

OTHER SAFETY CONSIDERATIONS

The above are usually regarded as the cardinal contraindications to treatment with LILT, but caution should be exercised in a number of other situations (Bazin et al 2006). Principally, for laser therapy, these include the following:

- **Treatment of infected tissue** (e.g. infected open wounds): as laser light has the potential to stimulate various bacteria in culture, including *Escherichia coli* (Karu 1998, Nussbaum et al 2002, 2003, Shields & O'Kane 1994), it would seem only prudent to recommend caution in the application of laser therapy to infected tissue, and especially infected open wounds. However, the situation is far from clear, as there is evidence to suggest that clinicians have successfully treated such conditions with laser therapy, and in some cases regard the presence of infection as an indication for such treatment (Baxter et al 1991).

- **Treatment over the sympathetic ganglia, vagus nerves and cardiac region in patients with heart disease**: the possibility of laser-mediated alterations in neural activity resulting in adverse effects upon cardiac function can represent an unacceptable risk for these patients.

- **Cognitive difficulties or unreliable patient**: the patient should be able to understand the explanation and mandatory warnings, and to comply with instructions.

- **Treatment over photosensitive areas**: patients with a history of photosensitivity (e.g. adverse reactions to sunlight) should be treated with care, and in such cases the use of a test dose is recommended. In addition, the concurrent use of photosensitizing drugs should also be excluded.

- **Treatment of patient with epilepsy**: care should be exercised when treating patients with a history of epilepsy.

- **Treatment of areas of altered skin sensation**: although laser treatment is athermic, and is recommended in the treatment of peripheral nerve lesions, care should be exercised in such cases.

References

Anders JJ, Geuna S, Rochkind S (2004) Phototherapy promotes regeneration and functional recovery of injured peripheral nerve. *Neurol Res* **26**: 233–239.

Baldry P (1993) *Acupuncture, Trigger Points and Musculoskeletal Pain*, 2nd edn. New York, Churchill Livingstone.

Basford JR (1995) Low intensity laser therapy: still not an established clinical tool. *Lasers Surg Med* **16**: 331–342.

Basford JR, Hallman JO, Matsumoto JY et al (1993) Effects of 830 nm laser diode irradiation on median nerve function in normal subjects. *Lasers Surg Med* **13**: 597–604.

Basford JR, Sheffield CG, Mair SD et al (1987) Low energy helium neon laser treatment of thumb osteoarthritis. *Arch Phys Med Rehab* **68**: 794–797.

Baxter GD (1989) Laser acupuncture analgesia: an overview. *Acupuncture Med* **6**: 57–60.

Baxter GD (1994) *Therapeutic Lasers: Theory and Practice*. New York, Churchill Livingstone.

Baxter GD, Bell AJ, Ravey J et al (1991) Low level laser therapy: current clinical practice in Northern Ireland. *Physiotherapy* **77**: 171–178.

Baxter GD, Walsh DM, Lowe AS et al (1994) Effects of low intensity infrared laser irradiation upon conduction in the human median nerve *in vivo*. *Exp Physiol* **79**: 227–234.

Bayat M, Delbari A, Almaseyeh MA et al (2005) Low-level laser therapy improves early healing of medial collateral ligament injuries in rats. *Photomed Laser Surg* **23**: 556–560.

Bayat M, Vasheghani MM, Razavi N (2006) Effect of low-level helium-neon laser therapy on the healing of third-degree burns in rats. *J Photochem Photobiol B – Biology* **83**: 87–93.

Bazin S, Kitchen S, Maskill D et al (2006) *Guidance for the Clinical Use of Electrophysical Agents*. London, Chartered Society of Physiotherapy.

Beckerman H, de Bie RA, Bouter LM et al (1992) The efficacy of laser therapy for musculoskeletal and skin disorders: a criteria-based meta-analysis of randomized clinical trials. *Phys Ther* **72**: 483–491.

Bjordal JM, Bogen B, Lopes-Martins RA et al (2005) Can Cochrane Reviews in controversial areas be biased? A sensitivity analysis based on the protocol of a Systematic Cochrane Review on low-level laser therapy in osteoarthritis. *Photomed Laser Surg* **23**: 453–458.

Bjordal JM, Couppe C, Ljungren AE (2001) Low level laser therapy for tendinopathy: evidence of a dose–response pattern. *Phys Ther Rev* **6**: 91–100.

Bolton P, Young S, Dyson M (1995) The direct effect of 860 nm light on cell proliferation and on succinic dehydrogenase activity of human fibroblasts in vitro. *Laser Ther* **7**: 55–60.

Brockhaus A, Elger CE (1990) Hypoalgesic efficacy of acupuncture on experimental pain in man. Comparison of laser acupuncture and needle acupuncture. *Pain* **43**: 181–186.

Brosseau L, Robinson V, Wells G et al (2005) Low level laser therapy (classes I, II and III) for treating rheumatoid arthritis. Cochrane Database Systematic Reviews, CD002049.

Brosseau L, Welch V, Wells G et al (2004) Low level laser therapy (classes I, II and III) for treating osteoarthritis. Cochrane Database Systematic Reviews, CD002046.

Byrnes KR, Wu X, Waynant RW et al (2005) Low power laser irradiation alters gene expression of olfactory ensheathing cells in vitro. *Lasers Surg Med* 37:161–171.

Chartered Society of Physiotherapy (CSP) (1991) Guidelines for the safe use of lasers in physiotherapy. *Physiotherapy* **77**: 169–170.

Chow R (2006) Laser acupuncture studies should not be included in systematic reviews of phototherapy. *Photomed Laser Surg* **24**: 69.

Chow RT, Barnsley L (2005) Systematic review of the literature of low-level laser therapy (LLLT) in the management of neck pain. *Lasers Surg Med* **37**: 46–52.

Devor M (1990) What's in a beam for pain therapy? *Pain* **43**: 139.

Douris P, Southard V, Ferrigi R et al (2006) Effect of phototherapy on delayed onset muscle soreness. *Photomed Laser Surg* **24**: 377–382.

Ferreira DM, Zangaro RA, Villaverde AB et al (2005) Analgesic effect of He-Ne (632.8 nm) low-level laser therapy on acute inflammatory pain. *Photomed Laser Surg* **23**: 177–181.

Gigo-Benato D, Geuna S, Rochkind S (2005) Phototherapy for enhancing peripheral nerve repair: a review of the literature. *Muscle Nerve* **31**: 694–701.

Gur A, Sarac AJ, Cevik R et al (2004) Efficacy of 904 nm gallium arsenide low level laser therapy in the management of chronic myofascial pain in the neck: a double-blind and randomized-controlled trial. *Lasers Surg Med* **35**: 229–235.

Hakguder A, Birtane M, Gurcan S et al (2003) Efficacy of low level laser therapy in myofascial pain syndrome: an algometric and thermographic evaluation. *Lasers Surg Med* **33**: 339–343.

Hawkins DH, Abrahamse H (2006) The role of laser fluence in cell viability, proliferation, and membrane integrity of wounded human skin fibroblasts following helium-neon laser irradiation. *Lasers Surg Med* **38**: 74–83.

Hopkins JT, McLoda TA, Seegmiller JG et al (2004) Low level laser therapy facilitates superficial wound healing in humans: a triple-blind, sham-controlled study. *J Athletic Training* **39**: 223–229.

Karu T (1998) *The Science of Low Power Laser Therapy*. Amsterdam, Gordon & Breach.

Khadra M, Kasem N, Haanaes HR et al (2004) Enhancement of bone formation in rat calvarial bone defects using low-level laser therapy. *Oral Surg Oral Med Oral Pathol Oral Radiol Endodontics* **97**: 693–700.

King PR (1990) Low level laser therapy: a review. *Physiother Theory Prac* **6**: 127–138.

Kopera D, Kokol R, Berger C et al (2005) Does the use of low-level laser influence wound healing in chronic venous leg ulcers? *J Wound Care* **14**: 391–394.

Lagan KM, Baxter GD, Ashford RL (1998) Combined phototherapy/low intensity laser therapy in the management of diabetic ischaemic and neuropathic ulceration: a single case series investigation. *Laser Ther* **10**: 103–110.

Logan ID, McKenna PG, Barnett YA (1995) An investigation of the cytotoxic and mutagenic potential of low intensity laser irradiation in Friend erythroleukaemia cells. *Mut Res* **347**: 67–71.

Lowe AS, Baxter GD, Walsh DM et al (1994) The effect of low intensity laser (830 nm) irradiation upon skin temperature and antidromic conduction latencies in the human median nerve: relevance of radiant exposure. *Lasers Surg Med* **14**: 40–46.

Lowe AS, McDowell BC, Walsh DM et al (1997) Failure to demonstrate any hypoalgesic effect of low intensity laser irradiation of Erb's point upon experimental ischaemic pain in humans. *Lasers Surg Med* **14**: 40–46.

Lucas C, Criens-Poublon LJ, Cockrell CT et al (2002) Wound healing in cell studies and animal model experiments by low level laser therapy; were clinical studies justified? A systematic review. *Lasers Med Sci* **17**: 110–134.

Medrado AR, Pugliese LS, Reis SR et al (2003) Influence of low level laser therapy on wound healing and its biological action upon myofibroblasts. *Lasers Surg Med* **32**: 239–244.

Mester AF, Mester A (1989) Wound healing. *Laser Ther* **1**: 7–15.

Mester E, Mester AF, Mester A (1985) The biomedical effects of laser application. *Lasers Surg Med* **5**: 31–39.

Navratil L, Kymplova J (2002) Contraindications in noninvasive laser therapy: truth and fiction. *J Clin Laser Med Surg* **20**: 341–343.

Nussbaum EL, Baxter GD, Lilge L (2003a) A review of laser technology and light tissue interactions as a background to therapeutic applications of low intensity lasers and other light sources. *Phys Ther Rev* **8**: 31–44.

Nussbaum EL, Lilge L, Mazzulli T (2003b) Effects of low-level laser therapy (LLLT) of 810 nm upon in vitro growth of bacteria: relevance of irradiance and radiant exposure. *J Clin Laser Med Surg* **21**: 283–290.

Nussbaum EL, Lilge L, Mazzulli T (2002) Effects of 630-, 660-, 810-, and 905 -nm laser irradiation delivering radiant exposure of 1–50 J/cm^2 on three species of bacteria *in vitro*. *J Clin Laser Med Surg* **20**: 325–333.

Nussbaum E, Van Zuylen V, Baxter GD (1999) Specification of treatment dosage in laser therapy: unreliable equipment and radiant power determination as confounding factors. *Physiother Canada* **51**: 159–167.

Ohshiro T, Calderhead RG (1988) *Low Level Laser Therapy: A Practical Introduction*. Chichester, UK, Wiley.

O'Kane S, Shields TD, Gilmore WS et al (1994) Low intensity laser irradiation inhibits tritiated thymidine incorporation in the haemopoietic cell lines HL-60 and U-937. *Lasers Surg Med* **14**: 34–39.

Ottawa Panel (2004) Evidence-based clinical practice guidelines for electrotherapy and thermotherapy interventions in the management of rheumatoid arthritis in adults. *Phys Ther* **84**: 1016–1043.

Pogrel MA, Chen JW, Zang K (1997) Effects of low-energy gallium-aluminium-arsenide laser irradiation on cultured fibroblasts and keratinocytes. *Lasers Surg Med* **20**: 426–432.

Ponnudurai RN, Zbuzek VK, Wu W (1987) Hypoalgesic effect of laser photobiostimulation shown by rat tail flick test. *Int J Acupuncture Electrother Res* **12**: 93–100.

Posten W, Wrone DA, Dover JS et al (2005) Low-level laser therapy for wound healing: mechanism and efficacy. *Dermatol Surg* **31**: 334–340.

Rabelo SB, Villaverde AB, Nicolau R et al (2006) Comparison between wound healing in induced diabetic and nondiabetic rats after low-level laser therapy. *Photomed Laser Surg* **24**: 474–479.

Rajaratnam S, Bolton P, Dyson M (1994) Macrophage responsiveness to laser therapy with varying pulsing frequencies. *Laser Ther* **6**: 107–112.

Robinson B, Walters J (1991) The use of low level laser therapy in diabetic and other ulcerations. *J Br Podiatr Med* **46**: 10.

Safavi-Farokhi Z, Bakhtiary AH (2005) The effect of infrared laser on sensory radial nerve electrophysiological parameters. *Electromyogr Clin Neurophysiol* **45**: 353–356.

Schindl M, Kerschan K, Schindl A et al (1999) Induction of complete wound healing in recalcitrant ulcers by low-intensity laser irradiation depends on ulcer cause and size. *Photodermatol Photoimmunol Photomed* **15**: 18–21.

Schindl A, Schindl M, Pernerstorfer-Schon H et al (2000) Low-intensity laser therapy: a review. *J Invest Med* **48**: 312–326.

Shields D, O'Kane S (1994) Laser photobiomodulation of wound healing. In Baxter GD (ed) *Therapeutic Lasers: Theory and Practice*. Edinburgh, Churchill Livingstone: 89–138.

Siebert W, Siechert N, Siebert B et al (1987) What is the efficacy of 'soft' and 'mid' lasers in therapy of tendinopathies? *Arch Orthop Traum Surg* **106**: 358–363.

Stasinopoulos DI, Johnson MI (2005) Effectiveness of low-level laser therapy for lateral elbow tendinopathy. *Photomed Laser Surg* **23**: 425–430.

Stein A, Benayahu D, Maltz L et al (2005) Low-level laser irradiation promotes proliferation and differentiation of human osteoblasts in vitro. *Photomed Laser Surg* **23**: 161–166.

Tuner J, Hode L (1999) *Low Level Laser Therapy. Clinical Practice and Scientific Background*. Spjutvagen, Sweden, Prima Books.

Vinck E, Cagnie B, Coorevits P et al (2006) Pain reduction by infrared light-emitting diode irradiation: a pilot study on experimentally induced delayed-onset muscle soreness in humans. *Lasers Med Sci* **21**: 11–18.

Walker MD, Rumpf S, Baxter GD et al (2000) Effect of low-intensity laser irradiation (660 nm) on a radiation-impaired wound-healing model in murine skin. *Lasers Surg Med* **26**: 41–47.

Waylonis GW, Wilkie S, O'Toole D et al (1988) Chronic myofascial pain: management by low output helium-neon laser therapy. *Arch Phys Med Rehab* **69**: 1017–1020.

Wedlock PM, Shephard RA (1996) Cranial irradiation with Gaalas laser leads to naloxone reversible analgesia in rats. *Psychol Reports* **78**: 727–731.

Wedlock P, Shephard RA, Little C, McBurney F (1996) Analgesic effects of cranial laser treatment in two rat nociception models. *Physiol Behav* **59**: 445–448.

Woodruff LD, Bounkeo JM, Brannon WM et al (2004) The efficacy of laser therapy in wound repair: a meta-analysis of the literature. *Photomed Laser Surg* **22**: 241–247.

World Association for Laser Therapy (WALT) (2005) *Recommended Anti-Inflammatory Dosage for Low Level Laser Therapy*. WALT. Online. Available: http://www.walt.nu

Chapter 12

Therapeutic ultrasound

Tim Watson and Stephen R. Young

INTRODUCTION

Ultrasound is almost certainly the most widely used of the 'electrotherapy' modalities in current clinical practice. In addition to its widespread use by physiotherapists (Pope et al 1995, ter Haar et al 1985), it is also commonly used by numerous therapists from other professional groups (e.g. osteopaths, chiropractors, sports therapists). Although widely considered as a form of electrotherapy, this is clearly not strictly the case in that ultrasound energy is a form of mechanical rather than electrical or electromagnetic energy (see Chapter 2), although the broader and in this case more accurate term 'electrophysical agent' would certainly encompass the modality comfortably.

Although therapeutic ultrasound has been used for over 40 years, its current use in the clinical environment has changed significantly over this period, and whereas in the past its use was primarily for its thermal effect, it is now more widely employed for its non-thermal effects, especially in relation to tissue repair and wound healing. There is a substantial volume of published evidence relating to the effects and use of ultrasound as a therapeutic modality, and this chapter aims to summarize this evidence.

The results of a survey carried out in Britain in 1985 (ter Haar et al 1985) showed that 20% of all physiotherapy treatments in NHS departments and 54% of all private treatments involved therapeutic ultrasound and the widely cited survey by Pope et al (1995) identified ultrasound as the most frequently employed modality (94%), with 64% of respondents reporting that they used the modality more than once a day (Fig. 12.1). In the 1985 survey, it was shown that there were large variations in the use of ultrasound including a range of intensities from 0.1 to $3.0\,W/cm^2$, giving a variation factor of 30 from the lowest to the highest applied intensity. The current application of ultrasound for fracture healing (see later) at even lower doses ($0.03\,W/cm^2$) would take that to a factor of 100. This is a very substantial variation on just one factor that affects the output of the machine, and it is not surprising, therefore, that some research evidence is supportive of the modality whereas other publications are clearly not. If the effects of 'electrotherapy' interventions are both modality specific and dose specific (see Chapter 1), it is entirely predictable that this would be the case. Further identification of the machine and its dose parameters is clearly needed.

BEHAVIOUR OF ULTRASOUND

The physics of therapeutic ultrasound is covered in Chapter 2 and is not repeated in this section; however, it is important to consider some crucial behavioural characteristics before considering therapeutic effects and clinical use.

ULTRASOUND TRANSMISSION

All materials (tissues) present an impedance to the passage of sound waves. The specific impedance

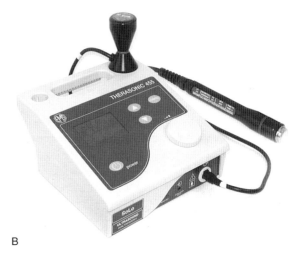

B

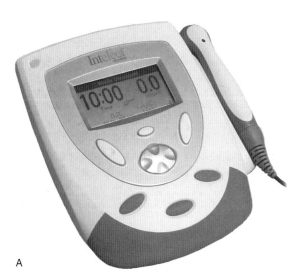

A

Figure 12.1 Modern therapeutic ultrasound machines. A, Chatanooga Intelect (PhysioMed, SKF Services); B, Therasonic (EMSPhysio); C, Enraf Sonopuls (Mobilis).

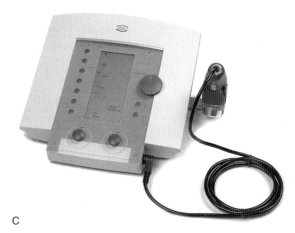

C

of a tissue will be determined by its density and elasticity. For the maximal transmission of energy from one medium to another, the impedance of the two media needs to be the same and thus the reflection that occurs at the interface will be minimized. Clearly, in the case of ultrasound passing from the generator to the body and then through the different tissue types, this cannot actually be achieved. The greater the difference in impedance at a boundary, the greater the reflection that will occur, and hence the smaller the amount of energy that will be transferred.

The difference in impedance is probably greatest for the steel–air interface, which is the first that the ultrasound has to overcome to reach the tissues. To minimize this difference, a suitable coupling medium has to be used. If an air gap exists between the transducer and the skin, the proportion of ultrasound that will be reflected approaches 99.998%, which means that there will be no effective transmission.

The coupling media used in this context include water, various oils, creams and gels. Ideally, the coupling medium should be sufficiently fluid to fill all available spaces; relatively viscous, so that it stays in place; have an impedance appropriate to the media it connects; and should allow transmission of ultrasound with minimal absorption, attenuation or disturbance (for extensive discussions regarding coupling media, see Casarotto et al 2004, Docker et al 1982, Klucinec et al 2000, Poltawski & Watson 2007a, Williams 1987). At the present time, the gel-based media are preferable to the oil- and cream-based media. Water is an effective medium and is a useful alternative but it fails to meet the above criteria in terms of its viscosity. A recent detailed study considering the effect of different coupling gels on ultrasound transmission demonstrated differences in transmission characteristics and absorption levels of commonly employed ultrasound gels, but there was no clinically significant difference between them (Poltawski & Watson 2007a).

In addition to the reflection that occurs at a boundary due to differences in impedance, there will also be some refraction if the wave does not strike the boundary surface at 90°. Essentially, the direction of the ultrasound beam through the second medium will not be the same as its path through the original medium – its pathway is angled. The critical angle for ultrasound at the skin interface appears to be about 15°. If the treatment head is at an angle of 15° or more to the plane of the skin surface, the majority of the ultrasound beam is predicted to travel through the dermal tissues (i.e. parallel to the skin surface) rather than penetrate the tissues as would be expected; it is therefore important to keep the treatment head as flat as possible to the skin surface.

PENETRATION AND ABSORPTION OF ULTRASOUND ENERGY

The absorption of ultrasound energy follows an exponential pattern, i.e. more energy is absorbed in the superficial tissues than in the deep tissues. For energy to have an effect, it must be absorbed. Transmission and attenuation of ultrasound energy are considered in detail in Chapter 2.

Because the absorption (penetration) of ultrasound energy is exponential, there is (in theory) no point at which all the energy has been absorbed, but there is certainly a point at which the energy levels are not sufficient to produce a therapeutic effect. As the ultrasound beam penetrates further into the tissues, a greater proportion of the energy will have been absorbed and therefore there is less energy available to achieve therapeutic effects.

The 'half value depth' is often quoted in relation to ultrasound. It represents the depth in the tissues at which half the surface energy is available. This will be different for each tissue and also for different ultrasound frequencies. As it is difficult (if not impossible) to know the thickness of each of these layers in an individual patient, average half value depths are employed for each frequency:

- 3 MHz   2.0 cm
- 1 MHz   4.0 cm.

These values are not universally accepted (see Ward 1986) and ongoing research suggests that in the clinical environment they may be significantly lower. To achieve a particular ultrasound intensity at depth, account must be taken of the proportion of energy that has been absorbed by the tissues in the more superficial layers (Watson 2002).

As the penetration (or transmission) of ultrasound is not the same in each tissue type, it is clear that some tissues are capable of greater absorption of ultrasound than others. Generally, the tissues with the higher protein content will absorb ultrasound to a greater extent. This means that tissues such as blood and fat, which have a high water content and a low protein content, absorb little of the ultrasound energy, whereas those with a lower water content and a higher protein content will absorb ultrasound far more efficiently. It has been suggested that tissues can therefore be ranked according to their tissue absorption (Fig. 12.2). Although cartilage and bone are at the upper end of this scale, the problems associated with wave reflection at the tissue surface mean that a significant proportion of ultrasound energy striking the surface of either of these tissues is likely to be reflected. The best-absorbing tissues in terms of clinical practice are those with high collagen content: ligament, tendon, fascia, joint capsule and scar tissue (Frizzel & Dunn 1982, Nussbaum 1998, ter Haar 1999, Watson 2000, 2002).

The application of therapeutic ultrasound to tissues with a low energy-absorption capacity is less likely to be effective than the application of the energy into a more highly absorbing material. Recent evidence of the ineffectiveness of such an intervention can be found in Wilkin et al (2004), whereas application in tissue that is a better absorber will, as expected, result in a more effective intervention (Leung et al 2004a, Sparrow et al 2005).

EFFECTS OF ULTRASOUND

When it enters the body, ultrasound exerts an effect on the cells and tissues via two physical mechanisms: thermal and non-thermal. It is important that these mechanisms are understood, as some are

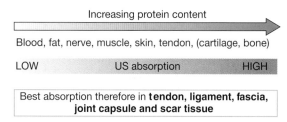

Best absorption therefore in **tendon, ligament, fascia, joint capsule and scar tissue**

Figure 12.2 Ranking of musculoskeletal tissues according to their relative absorption of ultrasound energy.

stimulatory in their effect on the tissue repair process whereas others are potentially dangerous (for further details of the physical principles that underlie the behaviour of ultrasound, see Chapter 2).

THERMAL EFFECTS

When ultrasound travels through tissue a percentage of it is absorbed, and this leads to the generation of heat within that tissue. The amount of absorption depends upon the nature of the tissue, its degree of vascularization, and the frequency of the applied ultrasound. Tissues with a high protein content absorb ultrasound more readily than those with a higher fat content, and also the higher the ultrasound frequency, the greater the absorption rate. A biologically significant thermal effect can be achieved if the temperature of the tissue is raised to between 40 and 45°C for at least 5 minutes. Controlled heating can produce desirable effects (Lehmann & De Lateur 1982), which include pain relief, decrease in joint stiffness and increased local blood flow. The therapeutic benefits of tissue heating are well established (see Chapters 7 and 9) but ultrasound is relatively inefficient at generating sufficient thermal change in the tissues to achieve this therapeutic effect.

Historically, ultrasound has been widely employed for its thermal effects but it has been argued more recently that the 'non-thermal' effects of this energy form are more effective (Watson 2000, 2006a), and currently the majority of clinical applications focus on these. Gallo et al (2004) demonstrated that both continuous and pulsed ultrasound interventions generated measurable thermal changes in the tissues (muscle) but that, considering the temperature changes achieved, they would be expected to be of minimal therapeutic value. Garrett et al (2000) compared the heating effect of a pulsed shortwave treatment with an ultrasound treatment; the pulsed shortwave intervention was clearly more effective at achieving the required thermal change for therapeutic benefit. A patient treated with ultrasound in continuous mode at a relatively high dose will feel a temperature change (mainly in the skin, which is where thermal receptors are predominantly located) but this is not the same as achieving a clinically significant thermal change in deeper tissues.

A possible complication can occur when an ultrasound beam strikes bone or a metal prosthesis. Because of the great acoustic impedance difference between these structures and the surrounding soft tissues at least 30% of the incident energy will be reflected back through the soft tissue. This means that further energy is deposited as heat during the beam's return journey. Therefore, heat rise in soft tissue could be higher when it is situated in front of a reflector. To complicate matters further, an interaction termed *mode conversion* occurs at the interface of the soft tissue and the reflector (e.g. bone or metal prosthesis). During mode conversion, a percentage of the reflected incident energy is converted from a longitudinal waveform into a transverse or shear waveform, which cannot propagate on the soft tissue side of the interface and is therefore absorbed rapidly, causing heat rise (and sometimes pain) at the bone–soft-tissue interface (periosteum). It is suggested that by maintaining a 'moving' treatment head approach and by using pulsed ultrasound, both of these effects will be minimized and will not constitute a clinical risk to the tissues. The greatest risk would be achieved with a high-dose, continuous ultrasound treatment using a stationary treatment applicator. The application of ultrasound over superficial bone or metal in the tissues is not contraindicated (see Chapter 21) although caution is advocated.

NON-THERMAL EFFECTS

There are many situations where ultrasound produces bioeffects and yet significant temperature change is not involved [e.g. low spatial-average temporal-average (SATA) intensity]. It is not strictly true to talk about 'non-thermal' mechanisms, in that the delivery and absorption of energy in the tissues will result in a temperature rise. The term 'non-thermal' in this context relates to the fact that there is no apparent thermal accumulation in the tissues (see Chapter 8) and is sometimes now referred to as a 'microthermal' effect. The term 'non-thermal' will be employed in the latter context throughout this section.

There is evidence indicating that non-thermal mechanisms play a primary role in producing a therapeutically significant effect: stimulation of tissue regeneration (Dyson et al 1968), soft-tissue repair (Dyson et al 1976, Watson 2006a), blood flow in chronically ischaemic tissues (Hogan et al 1982), protein synthesis (Webster et al 1978) and bone repair (Dyson & Brookes 1983, Malizos et al 2006).

The physical mechanisms thought to be involved in producing these non-thermal effects are one or more of the following: cavitation, acoustic streaming and standing waves (Baker et al 2001, ter Haar 1999, Williams 1987).

Cavitation

Ultrasound can cause the formation of micrometer-sized bubbles or cavities in gas-containing fluids. Depending on the pressure amplitude of the energy, the resultant bubbles can be either useful or dangerous. Low-pressure amplitudes result in the formation of bubbles that vibrate to a degree where reversible permeability changes are produced in cell membranes near to the cavitational event (Mortimer & Dyson 1988). Changes in cell permeability to various ions such as calcium can have a profound effect upon the activity of the cell (Sutherland & Rall 1968). High-pressure amplitudes can result in a more violent cavitational event (often called transient or collapse cavitation). During this event, the bubbles collapse during the positive pressure part of the cycle with such ferocity that pressures in excess of 1000 MPa and temperatures in excess of 10000 K are generated. This violent behaviour can lead to the formation of highly reactive free radicals. Although free radicals are produced by cells naturally (e.g. during cellular respiration), they are removed by free-radical scavengers. Production in excess of the natural free-radical scavenger system capacity could, however, be damaging. Avoidance of a standing-wave field and use of low intensities during therapy make it unlikely that transient cavitation will occur and there is no evidence that these effects are achieved in the tissues with therapeutic ultrasound when used appropriately. Some applications of ultrasound deliberately employ the unstable cavitation effect (high-intensity focused ultrasound; HIFU) but it is beyond the remit of this chapter (Wu 2006).

Acoustic streaming

This refers to the unidirectional movement of a fluid in an ultrasound field. High-velocity gradients develop next to boundaries between fluids and structures such as cells, bubbles and tissue fibres. Acoustic streaming can stimulate cell activity if it occurs at the boundary of the cell membrane and the surrounding fluid. The resultant viscous stress on the membrane, providing it is not too severe, can alter the membrane's permeability and second-messenger activity (Dyson 1982, 1985). This could result in therapeutically advantageous changes such as increased protein synthesis (Webster et al 1978), increased secretion from mast cells (Fyfe & Chahl 1982), fibroblast mobility changes (Mummery 1978), increased uptake of the second-messenger calcium (Mortimer & Dyson 1988, Mummery 1978), and increased production of growth factors by macrophages (Young & Dyson 1990a). All these effects could account for the acceleration of repair following ultrasound therapy.

Standing waves

When an ultrasound wave hits the interface between two tissues of different acoustic imped-ances (e.g. bone and muscle), reflection of a per-centage of the wave will occur. The reflected waves can interact with oncoming incident waves to form a standing-wave field in which the peaks of intensity (antinodes; see Chapter 2) of the waves are stationary and are separated by half a wave-length. Because the standing wave consists of two superimposed waves in addition to a travelling component, the peak intensities and pressures are higher than the normal incident wave. Between the antinodes, which are points of maximum and minimum pressure, are nodes, which are points of

fixed pressure. Gas bubbles collect at the antinodes and cells (if in suspension) collect at the nodes (National Council on Radiation Protection (NCRP) 1983). Fixed cells, such as endothelial cells, which line the blood vessels, can be damaged by micro-streaming forces around bubbles if they are situated at the pressure antinodes. Erythrocytes can be lysed if they are swept through the arrays of bubbles situated at the pressure antinodes. Reversible blood cell stasis has been demonstrated, the cells forming bands half a wavelength apart centred on the pres-sure nodes (Dyson et al 1974). The increased pres-sure produced in standing-wave fields can cause transient cavitation and consequently the forma-tion of free radicals (Nyborg 1977). It is therefore important to move the applicator continuously throughout treatment, and also use the lowest intensity required to cause an effect, to minimize the hazards involved in standing-wave field pro-duction (Dyson et al 1974).

The combination of stable cavitation and acoustic streaming is thought to be responsible for the cel-lular 'upregulation' that occurs during an ultra-sound treatment. The therapeutic effects (see below) of this type of intervention arise as a consequence of this stimulated cellular activity and, strictly speaking, the 'effects' of ultrasound are at a cell membrane level (Fig. 12.3).

TISSUE REPAIR

Following injury, a number of cellular and chemical events occur in soft tissues. Although these events

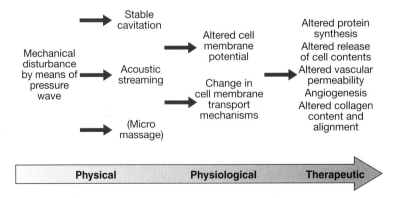

Figure 12.3 Summary of the mechanism by which ultrasound achieves therapeutic effects.

are explained in detail in Chapter 4, they are summarized here in the context of ultrasound therapy.

UNDERLYING REPAIR PROCESS

The major cellular components of the repair process include platelets, mast cells, polymorphonuclear leucocytes (PMNLs), macrophages, T lymphocytes, fibroblasts and endothelial cells. These cells migrate as a module into the injury site in a well-defined sequence that is controlled by numerous soluble wound factors. These wound factors originate from a various sources, such as inflammatory cells (e.g. macrophages and PMNLs), inflammatory cascade systems (e.g. coagulation and complement) and the breakdown products of damaged tissue.

For convenience, the whole repair process can be divided into several phases (Singer & Clark 1999, Watson 2006b), although it must be stated that these phases overlap considerably, lacking any distinct border between them. The three phases are:

1. inflammation
2. proliferation/granulation tissue formation
3. remodelling.

There is now overwhelming evidence to show that the effectiveness of therapeutic ultrasound depends on the phase of repair in which it is used. This will be discussed in more detail in subsequent sections.

Inflammation

This early, dynamic phase of repair is characterized initially by clot formation. Blood platelets are a major constituent of the blood clot and, in addition to their activities associated with clotting, platelets also contain numerous biologically active substances, including prostaglandins, and serotonin and platelet-derived growth factor (PDGF). These substances have a profound effect on the local environment of the wound and its subsequent repair (Singer & Clark 1999). Mast cells present another source of biologically active substances – or wound factors – which help orchestrate the early repair sequences.

Neutrophils are the first PMNLs to enter the wound bed, attracted by an array of wound factors present at the wound site. The function of the neutrophils is to clear the wound site of foreign particles such as bacteria and tissue debris. Macrophages enter the wound bed soon after the neutrophils, where they phagocytose bacteria (if present) and tissue debris. They also produce wound factors that stimulate the subsequent repair events.

Evidence will be presented later in this chapter to show that, when used appropriately, ultrasound can influence the release of these wound factors from the cells in and around the wound bed.

Proliferation/granulation tissue formation

During normal acute injury repair, the inflammatory phase is followed – within several days – by the formation of granulation tissue. During this stage, which is often referred to as the *proliferative phase*, the wound void is filled with cells (mainly macrophages and fibroblasts), numerous blood vessels (angiogenesis) and a connective tissue matrix composed of fibronectin, hyaluronic acid and collagen types I and III.

If skin is involved in the tissue damage, a new epidermis forms during this phase of repair. The new epidermal cells migrate from the edge of the wound (and also from around hair follicles within the injury site in the case of partial-thickness wounds) towards the centre of the wound.

Wound contraction occurs during this phase of repair and can be defined as the process by which the size of a wound decreases by the centripetal movement of the whole thickness of surrounding skin (Peacock 1984). Myofibroblasts appear to play an important role in this process (Desmouliere et al 2005).

The stimulus controlling all of these events comes from numerous sources, of which macrophages constitute a major one. The effect of ultrasound on the proliferative phase will be discussed in detail below.

Remodelling

Remodelling can continue for many months or years after the proliferative phase of repair. During remodelling, granulation tissue is gradually replaced by a scar composed of relatively acellular and avascular tissue. As the repair matures, the composition of the extracellular matrix changes.

Initially, it is composed of hyaluronic acid, fibronectin and collagens types I, III and V. The ratio of type I to III collagen changes during remodelling until type I is dominant. Scar tissue is a substitute for undamaged tissue. The rate at which wounds gain tensile strength is slow (Levenson et al 1965), and they are at only 20–25% of their maximum strength 3 weeks after injury. The increase in wound strength depends on two main factors: first, the rate of collagen deposition, remodelling and alignment, with the gradual formation of larger collagen bundles (Kischer & Shetlar 1974); second, alteration in the intermolecular cross-links (Bailey et al 1975). It will be shown later in this chapter that ultrasound can improve both the mechanical properties and functional capacity of the resulting scar tissue.

THE EFFECT OF ULTRASOUND ON THE INFLAMMATORY PHASE OF REPAIR

The inflammatory phase is extremely dynamic and numerous cell types (e.g. platelets, mast cells, macrophages and neutrophils) enter and leave the wound site. There is evidence to show that therapeutic ultrasound can interact with the above cells, influencing their activity and leading to the acceleration of repair (Fyfe & Chahl 1982, Maxwell 1992, Nussbaum 1997, ter Haar 1999, Watson, 2006a).

Acoustic streaming forces have been shown to produce changes in platelet membrane permeability leading to the release of serotonin (Williams 1974, Williams et al 1976). In addition to serotonin, platelets contain wound factors essential for successful repair (Ginsberg 1981). If streaming can stimulate the release of serotonin, it is proposed that it may also influence the release of these other factors.

One of the major chemicals that modifies the wound environment at this time after injury is histamine. The mast cell is the major source of this factor, which is normally released by a process known as mast cell degranulation. In this process, the membrane of the cell, in response to increased levels of intracellular calcium (Yurt 1981), ruptures and releases histamine and other products into the wound site. It has been shown that a single treatment of therapeutic ultrasound, if given soon after injury (i.e. during the early inflammatory phase),

can stimulate mast cells to degranulate, thereby releasing histamine into the surrounding tissues (Fyfe & Chahl 1982, Hashish 1986). It is possible that ultrasound is stimulating the mast cell to degranulate by increasing its permeability to calcium. Increased calcium ion permeability has been demonstrated by a number of researchers. Calcium ions can act as intracellular messengers; when their distribution and concentration change in response to environmental modifications of the plasma membrane they act as an intracellular signal for the appropriate metabolic response (Leung et al 2004a, Mortimer & Dyson 1988, Nussbaum 1997).

Reversible membrane permeability changes to calcium have been demonstrated using therapeutic levels of ultrasound (Dinno et al 1989, Mortimer & Dyson 1988, Mummery 1978). The fact that this effect can be suppressed by irradiation under pressure suggests that cavitation is the physical mechanism responsible. Changes in permeability to other ions such as potassium have also been demonstrated (Chapman et al 1979). Work by Dinno et al (1989) demonstrated that ultrasound can modify the electrophysiological properties of skin; this study reported an ultrasound-induced reduction in the sodium/potassium ATPase pump activity. A decrease in pump activity, if it occurs in neuronal plasma membranes, may inhibit the transduction of noxious stimuli and subsequent neural transmission, which may account in part for the pain relief that is often experienced following clinical exposure to therapeutic ultrasound, although as a modality, ultrasound is not often applied with the primary intention of achieving pain relief, and is considered to be a secondary benefit rather than of primary importance. It should be noted, however, that the mechanism of ultrasound-induced pain relief is still not fully understood and that it may be attributed, in part at least, to placebo effects.

As identified above, the evidence is clear: therapeutic ultrasound can alter membrane permeability to various ions. The ability to affect calcium transport through cell membranes is of considerable clinical significance as calcium, in its role as an intracellular or second messenger, can have a profound effect on cell activity, for instance by increasing synthesis and secretion of wound factors by cells involved in the healing process. This has been shown to occur in macrophages in response to therapeutic levels of ultrasound (Young & Dyson 1990a) and these are one of the key cells in the wound-healing system, being a source of numerous wound factors. This in-vitro study demonstrated that the ultrasound-induced change in wound factor secretion is frequency dependent. Ultrasound at an intensity of $0.5\,W/cm^2$ (SATA) and a frequency of $0.75\,MHz$ appeared to be most effective in encouraging the immediate release of factors already present in the cell cytoplasm, whereas the higher frequency $3.0\,MHz$ appeared to be most effective in stimulating the production of new factors, which were then released some time later by the cells' normal secretory processes. Therefore, there appeared to be a delayed effect when treating with the higher frequency; however, the resulting liberated factors, when compared with those liberated using $0.75\,MHz$, were more potent in their effect on the stimulation of fibroblast population growth. One possible reason why these two frequencies induce different effects relates to the physical mechanisms involved. At each frequency the peak pressure generated by the ultrasound was that necessary for cavitation to occur (Williams 1987). Cavitation is more likely to occur at the lower frequency, whereas heating is more likely to occur at the higher one. Therefore, the differing proportions of non-thermal to thermal mechanisms present in each of the two treatments may explain the difference seen in the resulting biological effects.

Hart (1993) also found that following the in vitro exposure of macrophages to ultrasound, a wound factor was released into the surrounding medium that was mitogenic for fibroblasts.

It has often been thought that ultrasound is an anti-inflammatory agent (Reid 1981, Snow & Johnson 1988). When viewed from a clinical standpoint – that is, rapid resolution of oedema (El Hag et al 1985) – this conclusion is understandable. However, research has shown that ultrasound is not anti-inflammatory in its action (Goddard et al 1983, Watson 2006a); rather, it encourages oedema formation to occur more rapidly (Fyfe & Chahl 1985, Hustler et al 1978) and then to subside more rapidly than control sham-irradiated groups, so accelerating the whole process and driving the wound into the proliferative phase of repair sooner.

Further confirmation of this has been shown experimentally in acute surgical wounds (Young &

Dyson 1990b). In this study, full-thickness excised skin lesions in rats were exposed to therapeutic ultrasound ($0.1\,W/cm^2$ SATA, $0.75\,MHz$ or $3.0\,MHz$) daily for 7 days (5 minutes per day per wound). By 5 days after injury, the ultrasound-treated groups had significantly fewer inflammatory cells in the wound bed and more extensive granulation tissue than the sham-irradiated controls. Also, the alignment of the fibroblasts – parallel to the wound surface – in the wound beds of the ultrasound-treated groups was indicative of a more advanced stage of tissue organization than the random alignment of fibroblasts seen in the sham-irradiated control wounds. The results obtained suggest that there had been an acceleration of the wounds through the inflammatory phase repair in response to ultrasound therapy. It was also noted that there were no abnormalities such as hypertrophy of the wound tissue seen in response to ultrasound therapy.

Therefore, ultrasound therapy appears to accelerate the process without the risk of interfering with the control mechanisms that limit the development of repair materials. By increasing the activity of these cells, the overall influence of therapeutic ultrasound is certainly pro- rather than anti-inflammatory. The benefit of this mode of action is not to 'increase' the inflammatory response as such (although, if applied with too great an intensity at this stage, it is a possible outcome; Ciccone et al 1991), but rather to act as an 'inflammatory optimizer'. The inflammatory response is essential to the effective repair of tissue, and the more efficiently the process can complete, the more effectively the tissue can progress to the next (proliferative) phase.

Employed at an appropriate treatment dose, with optimal treatment parameters (intensity, pulsing and time), the benefit of ultrasound is to make as efficient as possible the earliest repair phase, and thus have a promotional effect on the whole healing cascade. For tissues in which there is an inflammatory reaction, but in which there is no 'repair' to be achieved, the benefit of ultrasound is to promote the normal resolution of the inflammatory events, and hence resolve the 'problem' This will be most effectively achieved in the tissues that preferentially absorb ultrasound, i.e. the dense collagenous tissues.

THE EFFECT OF ULTRASOUND ON THE PROLIFERATIVE PHASE OF REPAIR

The main events occurring during this phase of repair include cell infiltration into the wound bed, angiogenesis, matrix deposition, wound contraction and re-epithelialization (for lesions involving the skin). During the proliferative phase (scar production) ultrasound also has a stimulative effect (cellular upregulation), although the primary active targets are now the fibroblasts, endothelial cells and myofibroblasts (Dyson & Smalley 1983, Maxwell 1992, Mortimer & Dyson 1988, Nussbaum 1997, 1998, Ramirez et al 1997, Young & Dyson 1990 a,b). These are all cells that are normally active during scar production and ultrasound is therefore pro-proliferative in the same way that it is pro-inflammatory – it does not change the normal proliferative phase but maximizes its efficiency, producing the required scar tissue in an optimal fashion.

Cells such as fibroblasts and endothelial cells are recruited to the wound site by a combination of migration and proliferation. Mummery (1978) showed in vitro that fibroblast motility could be increased when they were exposed to therapeutic levels of ultrasound. With regard to cell proliferation, there is little evidence in the literature to suggest that ultrasound has a direct stimulatory effect on fibroblast stimulation. Most of the in-vitro studies report either no effect or even an inhibitory effect on cell proliferation when exposed to therapeutic levels of ultrasound (Kaufman et al 1977, Loch et al 1971). However, the literature shows that when tissues are exposed to ultrasound in vivo a marked increase in wound bed cell numbers can be demonstrated (Dyson et al 1970, Young & Dyson 1990b). This anomaly can be explained if we examine the cellular interactions that occur during healing.

It was identified earlier that during wound repair much of the stimulus that controls the cellular events is derived from the macrophage. Therefore, it is highly likely that any increase in, for example, fibroblast proliferation, may be due in part to an indirect effect of ultrasound via the macrophage. Work by Young and Dyson (1990a) showed that if one exposes macrophages to therapeutic levels of ultrasound in vitro, then removes the surrounding culture medium and places it onto fibroblast cultures, there is a large stimulatory effect on the proliferation of the fibroblasts. It therefore appears that macrophages are sensitive to ultrasound and, in response to therapeutic levels, they release a factor, or factors, that stimulates fibroblasts to proliferate.

Ultrasound can also affect the rate of angiogenesis. Hogan et al (1982) showed that capillaries develop more rapidly in chronically ischaemic muscle when exposed to ultrasound. Other work has shown that the exposure of skin lesions to ultrasound can stimulate the growth of blood capillaries into the wound site (Hosseinpour 1988, Wang et al 2003, Young & Dyson 1990c).

When fibroblasts are exposed to ultrasound in vitro a marked stimulation in collagen secretion can be detected (Harvey et al 1975). It should be added that the degree of response is intensity dependent. When the fibroblasts were exposed to continuous ultrasound ($0.5\,\text{W/cm}^2$ SA), a 20% increase in collagen secretion was recorded; however, when the ultrasound was pulsed ($0.5\,\text{W/cm}^2$ SATA), a 30% increase was recorded. Webster et al (1978) demonstrated an increase in protein synthesis when fibroblasts were exposed to ultrasound.

Wound contraction can be accelerated with ultrasound. Work by Dyson and Smalley (1983) showed that pulsed ultrasound ($3\,\text{MHz}$, $0.5\,\text{W/cm}^2$ SATA) could stimulate the contraction of cryosurgical lesions. Hart (1993) showed that exposure of full-thickness excised skin lesions to low levels of pulsed ultrasound-stimulated contraction, leading to a significantly smaller scar. Interestingly, he also found that the same degree of contraction he induced using an intensity of $0.5\,\text{W/cm}^2$ (SATA) could also be achieved by using the much lower intensity of $0.1\,\text{W/cm}^2$ (SATA). This is a significant finding, which implies that reduced ultrasound treatment intensities can still achieve the desired results, via non-thermal effects.

The demonstration of enhanced fibroplasia and collagen synthesis by Harvey et al (1975) is supported by work conducted by Enwemeka (1989), Enwemeka et al (1990), Huys et al (1993), Ramirez et al (1997) and Turner et al (1989). Important work continues with regard to the influence of therapeutic ultrasound in relation to several chemical mediators affecting the proliferative phase (e.g. Reher et al 1999).

THE EFFECT OF ULTRASOUND ON THE REMODELLING PHASE OF REPAIR

During remodelling, the wound becomes relatively acellular and avascular, collagen content increases and the tensile strength of the wound increases. The remodelling phase can last from months to years, depending on the tissue involved and the nature of the injury. The mechanical properties of the scar are related to both the amount of collagen present and the arrangement or alignment of the collagen fibres within the repaired tissue.

The application of therapeutic ultrasound influences the remodelling of the scar tissue. It seems to enhance the appropriate orientation of the newly formed collagen fibres and to change the collagen profile from mainly type III to a more dominant type I construction, thus increasing tensile strength and enhancing scar mobility (Nussbaum 1998, Wang 1998). Ultrasound applied to tissues enhances the functional capacity of the scar tissues (Huys et al 1993, Nussbaum 1998).

The effects of ultrasound on the properties of the scar depend very much upon the time at which the therapy was first instigated. The most effective regimens appear to be those that are started soon after injury (i.e. during the inflammatory phase of repair). Webster (1980) found that when wounds were treated three times per week for 2 weeks after injury ($0.1 \, W/cm^2$ SATA) the resulting tensile strength and elasticity of the scar were significantly higher than those of the control group. Byl et al (1992, 1993) demonstrated an increase in tensile strength and collagen content in incised lesions whose treatment was commenced during the inflammatory phase. They also compared different ultrasound intensities and found that the lower intensity (1 MHz, pulsed, $0.5 \, W/cm^2$ SATA) was the most effective. Treatment with ultrasound during the inflammatory phase of repair not only increases the amount of collagen deposited in the wound but also encourages the deposition of that collagen in a pattern whose three-dimensional architecture more resembles that of uninjured skin than the untreated controls (Dyson 1981). Jackson et al (1991) showed that the mechanical properties of injured tendon can be improved with ultrasound if treatment starts early enough; however, the levels used were relatively high, at $1.5 \, W/cm^2$.

Enwemeka et al (1990) reported that increased tensile strength and elasticity can be achieved in injured tendons using much lower intensities ($0.5 \, W/cm^2$ SA).

The application of ultrasound during the inflammatory, proliferative and repair phases is not of value because it changes the normal sequence of events but because it has the capacity to stimulate or enhance these normal events and thus increase the efficiency of the repair phases (ter Haar 1999, Watson 2006a). It would appear that if a tissue is repairing in a compromised or inhibited fashion, the application of therapeutic ultrasound at an appropriate dose will enhance this activity. If the tissue is healing 'normally', the application appears to speed the process and thus enable the tissue to reach its endpoint faster than would otherwise be the case. The effective application of ultrasound to achieve these aims is dose dependent.

ULTRASOUND AND SPECIFIC TISSUE REPAIR

In addition to the general tissue repair issues identified in the previous sections, there are some specific areas that warrant further consideration.

ULTRASOUND AND WOUND HEALING

In humans, wound closure is due mainly to granulation tissue formation and re-epithelialization, whereas in animals, where the skin is more loosely connected to the underlying tissues, wound closure is due mainly to contraction. Dyson et al (1976) found that ultrasound therapy (3 MHz, pulsed, $0.2 \, W/cm^2$ SATA), accelerated the reduction in varicose ulcer area significantly. Similar findings were reported by Roche and West (1984).

Callam et al (1987) studied the effect of weekly ultrasound therapy (1 MHz, pulsed, $0.5 \, W/cm^2$ SATA) on the healing of chronic leg ulcers. They found a 20% increase in the healing rate of the ultrasound-treated ulcers. There have been negative reports as to the use of ultrasound treatment on these chronic conditions. Lundeberg et al (1990) did not demonstrate any statistically significant difference between ultrasound-treated and sham-treated venous ulcers. However, they noted a trend that suggested that ultrasound was more effective than placebo treatment. Interestingly, they stated that their experimental design, particularly their sample size, was such that an improvement of less than 30% could not be detected.

Accelerated wound closure has also been recorded in other chronic wounds, such as pressure sores (McDiarmid et al 1985, Paul et al 1960). McDiarmid et al also reported an interesting finding that microbiologically infected sores were more responsive to ultrasound therapy than uninfected sores. It is likely that the low-grade infection had in some way primed or further activated the healing system (e.g. recruiting more macrophages to the area), which in turn would produce an amplified signal to herald an early start to the other phases of repair.

A number of more recent studies have provided mixed evidence with regard to the effectiveness of ultrasound as part of the management of chronic wounds (predominantly venous leg ulcers and, to a lesser extent, pressure sores). Trials with positive outcomes include those by Ennis et al (2005) and Franek et al (2004, 2006); trials with no demonstrated advantage for ultrasound include that by Selkowitz et al (2002). An ongoing study in this area is reported by Watson and Nelson (2006) and useful reviews in this area can be found in Baba-Akbari et al (2006), Cullum et al (2001) and Flemming and Cullum (2000).

Although it is frustrating to review such evidence, it would appear that the mixed results may be attributed to a dose dependency (see Chapter 1; Uhlemann et al 2003, Uhlemann & Wollina 2003) and, with continuing research in this field, it is possible that the optimal treatment parameters will be identified. Furthermore, comparison of different 'electrotherapy' modalities is clearly needed. Ultrasound is only one of several modalities (e.g. laser, electrical stimulation) that have been demonstrated to have an effect on wound healing, and few studies have directly compared their effectiveness. Demir et al (2004) compared the effectiveness of laser therapy and ultrasound, identifying both as better than control intervention but stating that laser therapy was advantageous over ultrasound. Franek et al (2006) made a similar comparison between electrical stimulation, laser therapy and ultrasound. The electrical

stimulation and ultrasound were found to be significantly effective; laser therapy was not. This ambiguous evidence generates some confusion, but it is hoped that, with further comparative research, clarification can be achieved.

ULTRASOUND AND FRACTURE REPAIR

Bone repairs in much the same way as soft tissues. Both repair processes consist of three overlapping phases: inflammation, proliferation and remodelling. However, in bone repair, the proliferative phase is subdivided into soft and hard callus formation. The soft callus is an equivalent to granulation tissue in soft tissue injuries, and it is within this tissue that new bone regenerates to form the hard callus (see Chapter 4). Much work has been carried out investigating the effects of ultrasound therapy on this process. Amongst the earlier trials, Dyson and Brookes (1983) showed that it was possible to accelerate the repair of fibular fractures using therapeutic levels of ultrasound (1.5 or 3 MHz, pulsed, 0.5 W/cm^2 SATA). The treatments were for 5 minutes, four times per week. Treatments were carried out at different combinations of weeks after injury (e.g. during the first 2 weeks only, or during the third and fourth weeks only). The most effective treatments were found to be those which were carried out during the first 2 weeks of repair (i.e. during the inflammatory phase of repair). It was found that if treatment was delayed (i.e. started on weeks 3 to 4 after injury) the ultrasound appeared to stimulate cartilage growth, postponing bony union. Of the two frequencies used, 1.5 MHz was the more effective.

Pilla et al (1990) showed that low-intensity ultrasound (1.5 or 3 MHz, pulsed, 0.3 W/cm^2) could stimulate fracture repair to such a degree that maximum strength was gained in the treated limbs by 17 days after injury, compared with 28 days in the controls. Tsai et al (1992a) demonstrated an increase in femoral fracture repair when using low intensities of ultrasound (1.5 MHz, pulsed, 0.5 W/cm^2); however, when they tried 1.5 W/cm^2 they found that treatments inhibited repair. The same team (Tsai et al 1992b) found that, in the most effective output levels for stimulating repair, the production of endogenous prostaglandin E$_2$ (PGE$_2$) was highest. They suggested that bone healing stimulated by ultrasound may be mediated via the production of PGE_2.

In the last 10–12 years, there appears to have been a resurgence of research looking at the effect of ultrasound on fracture healing, using both animal and human models and considering normal (fresh) fractures, delayed and non-unions. As with the work on chronic wounds, other electrotherapy modalities have been demonstrated to be effective in terms of enhancing the repair of bone damage, but on balance the ultrasound evidence is less ambiguous in its outcome, and the majority of trials appear to be supportive of the intervention. Also in the same way as with chronic ulcer trials, there is little at the moment by way of direct comparative trials, and hence, although it is clearly demonstrated that fracture healing is enhanced by the appropriate application of ultrasound, it is difficult at the moment to be clear which electrotherapy intervention is most effective in this regard.

Low-intensity pulsed ultrasound (LIPUS), typically at 1.5 MHz, 0.03 W/cm² and using pulse regimens of 1 : 4 (20% duty cycle), are employed in most modern studies, commonly delivered with machines specifically designed for this purpose (Fig. 12.4). It is interesting to note, first, that the effective dose is lower than has been previously employed in relation to bone healing and, second, that it remains unclear whether this application dose can be effectively achieved with a 'standard' therapy device or whether specific machines need to be used. Warden et al (1999, 2006) provides an interesting analysis and review in this field.

Heckman et al (1994) investigated the effectiveness of low-intensity ultrasound on the healing of tibial fractures. The fractures were examined in a prospective, randomized, double-blind evaluation of low-intensity ultrasound. The treated group showed a significant decrease in the time to healing (86 days) compared to the control group (114 days). Similarly, Kristiensen et al (1997) conducted a similar trial with patients who had a distal radial fracture. Using almost identical intervention parameters, they too demonstrated a significant reduction in the time taken to reach consolidation in the ultrasound group compared to the controls. There are many similar trials with a predominance of positive outcomes and numerous reviews and

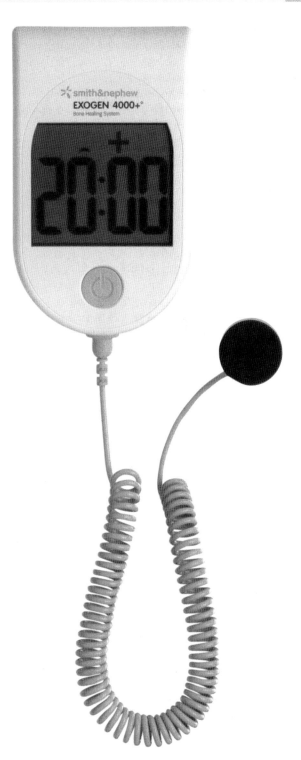

Figure 12.4 LIPUS (Exogen) device used to enhanced fracture healing (Smith & Nephew, Inc).

meta-analyses have been published in recent years, including Busse and Bhandari (2004), Busse et al (2002), Malizos et al (2006), Rubin et al (2001), Stein et al (2005) and Warden (2003).

In addition to the demonstrated benefits of ultrasound in terms of 'normal' fracture healing, additional experimental and review material considers its effective application for delayed and non-unions (Gebauer et al 2005, Lerner et al 2004, Leung et al 2004b, Mayr et al 2000, Nolte et al 2001). Furthermore, a range of recent publications demonstrates the application of LIPUS in the management of distraction osteogenesis (Dudda et al 2005, El-Mowafi & Mohsen 2005, Fujishiro et al 2005, Gebauer & Correll 2005).

The mechanisms through which the ultrasound appears to be effective relate primarily to osteoblast activation, prostaglandin synthesis and changes in chemically mediated repair events, and, in addition to the clinical trials and reviews identified above, many papers have examined the responses of cells and tissues in laboratory and animal model research.

It is interesting to note that the levels of ultrasound energy applied in these fracture-management programmes are at a lower level than commonly employed in therapy for soft-tissue healing enhancement, and it remains a possibility that future ultrasound doses may be even lower than those currently utilized, although, to date, detailed and quality investigation of this LIPUS intervention for soft-tissue treatment is not as far advanced as the work with fractures.

ULTRASOUND AND PAIN RELIEF

A number of studies have attempted to evaluate the use of ultrasound in the treatment of pain. However, analysis of available data shows that there is a lack of evidence from large controlled studies, which would indicate what effect ultrasound is having on pain relief, and by what mechanism (Gam & Johannsen 1995).

Ultrasound has been used by clinicians for the treatment of carpal tunnel syndrome (Ebenbichler et al 1998) and stress fractures (Brand et al 1999). Although not large trials, these studies do indicate that ultrasound may be an option worth trying when treating pain. It is known that ultrasound can accelerate the inflammatory phase of wound healing, leading to a rapid resolution of oedema (El Hag et al 1985), so it is possible that many of the reports of pain relief with ultrasound could be due to this – that is, get rid of swelling and you get rid of pain – and it is also possible that the reduction in local metabolite, toxin and chemical mediators may effectively reduce the irritation of nerve endings and hence pain. A large, randomized, controlled clinical trial is necessary to establish the efficacy and mechanism of ultrasound in the treatment of pain, although, at the present time, pain relief is commonly considered to be a secondary benefit of the therapy rather than a primary (intended) outcome.

PHONOPHORESIS

Phonophoresis is defined as the migration of drug molecules through the skin under the influence of ultrasound. Theoretically, phonophoresis is possible using the acoustic streaming forces that exist in the ultrasound field. However, it is debatable whether these forces are strong enough to produce a net forward movement capable of pushing all drugs through the skin to their target tissue. In addition, it is often difficult to determine whether a biological effect of a topically applied drug is a result of its direct action on the underlying target tissue or of a systemic effect. This could be one reason why there have been many mixed reports on the effectiveness of this modality for pushing drugs into the skin. It is likely that phonophoresis will be dependent not only on the frequency, intensity, duty cycle and treatment duration of the ultrasound (Mitragotri et al 2000), but also on the nature of the drug molecule itself.

Research is needed to clarify what parameters of ultrasound are most efficient for facilitating topical drug diffusion, and also which drugs can be most effectively used. In an interesting development, Rosim et al (2005) evaluated the effect of using ultrasound prior to the drug application on the skin rather than using the ultrasound to 'drive' the agent into the tissues. The outcome was positive and provides an interesting avenue for further work.

LOW-FREQUENCY ULTRASOUND

Since the early 1990s there has been an interest in the use of low-frequency (longwave) therapeutic ultrasound for the treatment of a variety of tissue injuries (Bradnock et al 1996) (Fig. 12.5). Typically, this modality operates at a frequency of around 44–48 kHz, which is significantly lower than the usual therapy range of 1–3 MHz. It is suggested that one benefit of using such a low frequency is that the depth of penetration is greatly enhanced and the risks of standing waves are minimized. There is considerable debate whether this 'greater penetration' benefit is of clinical relevance given, for example, the arguments made by Robertson and Ward (1997) illustrating the important relationship between the penetration depth and the relative proportion of longwave ultrasound energy that is absorbed in the superficial tissues. It is suggested that because the majority of the energy is absorbed in the superficial tissues, the immediate pain relief and extensibility changes are more akin to those seen as a result of thermal treatments. A recent study (Meakins & Watson 2006) compared the effect of longwave ultrasound and superficial contact heating on tissue extensibility and demonstrated that both were effective but that, although there was no statistically significant difference in their outcomes, there was a trend for the heat treatment to be more effective.

Apart from the Bradnock et al (1996) study, there have been few published clinical trials and one of

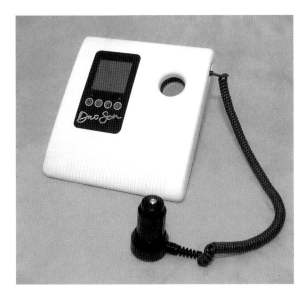

Figure 12.5 Low-frequency (longwave) ultrasound equipment (Orthosonics).

these (Basso & Pike 1998) demonstrated no therapeutic benefit when it was employed post wrist fracture in terms of mobility gains. Several studies have considered the effect of this intervention mode with regard to chronic wound management, wound infection and associated problems. Although not numerous, these studies do suggest that there may be a significant benefit of using the modality in these areas (Pavlov 2002, Sedov et al 1998).

There is a distinct lack of clinical or laboratory research in this field compared to 'traditional' ultrasound, and there is a need for large, controlled trials to establish where this relatively new modality can be used most effectively. It may be that there are circumstances or clinical conditions for which the low-frequency (longwave) ultrasound has 'better' effects than traditional (MHz) ultrasound, and the anecdotal evidence would support this contention to some extent. However, without quality published research it is a difficult contention to support from the evidence to date.

ULTRASOUND APPLICATION

A number of factors must be considered when using therapeutic ultrasound:

● choice of ultrasound machine
● calibration
● choice of coupling medium
● frequency
● intensity
● pulsed or continuous mode
● treatment intervals
● duration of treatment
● potential hazards to both therapist and patient.

CHOICE OF ULTRASOUND MACHINE

Most ultrasound machines have the same basic design, consisting of an ultrasound generator, which may be mains or battery powered (or have dual capability). The generator comprises an oscillator circuit, transformer and microcomputer, and is linked via a cable to the treatment applicator (see Fig. 12.1). The applicator houses the transducer, which produces ultrasound when stimulated by the oscillating voltage from the generator.

Machines may operate at single or multiple frequencies, most commonly 1 and 3 MHz. The intensity can be varied, as can the choice of output: from pulsed mode (a range of pulses is usually available) to continuous mode. It is also noted that some devices enable the operator to operate the machine at either frequency using the same treatment head, whereas others necessitate a change of applicator. Typically, 'large' (approximately 5 cm^2) and 'small' (approximately 1 cm^2) treatment applicators are available, although these may not be supplied as standard with the machine when purchased. The beam non-uniformity ratio (BNR) represents the difference between the peak and the mean power output across the transducer face, and the lower this value, the better for clinical applications. Typically, the values for modern machines range between 4 and 6.

CALIBRATION

The machine should be calibrated on a regular basis (at least annually) and the output checked at more frequent intervals (ideally once a week). The constant heavy usage that this type of equipment gets means it is likely that the power output set on the device may not correspond to the actual output. It is important to note that the reading on the machine power-output meter is not an accurate guide to what is actually coming out of the treatment head: the machine must be calibrated against a dedicated calibration device. It has been suggested that the effective calibration of therapy machines is currently inadequate (Artho et al 2002, Guirro et al 1997, Pye & Milford 1994, Sutton et al 2006), and although full technical calibration may not be realistic more than every 6 months, a regular weekly check of power output using a reasonably accurate power meter or water balance is advised.

CHOICE OF COUPLING MEDIUM

By its very nature, ultrasound cannot travel through air and so, without an adequate exit path, the sound generated by the transducer would reflect back from the interface between the air and the applicator treatment surface, which could damage the delicate transducer. To provide the generated ultrasound with an 'escape route' from the treatment head into the body, some form of coupling agent needs to be placed between the applicator face and the body.

The best coupling agent in terms of acoustic properties is water. The difference in acoustic impedance between water and soft tissue is small, which means that there is only approximately 0.2% reflection at the interface between the two. Alternatively, aqueous gels are almost as effective as water in terms of absolute transmission, but with the added advantage of higher viscosity, which means that they meet more of the 'essential requirements' for a clinical coupling medium (Dyson 1990).

As identified in an earlier section of this chapter, and also in Chapter 2, there is no clinically relevant difference between currently available coupling gels (Poltakski & Watson 2007a). Water is an effective coupling medium with some advantages, especially in relation to the treatment of small areas and body parts with significant bony protuberances, although with the advent of the 'small' treatment head this is now less of a clinical problem.

Treatment 'under water' has other advantages in that the treatment head need not actually touch the skin; this may be considered beneficial for patients with significant tenderness. Even with treatments applied in water, it is important to always keep the treatment head moving evenly over the treatment area.

For the treatment of open wounds, it is important to use a transmission system that will enable the ultrasound energy to reach the wound surface while not compromising the sterility of the area. Being able to treat through an existing wound dressing is considered to be advantageous in that there is less compromise to the wound environment and also less risk of introducing infective agents (Poltawski & Watson 2007b).

Some wound dressings demonstrate very good ultrasound transmission characteristics whereas others transmit very little, and still others absolutely no ultrasound energy at all. A recent review of 48 different wound dressings identified the characteristics and qualities of each. This is an important and necessary consideration and for any therapist working in this area (Poltawski & Watson 2007b).

FREQUENCY

Having control over the frequency of the ultrasound output gives the therapist control over the depth at which the energy can be targeted. The basic principle that the higher the frequency, the more superficial is the depth of penetration, leading to rapid attenuation of the ultrasound energy. Lower-frequency ultrasound energy has a lower absorption rate and thus a greater proportion of the energy reaches the deeper tissues. It is generally considered advantageous to have access to a dual-frequency device, and hence the capacity to be effective in both deep and superficial lesions. The average half value depths (previously in this chapter and in Chapter 2) will assist in determining the effective penetration of the energy in the clinical setting.

INTENSITY

Once the choice of frequency has been made so that the required depth of penetration can be achieved, the therapist has to make the decision as to what intensity level to use. There is no quantitative scientific or clinical information that indicates that 'high' levels of ultrasound [greater than $1\,W/cm^2$ (SATA)] need to be used to cause a significant biological effect in injured tissues. On the contrary, the data presented earlier in this chapter support the use of intensities of $0.5\,W/cm^2$ (SATA) and less to achieve maximum healing rates in damaged tissues. The evidence also showed that levels of ultrasound in excess of $1.5\,W/cm^2$ (SATA) may have an adverse effect on healing tissues.

There has been a trend over recent years towards the use of lower-intensity treatments. The advice is to always use the lowest intensity that produces the required therapeutic effect, as higher intensities may be damaging (Dyson 1990). Generally, with acute conditions the intensity used should be between 0.1 and $0.3\,W/cm^2$ and should not be higher than $0.5\,W/cm^2$ (SATA). For more chronic conditions, the levels would typically be between 0.3 and $0.8\,W/cm^2$, and should be no higher than $1\,W/cm^2$ (SATA). Although detailed information as regards treatment dose selection are beyond the remit of this section, the important point to consider is that these intensity values are those that are needed at the target, which clearly may not be the same as those delivered at the skin surface. Details of clinically effective intensities are available from numerous sources, including Watson (2002) and http://www.electrotherapy.org.

PULSED OR CONTINUOUS MODE?

Pulsing ultrasound has a major effect on reducing the amount of heat generated in the tissues. A controversy exists as to what the major mechanisms are by which ultrasound stimulates injuries to heal. It is unlikely that a specific bioeffect occurs as a result of the exclusive action of either thermal or non-thermal mechanisms; it is more likely to be as a mixture of both. Therefore, the area is rather a grey one. However, based on the literature available, the more acute the presentation, the more pulsed the machine output should be (start at around 1:4 or 20% duty cycle). With less acute (or more chronic) lesions, a lower pulse ratio (1:3, 1:2, duty cycles of 25% or 33%) is more effective. With truly chronic lesions, still lower pulse ratios (1:1 or continuous, duty cycles of 50% and 100%) appear to be most efficacious.

TREATMENT INTERVALS

The interval between successive treatments depends upon the nature of the injury. In general terms, the more acute the lesion, the better result will be achieved with low-dose treatments applied relatively frequently – daily in the ideal setting. Treatment more than once a day is a practice employed in some clinical areas (most commonly sports medicine, but also some acute orthopaedic units). There is no absolute evidence to demonstrate that treatment more than once a day is any more effective, and it is advised that if this practice is followed, then a gap of at least 6 hours is maintained between ultrasound interventions. With the less acute lesions, a higher but less frequent treatment dose (see above) seems to be effective and, as a general rule of thumb, three times a week for subacute and twice a week for chronic lesions appears to be effective. These are 'ideal' treatment frequencies and it is accepted that it might not be possible to achieve them in the clinical environment. It is also suggested that any level of intervention, with a treatment at the 'right' dose, will have a measurable benefit, although it may not be as effective as the ideal.

DURATION OF TREATMENT

The duration of treatment depends upon the area of the injury. Typically, the area should be divided into zones that are approximately the same size as the treatment head, and then each zone should be treated for 1 minute (Oakley 1978, Watson 2002, 2006a). Hoogland (1986) recommends a total maximal treatment time of 15 minutes, and that at least 1 minute should be spent in treating an area of 1 cm.

CONTRAINDICATIONS, DANGERS AND PRECAUTIONS

The detailed consideration of contraindications is found in Chapter 21 and will not be repeated here at length, but some additional salient issues are raised.

First, and importantly in the current clinical climate, the potential for the transmission of infective agents by means of ultrasound treatment devices has been considered recently by Schabrun et al (2006). It was demonstrated that a high proportion of ultrasound devices in clinical use demonstrated significant levels of nosocomial infective organisms (as did a high proportion of ultrasound gel containers). Importantly, the microbiological agents identified were those normally found on the skin rather than treatment-resistant varieties. Furthermore, the use of a 70% alcohol wipe on the treatment head significantly reduced the microorganism count. It is suggested, therefore, that the treatment head is wiped with a 70% alcohol wipe prior to each and every treatment, not just those involving broken skin or open wounds.

Ultrasound applied to a pregnant patient is deemed to be acceptable so long as the applied energy does not, or could not be reasonably expected to, reach the developing fetus. Although there is no definitive (human) evidence of adverse effects during pregnancy, some (limited) animal-model evidence demonstrates that ultrasound applied at therapeutic levels to the developing fetus can have adverse effects (e.g. Houghton & Radman 2000). The guideline (see Chapter 21) is that the lower thorax, trunk and pelvic regions are avoided throughout pregnancy to minimize the risk to the fetus. It is considered both safe and acceptable to apply ultrasound to the pregnant patient in areas outside this zone.

Similarly, other rapidly dividing tissues are considered best avoided with therapeutic ultrasound doses, although, again (understandably), the evidence is primarily derived from animal model experimentation. It has been shown that malignant tissue responds to the therapy with an increased rate of division at some doses (Lejbkowicz et al 1993, Sicard Rosenbaum et al 1995, 1998) and active epiphyseal regions have also been shown to change behaviour at some therapy doses and, until further detailed information is available, they too are probably best avoided (Lyon et al 2003, Nolte et al 2001, Wiltink et al 1995). Some experimental evidence contradicts these findings, adding to the current controversy (Ogurtan et al 2002).

It is a commonly held view that ultrasound is contraindicated when there is a fracture in the local area but, as can be seen from the evidence summarized above , ultrasound applied at the 'right' dose in local proximity to a fracture can have significantly advantageous effects. The use of high-dose continuous ultrasound as a diagnostic procedure for stress and other fractures is a clinically employed technique that appears to be discriminative and has some (limited) support from the literature. The provocation of pain over the fracture site (using continuous wave ultrasound at around $1.0\,\mathrm{W/cm^2}$) is not used in this sense for its therapeutic effects but as an indicator of the presence of a fracture in the immediate area.

Metal in the tissues need not constitute an absolute contraindication and it is considered acceptable to use low-power, pulsed ultrasound over metal in the tissues when the treatment is being applied for its non-thermal effects. There is no evidence of detrimental effect so long as the power is low, the output pulsed and the treatment head is kept in constant motion.

Other contraindications related to the use of ultrasound are considered in Chapter 21, along with all other modalities.

SUMMARY

Therapeutic ultrasound has the capacity to positively influence the normal processes of tissue repair following injury. Although the effects appear to be strongest during the inflammatory phase, they are certainly evident throughout all the other repair phases, although possibly to a lesser extent. The effect of this modality is not to change the process or repair but instead to enhance the normally occurring cascade of events such as to stimulate or enhance the events, resulting in a more efficient resolution of the clinical problem. The effects of the modality, like all others, appear to be dose dependent. It is important, therefore, to apply the energy at the 'right' time and at the 'right' dose in order to gain maximal benefit.

References

Artho PA, Thyne JG, Warring BP et al (2002) A calibration study of therapeutic ultrasound units. *Phys Ther* **82**(3): 257–263.

Baba-Akbari SA, Flemming K, Cullum NA et al (2006) Therapeutic ultrasound for pressure ulcers. Cochrane Database Syst Rev 3: CD001275.

Bailey AJ, Bazin S, Sims TJ et al (1975) Characterisation of the collagen of human hypertrophic and normal scars. *Biochem Biophys Acta* **405**: 412–421.

Baker KG, Robertson VJ, Duck FA (2001) A review of therapeutic ultrasound: biophysical effects. *Phys Ther* **81**(7): 1351–1358.

Basso O, Pike JM (1998) The effect of low frequency, long-wave ultrasound therapy on joint mobility and rehabilitation after wrist fracture. *J Hand Surg (Br)* **23**(1): 136–139.

Bradnock B, Law HT, Roscoe KA (1996) A quantitative comparative assessment of the immediate response to high frequency ultrasound and low frequency ultrasound (longwave therapy) in the treatment of acute ankle sprains. *Physiotherapy* **82**: 78–84.

Brand JC, Brindle T, Nyland J, et al DL (1999) Does pulsed low intensity ultrasound allow an early return to normal activities when treating stress fractures? A review of one tarsal navicular and eight stress fractures. *Iowa Orthop J* **19**: 26–30.

Busse JW, Bhandari M (2004) Therapeutic ultrasound and fracture healing: a survey of beliefs and practices. *Arch Phys Med Rehab* **85**(10): 1653–1656.

Busse JW, Bhandari M, Kulkarni AV et al (2002) The effect of low-intensity pulsed ultrasound therapy on time to fracture healing: a meta-analysis. *CMAJ* **166**(4): 437–441.

Byl NN, McKenzie AL, West JM et al (1992) Low-dose ultrasound effects on wound healing: a controlled study with Yucatan pigs. *Arch Phys Med Rehab* **73**: 656–664.

Byl NN, McKenzie AL, Wong T et al (1993) Incisional wound healing: a controlled study of low and high dose ultrasound. *J Orthop Sports Phys Ther* **18**: 619–628.

Callam MJ, Harper DR, Dale JJ et al (1987) A controlled trial of weekly ultrasound therapy in chronic leg ulceration. *Lancet* **July 25**: 204–206.

Casarotto RA, Adamowski JC, Fallopa F et al (2004) Coupling agents in therapeutic ultrasound: Acoustic and thermal behavior. *Arch Phys Med Rehab* **85**(1): 162–165.

Chapman IV, Macnally NA, Tucker S (1979) Ultrasound induced changes in the rates of influx and efflux of potassium ions in rat thymocytes *in vitro*. *Br J Radiol* **47**: 411–415.

Ciccone C, Leggin B, Callamaro J (1991) Effects of ultrasound and trolamine salicylate phonophoresis on delayed-onset muscle soreness. *Phys Ther* **71**: 666.

Cullum N, Nelson EA, Flemming K et al (2001) Systematic reviews of wound care management: (5) beds; (6) compression; (7) laser therapy, therapeutic ultrasound, electrotherapy and electromagnetic therapy. *Health Technol Assess* **5**(9): 1–221.

Demir H, Yarray S, Kirnap M et al (2004) Comparison of the effects of laser and ultrasound treatments on experimental wound healing in rats. *J Rehab Res Dev* **41**(5): 721–728.

Desmouliere A, Chaponnier C, Gabbiani G (2005) Tissue repair, contraction, and the myofibroblast. *Wound Repair Regen* **13**(1): 7–12.

Dinno MA, Dyson M, Young SR et al (1989) The significance of membrane changes in the safe and effective use of therapeutic and diagnostic ultrasound. *Phys Med Biol* **34**: 1543–1552.

Docker MF, Foulkes DJ, Patrick MK (1982) Ultrasound couplants for physiotherapy. *Physiotherapy* **68**(4): 124–125.

Dudda M, Pommer A, Muhr G et al (2005) Application of low intensity, pulsed ultrasound on distraction osteogenesis of the humerus. Case report. *Unfallchirurg* **108**(1): 69–74.

Dyson M (1981) The effect of ultrasound on the rate of wound healing and the quality of scar tissue. In Mortimer AJ, Lee N (eds) *Proceedings of the International Symposium on Therapeutic Ultrasound, Manitoba*. Winnipeg, Canadian Physiotherapy Association: 110–123.

Dyson M (1982) Nonthermal cellular effects of ultrasound. *Br J Cancer* **45**(suppl. V): 165–171.

Dyson M (1985) Therapeutic applications of ultrasound. In Nyborg WL, Ziskin MC (eds) *Biological Effects of Ultrasound. Clinics in Diagnostic Ultrasound*. New York, Churchill Livingstone: 121–133.

Dyson M (1990) Role of ultrasound in wound healing. In Kloth LC, McCulloch JM, Feedar JA (eds) *Wound Healing: Alternatives in Management*. Philadelphia, FA Davis: 259–285.

Dyson M, Brookes M (1983) Stimulation of bone repair by ultrasound. In Lerski RA, Morley P (eds) *Ultrasound 82, Proceedings 3rd Meeting World Federation of Ultrasound in Medicine and Biology*. Oxford, Pergamon Press: 232–236.

Dyson M, Smalley DS (1983) Effects of ultrasound on wound contraction. In Millner R, Rosenfeld E, Cobet U (eds)

Ultrasound Interactions in Biology and Medicine. New York, Plenum Press: 151.

Dyson M, Pond JB, Joseph J, Warwick R (1968) Stimulation of tissue repair by pulsed wave ultrasound. *IEEE Trans Sonics Ultrasonics* **SU-17**: 133–140.

Dyson M, Pond JB, Joseph J, Warwick R (1970) The stimulation of tissue regeneration by means of ultrasound. *Clin Sci* **35**: 273–285.

Dyson M, Pond JB, Woodward J, Broadbent J (1974) The production of blood cell stasis and endothelial cell damage in the blood vessels of chick embryos treated with ultrasound in a stationary wave field. *Ultrasound Med Biol* **1**: 133–148.

Dyson M, Franks C, Suckling J (1976) Stimulation of healing varicose ulcers by ultrasound. *Ultrasonics* **14**: 232–236.

Ebenbichler GR, Resch KL, Nicolakis P et al (1998) Ultrasound treatment for treating the carpel tunnel syndrome: randomised 'sham' controlled trial. *Br Med J* **316**(7133): 731–735.

El Hag M, Coghlan K, Christmas P et al (1985) The anti-inflammatory effects of dexamethasone and therapeutic ultrasound in oral surgery. *Br J Oral Maxillofac Surg* **23**: 17–23.

El-Mowafi H, Mohsen M (2005) The effect of low-intensity pulsed ultrasound on callus maturation in tibial distraction osteogenesis. *Int Orthop* **29**(2): 121–124.

Ennis WJ, Foremann P, Mozen N et al (2005) Ultrasound therapy for recalcitrant diabetic foot ulcers: results of a randomized, double-blind, controlled, multicenter study. *Ostomy Wound Manage* **51**(8): 24–39.

Enwemeka CS (1989) The effects of therapeutic ultrasound on tendon healing. *Am J Phys Med Rehab* **68**(6): 283–287.

Enwemeka CS, Rodriguez O, Mendosa S (1990) The biomechanical effects of low-intensity ultrasound on healing tendons. *Ultrasound Med Biol* **16**: 801–807.

Flemming K, Cullum N (2000) Therapeutic ultrasound for pressure sores (Cochrane Review). Cochrane Database Syst Rev 4.

Franek A, Chmielewska D, Brzezinska-Wcislo L et al (2004) Application of various power densities of ultrasound in the treatment of leg ulcers. *J Dermatol Treat* **15**(6): 379–386.

Franek A, Krol P, Chmielewska D et al (2006) [The venous ulcer therapy in use of the selected physical methods (Part 2) – the comparison analysis]. *Pol Merkur Lekarski* **20**(120): 691–695.

Frizzell LA, Dunn F (1982) Biophysics of ultrasound. In Lehmann JF (ed) *Therapeutic Heat and Cold*. Baltimore, MD, Williams & Wilkins. Chapter 9 p 397.

Fujishiro T, Matsui N, Yoshiya S et al (2005) Treatment of a bone defect in the femoral shaft after osteomyelitis using low-intensity pulsed ultrasound. *Eur J Orthop Surg Traumatol* **15**: 244–246.

Fyfe MC, Chahl LA (1982) Mast cell degranulation: A possible mechanism of action of therapeutic ultrasound. *Ultrasound Med Biol* **8**(suppl 1): 62.

Fyfe MC, Chahl LA (1985) The effect of single or repeated applications of 'therapeutic' ultrasound on plasma extravasation during silver nitrate induced inflammation of the rat hindpaw ankle joint *in vivo*. *Ultrasound Med Biol* **11**: 273–283.

Gallo JA, Draper DO, Brody LT et al (2004) A compari-son of human muscle temperature increases during 3-MHz continuous and pulsed ultrasound with equivalent temporal average intensities. *J Orthop Sports Phys Ther* **34**(7): 395–401.

Gam AN, Johannsen F (1995) Ultrasound therapy in musculoskeletal disorders: a meta-analysis. *Pain* **63**: 85–91.

Garrett CL, Draper DO, Knight KL (2000) Heat distribution in the lower leg from pulsed short-wave diathermy and ultrasound treatments. *J Athletic Training* **35**(1): 50–55.

Gebauer D, Correll J (2005) Pulsed low-intensity ultrasound: a new salvage procedure for delayed unions and nonunions after leg lengthening in children. *J Pediatr Orthop* **25**(6): 750–754.

Gebauer D, Mayr E, Orthner E et al (2005) Low-intensity pulsed ultrasound: effects on nonunions. *Ultrasound Med Biol* **31**(10): 1391–1402.

Ginsberg M (1981) Role of platelets in inflammation and rheumatic disease. *Adv Inflamm Res* **2**: 53.

Goddard DH, Revell PA, Cason J et al (1983) Ultrasound has no anti-inflammatory effect. *Ann Rheum Dis* **42**: 582–584.

Guirro R, Serrao F, Elias D et al (1997) Calibration of therapeutic ultrasound equipment. *Physiotherapy* **83**: 419–422.

Hart J (1993) *The Effect of Therapeutic Ultrasound on Dermal Repair with Emphasis on Fibroblast Activity*. PhD Thesis. University of London.

Harvey W, Dyson M, Pond JB, Grahame R (1975) The stimulation of protein synthesis in human fibroblasts by therapeutic ultrasound. *Rheum Rehab* **14**: 237.

Hashish I (1986) *The Effects of Ultrasound Therapy on Post Operative Inflammation*. PhD Thesis. University of London.

Heckman JD, Ryaby JP, McCabe J et al (1994) Acceleration of tibial fracture-healing by non-invasive, low-intensity pulsed ultrasound. *J Bone Joint Surg Am* **76**: 26–34.

Hogan RDB, Burke KM, Franklin TD (1982) The effect of ultrasound on the microvascular hemodynamics in skeletal muscle: effects during ischemia. *Microvasc Res* **23**: 370–379.

Hoogland R (1986) *Ultrasound Therapy*. Delft, the Netherlands, Enraf Nonius.

Hosseinpour AR (1988) *The Effects of Ultrasound on Angiogenesis and Wound Healing*. BSc Thesis. University of London.

Houghton PE, Radman A (2000) Effects of therapeutic ultrasound on fetal limb development in an organ culture system. *Physiother Theory Prac* **16**(3): 119–134.

Hustler JE, Zarod AP, Williams AR (1978) Ultrasonic modification of experimental bruising in the guinea pig pinna. *Ultrasonics* **16**(5): 223–228.

Huys S, Gan BS, Sherebrin M (1993) Comparison of effects of early and late ultrasound treatment on tendon healing in the chicken limb. *J Hand Ther* **6**: 58–59.

Jackson BA, Schwane JA, Starcher BC (1991) Effect of ultrasound therapy on the repair of achilles tendon injuries in rats. *Med Sci Sports Exer* **23**: 171–176.

Kaufman GE, Miller MW, Griffiths TD et al (1977) Lysis and viability of cultured mammalian cells exposed to 1 MHz ultrasound. *Ultrasound Med Biol* **3**: 21–25.

Kischer CW, Schetlar MR (1974) Collagen and mucopolysaccharides in the hypertrophic scar. *Conn Tiss Res* **2**: 205–213.

Klucinec B, Scheidler M, Denegar C et al (2000) Effectiveness of wound care products in the transmission of acoustic energy. *Phys Ther* **80**(5): 469–476.

Kristiansen TK, Ryaby JP, McCabe J et al (1997) Accelerated healing of distal radial fractures with the use of specific, low-intensity ultrasound. A multicenter, prospective, randomized, double-blind, placebo-controlled study. *J Bone Joint Surg Am* **79**(7): 961–973.

Lehmann JF, DeLateur BJ (1982) Therapeutic heat. In Lehmann JF (ed) *Therapeutic Heat and Cold*, 3rd edn. Baltimore, MD, Williams and Wilkins: 404.

Lejbkowicz F, Zwiran M, Salzberg S (1993) The response of normal and malignant cells to ultrasound in vitro. *Ultrasound Med Biol* **19**(1): 75–82.

Lerner A, Stein H, Soudry M (2004) Compound high-energy limb fractures with delayed union: our experience with adjuvant ultrasound stimulation (exogen). *Ultrasonics* **42**(1–9): 915–917.

Leung MC, Ng GY, Yip KK (2004a) Effect of ultrasound on acute inflammation of transected medial collateral ligaments. *Arch Phys Med Rehab* **85**: 963–966.

Leung KS, Lee WS, Tsui HF et al (2004b) Complex tibial fracture outcomes following treatment with low-intensity pulsed ultrasound. *Ultrasound Med Biol* **30**(3): 389–395.

Levenson SM, Geever EG, Crowley LV et al (1965) The healing of rat skin wounds. *Ann Surg* **161**: 293–308.

Loch EG, Fisher AB, Kuwert E (1971) Effect of diagnostic and therapeutic intensities of ultrasonics on normal and malignant human cells *in vitro*. *Am J Obstet Gynecol* **110**: 457–460.

Lundeberg T, Nordstrom F, Brodda-Jansen G (1990) Pulsed ultrasound does not improve healing of venous ulcers. *Scand J Rehab Med* **22**: 195–197.

Lyon R, Liu XC, Meier J (2003) The effects of therapeutic vs. high intensity ultrasound on the rabbit growth plate. *J Orthop Res* **21**: 865–871.

Malizos KN, Hantes ME, Protopappas V et al (2006) Low-intensity pulsed ultrasound for bone healing: An overview. *Injury* **37**(suppl 1): S56–S62.

Maxwell L (1992) Therapeutic ultrasound: Its effects on the cellular and molecular mechanisms of inflammation and repair. *Physiotherapy* **78**(6): 421–426.

Mayr E, Frankel V, Ruter A (2000) Ultrasound – an alternative healing method for nonunions? *Arch Orthop Trauma Surg* **120**(1–2): 1–8.

McDiarmid T, Burns PN, Lewith GT, Machin D (1985) Ultrasound and the treatment of pressure sores. *Physiotherapy* **71**: 66–70.

Meakins A, Watson T (2006) Longwave ultrasound and conductive heating increase functional ankle mobility in asymptomatic subjects. *Phys Ther Sport* **7**: 74–80.

Mitragotri S, Farrell J, Tang H et al (2000) Determination of threshold energy dose for ultrasound-induced transdermal drug transport. *J Cont Rel* **63**: 41–52.

Mortimer AJ, Dyson M (1988) The effect of therapeutic ultrasound on calcium uptake in fibroblasts. *Ultrasound Med Biol* **14**: 499–506.

Mummery CL (1978) *The Effect of Ultrasound on Fibroblasts in Vitro*. PhD Thesis. University of London.

National Council on Radiation Protection (NCRP) (1983) *Biological Effects of Ultrasound: Mechanisms and Implications*. Report No. 74, p 82.

Nolte PA, van der Krans A, Patka P et al (2001) Low-intensity pulsed ultrasound in the treatment of nonunions. *J Trauma* **51**(4): 693–702; discussion 702–703.

Nussbaum EL (1997) Ultrasound: to heat or not to heat – that is the question. *Phys Ther Rev* **2**: 59–72.

Nussbaum EL (1998) The influence of ultrasound on healing tissues. *J Hand Ther* **11**(2): 140–147.

Nyborg WL (1977) *Physical Mechanisms for Biological Effects of Ultrasound*. DHEW 78-8062. Washington, DC, US Government Printing Office.

Oakley EM (1978) Applications of continuous beam ultrasound at therapeutic levels. *Physiotherapy* **64**: 169–172.

Ogurtan Z, Celik I, Izci C et al (2002) Effect of experimental therapeutic ultrasound on the distal antebrachial growth plates in one-month-old rabbits. *Vet J* **164**(3): 280–287.

Paul BJ, Lafratta CW, Dawson AR et al (1960) Use of ultrasound in the treatment of pressure sores in patients with spinal cord injuries. *Arch Phys Med Rehab* **41**: 438–440.

Pavlov IV (2002) Use of low frequency ultrasonic technology in preventing and treating purulent wounds of the lung and pleura. *Khirurgiia (Mosk)* **5**: 64–67.

Pilla AA, Mont MA, Nasser PR et al (1990) Non-invasive low-intensity pulsed ultrasound accelerates bone healing in the rabbit. *J Orthop Trauma* **4**: 246–253.

Poltawski L, Watson T (2007a) Relative transmissivity of ultrasound coupling agents commonly used by therapists in the UK. *Ultrasound Med Biol* **33**(1): 120–128.

Poltawski L, Watson T (2007b) Transmission of therapeutic ultrasound by wound dressings. *Wounds* **19**(1): 1–12.

Pope GD, Mockett SP, Wright JP (1995) A survey of electrotherapeutic modalities: ownership and use in the NHS in England. *Physiotherapy* **81**(2): 82–91.

Pye S, Milford C (1994) The performance of ultrasound physiotherapy machines in Lothian Region. *Ultrasound Med Biol* **4**: 347–359.

Ramirez A, Schwane JA, McFarland C et al (1997) The effect of ultrasoundon collagen synthesis and fibroblast proliferation *in vitro*. *Med Sci Sports Exerc* **29**: 326–332.

Reher P, Doan N, Bradnock B et al (1999) Effect of ultrasound on the production of IL-8, basic FGF and VEGF. *Cytokine* **11**(6): 416–423.

Reid DC (1981) Possible contraindications and precautions associated with ultrasound therapy. In Mortimer AJ, Lee N (eds) *Proceedings of the International Symposium on Therapeutic Ultrasound*. Winnipeg, Canadian Physiotherapy Association: 274.

Robertson V, Ward A (1997) Longwave ultrasound reviewed and reconsidered. *Physiotherapy* **83**(3): 123–130.

Roche C, West J (1984) A controlled trial investigating the effect of ultrasound on venous ulcers referred from general practitioners. *Physiotherapy* **70**: 475–477.

Rosim GC, Barbieri CH, Lancas FM, Mazzer N (2005) Diclofenac phonophoresis in human volunteers. *Ultrasound Med Biol* **31**(3): 337–343.

Rubin C, Bolander M, Ryaby JP et al (2001) The use of low-intensity ultrasound to accelerate the healing of fractures. *J Bone Joint Surg Am* **83-A**(2): 259–270.

Schabrun S, Chipchase L, Rickard H (2006) Are therapeutic ultrasound units a potential vector for nosocomial infection? *Physiother Res Int* **11**(2): 61–71.

Sedov VM, Gordeev NA, Krivtsova GB et al (1998) Management of infected wounds and trophic ulcers by low frequency ultrasound. *Khirurgiia Mosk* **4**: 39–41.

Selkowitz DM, Cameron MH, Mainzer A et al (2002) Efficacy of pulsed low-intensity ultrasound in wound healing: a single-case design. *Ostomy Wound Manage* **48**(4): 40–44, 46–50.

Sicard Rosenbaum L, Lord D, Danoff JV et al (1995) Effects of continuous therapeutic ultrasound on growth and metastasis of subcutaneous murine tumors. *Phys Ther* **75**(1): 3–13.

Sicard-Rosenbaum L, Danoff JV, Guthrie JA et al (1998) Effects of energy-matched pulsed and continuous ultrasound on tumor growth in mice. *Phys Ther* **78**(3): 271–277.

Singer AJ, Clark RA (1999) Cutaneous wound healing. *N Engl J Med* **341**(10): 738–746.

Snow CJ, Johnson KJ (1988) Effect of therapeutic ultrasound on acute inflammation. *Physiother Canada* **40**: 162–167.

Sparrow KJ, Finucane SD, Owen JR et al (2005) The effects of low-intensity ultrasound on medial collateral ligament healing in the rabbit model. *Am J Sports Med* **33**(7): 1048–1056.

Stein H, Lerner A (2005) How does pulsed low-intensity ultrasound enhance fracture healing? *Orthopedics* **28**(10): 1161–1163.

Sutherland EW, Rall EW (1968) Formation of cyclic adenine ribonucleotide by tissue particles. *J Biol Chem* **232**: 1065–1076.

Sutton Y, McBride K, Pye S (2006) An ultrasound mini-balance for measurement of therapy level ultrasound. *Phys Med Biol* **51**(14): 3397–3404.

ter Haar G (1999) Therapeutic ultrasound. *Eur J Ultrasound* **9**: 3–9.

ter Haar G, Dyson M, Oakley EM (1985) The use of ultrasound by physiotherapists in Britain, 1985. *Ultrasound Med Biol* **13**: 659–663.

Tsai CL, Chang WH, Liu TK (1992a) Preliminary studies of duration and intensity of ultrasonic treatments on fracture repair. *Chin J Physiol* **35**: 21–26.

Tsai CL, Chang WH, Liu TK (1992b) Ultrasonic effect on fracture repair and prostaglandin E2 production. *Chin J Physiol* **35**: 168.

Turner S, Powell E, Ng C (1989) The effect of ultrasound on the healing of repaired cockerel tendon: is collagen cross-linkage a factor? *J Hand Surg* **14B**: 428–433.

Uhlemann C, Wollina U (2003) Physiological aspects of therapeutic ultrasound in wound- healing. *Phlebologie* **32**(4): 81–86.

Uhlemann C, Heinig B, Wollina U (2003) Therapeutic ultrasound in lower extremity wound management. *Int J Low Extrem Wounds* **2**(3): 152–157.

Wang CJ, Wang FA, Yang KD et al (2003) Shock wave therapy induces neovacularization at the tendon-bone junction. A study in rabbits. *J Orthop Res* **21**(6): 984–989.

Wang ED (1998) Tendon repair. *J Hand Ther* **11**(2): 105–110.

Ward AR (1986) *Electricity, Fields and Waves in Therapy.* Marrickville, Australia, Science Press.

Warden S (2003) A new direction for ultrasound therapy in sports medicine. *Sports Med* **33**(2): 95–107.

Warden S, Bennell K, McMeeken JM et al (1999) Can conventional therapeutic ultrasound units be used to accelerate fracture repair? *Phys Ther Rev* **4**: 117–126.

Warden SJ, Fuchs RK, Kessler CK et al (2006) Ultrasound produced by a conventional therapeutic ultrasound unit accelerates fracture repair. *Phys Ther* **86**(8): 1118–1127.

Watson J, Nelson EA (2006) An exploration of the use of ultrasound in the treatment of chronic venous leg ulcers. *J Wound Care* **15**(1): 39–41.

Watson T (2000) The role of electrotherapy in contemporary physiotherapy practice. *Man Ther* **5**(3): 132–141.

Watson T (2002) Ultrasound dose calculations. *In Touch* **101**: 14–17.

Watson T (2006a) Electrotherapy and tissue repair. *Sportex Med* **29**: 7–13.

Watson T (2006b) Tissue repair: the current state of the art. *Sportex Med* **28**: 8–12.

Webster DF (1980) *The Effect of Ultrasound on Wound Healing.* PhD Thesis. University of London.

Webster DF, Pond JB, Dyson M, Harvey W (1978) The role of cavitation in the *in vitro* stimulation of protein synthesis in human fibroblasts by ultrasound. *Ultrasound Med Biol* **4**: 343–351.

Wilkin LD, Merrick MA, Kirby TE et al (2004) Influence of therapeutic ultrasound on skeletal muscle regeneration following blunt contusion. *Int J Sports Med* **25**(1): 73–77.

Williams AR (1974) Release of serotonin from platelets by acoustic streaming. *J Acoustic Soc Am* **56**: 1640.

Williams AR (1987) Production and transmission of ultrasound. *Physiotherapy* **73**(3): 113–116.

Williams AR, Sykes SM, O'Brien WD (1976) Ultrasonic exposure modifies platelet morphology and function *in vitro.* *Ultrasound Med Biol* **2**: 311–317.

Wiltink A, Nijweide PJ, Oosterbaan WA et al (1995) Effect of therapeutic ultrasound on endochondral ossification. *Ultrasound Med Biol* **21**(1): 121–127.

Wu F (2006) Extracorporeal high intensity focused ultrasound in the treatment of patients with solid malignancy. *Minim Invasive Ther Allied Technol* **15**(1): 26–35.

Young SR, Dyson M (1990a) Macrophage responsiveness to therapeutic ultrasound. *Ultrasound Med Biol* **16**: 809–816.

Young SR, Dyson M (1990b) The effect of therapeutic ultrasound on the healing of full-thickness excised skin lesions. *Ultrasonics* **28**: 175–180.

Young SR, Dyson M (1990c) The effect of therapeutic ultrasound on angiogenesis. *Ultrasound Med Biol* **16**: 261–269.

Yurt RW (1981) Role of the mast cell in trauma. In Dineen P, Hildick-Smith G (eds) *The Surgical Wound.* Philadelphia, Lea and Febiger: 62.

SECTION 3

Electrical stimulation modalities

SECTION CONTENTS

Chapter 13

Introduction to low-frequency currents

Deirdre M. Walsh

INTRODUCTION

The term 'low-frequency currents' covers a range of electrical currents commonly used in clinical practice to stimulate muscles, nerves or a combination of both. The physiological effects of such stimulation are used therapeutically to strengthen muscle (Healy et al 2006, Stevens et al 2004), assist in wound healing (Bogie et al 2000, Kloth 2005), relieve pain (Khadilkar et al 2005) and reduce oedema (Man et al 2003). As the number of devices producing electrical currents for therapeutic applications has proliferated over the past few decades, the terminology relating to the output of these devices has become somewhat confusing. This introductory chapter will therefore provide an overview of the basic principles associated with these type of currents using standardized terminology; this will serve as a foundation for the subsequent chapters in this section that focus on individual currents: transcutaneous electrical nerve stimulation (TENS) and neuromuscular electrical stimulation. The chapter commences with a brief description of how an electrical current initiates an action potential in a nerve. This is followed by an explanation of the characteristics or stimulation parameters of the currents. Finally, a guide for the safe application of electrical currents is provided.

STIMULATION OF A NERVE USING ELECTRICAL CURRENTS

Chapter 5 describes the generation of an action potential in a nerve. This chapter gives a brief

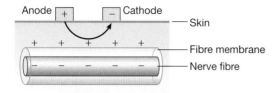

Figure 13.1 Stimulation of a nerve using an electrical current.

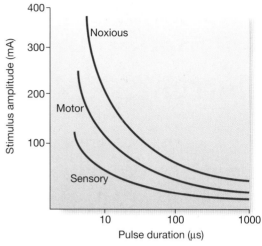

Figure 13.2 Strength duration curves for sensory, motor and noxious responses.

summary of stimulation of nerves using electrical currents as an introduction to the following chapters. An externally applied stimulus can cause depolarization of a nerve and thus initiate an action potential as long as the applied stimulus depolarizes the resting membrane potential to the threshold level. Depolarization means loss of the normal negative value of the resting membrane potential in a nerve ($-70\,\mathrm{mV}$). In an electrical circuit, one electrode is positively charged (anode) and the other is negatively charged (cathode). In the circuit, the current flows from anode to cathode (Fig. 13.1). Under the cathode, negative charges accumulate on the outer surface of the nerve fibre membrane as they are repelled by its negative charge; the outside of the membrane becomes relatively more negative. The inside of the membrane therefore becomes more positive, causing depolarization. For this reason, the cathode is commonly termed the 'active electrode'. Once the critical level of depolarization occurs (i.e. threshold level is reached), an action potential is initiated. Under the anode, negative charges move from the outside of the membrane towards the anode as they are attracted towards its positive charge. This makes the outside of the membrane more positive and therefore the inside of the membrane more negative, hence hyperpolarization occurs.

If the applied stimulus is electrical, the stimulation parameters of frequency, pulse duration and amplitude must correlate with the characteristics of the nerve fibre itself. The relationship between the stimulation parameters of pulse amplitude and duration of the stimulating current can be illustrated on a strength–duration (SD) curve. Basically, this curve illustrates the relationship between different combinations of pulse duration and amplitude that are required to optimally stimulate a specific fibre type and produce the response associated with

the fibre, i.e. motor, sensory or noxious response. Figure 13.2 illustrates SD curves for motor, sensory and nociceptive fibres. At any given pulse duration, the order of recruitment with increasing stimulus amplitude is sensory, then motor, then nociceptive fibres.

The SD curve itself is an indicator of the threshold required to cause depolarization of a specific type of nerve fibre. A subthreshold stimulus will have parameter combinations that fall to the left of the SD curve and will therefore not initiate an action potential. A suprathreshold stimulus will have parameter combinations that fall to the right of the curve and will initiate an action potential. If an electrical stimulus is applied over a mixed nerve, the order of response is first sensory (Aβ fibres); the patient will report a sensation of paraesthesia (pins and needles). Motor fibres are recruited next (Aα) with associated contractions, and finally nociceptive fibres (Aδ and C) are stimulated, producing a painful response.

STIMULATION PARAMETERS OF LOW–FREQUENCY CURRENTS

DOCUMENTATION OF PARAMETERS

One of the key factors associated with a poor treatment outcome is the use of inappropriate treatment

Table 13.1 Cochrane Systematic Reviews of low-frequency electrical currents

Author and year	Title
Khadilkar et al 2005	TENS for chronic low back pain
Cameron et al 2003	TENS for dementia
Brosseau et al 2003	TENS for treatment of rheumatoid arthritis of the hand
Proctor et al 2002	TENS and acupuncture for primary dysmenorrhoea
Pelland et al 2002	Electrical stimulation for the treatment of rheumatoid arthritis
Osiri et al 2000	TENS for knee osteoarthritis
Hosker et al 2007	Electrical stimulation for faecal incontinence in adults
Carroll et al 2000	TENS for chronic pain

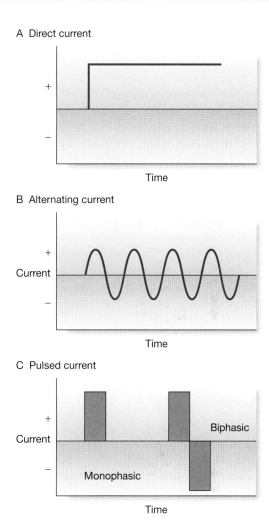

Figure 13.3 Three basic types of electrical current.

parameters (Sluka & Walsh 2003). Inadequate documentation of the stimulation parameters in clinical notes or research papers makes it inherently difficult to replicate that study by other clinical colleagues/researchers. Several Cochrane Systematic Reviews have been published on the efficacy of low-frequency currents for a variety of conditions (Table 13.1). A common observation by the authors of these reviews is the lack of standardized treatment regimens, which makes comparisons across clinical trials an impossible task.

The type of information required for documentation of any low-frequency current includes: type of current, frequency, pulse duration, amplitude, waveform, type of output, duty cycle, duration of treatment and electrodes (placement, size, shape). This section will briefly outline the basic stimulation parameters relevant to the electrical currents described in Chapters 14–18.

TYPES OF CURRENT

To avoid confusion, a definition of the three basic types of electrical current used for therapeutic purposes is provided first. Figure 13.3 illustrates these currents:

1. **Direct current (DC):** current flows continuously in one direction only (unidirectional) over time.

2. **Alternating current (AC):** current flows continuously in both directions (bidirectional) over time.

3. **Pulsed current:** the unidirectional or bidirectional flow of current periodically ceases over time. The basic element of this type of current is a pulse.

WAVEFORM

The waveform of a current refers to its shape as seen on a graph of current amplitude versus time. Common waveform shapes include square, rectangular and triangular. In a monophasic waveform, current flows in only one direction and therefore only one electrode acts as the cathode (Fig. 13.3C). A biphasic waveform means that current flows in both directions (see pulsed biphasic current, Fig. 13.3C). This type of waveform therefore has two components (or phases) – the positive and the negative components – which represent the change in current flow. A biphasic waveform is called symmetrical if the portion of the waveform in the first phase is an exact mirror image of, but opposite in direction to, the portion of the waveform in the second phase (i.e. current flow is equal in magnitude and duration in both directions). A biphasic symmetrical waveform results in each electrode acting as a cathode (i.e. the active electrode) during alternate phases of the pulse.

An asymmetrical biphasic waveform has two phases that are not equal in shape. This type of waveform can also be described as balanced or unbalanced. It is important to know if a biphasic waveform is balanced or unbalanced as this will determine whether both electrodes act as the cathode or only one. As depolarization occurs under the cathode, placement of this electrode is important to achieve the desired outcome. A balanced asymmetrical biphasic waveform means that there is equal flow of current in both directions. An unbalanced asymmetrical biphasic waveform means that the current flow is not equal between the two directions. Owing to this inequality, this typically means that only one direction of current flow (i.e. one phase of the waveform) is adequate to cause depolarization and therefore this waveform acts like a monophasic waveform in that only one electrode acts as the active electrode (cathode). It is important to note that an unbalanced asymmetrical biphasic waveform may therefore result in different sensations under each electrode. A lot of confusion can be avoided by determining the waveform of your current before you choose the position of your electrodes.

FREQUENCY

Frequency is measured in hertz (Hz) and refers to the number of pulses delivered per second for a pulsed current or the number of cycles delivered per second for an alternating current, e.g. a frequency of 100 Hz in a pulsed current means that 100 pulses are delivered by the device per second. Some manufacturers often label the frequency dial on an electrical stimulator as 'rate'. Figure 13.4 illustrates the calculation of frequency for a pulsed current (A) and an alternating current (B).

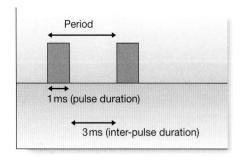

Pulsed current
Frequency = 1/period
= 1/4 ms
= 250 Hz

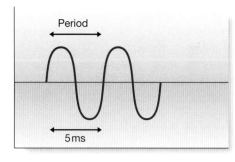

Alternating current
Frequency = 1/period
= 1/5 ms
= 200 Hz

Period
Pulsed current: period = pulse duration plus inter-pulse duration
Alternating current: period = time elapsed between a specific point on one cycle to the same point on the next cycle

Figure 13.4 Frequency calculations for a pulsed current and an alternating current.

PULSE DURATION

Pulse duration is a time-dependent characteristic and is often referred to as pulse width. The unit of pulse duration is usually given in milliseconds (ms) or microseconds (µs). Most texts tend to refer to the pulse duration as the duration of only the positive (i.e. depolarizing) component of the waveform. However, some sources refer to the pulse duration as the duration of both phases in the waveform, i.e. the sum of the duration of both positive and negative phases (Fig. 13.5). It is therefore important to check which definition the manufacturer uses to enable you to document this parameter accurately.

DUTY CYCLE

Duty cycle is the ratio of the 'on' time of the current to the total duration of the cycle (i.e. on time and off time), and is expressed as a percentage. For example, if a current has an 'on' time of 5 ms and the 'off' time is 10 ms, then the duty cycle is 33%:

$$\frac{5}{5 + 10} \times 100 = 33\%$$

AMPLITUDE/INTENSITY

Stimulators can be designed with either a constant current or constant voltage output, which means that either the voltage or current (respectively) will vary to maintain a constant current or voltage amplitude (within limits), as the impedance (resistance) of the electrode–patient system changes.

The amplitude (often referred to as intensity) of a constant current unit is measured in milliamps and the amplitude of a constant voltage unit is measured in volts. Current is the flow of electric charge and voltage is the driving force required to move this electric charge; it should be remembered that it is the level of the current and not the voltage that is ultimately responsible for depolarization of a nerve fibre membrane. Ohm's law describes the relationship between current and voltage: $V = IR$, where V is the voltage required to move an electric charge (I) across a resistance (R) that opposes the movement of electric charge. When an electrical current is applied to the skin, it will require a driving force because it will encounter impedance in the electrode–patient system (the driving force is supplied by the battery/mains supply). Peak amplitude is the maximum amplitude from the zero value in a phase (Fig. 13.6). Peak-to-peak amplitude is the amplitude measured from the peak of one phase to the peak of the second phase.

CONTINUOUS, BURST AND MODULATED OUTPUTS

Most devices offer a range of outputs. This describes the pattern in which the pulse is delivered, e.g. continuous, burst or modulated (Fig. 13.7). A continuous output means that the pulses are delivered in a continuous pattern over time. A burst or pulsed output indicates they are delivered in a group or train. The modulated output means that there is a variation in one or more of the pulse duration,

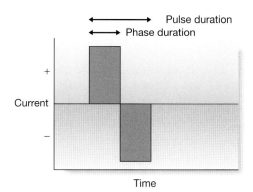

Figure 13.5 Pulse duration.

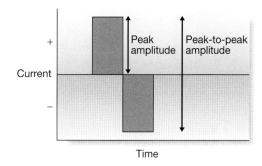

Figure 13.6 Amplitude.

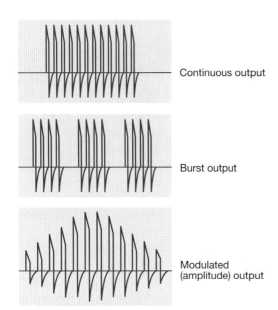

Continuous output

Burst output

Modulated (amplitude) output

Figure 13.7 Types of output.

frequency or amplitude parameters in a cyclical fashion.

DURATION OF TREATMENT

The duration of treatment is the time for which the treatment was applied, typically recorded in minutes.

ELECTRODES

Self-adhesive electrodes have largely replaced many of the old carbon rubber and gel applications. The size, shape and position of electrodes all play an important role in any treatment. It is important to note that current density is the amount of current per unit area and this is inversely proportional to the size of the electrode contact area. Therefore, the current density will increase if the size of the contact area decreases, e.g. if an electrode peels off the skin during treatment. If a small and a large electrode are used in one circuit, the current density will be greater under the small electrode and therefore the sensation will be greater under this electrode also. As previously indicated, the location of the cathode is important if you are using an unbalanced asymmetrical biphasic or monophasic

waveform, and care should be taken to document this in the treatment notes.

CHOICE OF STIMULATION PARAMETERS

The optimal stimulation parameters for any given type of low-frequency current remain elusive. A quick glance at the summaries of the Cochrane Systematic Reviews listed in Table 13.1 will confirm the common problem encountered in clinical trials of electrotherapy: lack of standardized treatment regimens. Research on various stimulation parameters over the years has provided some evidence upon which clinicians can base their applications, e.g. Bennie et al (2002) compared four waveforms (Russian, interferential, sine and square) on strengthening the quadriceps muscle (in a small number of healthy subjects) and concluded that the sine waveform produced the desired muscle tension with the least mean stimulation current. However, until definitive evidence is available, a degree of trial and error will still play a role in the selection process of stimulation parameters. In the following chapters, the latest evidence will be provided for each modality to assist the reader to make an informed decision.

PRINCIPLES OF CLINICAL APPLICATION

The application of any low-frequency current involves a common set of principles to ensure safe application. These are described below but each chapter will provide additional details:

1. Perform routine safety checks.

2. Ensure equipment is calibrated on a regular basis. Calibration of a device is relatively easy to do with an oscilloscope. Basically, calibration of the frequency of a unit determines whether, if the frequency dial is set to 50 Hz, this is what is being delivered by the unit.

3. Assess the patient.

4. Explain the treatment to the patient.

5. Check for contraindications and skin sensation (see relevant chapters).

6. Position patient comfortably.

7. Collect the equipment plus necessary items to prepare skin, e.g. soap and water.

8. Test the equipment on yourself.

9. Demonstrate the treatment to the patient.

10. Prepare the skin and attach electrodes.

11. Ensure all leads are attached correctly to the device and to the electrodes.

12. Select the appropriate stimulation parameters (see relevant chapters).

13. Check that the amplitude dial is at zero.

14. Warn the patient with regard to what he/she should expect to feel and what he/she should not feel. If, for example, you are trying to stimulate a muscle, it is important to let the patient know that he/she should expect to feel the muscle contracting, otherwise this can be very disconcerting.

15. Increase the amplitude *slowly*. The rate of increase of current will vary between different machines.

16. Monitor treatment.

17. Terminate treatment by slowly decreasing the intensity. Never lift an electrode before turning the amplitude to zero and switching the device off.

18. Check the skin for any adverse effects after removal of electrodes.

19. Document the treatment, including all treatment parameters and any adverse effects.

SUMMARY

Nerve fibres can be stimulated by the external application of low-frequency electrical currents. To elicit the desired response (sensory, motor, noxious), the electrical stimulus must have certain characteristics that are compatible with those of the nerve if an action potential is to be elicited. These characteristics or stimulation parameters should be documented carefully for any given clinical or research application.

References

Bennie SD, Petrofsky JS, Nisperos J et al (2002) Toward the optimal waveform for electrical stimulation of human muscle. *Eur J Appl Physiol* **88**(1–2): 13–19.

Bogie KM, Reger SI, Levine SP et al (2000) Electrical stimulation for pressure sore prevention and wound healing. *Assistive Technol* **12**(1): 50–66.

Brosseau L, Yonge KA, Robinson V et al (2003) Transcutaneous electrical nerve stimulation (TENS) for the treatment of rheumatoid arthritis in the hand. The Cochrane Database of Systematic Reviews: Issue 2. John Wiley & Sons Ltd, Chichester.

Cameron M, Lonergan E, Lee H (2003) Transcutaneous electrical nerve stimulation (TENS) for dementia. The Cochrane Database of Systematic Reviews: Issue 3. John Wiley & Sons, Chichester.

Carroll D, Moore RA, McQuay HJ et al (2000) Transcutaneous electrical nerve stimulation (TENS) for chronic pain. The Cochrane Database of Systematic Reviews: Issue 4. John Wiley & Sons Ltd, Chichester.

Healy CF, Brannigan AE, Connolly EM et al (2006) The effects of low-frequency endoanal electrical stimulation on faecal incontinence: a prospective study. *Int J Colorectal Dis* **21**: 802–806, Epub 2006 March 17.

Hosker G, Cody JD, Norton CC (2007) Electrical stimulation for faecal incontinence in adults. The Cochrane Database of Systematic Reviews 2007: Issue 3. John Wiley & Sons Ltd, Chichester.

Khadilkar A, Milne S, Brosseau L et al (2005) Transcutaneous electrical nerve stimulation (TENS) for chronic low-back pain. The Cochrane Database of Systematic Reviews: Issue 3. John Wiley & Sons Ltd, Chichester.

Kloth LC (2005) Electrical stimulation for wound healing: a review of evidence from in vitro studies, animal experiments, and clinical trials. *Int J Lower Extrem Wounds* **4**(1): 23–44.

Man IO, Lepar GS, Morrissey MC et al (2003) Effect of neuromuscular electrical stimulation on foot/ankle volume during standing. *Med Sci Sports Exer* **35**(4): 630–634.

Osiri M, Welch V, Brosseau L et al (2000) Transcutaneous electrical nerve stimulation for knee osteoarthritis. The Cochrane Database of Systematic Review 2000: Issue 4. John Wiley & Sons Ltd, Chichester.

Pelland L, Brosseau L, Casimiro L et al (2002) Electrical stimulation for the treatment of rheumatoid arthritis. The Cochrane Database of Systematic Reviews: Issue 2. John Wiley & Sons Ltd, Chichester.

Proctor ML, Smith CA, Farquhar CM et al (2002) Transcutaneous electrical nerve stimulation and acupuncture for primary dysmenorrhoea. The Cochrane Database of Systematic Reviews: Issue 1. John Wiley & Sons Ltd, Chichester.

Sluka KA, Walsh D (2003) TENS: basic science mechanisms and clinical effectiveness. *J Pain* **4**(3): 109–121.

Stevens JE, Mizner RL, Snyder-Mackler L (2004) Neuromuscular electrical stimulation for quadriceps muscle strengthening after bilateral total knee arthroplasty: a case series. *J Orthop Sports Phys Ther* **34**(1): 21–29.

Chapter 14

Neuromuscular electrical stimulation: nerve–muscle interaction

Mary Cramp and Oona Scott

INTRODUCTION

It is well known that physical performance capabilities are affected by the amount and types of daily physical exercise. Someone who exercises on a regular basis has a leaner body mass and greater strength than someone who takes little or no exercise (Enoka 1997). Andersen and colleagues (1999), looking ahead to the possibilities of genetic enhancement, raised the issue of whether elite runners, swimmers, cyclists and cross-country runners are born different from the rest of us or whether 'proper' training and determination could turn almost anyone into a champion.

Recent findings have contributed to our understanding of how human muscle adapts to exercise or the lack of it and the extent to which muscle alters in response to different challenges. Voluntary muscle strength increases with training but the mechanisms involved remain controversial (Gandevia 2001) and there is marked intersubject variation (Enoka 1997). Detraining effects have been shown to affect cardiorespiratory endurance, muscle endurance, muscle strength and power (see the section Effect of immobilization, below).

Selecting appropriate electrical stimulation and exercise regimens are two of the ongoing challenges in rehabilitation in the twenty-first century. In respect of electrical stimulation, much has been gained from animal studies, in which variables can be controlled and extensive investigations undertaken. In drawing evidence from existing human studies, there is a need to distinguish between evidence drawn from studies involving normal healthy individuals and studies on the many different patient groups (Bax et al 2005).

BACKGROUND

Differences in the distribution of fibre types in whole human muscles were first established in autopsy studies (Johnson et al 1973). Advances in histochemical techniques (see Chapter 5), together with more acceptable methods of taking muscle biopsies from human subjects (Edwards et al 1977), were complemented by the examination of contractile properties using electrophysiological techniques. Increasingly, teams of researchers from a range of scientific and clinical backgrounds have become involved in studies to monitor the changes that occur in the genetic, molecular, physiological, and biochemical components of living human muscle (see Chapter 5).

Investigation of changes in fundamental characteristics of human skeletal muscles are often accompanied by measurements of individual or group muscle performance in either isometric or isokinetic contractions or using kinemetric technology (Hortobagyi et al 2000, Liu et al 2003, Short et al 2005). These can, or possibly should, at least include measurements of peripheral fatigue and the time course of muscle contraction in addition to monitoring changes in electrophysiological activity using surface EMG (see below).

MONITORING AND MEASUREMENT

Recent years have seen a growing elucidation of peripheral and central electrophysiological responses and objective documentation of the clinical benefits that neuromuscular electrical stimulation (NMES) can provide (Alon 2003). Evidence has shown that these changes are extensive and occur at a number of levels (including changes at a molecular level in the contractile proteins, and at a biochemical level in respect of the metabolic enzymes) affecting the structural and physiological characteristics of skeletal muscle. So far in clinical studies of electrical stimulation, the tendency has been to focus on changes in maximum voluntary strength (MVC) and levels of muscle activation (see below).

There is a pressing need to continue to explore and evaluate the underlying changes that result in loss of and recovery of strength. At the same time, with regard to measures of functional performance, the tendency has been to assume that once subjects have regained some strength, they will achieve restoration of more normal function and not to take into account aspects of detraining and lack of motivation.

Assessment of any aspect of muscle strength in clinical and experimental situations usually requires the full cooperation and motivation of the subject. Gandevia (2001) provided a summary of the well-established experimental details and critical procedures that should always be in place when measuring muscle strength. These include:

- All maximal efforts should be accompanied by some instruction and practice.

- Feedback of performance should be given during the efforts (e.g. by visual display) and not delayed until afterwards.

- Appropriate verbal encouragement should be given by the investigators, preferably *not* by audio tape.

- Subjects must be allowed to reject efforts that they do not regard as maximal, although with care this rarely happens.

- In studies that include repeated testing or patients in whom there might have been a decline in strength, real-time feedback should be varied so that the subject or patient is not aware of any decline. The aim is to maximize performance without providing a calibrated indicator.

- For repeat testing over a number of sessions, rewards should be considered.

MAXIMUM VOLUNTARY CONTRACTION (MVC)

Maximum or maximal voluntary strength or contraction (MVC) sometimes known as maximum voluntary isometric contraction (MVIC) is the maximum tension developed against an unyielding resistance in a single contraction. Determined by a combination of neural, mechanical and muscular factors, an MVC is typically generated for a short duration over 5 seconds. The measurement recorded is either peak force or torque generated or, on occasion, mean force or torque over a shorter period, say 3 seconds.

VOLUNTARY MUSCLE ACTIVATION

The ability to activate all of the motor units of a muscle can be tested using twitch superimposition, now often know as twitch interpolation (Enoka & Fuglevand 1993, Herbert & Gandevia 1999, Rutherford et al 1986). Figure 14.1 shows that twitch interpolation occurs during an MVC when a single pulse or, as in this case, a series of single twitches are delivered to the intramuscular branches of the femoral nerve. In Figure 14.1B, a twitch-like increment in force can be detected on the force output as the subject attempts to achieve a maximal voluntary contraction of their muscles but fails to recruit all of their quadriceps femoris motor units to a maximal level (Behm & St Pierre 1997, Merton 1954, Todd et al 2004).

Other researchers have used a ten-pulse electrical train at 100 Hz on a maximal effort contraction and compared volitional to electrically augmented effort (Chmielewski at al 2001, Stackhouse et al 2001, Synder-Mackler et al 1994). The resulting deflection in torque is used to measure the 'level' of excitation of muscle. Most normal healthy subjects have the ability to activate their muscles to a high level (voluntary activation scores ≈95%); the level is not consistently 100% (Gandevia 2001).

Maximum activation can be brought about through greater motor unit recruitment or a higher rate of motor unit firing. In healthy subjects, early gains of muscle strength have been attributed to altered neural drive, sometimes known as the learning effect (Jones et al 1989, Komi 1986). In untrained subjects, increases in muscle strength on repeated assessment and in the first few weeks of training may be due to this learning effect.

FATIGUE AND ENDURANCE

The term 'fatigue' (the opposite of endurance) has many different meanings, often associated with exhaustion and overuse. Fatigue can be a symptom reported by someone with no apparent physiological or pathological state, where performance is below expected maximum. For the physiologist, muscle fatigue has been defined as the failure to maintain the required force or power output during sustained or repeated voluntary or electrically elicited contractions (Edwards 1981). The rate of fatigue depends on the muscles employed and whether the contractions are continuous or intermittent. Fatigue has both central and peripheral components. Failure at any point in the chain of command from the higher centres in the brain via the spinal cord, motor neurons and neuromuscular junctions to the individual cross-bridges can lead to loss of force and slower rates of relaxation. The central components occur proximal to the anterior horn cell. Supraspinal fatigue, a subset of central fatigue is the failure to generate output from the motor cortex (for a review, see Gandevia 2001). Peripheral fatigue occurs at or beyond the neuromuscular junction and within the muscle fibres themselves.

The response of skeletal muscle to sustained electrical stimulation is one way used to study peripheral fatigue in human skeletal muscle (Fig. 14.2). The protocol based on fatigue testing by Burke (1967) monitors the decline in tension of between 20 and 30% MVC during repeated tetanic stimulation at 40 Hz for 250 ms over a period of 3–5 minutes. This form of testing allows peripheral fatigue to be measured independently of volition and of failure of the central neural processes, and has established validity and reliability in both adult and children's muscles (Hanchard et al 1998, Scott et al 1985).

TIME COURSE OF CONTRACTION AND FORCE–FREQUENCY RESPONSES

The contractile properties are assessed within the same protocol (see Fig. 14.2). Force–frequency responses to short trains of stimuli (1, 10, 20 and 40 Hz) can be determined and the response calculated by relating the force generated at the lower frequencies to that generated at 40 Hz both before and after the fatigue test. The time course of contraction can be monitored throughout and changes in the half-time of relaxation ($\frac{1}{2}RT_{40}$) defined as the time for the force to drop from peak force to half peak force recorded (Scott et al 1990).

SUMMARY

In summary, using standardized equipment and a simple strain gauge arrangement, it is possible to measure the:

● MVC with and without superimposed twitches or short trains of 100 Hz stimulation

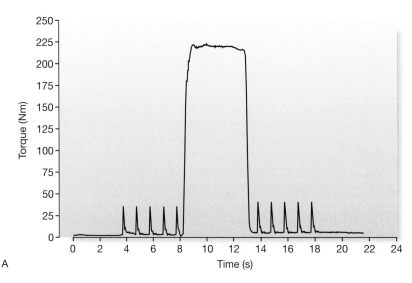

A

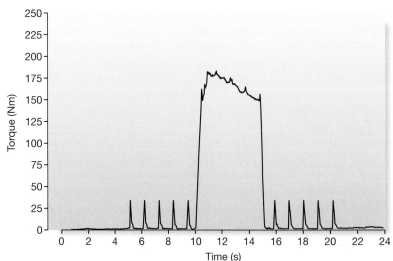

B

Figure 14.1 Maximum voluntary contraction (MVC) of the quadriceps femoris with superimposed twitches. A, full activation; B, detectable force – less than full activation.

- response to short trains of stimulation at different frequencies of electrical stimulation

- response to fatigue testing by stimulation, e.g. at 40 Hz for 250 ms/s, for 3 minutes

- time course of muscle relaxation during twitch, short trains and fatigue testing.

These measurements of muscle strength, fatigue resistance and contractile properties provide valuable information reflecting muscle composition and function which can then be used both to guide selection of the appropriate parameters for electrical stimulation and as a means of monitoring the efficacy of intervention.

CENTRAL MOTOR PATHWAY CONDUCTIVITY AND INFLUENCES OF DESCENDING NERVE PATHWAYS

Magnetic stimulation is one of the most recent developments in the field of electrodiagnosis. Originally designed for the stimulation of peripheral nerves (Merton et al 1982), magnetic stimulation has been applied widely for painless stimulation of the brain, spinal cord and nerve roots. It is currently used to examine central motor pathway conductivity and to assess excitatory and inhibitory influences of descending neural pathways. Magnetic stimulators use a magnetic field that varies over time and passes unchanged through skin and bone to induce currents in excitable tissue. When such

activation is applied to the brain, neurons in the cortex can be activated and a motor response elicited in the form of electromyographic (EMG) recordings in the targeted muscle. Recent work using transcranial magnetic stimulation (TMS) has demonstrated impaired voluntary activation both during maximal effort and in sustained maximal fatiguing contractions in the elbow flexors and provides a potential means to identify the 'site' of failure of voluntary drive, i.e. central fatigue (Todd et al 2004).

ELECTRICAL ACTIVITY OF MUSCLES: SURFACE ELECTROMYOGRAPHY RECORDINGS

Surface EMG recordings represent the summation of electrical activities of all of the active motor units in the muscle at that instant (Akataki et al 2004, Kamen & Caldwell 1996). Figure 14.3 illustrates – schematically – a single action potential (AP) being recorded from a muscle fibre by two external electrodes. The muscle cell membrane is

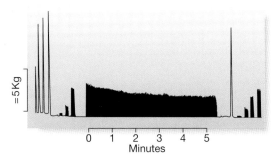

Figure 14.2 A typical trace of force measurements of the human tibialis muscle showing maximum voluntary contraction and the response to stimulation at 1, 10, 20 and 40 Hz, before and after fatigue testing, and the response to fatigue testing by stimulation at 40 Hz for 250 ms, every second for 5 minutes.

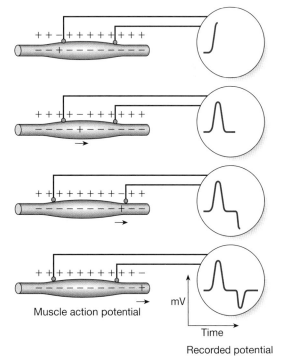

Figure 14.3 Representation of the changes in action potentials being recorded by external electrodes.

electrically excitable so that it caries the all-or-none action potentials just as in the nerve action potential (see Chapter 5). The muscle fibres from which activation is recorded vary considerably in temporal and spatial dimensions. The APs from the numerous muscle fibres innervated by a single motor neuron summate to produce a motor unit action potential (MUAP). Surface electrodes (either silver–silver-chloride discs or more malleable self-adhesive electrodes) are attached to the skin overlying the muscle from which activity is to be recorded. The potential difference between two electrodes is recorded through a differential amplifier; a third more remote electrode is used as reference. The recorded signal represents the sum of the individual potentials of all the muscle fibres that are being activated.

Surface EMG signals can be analysed in terms of two variables: amplitude and frequency. The first step in determining amplitude involves full-wave rectification. *Rectification* means that the EMG signal is converted into a signal containing only positive voltages. The rectified signal is then filtered with a low-pass filter (Winter 1990). This provides a linear envelope or 'moving average' because it follows the trend of the EMG. The area of the linear envelope can then be computed providing an assessment of the amplitude of the signal. Sometimes known as the *time domain*, the amplitude or root mean square (RMS) of this integrated signal has been documented as being positively correlated to muscle force. Loss of force and changes in integrated signal, together with changes in median frequency (see below), can also be used to monitor fatigue during a sustained voluntary contraction. However, care has to be taken in interpreting the relationship between tension generated by the muscle and this signal. A known standard such as the amplitude of the signal in a maximum contraction should be used for purposes of comparison.

The frequency content of the recorded signal is related to the number of active motor units as well as to their constituent firing rates. Recruitment of an individual motor unit results in the generation of an MUAP of specific size, shape and frequency. Because of their higher conduction velocities, MUAPs travelling on fast-twitch fibres have inherently higher frequency content than those of slow-twitch fibres (Kamen & Caldwell 1996).

A fast Fourier transform function is used to determine the power density spectrum – the frequency domain of the EMG. This function determines the power of frequencies in any set period of time. Three parameters provide useful measures of the spectrum:

1. Median frequency (MDF): the frequency that divides the power density spectrum into two regions of equal power.

2. Mean power or average frequency (MPF).

3. Bandwidth of the spectrum sets range of frequencies to be recorded and analysed (for further information see Basmajian & Luca 1985).

Studies have suggested that the MDF is least susceptible to noise (see Kollmitzer et al 1999) and, increasingly, MDF is used to identify motor neuron recruitment strategies during muscle contractions (Bernardi et al 1995, Gerdle et al 2000).

FUNCTIONAL ASPECTS OF CHANGES IN ARCHITECTURAL STRUCTURE

Skeletal muscle architecture can be defined as 'the arrangement of muscle fibres within a muscle relative to the axis of force generation' (Lieber & Friden 2000). There are three general classes of muscle fibre architecture:

1. Those with fibres that extend parallel to the muscle's generating axis: these are described as fusiform (e.g. biceps brachii).

2. Those with fibres oriented at a single angle relative to the force-generating axis; these are described as being unipennate (e.g. vastus lateralis).

3. Those with fibres where the angle between the fibre and the force-generating axis varies; these are described as multipennate muscles.

Most skeletal muscles are multipennate (e.g. gluteus medius). Body mass and muscle cross-sectional area (CSA) strongly influence muscle strength. In terms of *muscle CSA*, the phenomenon of muscle fibre pennation allows *physiological muscle CSA*, which is defined as the magnitude of muscle fibre area perpendicular to the longitudinal axis of individual muscle fibres multiplied by the cosine of the angle of pennation exceed the *anatomical muscle CSA* measured in a plane axial to the longitudinal axis of the muscle (Aagaard et al 2001). Measurements of muscle thickness, fibre length and pennation angle provide additional data for understanding both strength deficits and the effects of training, and can be calculated using ultrasound (Aagaard et al 2001, Fukunaga et al 1997, Leiber & Friden 2000). These measures are non-invasive and not dependent on the ability to perform a maximum muscle contraction (Aagaard et al 2001). Understanding the underlying macroscopic arrangement of muscle fibres and the changes in muscle size and shape that can occur, for example following immobilization and training, or in children with Duchenne muscular dystrophy (DMD), are important in understanding the mechanisms underlying loss of muscle strength.

EFFECTS OF IMMOBILIZATION

Most people are very aware of the effects of disuse, immobilization and prolonged bed rest. An individual confined to bed for a few weeks or who has had a limb immobilized in a cast will experience muscle atrophy and loss of muscle strength. Duchateau and Hainaut (1990), looking at the effects of plaster cast immobilization on the adductor pollicis, showed loss of strength and EMG and an inability to activate fully on voluntary command after 6 weeks of immobilization, with a rapid return to normal activity on remobilization. A similar experiment of immobilization for 4 weeks by Yue et al (1994) resulted in loss of strength and an inability to activate the elbow flexor muscles. Immobilization reduces motor firing rate (Duchateau & Hainaut 1990) and affects the mechanical properties of the muscle (Davies et al 1987).

Williams and Goldspink (1984) showed that reduction in fibre length of muscles immobilized in a shortened position is accompanied by reduced compliance of the muscle and an increase in the proportion of connective tissue. But if the muscle was then stretched for short periods, this prevented the connective tissue changes but did not prevent the reduction in muscle length (Williams et al 1986). Cotter and Phillips (1986) found that the transition from fast to slow muscle

fibres was accelerated in rabbit tibialis anterior muscle with immobilization in the neutral position; Williams et al (1986) found greater increases in sarcomeres when a muscle was immobilized in a stretched position. Later, links were established between gene expression and mechanical signals, including muscle fibre phenotype expression (Goldspink et al 1992). Cast immobilization in either the lengthened or the shortened position and with or without electrical stimulation caused regression of fast type and activation of slow myosin genes.

St-Pierre and Gardiner (1987), reviewing the effects of immobilization and exercise in both animal and human skeletal muscle studies, summarized their conclusions as follows:

- The amount of atrophy depends on the length at which the muscle has been fixed (short > neutral > lengthened).

- As muscle atrophies, its ability to generate tension decreases and possible dysfunction in the contractile proteins is seen.

- Atrophy has been reported to affect all muscle fibres to some extent, or mainly type I or type II fibres

- Muscle metabolism is affected by immobilization.

St-Pierre and Gardiner concluded that the efficacy of exercises (voluntary or electrically stimulated) in immobilized limbs to reduce muscle atrophy had not been demonstrated conclusively and, furthermore, that the beneficial effect of post-immobilization training was equivocal.

Changes in strength, size of muscle fibre and *MHC* gene expression were monitored in 48 previously sedentary young men and women after 3 weeks of unilateral knee splint immobilization followed by 12 weeks of retraining (Hortobágyi et al 2000). Immobilization significantly but uniformly reduced eccentric, concentric and isometric strength by 47%, whereas no changes in strength occurred in the control group; fibre type I, IIa and IIx muscle fibre areas were reduced by 13, 10 and 10%, respectively, but fibre type did not alter; EMG activity (RMS) altered in parallel with the force data and did not change in the non-immobilized knee. After 2 weeks of spontaneous

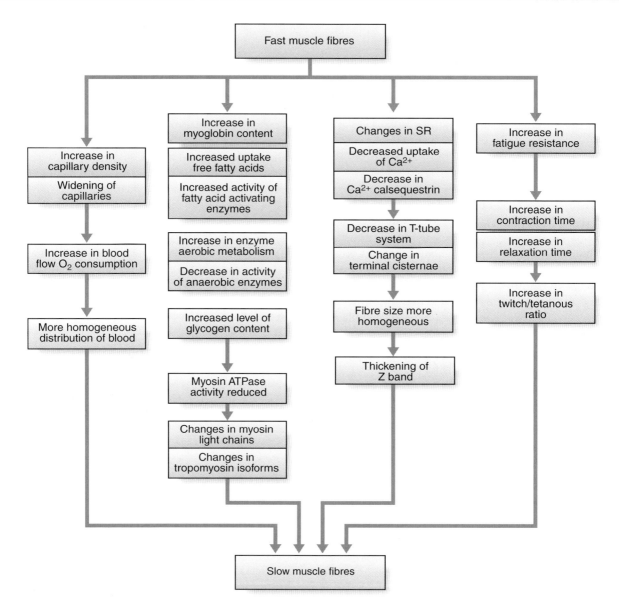

Figure 14.4 Schematic representation of effects of chronic low-frequency stimulation on fast muscle fibres.

recovery, all fibres were 5% smaller than at base-line. The subjects were then randomly assigned to a control group and three exercise groups for 12 weeks, three sessions/week. Hypertrophy of type I, IIa and IIx fibres relative to baseline was 10, 16 and 16% after eccentric and 11, 9 and 10% after mixed training, exceeding the 4, 5 and 5% gains after concentric training. Immobilization down-regulated the expression of type I MHC mRNA to 0.72 of baseline and exercise training upregulated

it to 0.95 of baseline, whereas immobilization and exercise training upregulated type IIa MHC mRNA 2.9-fold and 1.2-fold, respectively. Significantly greater hypertrophy of the muscle fibres was found after eccentric training together with upregulation of type IIx myosin heavy-chain messenger RNA. The suggestion was that the faster rate of strength recovery and greater strength gains were due to the unique aspects of the muscle lengthening of eccentric training.

Studies (Andersen et al 1999) of bed rest in normal healthy subjects for a similar period using both ATPase histochemistry and immunocytochemistry observed overall fibre atrophy together with an increase in fibres in a 'transitional' state from phenotypic type I → IIa and Ia → Ix. Atrophy of the quadriceps femoris was investigated in nine patients after anterior cruciate ligament reconstruction (ACLR) and immobilization in a long leg plaster (Häggmark et al 1981). Allowed to walk on the operated leg as soon as pain permitted, standard isometric training consisted of 3–6 seconds maximal hold relaxed for 6 seconds until training could be sustained for 1 hour. Muscle biopsies were taken before surgery, 1 week after surgery and after 5 weeks but before the cast was removed. Selective atrophy was found with reduction of cross-cut area and oxidative enzymic activity in the slow-twitch type I fibres. The inhibiting role of postoperative pain was raised as a critical factor in inhibiting muscle activity in this acute postoperative period. A recent review (Risberg et al 2004) showed that recovery of muscle strength following traumatic knee injury and restoration of performance capabilities can in some instances take many months despite intensive rehabilitation.

Studies by Snyder-Mackler and colleagues (1993) on the activity of the quadriceps femoris muscle following ACLR using a modified Burke fatigue test showed weakness of the involved muscles but a less marked rate of fatigue over the first 60 seconds of the test than occurred in the stronger, uninvolved muscles. These were surprising results and suggest that there had been selective type II fibre atrophy in the involved muscles.

MUSCLE WEAKNESS AND ENDURANCE IN ELDERLY PEOPLE

Ageing is associated with reduced muscle strength and atrophy of type II muscle fibres (Bazzucchi et al 2004, Frontera et al 2000, Roos et al 1999, Short et al 2005, Suetta et al 2004, Williams et al 2002, Williamson et al 2000). Age-related declines in muscle strength and power, an inactive lifestyle, increasing difficulty with functional tasks requiring rapid power output, such as climbing stairs or rising from a chair, and an increased incidence of falls are well documented in older people (for a review, see Thompson 1994). Loss of strength is most marked in the lower limb muscles. Studies of the quadriceps femoris show age-related reductions in muscle mass, although there is some doubt about the ability of elderly people to fully activate this muscle.

The differences in strength between young women and fit elderly women have been associated with increased fatigue resistance together with slowing of relaxation times but with no differences in their ability to activate their quadriceps femoris muscles fully (O'Connor et al 1993). Roos and colleagues (1999), in a study of the muscles of young and old men, reported a similar 50% loss of strength, slower contractile speeds and higher tetanic fusion at lower frequencies of stimulation with full activation of quadriceps femoris muscles in the older men. They found no age-related difference in motor unit firing rates. This suggests that the loss of strength was not related to central activation or changes in motor neuron firing rates but rather to detraining through lack of exercise.

Progressive resistance training has been shown to be an effective means of improving muscle strength in very elderly people; the 'neural' changes specific to the training tasks played an important role in the initial strength gains (Harridge et al 1999). None of the women were able to activate the quadriceps femoris muscles fully either before, or indeed after, progressive exercise training. However, there was an increase in muscle mass after training, together with increased strength and ability to lift weights.

CHANGES IN MUSCLE PROPERTIES FOLLOWING SPINAL CORD INJURY

Early work at the Rehabilitation Engineering Centre in Ljubljana and at Rancho Los Amigos Hospital, Rehabilitation Engineering Center, Los Angeles, California, set the scene for using electrical stimulation to assist people with spinal cord injury (SCI) to undertake functional activities. Preprogrammed multistimulators were developed to assist in walking, to increase the strength of hypotrophic skeletal muscle and to reduce spasticity (Bajd 2004, Vodovnik et al 1985). The concept was that of *restorative neurology*: the possibility of improving the function of an impaired nervous system by selective modification of abnormal neurocontrol according to underlying mechanisms and clinically unrecognized residual functions (Dimitrijevic 1994).

The literature on muscle alterations following denervation is extensive. A historical account and the salient aspects of progressive atrophy and accompanying structural and ultrastructural alterations have been reviewed by Midrio (2006).

Recovery in motor function is thought to be defined to a significant degree by the level and types of motor training or experience following the injury (Edgerton et al 2004, 2006). Understanding the automaticity of walking and how it is possible to carry out complex but routine motor tasks without 'conscious' thought is beyond the scope of this chapter but is explored in greater depth elsewhere (see Edgerton et al 2006).

Collaborative work under Professors Donaldson and Hunt and their colleagues at University College London and Glasgow University, respectively, led to the development of implanted motor root stimulators (Donaldson et al 2003) and to the engineering development of systems such as commercially available tricycles that restore function and enable effective exercise for people with SCI (Donaldson et al 2003, Hunt 2005, Perkins et al 2002). Earlier rehabilitation strategies combined with continuous electrical stimulation (pulse duration 0.3 ms at 20 Hz) when standing are directed towards recovery of muscle contractile properties, maintenance of the standing position and later walking (Badj 2004, Scelsi 2001); the routine is seen as being key to maintaining blood circulation, calcium content in bones, renal function, and for reducing spasticity. Morphological investigations post SCI show that, when deprived of neural activation, muscle fibres begin to alter their histopathological and enzyme– histochemical characteristics 1 month after injury (Scelsi 2001, Scott et al 2006). Several studies have explored these changes in quadriceps femoris (Gerrits et al 1999, Scelsi 2001, Scott et al 2006). Ongoing weakness and fatiguability of the knee extensors can limit standing and walking (Gerrits et al 1999). For the first year after injury, fibre diameter in young patients decreases progressively. Scott and colleagues (2006) reported preferential atrophy of

rectus femoris within the first 2 months. Over the first year, this was directly proportional to the age of the cord lesion (Scelsi 2001). Mitochondrial size and percentage distribution decreases and there is a six fold increase in the percentage of lipid droplets per fibre area 7–12 months post-SCI (Scelsi 2001). There is general agreement that in the first few months after SCI, fibre-type transitions occur mostly within fast-twitch, fatiguable fibres, with myosin heavy chain MHCIIa being replaced by MHCIIx. These changes are most evident at 4 months post SCI. As time from injury increases (4–9 months), transitions from type I to type II also occur as MHCI is replaced by MHCIIa. The proteins associated with Ca^{2+}-ATPase of the sarcoplasmic reticulum, which is responsible for re-sequestering Ca^{2+} into the sarcoplasmic reticulum from the myoplasm, also undergo transitions. The oxidative capacity of the muscle is reduced as enzymes associated with the oxidative production of energy and blood flow to the muscles decreases (Gerritts et al 1999, Scott et al 2006).

Marked changes in contractile properties have been reported in quadriceps femoris, soleus, tibialis anterior and thenar muscles of patients paralysed with chronic (12 months or longer) SCI compared to age-matched able-bodied controls (Gerrits et al 1999, Scott et al 2006, Shields et al 1997, Thomas 1997). When stimulated, the paralysed muscles have increased twitch height, contract and relax faster and fatigue more readily than control muscles. Differences in force frequency ratios in quadriceps femoris are attributed to the shift in fibre type (Gerritts et al 1999). However, Scott and colleagues (2006) cited fat infiltration, endomysial fibrosis and diffuse muscle atrophy associated with later stages of paraplegia (10–17 months) post SCI and suggested that increased forces at higher rates of stimulation were due to increased muscle stiffness and shortening. In two sequential studies, Klein et al (2006) and Häger-Ross et al (2006) show that the exaggerated fatiguability of paralysed thenar muscles was due to impairments within the muscle fibres and not to failure of neuromuscular transmission or membrane excitability. Muscles that lose all their innervation undergo drastic and rapid wasting, leading to muscle degeneration, if reinnervation does not take place (Midiro 2006). Considerable reductions in motor unit numbers were found in paralysed thenar muscles after complete cervical injuries, indicating that motor neuron loss is an important contributor to muscle atrophy after brain injury. However, the remaining motor units demonstrate a high capacity to sprout and reinnervate muscle fibres (Gordon & Mao 1994) and there is evidence that high fatiguability and the associated switch in muscle phenotype can be prevented or reversed by low levels of sustained stimulation (Gordon 1998, Pette & Vrbová 1999).

CHANGES IN CONTRACTILE PROPERTIES FOLLOWING STROKE

Muscle weakness is an immediate consequence of stroke. Strength is impaired bilaterally, but more so on the side contralateral to the brain lesion (Adams et al 1990, Andrews & Bohannon 2000, Colebatch & Gandevia 1989). Although the weakness is widely attributed to upper motor neuron deficits, secondary changes may occur and contribute to muscle dysfunction (Ryan et al 2002). Muscle on the hemiparetic side is subject to both disuse and abnormal neural innervation, and it is not yet clear whether disuse or abnormal neurological innervation patterning drives the underlying changes (de Deyne et al 2004).

A number of studies have looked at recovery of muscle strength together with alterations in contractile properties and central control mechanisms following stroke (Cramp 1998). As expected, affected muscles were weaker than unaffected muscles and reciprocal inhibition mediated by Ia recovery was reduced in affected limbs in the early stages after stroke. Increased fatiguability and similar patterns of change were seen in affected and unaffected muscles of stroke patients compared to age-matched controls, suggesting that extraneous factors such as inactivity had affected muscle function. This view was supported by the observed differences in muscle strength, fatigue resistance and reciprocal inhibition between patients with good walking function (and who were assumed to be more active) and those with poor walking function (Cramp 1998).

A later study by de Deyne and colleagues (2004) explored changes in molecular phenotype with gait speed in patients 6 months after stroke. They found both a major shift towards an increased proportion of fast MHC isoforms in the paretic vastus lateralis and a striking negative correlation between self-selected walking speed and the percentage of fast myosin heavy-chain isoform.

Muscle spasticity, or an increased resistance to passive movement, is not an inevitable consequence of stroke. In physiological terms, spasticity can be defined as a motor disorder characterized by a velocity-dependent increase in tonic stretch reflexes with exaggerated tendon jerks resulting from hyperexcitability of the stretch reflex. There is some evidence that changes in muscle structure, as a consequence of defective muscle activation or disuse, are responsible for the increased resistance associated with muscle spasticity. Dietz et al (1986) found fibre-type transformation, type II atrophy and structural changes in spastic gastrocnemius medialis muscle and muscle changes correlated with alterations in muscle activation. O'Dwyer et al (1996) found that increased resistance to passive stretch was associated with muscle contracture but not with reflex hyperexcitability in 24 patients with stroke. There is a general opinion that both neural and non-neural mechanisms underlie the development and presence of spasticity in stroke patients.

Subluxation of the shoulder joint occurs in 15–81% of hemiplegic patients after stroke and is accompanied by problems such as pain, brachial plexus nerve injury, rotator cuff tear and joint capsulitis. A meta-analysis (Ada & Foongchomcheay 2002) to evaluate the efficacy of surface electrical stimulation that produced a motor response in supraspinatus and/or deltoid showed evidence to support early intervention with electrical stimulation. Seven [four early (<2 months after stroke) and three late (>2 months after stroke)] studies met the criteria for inclusion; the evidence supports the use of electrical stimulation early but not late after stroke for the reduction of shoulder subluxation. Stimulation prevented on average 6.5 mm of shoulder subluxation (weighted mean difference, 95% CI 4.4–8.6) but reduced it by only 1.9 mm (weighted mean difference 95% CI –2.3 to 6.1) compared with conventional therapy alone. All of the four early studies used electrical stimulation as an adjunct to conventional therapy; intervention ranged from 4–6 weeks, 5–7 days/week and, after a preliminary period, from 0.5 to 6 hours/day; most used frequencies greater than 30 Hz. The evidence from this study builds on earlier Australian calls for systematic evaluation combined with methodological rigor (Singer 1987).

CHANGES IN MUSCLE PROPERTIES IN CHILDREN WITH NEUROMUSCULAR DISEASES

'As children grow older, they become stronger'. This well-established fact is characterized in the linear relationship between the strength of the trunk and the limb musculature in fit, healthy young children. Interestingly, the muscles of young children before puberty show a high resistance to fatigue, with a significant slowing of relaxation time during electrically stimulated fatigue testing. By contrast, children with Duchenne muscular dystrophy (DMD), a progressive muscular disease, show no increase in strength of their muscles as they grow older. Histochemically, there is a predominance of type I fibres and few if any type II fibres. Immunocytochemical techniques have shown the persistence of fetal and slow myosin in many of these fibres. As in healthy children's muscles, dystrophic muscles have a high resistance to fatigue but, unlike the muscles of healthy children, do not show any change in their contractile characteristics during or after fatigue testing (Scott et al 1986, 1990).

TRAINING SKELETAL MUSCLE: EXERCISE AND ELECTRICAL STIMULATION

It is well known that muscle strength can be increased by almost any method provided the frequency of the exercise and loading intensities sufficiently exceed those of the normal or current level of activation of an individual muscle (Komi 1986). Training at high forces (i.e. with loads greater than 60–70% of maximum strength) repeated as few as 10 times per day, where each contraction is held for 2–5 seconds, recruits both high- and low-threshold motor units and increases maximum voluntary strength by about 0.5–1% per day (Jones et al 1989). In lower-intensity training regimens of about 30% of maximum strength, increases in strength have

also been recorded when each contraction is held for longer (say 60 seconds). This may be because the higher-threshold units can be recruited as the lower-threshold units become fatigued (for reviews, see Edström & Grimby 1986, Jones et al 1989). It has been claimed that, prior to training, muscle cannot be maximally activated by voluntary activity and that large, fast motor units are recruited only when higher forces are applied. It is possible that some of these fast units are never recruited in the untrained state and there is evidence to show that in trained muscle there is increased synchronization (Komi 1986).

In the first 6–8 weeks before changes in muscle size become apparent, activation and therefore strength increases as a result of establishing appropriate motor patterns of control of the muscles and of increased neural drive. If training is continued beyond about 12 weeks, a steady and slow increase occurs in both size and strength of the exercised muscles (Jones et al 1989). Training studies tend to be of short duration (less than 5 weeks) and confined to a period when neural adaptations are thought to underlie the increases in strength, so at present it is still unclear whether the gains in strength with short-term electromyostimulation are superior to voluntary training (see Chapter 15).

Excitability of nerve and muscle tissue provides a basis for the therapeutic application of electrical stimulation, which was used throughout the twentieth century (Midiro 2006). Imposed electrical stimulation is seen to have certain advantages in increasing muscle activity compared with exercise. It has been suggested that the hierarchical order of recruitment of the motor units in electrical stimulation is the reverse of the natural sequence (Trimble & Enoka 1991; see the section Recruitment of motor units in voluntary contractions, in Chapter 5. Because of their large-diameter axons and low activation threshold, the larger, normally inactive motor units are recruited first and may experience the most profound change in their use. These fast-contracting, high-tension-generating, easily fatiguable motor units are often found in the superficial layers of a muscle and are closer to the stimulating electrodes. The stimulation will also be conducted antidromically, that is, going towards the spinal cord, along the motor nerve and by the afferent sensory nerves. This has also been shown to cause a reversal of the normal order of motor unit recruitment (Garnett et al 1978). However, doubts have been raised about the reversal of the size principle (Gregory & Bickel 2005). The contention is that although this neurophysiological phenomenon may hold true for direct stimulation of the motor nerve, the orientation of the peripheral nerves does not favour preferential fast-fibre recruitment with cutaneous electrical stimulation. Their interpretation is supported by evidence drawn from a number of studies in respect of voluntary and electrically stimulated fatigue testing, metabolic data on total glycogen content, and the finding that twitch contraction speeds do not alter as an increasing percentage of MVC is elicited.

With electrical stimulation, unlike exercise, activity is restricted to the stimulated muscle and the muscle is less influenced by other systemic changes that occur during exercise (Pette & Vrbová 1992). Superimposed electrical stimulation bypasses the central neuronal control mechanisms. Provided that stimuli (pulses) are of sufficient intensity and duration to depolarize the nerve membrane, action potentials are generated, the motor units are activated synchronously and muscle contraction occurs. There is now overwhelming evidence that an important factor in determining the properties of a skeletal muscle is the amount of neuronal or impulse activity relative to the activity that is usual for that muscle (for a review, see Pette & Staron 1997, Pette & Vrbová 1992). Electrical stimulation manipulates the output activity pattern from the motor neuron by adding to its inherent activity; in contrast, during voluntary exercise, individual motor units are activated in a graded and hierarchical manner (see the section Recruitment of motor units in voluntary contractions in Chapter 5.

In the past 20 years, the ability of human skeletal muscle to alter both its functional and contractile properties in response to long-term or chronic low-frequency stimulation has been investigated and applied to clinical practice.

LOW-FREQUENCY ELECTRICAL STIMULATION

Low-frequency electrical stimulation in human studies, in which the impulses are no faster than 1000 Hz and usually lower than 100 Hz, has traditionally been used to facilitate or to mimic voluntary contractions of skeletal muscle and as a supplement to normal training procedures. Not surprisingly, the focus in animal studies has been on the effect of long-term, low-frequency electrical stimulation, where there is no need for active cooperation. More surprising is the continuing paucity of human studies that evaluate any physiological changes other than increases in strength that may occur.

Selkowitz (1989) identified two major categories of electrical stimulation: low-frequency, 'endurance-training' programmes in which the underlying aim is to harness muscle; plasticity and the possibility of changing the underlying molecular and genetic properties of skeletal muscle; and strength training using interferential stimulation. He suggested that short-term, low-frequency muscle regimens have relatively short intervals between contractions, with the contraction durations approximately equal to the rest periods (usually {4/15} seconds on/off) and lasting for a total of 6–15 minutes for each treatment session. Nowadays, this form of electrical stimulation may be seen in the context of re-establishing full activation through greater muscle recruitment (see earlier) and will be addressed in Chapter 15.

LONG–TERM (CHRONIC) ELECTRICAL STIMULATION OF SKELETAL MUSCLE

Investigations in animals and recent studies in human muscle have confirmed that it is possible to modify the properties of mammalian skeletal muscle by long-term electrical stimulation. Skeletal muscle has a remarkable ability to change its properties in response to demand, so much so that it is now recognized that appropriate use of chronic low-frequency stimulation can change most cellular elements of a muscle in an orderly sequence. This model has provided a means for researchers to correlate functional changes with changes at the molecular level and has enabled investigations to be undertaken that explore the extent of muscle plasticity. Observation of the time course of changes has led to the study of gene expression of different functional elements in muscle fibres and transformation of their phenotype (Pette & Vrbová 1999).

A number of reviews have summarized the major effects of long-term low-frequency electrical stimulation (Enoka 1988, Lieber 1986, Pette & Vrbová 1992, Salmons & Henriksson 1981). Variation in the parameters used in animal studies, inherent differences between species and the varying condition of animals prior to stimulation have made it difficult to compare results from different studies. Nevertheless, the findings are largely complementary and an overall pattern of transformation has been established.

Although we know that the neuronal control and patterns of activation are different for each activity and for each muscle, and even for the constituent motor units, we do not yet know how best to exploit this ability to change muscle properties. The time course of reversal of induced changes when stimulation is discontinued appears to be different for each muscle property but, in general terms, it is comparable to the time course of transformation.

CHANGES IN CONTRACTILE PROPERTIES

In response to chronic, low-frequency stimulation in both rabbit and cat fast-contracting muscles, the first effect noted was an increase in both contraction and relaxation times of stimulated muscles compared to those of control muscles (Pette et al 1973, Salmons & Vrbová 1969, Vrbová 1966). There was also an alteration in the ratio of twitch to tetanic force, in that the twitch tension was very similar to that of the control muscle but the maximal tetanic tension was considerably reduced. The slowing effect became apparent after 9–12 days of stimulation.

Similar changes within 3 weeks of superimposed stimulation have been reported in chronically stimulated tibialis anterior muscle, adductor pollicis human adult muscles (Scott et al 1985, Rutherford & Jones 1988) and, more recently, in quadriceps femoris muscle (Cramp et al 1995). A consistent finding in both animal and human studies in response to long-term stimulation has been an increased resistance to fatigue.

METABOLIC CHANGES

In animal muscles, the increased resistance to fatigue has been associated with increases in aerobic–oxidative capacity and with a marked decrease in glycolytic enzyme activities. Transformation of fast-twitch muscle fibres into slow ones by chronic stimulation at 10 Hz is well documented (see the section Matching motor newtons to the muscle fibres, in Chapter 5). It is associated with changes in contractile characteristics, shifts in metabolic enzyme patterns, Ca^{2+} uptake by the sarcoplasmic reticulum and eventual changes in myosin heavy and light chains. These changes in metabolic, histochemical and structural properties have been extensively reviewed (Enoka 1988, Pette & Vrbová 1992, 1999, Salmons & Henrikson 1981) and are shown schematically in Figure 14.3 (p. 215).

CIRCULATORY CHANGES

The earliest changes recorded in animal muscles can be identified as changes in the sarcoplasmic reticulum, an increase in blood supply followed by an increase in capillary density surrounding the stimulated muscle fibres, and a decrease in muscle fibre diameter (Cotter et al 1973). Hudlická et al (1977) found that, after 4 days, the stimulated muscles fatigued less than the control muscles, suggesting that increased capillary density provided a more homogeneous distribution of blood and better diffusion of oxygen. It was suggested that this might be because a greater number of muscle fibres would have access to oxygen, which would facilitate re-phosphorylation of ATP and creative phosphate (see the section The sliding-filament hypothesis, Chapter 5).

STRUCTURAL CHANGES

Heilmann and Pette (1979), investigating the effects of continuous 10 Hz stimulation on rabbit fast-twitch muscles, found that one of the earliest changes was a reduction in both the initial and total Ca^{2+} uptake, accompanied by a change in the polypeptide patterns of the sarcoplasmic reticulum. Stimulation-induced changes in muscle fibres include a more homogeneous population of fibres with a smaller cross-sectional area, but no loss of muscle fibres.

Myofibrillar ATPase histochemistry has shown a stimulation-induced increase in the number of type I muscle fibres in many species, and detailed analysis of chronically stimulated extensor digitorum longus and tibialis anterior in rabbit muscles has shown an overall transition of fast-type muscle to slow, including changes in the myosin molecule.

Particular attention has been paid to changes in the myofibrillar protein myosin, and to the regulatory proteins tropomyosin and troponin, which are associated with actin. Changes in the myosin molecule were first observed after 2–4 weeks but the complete fast-to-slow transition of the myosin light chains appears to take several months (for further details, see Pette & Vrbová 1992, 1999).

DIFFERENT PATTERNS OF STIMULATION

Much less research has been carried out into the transformation of slow muscle to fast (apart from early work on the soleus muscle; Vrbová 1963) but in recent years more work has been done on the effect of different patterns of stimulation in human muscle. In many of these studies, the investigators have been concerned to consider the effect of external factors on the changes that have been observed in response to stimulation. Such external factors may be of importance when considering the possible effect of long-term stimulation in human muscles. In animal studies it is usual for the entire muscle to be stimulated using implanted electrodes. In human studies, by contrast, muscles are generally stimulated using surface electrodes (rather than through implants), and so it is important to be aware of the percentage of a muscle that is being stimulated. As already observed, the position and loading of the muscle during stimulation are likely to affect the changes that occur.

STUDIES ON HEALTHY HUMAN MUSCLES

In 1985, Scott et al investigated the effect on contractile properties of tibialis anterior by stimulating the intramuscular branches of the deep peroneal nerve at 10 Hz for 1 hour, three times a day for 6 weeks. Using an asymmetrical biphasic waveform of sufficient intensity to give a visible contraction of the tibialis anterior accompanied by movement of the foot, they monitored the effect of chronic low-frequency stimulation and showed that it was possible to change the contractile characteristics of this muscle in human subjects. As in animal studies, long-term low-frequency stimulation induced a significant increase in resistance to fatigue in the stimulated muscles compared to unstimulated controls, suggesting a change in properties of the type II, fast-contracting, easily fatiguable, glycolytic fibres.

Comparing the effect of long-term, low-frequency stimulation with a non-uniform pattern of stimulation incorporating a range of low through to high frequencies (5–40 Hz), Rutherford and Jones (1988) found similar changes in the fatigue characteristics in response to both patterns of stimulation. However, those subjects whose muscles were stimulated with a low-frequency pattern lost muscle strength, whereas those subjects whose muscles were stimulated using a mixed pattern of stimulation became stronger. The reduction in muscle bulk as well as strength that was reported may have been due to reduction of fibre diameter of the largest and most fatiguable muscle fibres being exposed to sudden excessive activity.

More recently Cramp et al (1995) explored the effects of selected patterns of long-term electrical stimulation on quadriceps femoris muscle of 21 healthy subjects. Stimulated muscles showed significant increases in strength, fatigue resistance and relaxation times after 3 weeks and in force-frequency output after 6 weeks. Significant changes were observed in those muscles stimulated with a mixed or random pattern of activation, indicating that a mixed or random pattern of activation induced greater changes than a uniform 8 Hz pattern.

CLINICAL STUDIES
Facial paralysis (Bell's palsy)

In some studies, attempts were made to simulate motor neuron discharge patterns on the basis that the natural pattern of discharge of a single, slow motor unit is not a uniform one. Farragher et al (1987) described this form of stimulation as 'eutrophic stimulation', identifying a 'neurotrophic effect' of the simulated pattern, and reported considerable clinical merit for patients suffering from intractable Bell's palsy.

Rheumatoid arthritis

Kidd and Oldham (1988) and Oldham and Stanley (1989) gave accounts of the benefits of using chronic 'eutrophic' or 'physiological' stimulation versus fixed 10 Hz (300 μs square wave for 3 hours daily) for 10 weeks (168 hours) on the small muscles of the hand of 12 patients with rheumatoid arthritis. The physiological pattern of stimulation was derived from a fatigued motor unit from the first dorsal interosseus muscle in a normal hand. The most favourable results were for the patterned electrical stimulation, which had a clinically favourable effect on grip strength and voluntary fatigue (Pelland et al 2002). However, issues of study design (including details of stimulation parameters), the small number of control subjects, compliance and longer-term follow-up raised concern, and two recent review studies of electrical stimulation in treatment of rheumatoid arthritis (Ottawa Panel 2004, Pelland et al 2002) concluded that these earlier studies were unable to gauge the efficacy of electrical stimulation in rheumatoid arthritis.

Chronic heart failure

Exercise intolerance is generally recognized as the most devastating consequence of chronic obstructive pulmonary disease (COPD), and electrical stimulation has been shown to be a useful adjunct to comprehensive pulmonary rehabilitation. Whittom and colleagues (1998), exploring the factors that impact on muscle aerobic capacity, found reductions in type I and increases in type IIb fibre proportions, together with a decrease in types I, IIa and IIb fibre CSA and relatively well-preserved capillarization in vastus lateralis. After comprehensive aerobic endurance training (30 minutes, three times a week for 12 weeks) they found a significant increase in type I and IIa CSA. But for nine patients with severe disease, electrical stimulation (200 ms at 50 Hz every 1500 ms, 20 minutes each limb, three times a week for 6 weeks, no details of pulse shape/width) significantly improved both the MVC of their quadriceps femoris and hamstring muscles and their shuttle walking distance compared to the control group (Bourjeily-Habr et al 2002).

Duchenne muscular dystrophy

Studies using different patterns of long-term electrical stimulation on the muscles of boys with Duchenne muscular dystrophy (DMD) identified the importance of the pattern of stimulation (Scott et al 1986, 1990). The application of a uniform 8-Hz pattern to stimulate the tibialis anterior and quadriceps femoris of young boys with DMD resulted in improvements in maximum voluntary contraction of stimulated muscles in comparison with unstimulated controls. By contrast, use of a 30-Hz pattern of stimulation on a group of six boys with DMD resulted in a decrease in maximum voluntary contraction. Three of the latter group subsequently stimulated their muscles with the uniform 8-Hz pattern and gained voluntary strength.

SHORT–TERM ELECTRICAL STIMULATION

This form of electrical stimulation is sometimes known as electromyostimulation or faradic-type (i.e. shorter pulses usually between 0.1 and 1 ms duration and applied at between 30 and 100 Hz) stimulation. The therapeutic rationale is based on the assumption that the output of the motor system is insufficient and needs to be supplemented by artificial means. This seems reasonable, particularly when the function of the nervous system might have been compromised by a traumatic event. Chapter 15 discusses these forms of electrical stimulation.

SUMMARY

Concern has rightly been expressed concerning the many methodological flaws in the current published literature and the major barrier this may pose to our ability to transform scientific knowledge into a working and patient-based technology (Alon 2003). There is still a striking disproportion between our need to take into account the underlying knowledge of the physiological properties of human skeletal muscle, but also than of the operation of the nervous system as the coordinator of these elemental activities. There is still uncertainty over optimum patterns of electrical stimulation in different physiological circumstances. Another area that has not yet been addressed is the need to consider the effect of loading and normal use of the muscle during periods of stimulation.

References

Aagaard P, Andersen JL, Dyhre-Poulsen P et al (2001) A mechanism for increased contractile strength of human pennate muscle in response to strength training: changes in muscle architecture. *J Physiol* **534**: 613–623.

Ada L, Foongchomcheay A (2002) Efficacy of electrical stimulation in preventing or reducing subluxation of the shoulder after stroke: a meta-analysis. *Aust J Physiother* **48**: 257–267.

Adams RW, Gandevia SC, Skuse NF (1990) The distribution of muscle weakness in upper motor neuron lesions affecting the lower limb. *Brain* **113**: 459–476.

Akataki K, Mita K, Watakabe M (2004) Electromyographic and mechanomyographic estimation of motor unit activation strategy in voluntary force production. *Electromyogr Clin Neurophysiol* **44**: 489–496.

Alon G (2003) Use of neuromuscular electrical stimulation in neurorehabilitation: a challenge to all. *Res Dev* **40**(6): ix–xii.

Andersen JL, Cruschy-Knudsen T, Sandri C et al (1999) Bed rest increases the amount of mismatched fibres in human skeletal muscle. *J Appl Physiol* **86**(2): 455–460.

Andrews AW, Bohannon R (2000) Distribution of muscle strength impairments following stroke. *Clin Rehab* **14**: 79–87.

Bajd T (2004) Neurorehabilitation of standing and walking after spinal cord injury. In Rosch PJ, Markov MS (eds) *Bioelectromagnetic Medicine*. New York, Marcel Dekker: 439–459.

Basmajian JV, Luca CJ (1985) *Muscles Alive. Their Functions Revealed by Electromyography*, 5th edn. Baltimore, MD, Williams & Wilkins.

Bax L, Staes F, Verhagen A (2005) Does neuromuscular electrical stimulation strengthen the quadriceps femoris? *Sports Med* **35**(3): 191–212.

Bazzucchi I, Felici F, Macaluso A, de Vito G (2004) Differences between young and older women in maximal force, force fluctuations, and surface EMG during isometric knee extension and elbow flexion. *Muscle Nerve* **30**: 626–635.

Behm DG, St Pierre DMM (1997) Effects of fatigue duration and muscle type on voluntary and evoked contractile properties. *J Appl Physiol* **82**(5): 1654–1661.

Bernardi M, Solomonov M, Sanchez JH et al (1995) Motor unit recruitment strategy of knee antagonist muscles in step-wise increasing contractions. *Eur J Appl Physiol* **70**: 493–501.

Bourjeily-Habr G, Rochester CL, Palermo F et al (2002) Randomised controlled trial of transcutaneous electrical muscle stimulation of the lower extremities in patients with chronic obstructive pulmonary disease. *Thorax* **57**: 1045–1049.

Burke RE (1967) Motor unit types of cat triceps surae muscle. *J Physiol* **193**: 14–150.

Chmielewski TL, Rudoloph KS, Fitzgerald GK et al (2001). Biomechanical evidence supporting a differential response to acute ACL injury. *Clin Biomech* **16**(7): 586–591.

Colebatch JG, Gandevia SC (1989) The distribution of muscular weakness in upper motor neuron lesions affecting the upper limb. *Brain* **112**: 749–763.

Cotter M, Phillips P (1986) Rapid fast to slow fiber transformation in response to chronic stimulation of immobilized muscles of the rabbit. *Exp Neurol* **93**: 531–545.

Cotter M, Hudlická O, Vrbová, G (1973) Growth of capillaries during long-term activity in skeletal muscle. *Bibliogr Anat* **11**: 395–398.

Cramp MC (1998) *Alterations in Human Muscle and Central Control Mechanisms*. PhD thesis. University of East London.

Cramp MC, Manuel JA, Scott OM (1995) Effects of different patterns of long-term electrical stimulation on human quadriceps femoris muscle. *J Physiol* **483**: 82P.

Davies CT, Rutherford I C, Thomas DO (1987). Electrically evoked contractions of the triceps surae during and following 21 days of voluntary leg immobilization. *Eur J Appl Physiol Occup Physiol* **56**: 306–312.

de Deyne PG, Hafer-Macko CE, Ivey FM et al (2004) Muscle molecular phenotype after stroke is associated with gait speed. *Muscle Nerve* **30**: 209–215.

Dietz V, Ketelsen UP, Berger W, Quintern J (1986) Motor unit involvement in spastic paresis: relationship between leg activation and histochemistry. *J Neurol Sci* **75**: 89–103.

Dimitrijevic MR (1994) Motor control in spinal chord injury patients. *Scand J Rehab Med suppl* **30**: 53–62.

Donaldson N de N, Rushton DN, Perkins TA et al (2003) Recruitment by motor nerve root stimulators: significance for implant design *Med Eng Phys* **25**: 527–537.

Duchateau J, Hainaut K (1990) Effects of immobilisation on contractile properties, recruitment and firing rates of human motor units. *J Physiol* **422**: 55–65.

Edgerton VR, Tillakaratne NJK, Bigbee AJ et al (2004) Plasticity of the spinal neural circuitry after injury. *Ann Rev Neurosci* **27**:145–167.

Edgerton VR, Kim SJ, Ichiyama RM et al (2006) Rehabilitative therapies after spinal cord injury. *J Neurotrauma* **23**(3/4): 560–570.

Edström L, Grimby L (1986) Effect of exercise on the motor unit. *Muscle Nerve* **9**: 104–126.

Edwards RHT (1981) *Human Muscle Function and Fatigue*. Ciba Foundation Symposium 82: 1-18. Pitman, London.

Edwards RHT, Young A, Hoskings GP, Jones DA (1977) Human skeletal muscle function: Description of tests and normal values. *Sci Mol Med* **52**: 283–290.

Enoka RM (1988) Muscle strength and its development: new perspectives. *Sports Med* **6**: 146–168.

Enoka RM (1997) Neural adaptations with chronic physical activity. *J Biomecha* **30**(5): 447–455.

Enoka RM, Fuglevand AJ (1993) Neuromuscular basis of the maximum force capacity of a muscle. In Grabiner MD (ed) *Current Issues in Biomechanics*. Champaign, IL, Human Kinetics: 215–235.

Farragher D, Kidd GL, Tallis RC (1987) Eutrophic electrical stimulation for Bell's palsy. *Clin Rehab* **1**: 265–271.

Frontera WR, Hughes VA, Fielding RA et al (2000) Aging of skeletal muscle: a 12-year longitudinal study. *J Appl Physiol* **88**: 1321–1326.

Fukunaga T, Ichinose Y, Masamitsu I et al (1997) Determination of fasicle length and pennation in a contracting human muscle in vivo. *J Appl Physiol* **82**(1): 354–358.

Gandevia SG (2001) Spinal and supraspinal factors in human muscle fatigue *Physiol Rev* **81**(4): 1725–1789.

Garnett RAF, O'Donnovan MJ, Stephens JA, Taylor A (1978) Motor unit organisation of human medial gastrocnemius. *J Physiol (Lond)* **287**: 33–43.

Gerdle B, Larsson B, Karlsson S. (2000) Criterion validation of surface EMG variables as fatigue indicators using peak torque. A study of repetitive maximum isokinetic knee extensions. *J Electromyogr Kinesiol* **10**: 225–232.

Gerrits HL, de Hann A, Hopman MTE et al (1999) Contractile properties of the quadriceps muscle in individuals with spinal cord injury. *Muscle Nerve* **22**: 1249–1253.

Goldspink G, Scutt A, Loughna PT et al (1992) Gene expression in skeletal muscle in response to stretch and force generation. *Am J Physiol* **262**: R356–R363.

Gordon T (1998) *Adaptability of Paralysed Muscles after Spinal Cord Injury*. Presented to the scientific meeting 'Human motor performance: the interaction between science and therapy', University of East London.

Gordon T, Mao J (1994) Muscle atrophy and procedures for training after spinal chord injury. *Phys Ther* **74**(1): 50–60.

Gregory CM, Bickel CS (2005) Recruitment patterns in human skeletal muscle during electrical stimulation. *Phys Ther* **85**(4): 35–364.

Hager-Ross CK, Klein CS, Thomas CK (2006). Twitch and tetanic properties of human thenar motor units paralyzed by chronic spinal cord injury. *J Neurophysiol* **96**(1): 165–174.

Häggmark T, Jansson E, Eriksson E (1981) Fiber type area and metabolic potential of the thigh muscle in man after knee surgery and immobilisation. *Int J Sports Med* **2**: 12–17.

Hanchard NCA, Williamson M, Caley RW Cooper RG (1998) Electrical stimulation of human tibialis anterior: (A) contractile properties are stable over a range of submaximal voltages; (B) high and low-frequency fatigue are inducible and reliably assessable at submaximal voltages. *Clin Rehab* **12**: 413–427.

Harridge SDR, Kryger A, Stensgaard A (1999) Knee extensor strength, activation and size in very elderly people following strength training. *Muscle Nerve* **22**: 831–839.

Heilmann C, Pette, D (1979) Molecular transformations in sarcoplasmic reticulum of fast twitch muscle by electrostimulation. *Eur J Biochem* **93**: 437–446.

Herbert RD, Gandevia SC (1999) Twitch interpolation in human muscles: mechanisms and implications for measurement of voluntary activation. *J Neurophysiol* **82**: 2271–2283.

Hortobágyi T, Dempsey D, Fraser D et al (2000) Changes in muscle strength, muscle fibre size and myofibrillar gene expression after immobilisation and retraining in humans. *J Physiol* **524**(1): 293–304.

Hudlická O, Brown M, Cotter M et al (1977) The effect of long-term stimulation on fast muscles on their blood flow, metabolism and ability to withstand fatigue. *Pflugers Arch* **369**: 141–149.

Hunt RJ (2005) *Control Systems for Function Restoration, Exercise, Fitness and Health in Spinal Cord Injury*. DSc thesis, University of Glasgow.

Johnson MA, Polgar J, Weightman D et al (1973) Data on the distribution of fibre types in thirty-six human muscles. *J Neurol Sci* **18**: 111–129.

Jones DA, Rutherford OM, Parker DF (1989) Physiological changes in skeletal muscle as a result of strength training. *Qu J Exp Physiol* **74**: 233–256.

Kamen G, Caldwell GE (1996) Physiology and interpretation of the electromyogram. *J Clin Neurophysiol* **13**(5): 366–384.

Kidd GL, Oldham JA (1988) Eutrophic electrotherapy and atrophied muscle: a pilot clinical study. *Clin Rehab* **2**: 219–230.

Klein CS, Häger-Ross CK, Thomas CK (2006) Fatigue properties of human thenar motor units paralysed by chronic spinal chord injury. *J Physiol* **573**(1): 161–171.

Kollmitzer J, Ebenbichler GR, Kopf A (1999) Reliability of surface electromyographic measurements. *Clin Neurophysiol* **110**: 725–734.

Komi PV (1986) Training of muscle strength and power: Interaction of neuromotoric, hypertrophic and mechanical factors. *Int J Sports Med* **7**: 10–15.

Lieber RL (1986) Skeletal muscle adaptability: muscle properties following chronic electrical stimulation. *Dev Med Child Neurol* **28**: 662–670.

Lieber RL, Friden J (2000) Functional and clinical significance of skeletal muscle architecture *Muscle Nerve* **23**: 1647–1666.

Liu Y, Schlumberger A, Wirth K et al (2003) Different effects on human skeletal myosin heavy chain isoform expression: strength vs. combination training. *J Appl Physiol* **94**: 2282–2288.

Merton PA (1954) Voluntary strength and fatigue. *J Physiol* **123**: 553–564.

Merton PA, Morton HB, Hill DK, Marsden CD (1982) Scope of a technique for electrical stimulation of human brain, spinal cord and muscle. *Lancet* **ii**: 597–600.

Midiro M (2006) The denervated muscle: facts and hypotheses. A historical review. *J Appl Physiol* **98**: 1–21.

O'Connor MC, Carnell P, Manuel JM, Scott OM (1993) Characteristics of human quadriceps femoris muscle during voluntary and electrically induced fatigue. *J Physiol* **473**: 71P.

O'Dwyer NJ, Ada L, Neilson PD (1996) Spasticity and muscle contracture in relation to spastic hypertonia. *Curr Opin Neurol* **9**: 451–455.

Oldham JA, Stanley JK (1989) Rehabilitation of atrophied muscle in the rheumatoid arthritic hand: a comparison of two methods of electrical stimulation. *J Hand Surg (Br)* **14B**: 294–297.

Ottawa Panel (2004) Evidence-based clinical practice guidelines for electrotherapy and thermotherapy interventions in the management of rheumatoid arthritis in adults (2004). *Phys Ther* **84**: 1016–1043.

Pelland L, Brosseau L, Casimiro L et al (2002) Electrical stimulation in the treatment of rheumatoid arthritis. Cochrane Database of Systematic Reviews Issue 2 Art. No. DOI: 10.1002/14651858.CD003687.

Perkins TA, Donaldson N de N, Hatcher NAC et al (2002) Control of leg powered paraplegic cycling using stimulation of the lumbo-sacral anterior spinal roots. IEEE Trans Rehab 10: 158–164.

Pette D, Staron RS (1997) Mammalian skeletal muscle fiber type transitions. Int Rev Cytol 170: 143–223.

Pette D, Vrbová G (1992) Adaptation of mammalian skeletal muscle fibres to chronic electrical stimulation. Rev Physiol Biochem 120: 116–202.

Pette D, Vrbová G (1999) What does chronic electrical stimulation teach us about muscle plasticity? Muscle Nerve 22: 666–677.

Pette D, Smith ME, Staudte HW, Vrbová G (1973) Effects of long-term electrical stimulation on some contractile and metabolic characteristics of fast rabbit muscles. Pflugers Arch 338: 257–272.

Risberg MA, Lewek M, Synder-Mackler (2004) A systematic review of evidence for anterior ligament rehabilitation: how much and what type? Phys Ther Sport 5: 125–145.

Roos MR, Rice CL, Connelly DM, Vandervoot AA (1999) Quadriceps muscle strength, contractile properties, and motor unit firing rates in young and old men. Muscle Nerve 22: 1094–1103.

Rutherford OM, Jones DA (1988) Contractile properties and fatigability of the human adductor muscle and first dorsal interosseus: a comparison of the effects of two chronic stimulation patterns. J Neurol Sci 85: 319–331.

Rutherford OM, Jones DA, Newham DJ (1986) Clinical and experimental application of the percutaneous twitch superimposition technique for the study of human muscle activation. J Neurol Neurosurg Psychiatry 49: 1288–1291.

Ryan AS, Dobrovolny L, Smith GV et al (2002) Hemiparetic muscle atrophy and increased intramuscular fat in stroke patients. Arch Phys Med Rehab 83(12): 1703–1707.

Salmons S, Henriksson J (1981) The adaptive response of skeletal muscle to increased use. Muscle Nerve 4: 94–105.

Salmons S, Vrbová G (1969) The influence of activity on some contractile characteristics of mammalian fast and slow muscles. J Physiol 201: 535–549.

Scelsi R (2001) Skeletal muscle pathology after spinal chord injury: Our 20 year experience and results on skeletal muscle changes in paraplegics, related to functional rehabilitation Basic Appl Myol 11(2): 75–85.

Scott OM, Vrbová G, Hyde SA, Dubowitz D (1985) Effects of chronic, low-frequency electrical stimulation on normal tibialis anterior muscle. J Neurol Neurosurg Psychiatry 48: 774–781.

Scott OM, Vrbová G, Hyde SA, Dubowitz D (1986) Responses of muscles of patients with Duchenne muscular dystrophy to chronic electrical stimulation. J Neurol Neurosurg Psychiatry 49: 1427–1434.

Scott OM, Hyde SA, Vrbová G, Dubowitz V (1990) Therapeutic possibilities of chronic low frequency electrical stimulation in children with Duchenne muscular dystrophy. J Neurol Sci 95: 171–182.

Scott WB, Lee SCK, Johnston TE et al (2006) Contractile properties and the force-frequency relationship of the paralyzed human quadriceps femoris muscle. Phys Ther 86: 788–799.

Selkowitz DM (1989) High frequency electrical stimulation in muscle strengthening: a review and discussion. Am J Sports Med 17(1): 103–111.

Shields RK, Dudley-Javoroski S, Law LA (1997) Electrically induced muscle contractions influence bone density decline after spinal chord injury. Spine 31(5): 548–553.

Short KR, Vittone JL, Bigelow ML et al (2005) Changes in myosin heavy chain mRNA and protein expression in human skeletal muscle with age and endurance exercise training J Appl Physiol 99: 95–102.

Singer B (1987) Functional electrical stimulation of the extremities in the neurological patient: a review. Aust J Physiother 33(1): 33–42.

Snyder-Mackler L, Binder-Macleod SA, Williams PR (1993) Fatigability of human quadriceps femoris muscle following anterior cruciate ligament reconstruction. Med Sci Sports Exer 25(7): 783–789.

Snyder-Mackler L, Delitto A, Stralka SW, Bailey SL (1994) Use of electrical stimulation to enhance recovery of quadriceps femoris muscle force production in patients following anterior cruciate ligament reconstruction. Phys Ther 74(10): 901–907.

Stackhouse SK, Stevens KE, Lee SCK et al (2001) Maximum voluntary activation in nonfatigued and fatigues muscle of young and elderly individuals. Phys Ther 81(5): 1102–1109.

St-Pierre D, Gardiner PF (1987) The effect of immobilization and exercise on muscle function: a review. Physiother Canada 39(1): 24–35.

Suetta C, Aagaard P, Rosted A et al (2004) Training induced changes in muscle CSA, muscle strength, EMG and rate of force development in elderly subjects after disuse. J Appl Physiol 97: 1954–1961.

Thomas CK (1997) Fatigue in human thenar muscles paralysed by spinal cord injury. J Electromyogr Kinesiol 7(1): 15–26.

Thompson LV (1994) Effects of age and training on skeletal muscle physiology and performance. Phys Ther 74: 71–81.

Todd G, Gorman R, Gandevia S (2004) Measurement and reproducibility of strength and voluntary activation of lower limb muscles. Muscle Nerve 29: 834–842.

Trimble MH, Enoka RM (1991) Mechanisms underlying the training effects associated with neuromuscular electrical stimulation. Phys Ther 71(4): 273–282.

Vodovnik L, Kralj A, Bajd T (1985) Modification of abnormal motor control with functional electrical stimulation of peripheralnerves. In Eccles, Dimitrijevic (eds) Recent Achievements in Restorative Neurology 1: Upper Motor Neuron Functions and Dysfunctions. Basel. S. Karger. Chapter 5, 42–55.

Vrbová G (1963) The effect of motor neuron activity on the speed of contraction of striated muscle. J Physiol (Lond) 169: 513–526.

Vrbová G (1966) Factors determining the speed of contraction of striated muscle. *J Physiol (Lond)* **185**: 17P–18P.

Whittom F, Jobin J, Peirre-Michel S et al (1998) Histochemical and morphological characteristics of the vastus lateralis muscle in patients with chronic obstructive disease. *Med Sci Sports Exerc* **30**(10): 1467–1474.

Williams PE, Goldspink G (1984) Connective tissue changes in immobilized muscle. *J Anat* **138**(2): 343–350.

Williams PE, Watt P, Bicik V, Goldspink G (1986) Effects of stretch combined with electrical stimulation on the type of sarcomeres produced at the ends of muscle fibres. *Exp Neurol* **93**: 500–509.

Williams GN, Higgins MJ, Lewek MD (2002) Aging skeletal muscle: physiologic changes and the effects of training. *Phys Ther* **82**(1): 62–68.

Williamson DL, Godard MP, Porter DA et al (2000) Progressive resistance training reduces myosin heavy chain co expression in single muscle fibres from older men. *J Appl Physiol* **88**: 627–633.

Winter DA (1990) *Biomechanics and Motor Control of Human Movement*, 2nd edn. New York, John Wiley & Sons.

Yue GH, Bilodeau M, Enoka RN (1994) Elbow joint immobilisation decreases fatigability and alters the pattern of activation in humans. *Soc Neurosci Abstr* **20**: 1205.

Chapter **15**

Neuromuscular and muscular electrical stimulation

Suzanne McDonough

INTRODUCTION

To apply electrical stimulation effectively it is important to revise some basic principles on how nerves are activated by electrical signals and how muscle contracts in response to these signals (see Chapter 5). It is also important to understand types of muscle fibre, patterns of normal recruitment of muscle fibres and how these are reversed when electrical stimulation is used. This is covered in Chapter 13, which also identifies the differences between electrical stimulation and voluntary exercise and discusses the mechanisms underlying increases in strength with electrical stimulation. Chapter 13 also discusses the types of current that can be used to produce an electrical response in muscle and nerve and the parameters that can be varied to produce different responses.

This chapter examines the clinical areas in which electrical stimulation has been used and reviews

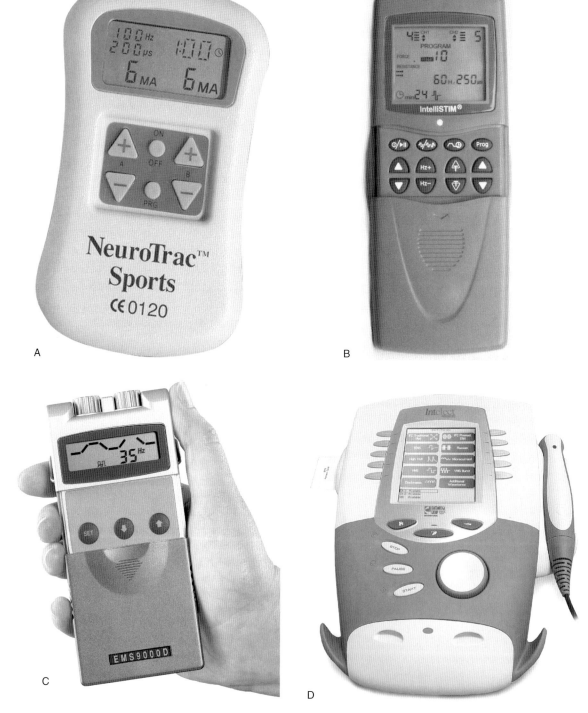

Figure 15.1 A range of battery and mains powered muscle stimulation units. A, NeuroTrac Sports (SKF); B, IntelliSTIM (Natures Gate); C, DigiStim (PhysioMed); D, Chatanooga Multimodal system (PhysioMed, SKF).

the relevant literature to identify what is known about the clinical effects of treatment and why these may occur. The practical application of neuromuscular electrical stimulation (NMES) for innervated muscle and electrical muscular stimulation (EMS) for denervated muscle will be discussed.

TYPES OF UNIT

A multitude of commercially available electrical stimulation units (using a variety of current types) are marketed under a variety of names. Units can either be portable (battery operated) or line powered and there has been some debate as to which type of unit is better for muscle strengthening. Some investigators have argued that line-powered units can produce greater strength gains as these units can cause higher training contraction force levels, particularly when used for larger muscle groups such as quadriceps (Robinson 1995). However, more recent evidence suggests that both types of unit can produce similar increases in peak torque along with comparable levels of discomfort (Fitzgerald et al 2003). It is essential that the user checks that the machine to be used has available the parameters required for treatment, although this chapter will show that there is some lack of clarity about the most effective to use on all occasions. Figure 15.1 illustrates a range of portable, battery-powered muscle stimulation units and a typical mains powered multimodal device that includes muscle-stimulating currents.

NOMENCLATURE AND TYPES OF ELECTRICAL STIMULATION IN NERVE AND MUSCLE

The Clinical Electrophysiology Section of the American Physical Therapy Association established a unified terminology for clinical electrical currents: direct current, alternating current and pulsed current (American Physical Therapy Association (APTA) 1990). Although the use of this terminology would make the task of classifying commercial stimulators and interpreting the results of research studies more straightforward, it does not appear to have been widely adopted and inconsistencies remain in the literature with regard to nomenclature. Investigators use terms interchangeably and sometimes the precise form of electrical stimulation can be gleaned only by careful review of the particular paper. The following terms tend to be used interchangeably.

NEUROMUSCULAR ELECTRICAL STIMULATION (NMES)

This form of electrical stimulation is commonly used at sufficiently high intensities to produce muscular contraction and may be applied to the muscle during movement or without functional movement occurring.

FUNCTIONAL ELECTRICAL OR NEUROMUSCULAR STIMULATION (FES/FNS)

This term is used when the aim of treatment is to enhance or produce functional movement. The level of complexity of FES can range from its use (with dual-channel stimulators) to enhance dorsiflexion during gait in children with cerebral palsy (Atwater et al 1991) to multichannel FES to activate many muscles to restore stance and gait in patients with paraplegia (Hömberg 1997). FES is covered in detail in Chapter 18.

THERAPEUTIC ELECTRICAL STIMULATION (TES)

This term has been used specifically to describe a form of electrical stimulation that produces sensory effects only (Beck 1997, Pape 1997, Steinbok et al 1997). Unfortunately, the term 'therapeutic electrical stimulation' has also been used by some investigators to differentiate between electrical stimulation applied to promote function (FES) and that applied for some other therapeutic function, for example NMES for children with cerebral palsy (Hazlewood et al 1994) and adults with spasticity and spinal cord injury (Chae et al 2000, Pease 1998).

ELECTRICAL STIMULATION (ES)

The meaning of the generic term 'electrical stimulation' is further complicated by the expanding use of electrical stimulation. Some investigators may not simply be applying it to strengthen weakened muscles but may also be investigating its role in promoting functional recovery (Pandyan et al 1997, Powell et al 1999, Steinbok et al 1997) and reducing spasticity in neurological conditions (Alfieri 1982, Hesse et al 1998, Vodovnik et al 1984).

EVIDENCE OF CLINICAL EFFICACY

Although there is an abundance of literature in this area, reviews reveal inconsistent findings on what effects can be produced with electrical stimulation, the specific parameters to produce these effects and what the underlying principle of these effects might be. This may be due to certain underlying problems with the literature rather than an intrinsic lack of efficacy. The following paragraphs outline some of the shortcomings in the literature.

Some early studies do not include a comparison group and therefore have not identified the benefit of electrical stimulation over other forms of intervention. For example, electrical stimulation has been shown to strengthen atrophied muscle significantly (Singer et al 1983, William & Street 1976) but in some studies with a matched voluntary exercise group had no additional benefit (Grove-Lainey et al 1983).

The subject numbers in some studies are too small. Small studies produce findings both for (Delitto et al 1988, Snyder-Mackler et al 1991) and against (Grove-Lainey et al 1983, Sisk et al 1987) a modality, neither of which provides reliable evidence.

Even some well-designed randomized controlled trials (RCT) make interpretation of the findings difficult as there is no consistency between electrical stimulation, exercise protocols or both. An example is differences in the 'intensity' used for NMES ('intensity' here applies to several parameters, i.e. not only the intensity of the applied current but also the frequency and duty cycle), which may account for the conflicting findings about the effectiveness of NMES to strengthen muscle. NMES has been found by Robinson (1995) to be significantly more effective at strengthening quadriceps than voluntary exercise, whereas Lieber et al (1996) and Paternostro-Sluga et al (1999) demonstrated that NMES was no more effective

than voluntary exercise. However, the parameters used in the latter two studies were considered 'low intensity' by Robinson (1995), and so possibly not suitable for strengthening.

Even in studies in which the aim was to compare different types of electrical stimulation there are a number of varying factors, which makes it very difficult to establish which factor may be the important variable that leads to strengthening in a trial. Robinson (1995) showed that 'high-intensity' NMES (as defined above) caused significantly more strengthening than both 'low-intensity' NMES and voluntary exercise. Robinson (1995) argue that the difference in results can be accounted for by the fact that the 'high-intensity' group trained harder than the 'low-intensity' group. There is evidence that the higher the training contraction force, the greater the improvement in quadriceps strength (Robinson 1995) and these authors concluded that these results supported the use of line-powered units. However, it is important to note that the protocols for battery-operated and line-powered units in this study were very different. Some of the differences may be explained by the placebo effect of a bigger line-powered unit or the therapist–patient interaction, which was absent when patients used a portable unit at home.

Nevertheless, there does appear to be evidence for the clinical effectiveness of electrical stimulation for strengthening muscle, improving function and reducing tone in patient populations. The shortcomings in the research base, however, mean it is not possible to assign particular effects to certain interactions of parameters and only broad guidelines can be given. The following section examines the evidence for clinical efficacy in a number of areas; possible treatment parameters to achieve these effects are presented in the section on practical application (p. 238).

STRENGTHENING IN NON–NEUROLOGICAL CONDITIONS

Two mechanisms for strengthening muscle with NMES have been proposed. First, strength gains may be achieved in the same manner as standard voluntary strengthening programmes, which use a low number of repetitions with high external loads and a high intensity of muscle contraction (at least 75% of maximum). The second mechanism by which strengthening can occur is the preferential recruitment of type II phasic muscle fibres, which have a lower threshold for NMES (Delitto 7 Snyder-Mackler 1990, Lake 1992).

Electrical stimulation of healthy muscle

In general, the research evidence does not support the use of electrical stimulation for increasing either strength or endurance in healthy muscle. Although there is evidence that electrical stimulation is more effective than no exercise, it has been clearly shown that the combination of electrical stimulation and exercise is no more effective than exercise alone (Bax et al 2005). This systematic review of 17 articles (published between 1983 and 2000) investigated the effect of NMES on healthy quadriceps muscle; 14 of these articles compared NMES to no exercise and 10 compared it to volitional exercise. The results of the meta-analysis of 12/14 studies (235 subjects) confirmed the view from previous single studies that NMES is more effective than no exercise whereas there is no difference (or indeed volitional exercise may be better) than NMES (meta-analysis, 8/10, $n = 155$ subjects) in unimpaired quadriceps. Further systematic review work is planned in this area and will update these findings in due course (Mizusaki et al 2006).

There is, however, some controversy over whether NMES is more effective for strengthening abdominal muscles than voluntary exercise. Although multiple-muscle-group NMES (which includes stimulation of the abdominal muscles) as used in muscle-toning clinics has proved totally ineffective in muscle strengthening (Lake 1988, Lake & Gillespie 1988), there is some evidence that NMES combined with voluntary exercise can be more effective than exercise alone for abdominal training in healthy subjects (Alon et al 1987, Alon & Taylor 1997). This latter finding may be explained by the fact that in many healthy adults the abdominal muscles are atrophic, or that use of NMES makes it easier to learn the correct activation of the abdominal muscles. A similar argument could be put forward for the fact that one study has shown that NMES is more effective than exercise for

strengthening of the back musculature (Kahanovitz et al 1987). Further trials are therefore required to clarify these results but it is worth highlighting here that future trials should identify whether NMES is superior to voluntary exercise rather than showing NMES to be superior to no exercise, as in Porcari's recent trial (2005).

Electrical stimulation of atrophied muscle

Electrical stimulation for strengthening is useful clinically in cases involving immobilization or contraindications to dynamic exercise to prevent disuse atrophy (Selkowitz 1989), in early rehabilitation by facilitating muscle contraction, and in selective muscle strengthening or muscle re-education (Lake 1992).

Quadriceps Recent review evidence concludes that there is evidence that high-intensity neuromuscular electrical stimulation in addition to volitional exercises significantly improves isometric quadriceps muscle strength compared to volitional exercises alone (Arna Risberg et al 2004) and that voluntary muscle training programmes were only able to produce equivalent results when the latter's intensity was higher (Lieber et al 1996, Paternostro-Sluga et al 1999). This would suggest that NMES is a very useful modality when the patient is unable to exercise voluntarily at high levels. However, in order to produce therapeutic strength changes the patient will need to tolerate intensive NMES training regimens and the clinician needs to use high power outputs to produce more positive results (Bax et al 2005).

Rheumatoid arthritis A Cochrane Review by Pelland et al (2002) identified one RCT that showed that a patterned form of NMES (derived from the fatigued motor unit of the first dorsal interosseous in a normal hand) and NMES at 10 Hz had a significant effect on hand function compared to a control no-treatment group. However, these conclusions are limited by the low methodological quality of the single trial. More well-designed studies are therefore needed to provide further evidence of the benefits in the management of rheumatoid arthritis.

Pelvic floor muscles Although studies examining the effect of NMES have focused largely on rehabilitation of knee injuries, it has also been shown to be useful in rehabilitation of patients with pelvic floor dysfunction, which can lead to faecal (Fynes et al 1999) and urinary incontinence (Sand et al 1995).

Urinary incontinence A recent review in *Clinical Evidence* (Onwude 2005) included RCTs and three systematic reviews (Berghmans et al 1998, Herbison et al, 2002, Moehrer et al 2002) that investigated the effects of NMES on female urinary stress incontinence. Onwude (2005) concluded that there was no evidence for a difference between NMES + exercise, NMES + weighted cones or NMES + oestrogen supplements. However, NMES was significantly better than no treatment or sham treatment. It was noted that some of the included RCTs might have lacked the power to detect a clinically important difference (Onwude 2005) and therefore it would still be pertinent to use the parameters from a positive study to guide treatment. For example, significant improvements in urinary stress incontinence were found after 15 weeks of pelvic floor muscle stimulation (Sand et al 1995). A protocol pertinent to this topic can be found in the Cochrane library, which will provide an update on stress, urge and mixed urinary continence in due course (Berghmans et al 2004).

Faecal incontinence There have been two Cochrane Systematic Reviews in this area (Hosker et al 2000, Norton et al 2006), which identified only two RCTs (Fynes et al 1999, Mahony et al 2004) that evaluated the effectiveness of NMES on faecal incontinence. In the study by Fynes et al (1999), electrical stimulation was performed via an endoanal probe using low-frequency (20 Hz) and high-frequency (50 Hz) settings to target static (slow-twitch) and dynamic (fast-twitch) fibre activity with a 20% ramp modulation time. Over 12 weeks of treatment (one session per week), electrical stimulation combined with audiovisual biofeedback of muscle activity significantly improved continence scores (Fynes et al 1999). Mahony et al (2004) compared EMG biofeedback with biofeedback plus anal electrical stimulation at 35 Hz and a 20% modulation ramp over 12 weeks, and showed no differences between the two groups. Further work is therefore required to establish the effectiveness of NMES for this condition.

Electrical stimulation of denervated muscle

Despite more than a century of using EMS to stimulate denervated muscle, controversy over its use and efficacy continues (Davies 1983, Delitto et al 1995). This is primarily due to the variety of treatment protocols that have been used to assess care. Although there is no current consensus about the duty cycle that should be used, the frequency of stimulation or the number of contractions that should be employed, Snyder-Mackler and Robinson (1995) suggest that EMS can delay atrophy and its associated changes. However, they also note that there is no evidence to suggest that such a delay is significant in terms of final recovery.

USE OF ELECTRICAL STIMULATION IN ADULTS WITH NEUROLOGICAL CONDITIONS

The effects of electrical stimulation in neurological rehabilitation can be divided into improved motor function (Barecca et al 2003, de Kroon et al 2005), reduction in spasticity (Alfieri 1982, Hesse et al 1998, Vodovnik et al 1984, Weingarden et al 1998), increase in muscle strength (Glanz et al 1996, Powell et al 1999), increase in range of movement of the wrist (Pandyan et al 1997, Powell et al 1999) and reduction of shoulder subluxation in stroke patients (Ada & Foongchomcheay 2002). Some of these trials use FES, which is explored in more detail in Chapter 18.

Motor recovery

de Kroon et al (2005) reviewed 19 trials that evaluated the effect of electrical stimulation on motor control. Several types of electrical stimulation were explored: (1) the patient was not actively involved in the muscle contraction; (2) two forms of stimulation that relied on the patients either voluntarily contracting their muscle to a predefined level to trigger the electrical stimulation (EMG-triggered electrical stimulation) or moving the joint to a predefined position for the electrical stimulation to be triggered (positional feedback training). Twelve trials were RCTs, two non-RCTs, two had a multiple baseline design and three were case series (de Kroon et al 2005). Thirteen comparisons produced results in favour of electrical stimulation, whereas nine comparisons were in favour of the control group or showed no difference. So, on balance, the results would appear to be positive, although this needs to be tempered by the methodological shortcomings of some of these trials.

Strength

A meta-analysis of studies that used various forms of electrical stimulation in stroke patients showed that the strength of wrist, knee and ankle extensors was significantly increased after 3–4 weeks of treatment (Glanz et al 1996). More recent randomized controlled trials confirmed this finding of increased strength (de Kroon et al 2005).

Shoulder subluxation after stroke

A meta-analysis of seven trials found that early use of electrical stimulation (within 28 days of onset of stroke) may reduce the degree of shoulder subluxation and prevent further capsular stretch in acute stroke patients (Ada & Foongchomcheay 2002). These studies applied NMES to the posterior deltoid (active electrode) and supraspinatus muscles (passive electrode) at an intensity level sufficient to produce muscular contraction. Only one study – that by Faghri et al 1994 – specified the movement (humeral elevation and some abduction and extension). Further consideration of NMES in relation to post-stroke shoulder problems can be found in Chapters 14 and 18.

Reducing spasticity in adults with neurological conditions

The term 'spasticity' is used in a variety of circumstances to describe impaired movement execution, enhanced muscular resistance against passive movement or abnormal limb postures (Hummelsheim & Mauritz 1993). Spasticity has been explained by enhanced motor neuron excitability to the muscle (Artieda et al 1991) and altered mechanical properties of the muscle (Dietz et al 1981). Hömberg (1997) reviewed some evidence for the effectiveness of electrical stimulation in reducing spasticity (of spinal or cerebral origin). He discussed both FES and NMES interchangeably under the heading of FES. There was evidence for a reduction in

spasticity of the agonist when NMES was applied to the antagonist muscle (Alfieri 1982) or to both agonist and antagonist muscles (Hesse et al 1998, Vodovnik et al 1984, Weingarden et al 1998); however, the mechanisms underpinning these effects are still unclear. In one randomized controlled trial, NMES had no effect on spasticity when it was applied to the agonist only (Powell et al 1999).

It has been proposed that stimulation of the antagonist reduces spasticity in the agonist via the group Ia reciprocal inhibitory pathway (Hömberg 1997, Levine et al 1952) or via polysynaptic pathways mediated by flexion reflex afferents (Apkarian & Naumann 1991). Stimulation of the spastic agonist may lead to a reduction in activity via recurrent inhibition of its own α motor neuron (Granit et al 1957, Ryall et al 1972). It is also possible that, by stretching the agonist or the antagonist muscles through their available range of movement, mechanical factors are altered, so leading to a reduction in spasticity (Botte et al 1988). Indeed, electrical stimulation for motor relearning after stroke may produce its desired effects by virtue of the fact it produces a desired muscle contraction in muscles that are otherwise not activated at all, abnormally activated, or responding abnormally (Daly & Ruff 2000).

Regardless of the method used, there is evidence of positive effects, although further controlled studies are required to confirm these findings. The evidence also suggests that use of NMES in a nonfunctional way can produce effects so that if the clinician only has access to a very simple battery-operated NMES device it is possible to use it to reduce spasticity (Alfieri 1982).

CHILDREN: STRENGTHENING ATROPHIED MUSCLE IN NEUROLOGICAL CONDITIONS

In a systematic review by our group we identified 18 articles that applied electrical stimulation to the trunk, or upper and lower limb muscles in children with cerebral palsy (Kerr et al 2004). Two main forms of electrical stimulation were used in the former studies: either TES or NMES. Of the 12 studies investigating the efficacy of NMES, one reported no improvement with treatment, one reported inconclusive findings and the remaining 10 all described improvements in function and/or

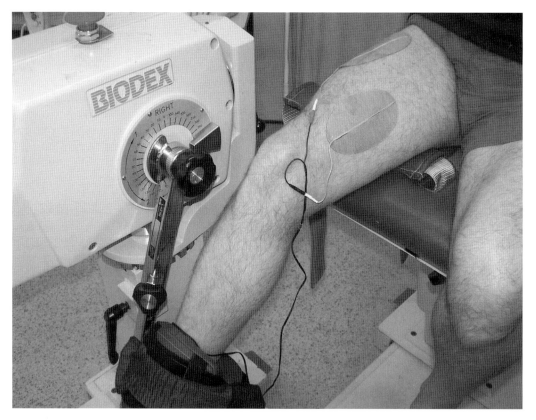

Figure 15.2 Electrode positioning for quadriceps stimulation (after Alon & Smith 2005).

strength. However, it is notable that the findings in the RCTs, of which there were only three, were less positive than the uncontrolled studies and case reports. For TES there was less evidence, with only one of three RCTS supporting its use. In conclusion, this review highlighted the scarcity of well-controlled trials in this area and makes it difficult to definitively support or discard the use of electrical stimulation in the paediatric cerebral palsy population (Kerr et al 2004).

To address the lack of suitably powered RCTs, our group investigated the efficacy of NMES and TES versus placebo electrical stimulation in 60 children with cerebral palsy. No statistically significant differences were demonstrated between NMES or TES versus placebo for strength or function. In conclusion, further evidence is required to show whether NMES and/or TES might be useful as an adjunct to therapy in ambulatory children with diplegia who find resistive programmes difficult (Kerr et al 2006).

PRACTICAL APPLICATION

Although both innervated and denervated muscle can be made to contract by current applied to the skin, most studies today focus on the use of electrical currents to stimulate innervated muscle. The method of application of treatment for both is, however, identical. Chapter 15 provides basic details of practical application; additional details follow.

PATIENT POSITION

The patient should be positioned comfortably, so that the muscle is completed relaxed and can easily be stimulated and so that there is no danger of the patient voluntarily contracting the stimulated muscle. The majority of trials with the quadriceps muscle have used isometric training methods with the knee flexed at a 30–90° angle (Fig. 15.2). This can easily be achieved using an isokinetic machine or by getting the patient to sit over a plinth with

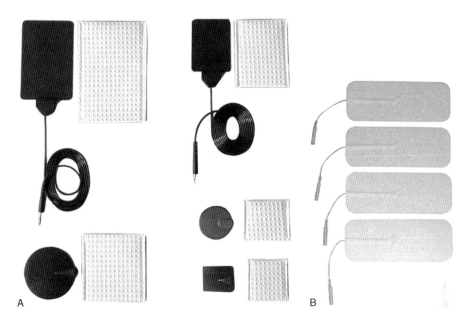

Figure 15.3 A, Carbon–rubber electrodes and B, pre-gelled self-adhesive electrodes (SKF Services Ltd).

the foot not fixed (see the section Electrode placement, p. 240, for positioning of electrodes for quadriceps activation). It is worth noting that using NMES with the knee flexed to 65° eliminates undesirable strain on the anterior cruciate ligament (Fitzgerald et al 2003).

SKIN PREPARATION

Prior to treatment, the skin should either be washed with soap and water or cleaned with a proprietary, alcohol-based wipe. This removes skin debris (including dead epithelial cells and sebum), sweat and dirt and is necessary to facilitate good contact between the electrode and the skin and thus reduce the electrical resistance of the interface.

ELECTRODES

Types and attachment

Carbon–rubber electrodes have been introduced on to the market in recent years and are currently the most popular type of polymer-based electrode as a result of their ease of use. They consist of carbon-impregnated silicone rubber (Fig. 15.3A). Such electrodes are reusable, can be cut to size and can be moulded to the skin surface provided this is

not too irregular. They are normally coupled to the skin by an electrically conductive gel and must be taped securely into place. Other polymer-based electrodes are also available but are generally less efficient at transmitting electrical stimuli to the tissue (Nolan 1991). Recent advances in electrode design have further increased the ease with which they can be applied and have improved their electrical contact with the skin. Such electrodes are considerably more malleable than those previously available and have an even layer of conductive material already in place; it is these particular qualities that allow them to make more effective contact with the skin. In addition, they are self-adhesive and reusable, factors which make them quick, easy and economical to use.

A number of authors, including Nelson et al (1980) and Nolan (1991), have compared the efficiency with which various electrodes conduct stimuli to the tissues. Nelson et al (1980) demonstrated that metal electrodes are most efficient, whereas Nolan (1991) showed that carbon–rubber electrodes are generally more efficient than many other polymer-based types. However, the final choice is determined by assessing all the factors mentioned above.

Both hand-held and pad electrodes are available. The first facilitates rapid movement of the electrode, which may be particularly useful when searching for the optimal stimulation point. The second is more useful for a prolonged period of stimulation.

Electrode size

Fundamentally, the choice of electrode size depends on the size of the muscle to be stimulated and the intensity of the contraction to be elicited. Small electrodes may be used to localize stimulation to small muscles or to apply a stimulus over a nerve that supplies a muscle. Larger electrodes are needed to stimulate larger muscles and muscle groups and to act as dispersive terminals (see below). It should be noted here that for the quadriceps muscle it is recommended that electrodes cover the bulk of the muscle (e.g. 7.6 × 12.7 cm) and that the standard-sized electrodes that come with most battery-powered and line-powered units are likely to be too small.

Although the spread of the electrical current over the surface of electrodes may be irregular (e.g. the intensity is often greater at the point where the current enters the electrode), it is generally true to say that the larger the electrode, the lower the current density. Thus, small electrodes tend to lead to stronger muscle contractions. However, it should be remembered that the final stimulus received by the tissue is also dependent on other factors, such as the point at which the current enters the electrode and the nature and efficiency of the contact medium.

Electrode placement

Electrodes may be sited on muscles in a number of ways. First, a primary electrode may be placed over the 'motor point' of a muscle. This may be defined as the point on the surface of the skin that allows a contraction to occur using the least energy. In general, the motor point of a muscle is located over the muscle's belly, often, but not always, at the junction between the upper and middle thirds of the belly. It is worth noting here that there are multiple 'motor points' in each muscle and this technique simply locates the most superficial motor point. Figures 15.4–15.13 show

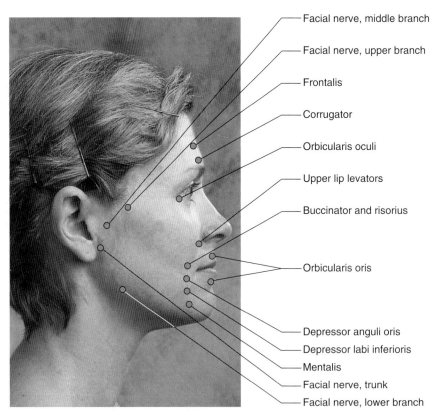

Facial nerve, middle branch

Facial nerve, upper branch

Frontalis

Corrugator

Orbicularis oculi

Upper lip levators

Buccinator and risorius

Orbicularis oris

Depressor anguli oris

Depressor labi inferioris

Mentalis

Facial nerve, trunk

Facial nerve, lower branch

Figure 15.4 Motor points of some of the muscles supplied by the facial nerve.

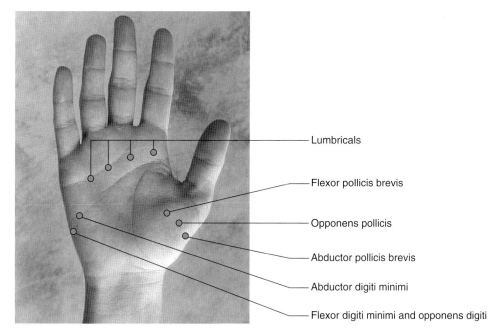

Lumbricals

Flexor pollicis brevis

Opponens pollicis

Abductor pollicis brevis

Abductor digiti minimi

Flexor digiti minimi and opponens digiti

Figure 15.5 Approximate positions of some of the motor points on the anterior aspect of the hand.

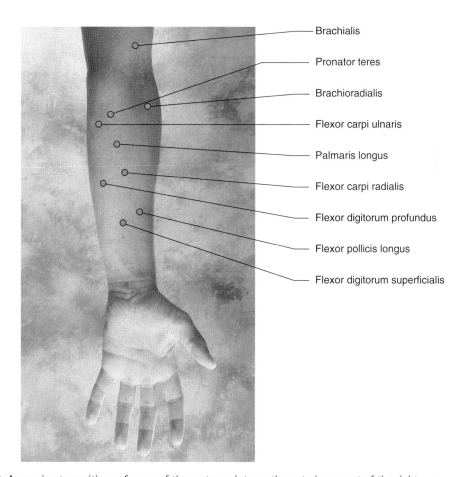

Brachialis

Pronator teres

Brachioradialis

Flexor carpi ulnaris

Palmaris longus

Flexor carpi radialis

Flexor digitorum profundus

Flexor pollicis longus

Flexor digitorum superficialis

Figure 15.6 Approximate positions of some of the motor points on the anterior aspect of the right arm.

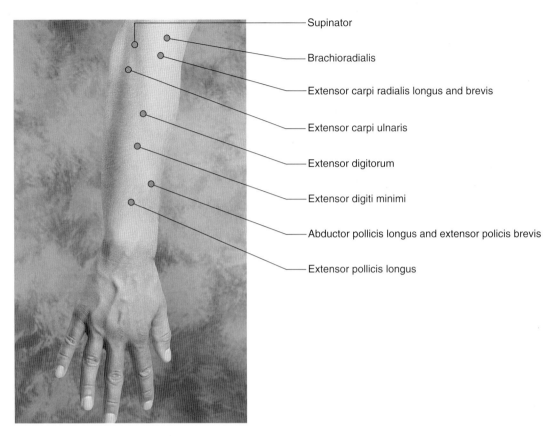

Figure 15.7 Approximate positions of some of the motor points on the posterior aspect of the right arm.

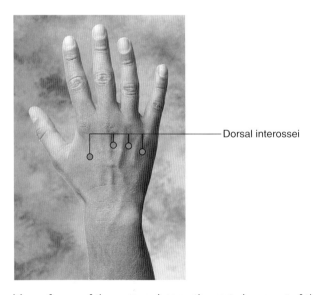

Figure 15.8 Approximate positions of some of the motor points on the posterior aspect of the hand.

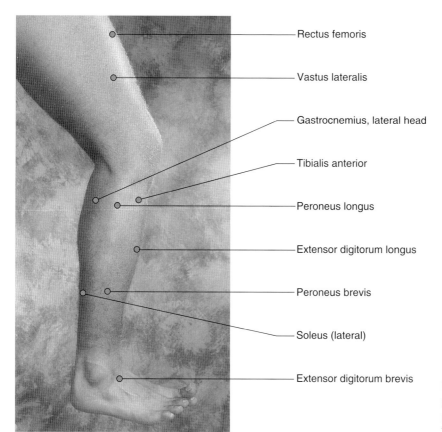

- Rectus femoris
- Vastus lateralis
- Gastrocnemius, lateral head
- Tibialis anterior
- Peroneus longus
- Extensor digitorum longus
- Peroneus brevis
- Soleus (lateral)
- Extensor digitorum brevis

Figure 15.9 Approximate positions of some of the motor points on the anterior aspect of the right leg.

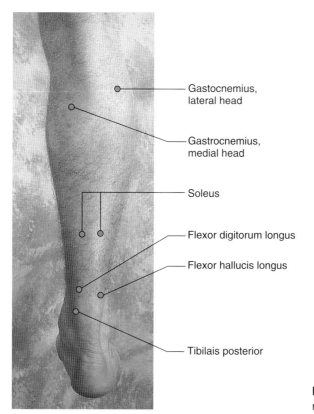

- Gastocnemius, lateral head
- Gastrocnemius, medial head
- Soleus
- Flexor digitorum longus
- Flexor hallucis longus
- Tibilais posterior

Figure 15.10 Approximate positions of some of the motor points on the posterior aspect of the right leg.

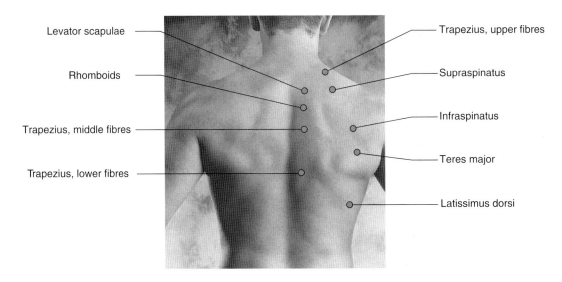

Levator scapulae

Rhomboids

Trapezius, middle fibres

Trapezius, lower fibres

Trapezius, upper fibres

Supraspinatus

Infraspinatus

Teres major

Latissimus dorsi

Figure 15.11 Approximate positions of some of the motor points of the back.

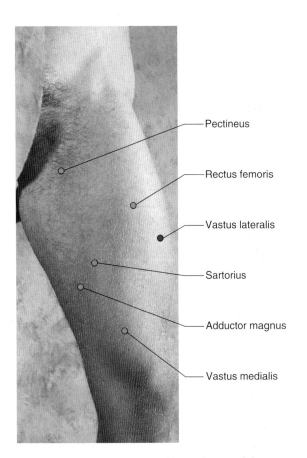

Pectineus

Rectus femoris

Vastus lateralis

Sartorius

Adductor magnus

Vastus medialis

Figure 15.12 Approximate positions of some of the motor points of the left anterior thigh.

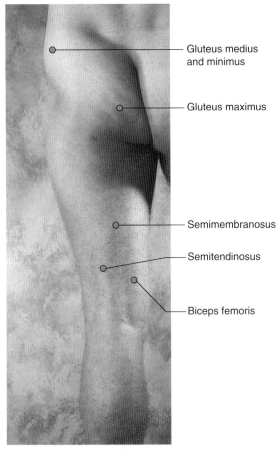

Gluteus medius and minimus

Gluteus maximus

Semimembranosus

Semitendinosus

Biceps femoris

Figure 15.13 Approximate positions of some of the motor points of the posterior thigh.

the approximate positions of these points. It is important to remember, however, that these points act only as a guide: alternative placements may be both more effective and more comfortable for certain individuals. When using this technique, a second dispersive or indifferent electrode must be placed elsewhere on the body part, at a convenient location near to the muscle being treated. This electrode should be larger, so that the current density across it is lower and it is therefore unlikely to elicit either motor or sensory responses. This method is suitable for innervated muscle and is sometimes called a *unipolar* technique.

An alternative electrode positioning system would be the use of electrodes of a similar size placed at either end of a muscle belly or over the bulk of the muscle. This method is suitable for both innervated and denervated muscle and is termed *bipolar*. In this method, location of the motor point is not important but, to identify where best to place the electrodes, it is important to have a good knowledge of the anatomy of the muscle. The easiest way to confirm location is to ask the patient to contract the muscle to be stimulated so that the bulk of the muscle can be located. If it is not possible to contract the muscle in question, the patient can contract the contralateral muscle which can guide placement.

Example: quadriceps and triceps surae placement Electrodes (ranging in size from 3.8×6.35 cm to 7.6×12.7 cm) can be placed transversely across the width of the proximal and distal quadriceps femoris, or across the width of the proximal portion of the medial and lateral gastrocnemius muscles just below the joint line, and longitudinally over the distal portion of the soleus superior to the Achilles tendon (Stackhouse et al 2005). An alternative method of electrode placement is identified by Alon et al (2005), who placed the two electrodes (7.7×12.7 cm) in parallel to the quadriceps muscle (see Fig. 15.2).

Treatment parameters

The treatment parameters affecting muscle and nerve response are described in Chapter 13. These include current waveform, pulse amplitude and duration, pulse frequency, duty cycle, ramp modulation and duration of treatment. Patient preference must also be borne in mind, although it is not clear from the literature which waveforms are most acceptable. Bowman and Barker (1985) suggest that symmetrical, biphasic waves are generally preferred, whereas Delitto and Rose (1986) reported no significant differences between sinusoidal, rectangular and triangular waves. The therapist should therefore adjust the waveform to produce a satisfactory contraction in as comfortable a fashion as possible. To produce a contraction of a designated intensity, it should be remembered that the shorter the pulse duration, the greater the pulse amplitude needed; this is demonstrated in the strength–duration curve shown in Figure 13.2. Figure 15.14B shows that the same relationship between pulse duration and amplitude exists for denervated muscle; however, the figure also shows that the whole curve is shifted to the right, such muscle requiring pulses of longer duration and greater amplitude than innervated tissue.

Force of contraction is determined by the amplitude, frequency, duration and shape of the stimulating waveform (these factors are discussed in Chapter 13). A considerable number of researchers have examined the ways in which these parameters can be combined to produce optimal contractions; to date, no single combination of parameters has been shown to be most effective (see the discussion below).

In summary, and regardless of the reason for using electrical stimulation, Table 15.1 provides a guide to the range of parameters that can be used.

STRENGTHENING/RE-EDUCATION

There is a comprehensive review of the parameters that should be used for strengthening muscle in Lake (1992); some of the key details are identified here. The same parameters can be used for re-education as for strengthening, but there is no evidence that high-stimulus intensities are required (Lake 1992). If the aim of treatment is facilitation of muscle contraction, for example in the case of painful inhibition of the quadriceps complex it is important to progress treatment by instructing the patient to 'feel' the muscle action and then try to contract along with the electrical stimulation. Once the patient starts to contract the muscle voluntarily the intensity of NMES can be gradually reduced.

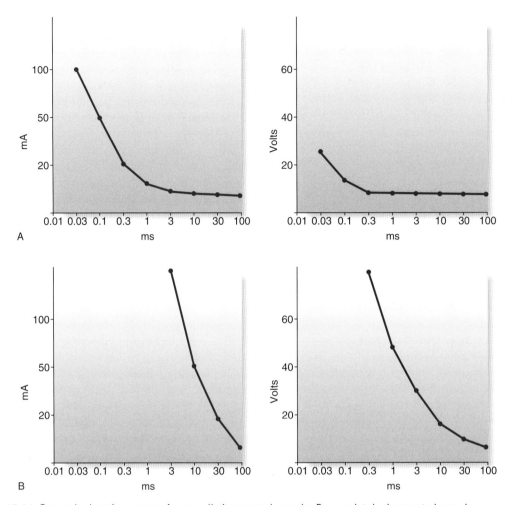

Figure 15.14 Strength–duration curves. A, normally innervated muscle; B, completely denervated muscle.

Table 15.1 Parameters for electrical stimulation

Type of current	Pulsatile or burst-modulated alternating current
Amplitude of stimulation	Maximum tolerable to produce maximum range of movement
Pulse duration	100–300 ms
Waveform	Subject preference
Frequency of stimulation	20–100 pulses or bursts/s
Duty cycle	Start with on : off of 2 s : 10 s or 5 s : 15 s
Type of contractions	Isometric
Number of contractions per session	10–20 at maximum tolerable intensity or 15 minutes per session 2–3 times daily
Frequency of sessions	3–7 times/week

AMPLITUDE

Alon and Smith (2005) provide an excellent overview of the issues surrounding amplitude and NMES. Based on their review of the literature, muscle contraction of between 25 and 50% of maximum voluntary isometric contractions (MVIC) may be required to realize clinically meaningful outcomes. They suggest that conditioning over time is required if participants are to tolerate such levels of MVIC. However, it is worth noting that some participants may not reach the desired stimulation goal (25–50% MVIC) in six sessions and females in particular may require a greater number of conditioning sessions to reach contraction levels of therapeutic benefits (Alon & Smith 2005).

FREQUENCY OF CURRENT

Initially, low frequencies (20 Hz) and short contraction/long relaxation times can be used to minimize muscle fatigue (Jones et al 1979). It is worth noting that the rate of muscle fatigue during NMES is greater than that seen during voluntary contraction (Binder-Macleod & Snyder-Mackler 1993). Lake (1992) suggests 60 Hz as a starting frequency with an on : off ratio of 1 : 3. However, comparison of strength gains produced at 20 Hz, 45 Hz and 80 Hz in normal quadriceps femoris showed no significant difference (Balogun et al 1993).

DUTY CYCLES/RAMP TIMES

The on : off ratio should be modified to match the fatigue characteristics of the muscle being stimulated. A moderate ramp of 2–3 seconds should be used except in cases of high current intensities, where longer ramp-up and ramp-down times (5 seconds) may be more appropriate (Lake 1992). There is evidence that if the on-time is 10 seconds then the off-time must be at least 60 seconds to avoid fatigue (Binder-Macleod & Snyder-Mackler 1993). If the aim of treatment is to strengthen muscle then treatment can be progressed over a number of sessions by increasing the frequency up to 100 Hz (Binder-Macleod & Guerin 1990) and altering the duty cycle so that the contraction time is lengthened and the relaxation time reduced. Evidence suggests that the stronger the induced contraction force in the muscle the greater are the strength gains (Snyder-Mackler et al 1995). In addition, inducing fatigue is an important component of any strengthening regimen (by altering the duty cycle), although in early treatment sessions of weakened muscle the parameters are chosen to minimize fatigue (Lake 1992).

FREQUENCY OF TREATMENT

The frequency of sessions and the number of contractions can also be increased over time and generally follow the same principles used in voluntary exercise strengthening programmes, that is, 8–15 maximum contractions per session, for three to five sessions per week, over 3–6 weeks of training (Bax et al 2005, Lake 1992).

MOTOR RECOVERY FOLLOWING NEUROLOGICAL DAMAGE

Comparison of parameters used between studies reveals a wide range (Chae et al 1998, Fransisco et al 1998, Hesse et al 1998, Pandyan et al 1997, Powell et al 1999, Weingarden et al 1998). However, in general the parameter ranges were: frequency 20–100 Hz, pulse duration 200–300 ms, short ramp-up and ramp-down and intensities set to produce a maximum range of movement. NMES was most commonly applied for 30 minutes two to three times daily, although in one study this was increased to several hours a day (Weingarden et al 1998). Treatment was applied for varying periods of time ranging from 8 weeks (Powell et al 1999) to 6 months (Weingarden et al 1998). Although no studies have been carried out in this group of subjects to identify whether an optimum range of parameters exists, a recent review by de Kroon et al (2005) helps to inform the reader. The authors attempted to explore the relationship between outcome and stimulation characteristics. Unfortunately, there were insufficient data to make any judgement on outcome and pulse duration, amplitude or the number of muscles stimulated. Moreover, there was no relationship between the frequency of stimulation or the total/weekly dose (in hours) and positive or negative trials. However, those trials that used some method of linking the patient's voluntary activity to the triggering of electrical stimulation produced more positive results (de Kroon et al, 2005).

SHOULDER SUBLUXATION AFTER STROKE

Ada & Fonchomcheay (2002) provide an overview of the parameters used in subluxation trials. Most trials used frequencies of around 30 Hz, pulse duration of 350 ms, duty cycle ratios initially of 1:3 and 1:5 with very brief contraction times of 2 seconds; these were gradually increased up to 12–24 seconds and the relaxation time was reduced to 2 seconds. Intervention was given over 4–6 weeks, 5–7 days/week. The length of application changed from 90 minutes to 6 hours daily. All trials applied electrical stimulation to supraspinatus and deltoid muscles.

REDUCTION OF SPASTICITY

Based on the studies cited above, the following parameters have been used most often to produce a reduction in spasticity: frequency of 20–50 Hz; pulse duration 200–500 ms; ramp of 0.1–05 ms; on:off time with equal short contraction and rest times (i.e. 2 s:2 s or 5 s:5 s); intensity with just minimal movement to full available range of movement; session time of 30 minutes for 3–5 days up to 2–6 months and frequency of sessions two to three times daily.

Children: strengthening atrophied muscle in neurological conditions

Regardless of the type of electrical stimulation used, most authors in the studies discussed above used similar parameters (i.e. frequencies of 30–45 Hz, pulse durations of 100–300 ms, ramp pulse shapes with rise times of 0.5–2 seconds). There was some variation in on:off times but most studies used equal on:off times (Carmick 1993a, b, 1995, 1997, Comeaux et al 1997, Pape et al 1993, Steinbok et al 1997). Intensity and the total treatment time depended on the type of stimulation required. TES tended to be applied for at least 48 hours per week for 6–14 months whereas NMES was most commonly applied for 1–3 hours per week in short daily sessions over a 2-month period (Kerr et al 2004).

CONTRAINDICATIONS AND HAZARDS

A more detailed consideration of the contraindications is included in Chapter 21. The key issues are listed below.

NMES should not be used, or should be used with caution, in patients with:

- pacemakers
- peripheral vascular disease, especially when there is the possibility of loosening thrombi
- hypertension and hypotension, because NMES may affect the autonomic responses of these patients
- areas of excess adipose tissue, e.g. obese subjects, because they require high levels of stimuli, that may lead to autonomic changes
- neoplastic tissue
- areas of active tissue infection
- devitalized skin, e.g. after treatment with deep X-ray therapy
- cognitive difficulties making them unable to understand the nature of the intervention or provide feedback about the treatment.

In addition, treatment should not be applied over the following areas:

- carotid sinus
- thoracic region: it has been suggested that transthoracic NMES may interfere with the function of the heart
- phrenic nerve
- trunk: in a pregnant subject.

The hazards that should be guarded against when using NMES include:

- chemical damage due to inadequate skin protection when direct or interrupted direct current is used
- disruption of stimulating devices due to the proximity of diathermy equipment, which can result in altered output.

CONCLUSION

Electrical stimulation of innervated muscle continues to be a popular form of treatment; stimulation of denervated muscle is less popular. As with many other electrophysical agents, there are still major gaps in our knowledge about the effects of electrical stimulation, the most effective parameters for its use and its long-term efficacy.

References

Ada L, Foongchomcheay A (2002) Efficacy of electrical stimulation in preventing or reducing subluxation of the shoulder after stroke: a meta-analysis. *Aust J Physiother* **48**: 257–267.

Alfieri V (1982) Electrical treatments of spasticity: reflex tonic activity in hemiplegic patients and selected specific electrostimulation. *Scand J Rehab Med* **14**: 177–182.

Alon G, Smith GV (2005) Tolerance and conditioning to neuromuscular electrical stimulation within and between sessions and gender. *J Sports Sci Med* **4**: 395–405.

Alon G, Taylor DJ (1997) Electrically elicited minimal visible tetanic contraction and its effect on abdominal muscles strength and endurance. *Eur J Phys Med Rehab* **7**: 2–6.

Alon G, McCombe SA, Koutsantonis S et al (1987) Comparison of the effects of electrical stimulation and exercise on abdominal musculature. *J Orthop Sports Phys Ther* **8**: 567–573.

Apkarian JA, Naumann S (1991) Stretch reflex inhibition using electrical stimulation in normal subjects and subjects with spasticity. *J Biomed Eng* **13**: 67–73.

American Physical Therapy Association (ATPA) (1990). *Electrotherapeutic Terminology in Physical Therapy*. Section on Clinical Electrophysiology, Alexandria, VA: American Physical Therapy Association, 1990.

Arna Risberg M, Lewek M, Snyder-Mackler L (2004) A systematic review of evidence for anterior cruciate ligament rehabilitation: how much and what type? *Phys Ther Sport* **5**(3): 125–145.

Artieda J, Quesada P, Obeso J (1991) Reciprocal inhibition between forearm muscles in spastic hemiplegia. *Neurology* **41**: 286–289.

Atwater SW, Tatarka ME, Kathrein JE, Shapiro S (1991) Electromyography-triggered electrical muscle stimulation for children with cerebral palsy: a pilot study. *Pediatr Phys Ther* **3**: 190–199.

Balogun JA, Onilari OO, Akeju OA et al (1993) High voltage electrical stimulation in the augmentation of muscle strength: effects of pulse frequency. *Arch Phys Med Rehab* **74**: 910–916.

Barecca S, Wolf SL, Fasoli S et al (2003) Treatment interventions for the poetic upper limb of stroke survivors: a critical review. *Neurorehabil Neural Repair* **17**(4):220–226.

Bax L, Staes F, Verhagen A (2005) Does neuromuscular electrical stimulation strengthen the quadriceps femoris? A systematic review of randomised controlled trials. *Sports Med* **35**(3): 191–212.

Beck S (1997) Use of sensory level electrical stimulation in the physical therapy management of a child with cerebral palsy. *Pediatr Phys Ther* **9**: 137–138.

Berghmans LCM, Hendriks HJM, Bo K et al (1998) Conservative treatment of stress urinary incontinence in women: a systematic review of randomized clinical trials. *Br J Urol* **82**:181–191.

Berghmans B, Bo K, Hendriks E et al (2004) Electrical stimulation with non-implanted electrodes for urinary incontinence in adults. (Protocol) Cochrane Database of Systematic Reviews 3. Art. No.: CD001202. DOI: 10.1002/14651858.CD001202.pub2.

Binder-Macleod SA, Guerin T (1990) Preservation of force output through progressive reduction of stimulation frequency in human quadriceps femoris muscle. *Phys Ther* **70**: 619–625.

Binder-Macleod SA, Snyder-Mackler L (1993) Muscle fatigue: clinical implications for fatigue assessment and neuromuscular electrical stimulation. *Phys Ther* **73**(12): 902–910.

Botte MJ, Nickel VL, Akeson WH (1988) Spasticity and contractures. Physiologic aspects of formation. *Clin Orthop* **233**: 7–18.

Bowman BR, Barker LL (1985) Effects of waveform parameters on comfort during transcutaneous neuromuscular electrical stimulation. *Ann Biomed Eng* **13**: 59–74.

Carmick J (1993a) Clinical use of neuromuscular electrical stimulation for children with cerebral palsy, part 1: lower extremity. *Phys Ther* **73**: 505–513.

Carmick J (1993b) Clinical use of neuromuscular electrical stimulation for children with cerebral palsy, part 2: upper extremity. *Phys Ther* **73**: 514–520.

Carmick J (1995) Managing equinus in children with cerebral palsy: electrical stimulation to strengthen the triceps surae muscle. *Dev Med Child Neurol* **37**: 965–975.

Carmick J (1997) Use of neuromuscular electrical stimulation and a dorsal wrist splint to improve the hand function of a child with spastic hemiparesis. *Phys Ther* **77**: 661–671.

Chae J, Bethoux F, Bohinc T et al (1998) Neuromuscular stimulation for upper extremity motor and functional recovery in acute hemiplegia. *Stroke* **19**: 975–979.

Chae J, Kilgore K, Triolo R et al (2000) Neuromuscular stimulation for motor neuroprosthesis in hemiplegia. *Crit Rev Phys Rehab Med* **12**: 1–23.

Comeaux P, Patterson N, Rubin M et al (1997) Effect of neuromuscular electrical stimulation during gait in children with cerebral palsy. *Pediatr Phys Ther* **9**: 103–109.

Daly JJ, Ruff RL (2000) Electrically induced recovery of gait components for older patients with chronic stroke. *Am J Phys Med Rehab* **79**(4): 349–360.

Davies HL (1983) Is electrostimulation beneficial to denervated nerve? A review of results from basic research. *Physiotherapy (Canada)* **35**: 306–310.

de Kroon JR, Ijzerman MJ, Chae J et al (2005) Relation between stimulation characteristics and clinical outcome in studies using electrical stimulation to improve motor control of the upper extremity in stroke. *J Rehab Med* **37**(2): 65–74.

Delitto A, Rose SJ (1986) Comparative comfort of three wave forms used in electrically elicited quadriceps femoris contractions. *Phys Ther* **66**: 1704–1707.

Delitto A, Snyder-Mackler L (1990) Two theories of muscle strength augmentation using percutaneous electrical stimulation. *Phys Ther* **70**: 158–164.

Delitto A, Rose SJ, McKowen JM et al (1988) Electrical stimulation versus voluntary exercise in strengthening thigh musculature after anterior cruciate ligament surgery. *Phys Ther* **68**: 660–663.

Delitto A, Snyder-Mackler L, Robinson AJ (1995) Electrical stimulation of muscle: techniques and applications. In Robinson AJ, Snyder-Mackler L (eds) *Clinical Electrophysiology: Electrotherapy and Electrophysiological Testing*. Baltimore, MD, Williams & Wilkins.

Dietz V, Quintern J, Berger W (1981) Electrophysiological studies of gait in spasticity and rigidity. Evidence that altered mechanical properties of muscle contribute to hypertonia. *Brain* **104**: 431–449.

Faghri D, Rodgers M, Glaser R et al (1994) The effects of functional electrical stimulation on shoulder subluxation, arm function recovery, and shoulder pain in hemiplegic stroke patients. *Arch Phys Med Rehab* **75**: 73–79.

Fitzgerald GK, Piva SR, Irrgang JJ (2003) A modified neuromuscular electrical stimulation protocol for quadriceps strength training following anterior cruciate ligament reconstruction. *J Orthop Sports Phys Ther* **33**: 492–501.

Fransisco G, Chae J, Chawla H et al (1998) Electromyogram-triggered neuromuscular stimulation for improving the arm function of acute stroke survivors: a randomised pilot study. *Arch Phys Med Rehab* **79**: 571–575.

Fynes M, Marshall K, Cassidy M et al (1999) A prospective, randomised study comparing the effect of augmented biofeedback with sensory biofeedback alone on fecal incontinence after obstetric trauma. *Dis Colon Rectum* **42**(6): 753–758.

Glanz M, Klawansky S, Stason W et al (1996) Functional electrostimulation in poststroke rehabilitation: a meta-analysis of the randomised controlled trials. *Arch Phys Med Rehab* **77**: 549–553.

Granit R, Pascoe JE, Steg G (1957) The behaviour of tonic alpha and gamma motor neurones during stimulation of recurrent collaterals. *J Physiol* **13**(8): 381–400.

Grove-Lainey C, Walmsley RP, Andrew GM (1983) Effectiveness of exercise alone versus exercise plus electrical stimulation in strengthening the quadriceps muscle. *Physiotherapy (Canada)* **35**: 5–11.

Hazlewood ME, Brown JK, Rowe PJ et al (1994) The use of therapeutic electrical stimulation in the treatment of hemiplegic cerebral palsy. *Dev Med Child Neurol* **36**: 661–673.

Herbison P, Plevnik S, Mantle J (2002) Weighted vaginal cones for urinary incontinence. Cochrane Database of Systematic Reviews 1. Art. No.: CD002115. DOI: 10.1002/14651858.CD002115.

Hesse S, Reiter F, Konrad M et al (1998) Botulinum toxin type A and short term electrical stimulation in the treatment of upper limb flexor spasticity after stroke: a randomised, double-blind, placebo-controlled trial. *Clin Rehab* **12**: 381–388.

Hömberg V (1997) Is rehabilitation effective in spastic syndromes? In Thilmann F et al (eds) *Spasticity Mechanisms and Management*. Berlin, Springer-Verlag: 439–450.

Hosker G, Norton C, Brazzelli M (2000) Electrical stimulation for faecal incontinence in adults. Cochrane Database of Systematic Reviews, 1. Art. No.: CD001310. DOI: 10.1002/14651858.CD001310.

Hummelsheim H, Mauritz KH (1993) Neurological mechanisms of spasticity. Modification by physiotherapy. In Thilmann F et al (eds) *Spasticity Mechanisms and Management*. Berlin, Springer-Verlag: 427–437.

Jones DA, Bigland-Ritchie B, Edwards RHT (1979) Excitation frequency and muscle fatigue: mechanical responses during voluntary and stimulated contractions. *Exper Neurol* **64**: 401–413.

Kahanovitz N, Nordin M, Verderame R et al (1987) Normal trunk muscle strength and endurance in woman and the effects of exercises and electrical stimulation, part 2: comparative analysis of electrical stimulation and exercises to increase trunk muscle strength and endurance. *Spine* **12**: 112–118.

Kerr C, McDowell B, McDonough SM (2004). Electrical stimulation: effects on muscle strength and motor function. *Dev Med Child Neurol* **46**: 205–213.

Kerr C, McDowell B, McDonough S et al (2006) Electrical Stimulation for muscle strengthening in cerebral palsy: a randomized placebo controlled trial. *Dev Med Child Neurol* **48**: 870–876.

Lake DA (1988) The effects of neuromuscular stimulation as applied by 'toning salons' on muscle strength and body shape. *Phys Ther* **68**: 789. Abstract RO77.

Lake DA (1992) Neuromuscular electrical stimulation. An overview of its application in the treatment of sports injuries. *Sports Med* **15**(5): 320–336.

Lake DA, Gillespie WJ (1988) Electrical stimulation (NMES) does not decrease body fat. *Med Sci Sports Exerc* **20** (suppl): S22. Abstract 131.

Levine MG, Knott M, Kabot H (1952) Relaxation of spasticity by electrical stimulation of antagonist muscles. *Arch Phys Med* **33**: 668–673.

Lieber RL, Silva PD, Daniel DM (1996) Equal effectiveness of electrical and volitional strength training for quadriceps femoris muscles after anterior cruciate ligament surgery. *J Orthop Res* **14**: 131–138.

Lyons CL, Robb JB, Irrgang JJ et al (2005) Differences in quadriceps femoris muscle torque when using a clinical electrical stimulator versus a portable electrical stimulator. *Phys Ther* **85**(1): 44–51.

Mahony R, Malone P, Nalty J et al (2004) Prospective randomized comparison of intra-anal electromyographic biofeedback and intra-anal electromyographic feedback augmented with electrical stimulation of the anal sphincter. *Am J Obstet Gynecol* **191**(3): 885–890.

Mizusaki A, Almeida GJM, Atallah AN et al (2006) Electrical stimulation for rehabilitation after soft tissue injury of the knee in adults (Protocol). The Cochrane Database of Systematic Reviews 4 Art. No.:CD001826.pub2. DOI:10.1002/14651858.CD001826.pub2.

Moehrer B, Hextall A, Jackson S (2002) Oestrogens for urinary incontinence in women. In *The Cochrane Library*, Issue 1. Oxford: Update Software.

Nelson H, Smith M, Bowman B et al (1980) Electrode effectiveness during transcutaneous motor stimulation. *Arch Phys Med Rehab* **61**: 73–77.

Nolan MF (1991) Conductive differences in electrodes used with transcutaneous electrical nerve stimulation devices. *Phys Ther* **71**: 746–751.

Norton C, Cody JD, Hosker G (2006) Biofeedback and/or sphincter exercise for the treatment of faecal incontinence in adults. Cochrane database of systematic reviews, 3. Art. No.: CD002111. DOI:10.1002/14651858. CD002111.pub2.

Onwude JL (2005) Stress incontinence. Pelvic floor electrical stimulation. *Clinical Evidence*. Online. Available: http://www.clinicalevidence.org/ceweb/conditions/woh/0808/0808_I2.jsp [accessed 20th July 2006].

Pandyan AD, Granat MH, Stott DJ (1997) Effects of electrical stimulation on flexion contractures in hemiplegic wrist. *Clin Rehab* **11**: 123–130.

Pape K (1997) Therapeutic electrical stimulation (TES) for the treatment of disuse muscle atrophy in cerebral palsy. *Pediatr Phys Ther* **9**: 110–112.

Paternostro-Sluga T, Fialka C, Alacamliogliu Y et al (1999) Neuromuscular electrical stimulation after anterior cruciate ligament surgery. *Clin Orthop Rel Res* **368**: 166–175.

Pease W (1998) Therapeutic electrical stimulation for spasticity. Quantitative gait analysis. *Am J Phys Med Rehab* **77**: 351–355.

Pelland L, Brosseau L, Casimiro L et al (2002) Electrical stimulation for the treatment of rheumatoid arthritis. The Cochrane database of systematic reviews. 2, Art. No.: CD003687. DOI: 10.1002/14651858.CD003687.

Porcari JP, Miller J, Cornwell K et al (2005) The effects of neuromuscular electrical stimulation training on abdominal strength, endurance, and selected anthropometric measures. *J Sports Sci Med* **4**: 66–75.

Powell J, Pandyan D, Granat M et al (1999) Electrical stimulation of wrist extensors in poststroke hemiplegia. *Stroke* **30**: 1384–1389.

Robinson AJ (1995) Instrumentation for Electrotherapy, p 64. In *Electrotherapy and Electrophysiological Testing*. Robinson AJ, Snyder-Mackler L (eds). Baltimore, MD, Williams & Wilkins.

Ryall RW, Piercy MF, Polosa C et al (1972) Excitation of Renshaw cells in relation to orthodromic and antidromic excitation of motor neurons. *J Neurophysiol* **35**: 137–148.

Sand PK, Richardson DA, Staskin DR et al (1995) Pelvic floor electrical stimulation in the treatment of genuine stress incontinence: a multicenter, placebo-controlled trial. *Am J Obstet Gynecol* **173**: 72–79.

Selkowitz DM (1989) High frequency electrical stimulation in muscle strengthening. A review and discussion. *Am J Sports Med* **17**(1): 103–111.

Singer KP, Gow PJ, Otway WF et al (1983) A comparison of electrical muscle stimulation isometric, isotonic and isokinetic strength training programmes. *NZ J Sports Med* **11**: 61–63.

Sisk TD, Stralka SW, Deering MB et al (1987) Effects of electrical stimulation on quadriceps strength after reconstructive surgery of the anterior cruciate ligament. *Am J Sports Med* **15**: 215–219.

Snyder-Mackler L, Ladin Z, Schepsis A et al (1991) Electrical stimulation of the thigh muscles after reconstruction of the anterior cruciate ligament. Effect of electrically elicited contractions of the quadriceps femoris and hamstring muscles on gait and strength of the thigh muscles. *J Bone Joint Surg (Am)* **73**: 1025–1036.

Stackhouse SK, Binder-Macleod SA, Lee SCK (2005) Voluntary muscle activation, contractile properties, and fatigability in children with and without cerebral palsy. *Muscle Nerve* **31**: 594–601.

Steinbok P, Reiner A, Kestle JR (1997) Therapeutic electrical stimulation following selective posterior rhizotomy in children with spastic diplegic cerebral palsy: a randomized clinical trial. *Dev Med Child Neurol* **39**: 515–520.

Vodovnik L, Bowman BR, Hufford P (1984) Effects of electrical stimulation on spinal spasticity. *Scand J Rehab Med* **16**: 29–34.

Weingarden HP, Zeilig G, Heruti R (1998) Hybrid functional electrical stimulation orthosis system for the upper limb. Effects on spasticity in chronic stable hemiplegia. *Am J Phys Med Rehab* **77**(4): 276–281.

William JG, Street M (1976) Sequential faradism in quadriceps rehabilitation. *Physiotherapy* **62**: 252–254.

Chapter 16

Transcutaneous electrical nerve stimulation (TENS)

Mark I. Johnson

INTRODUCTION

Transcutaneous electrical nerve stimulation (TENS) is a simple, non-invasive analgesic technique that is used for the symptomatic management of acute and non-malignant chronic pain (Box 16.1; Barlas & Lundeberg 2006, Walsh 1997a, Woolf & Thompson 1994). TENS is also used in palliative care to manage pain caused by metastatic bone disease and neoplasms (Berkovitch & Waller 2005, Stannard 2002, Thompson & Filshie 1993). It is claimed that TENS also has antiemetic and tissue-healing effects, and that it can improve some of the neurophysiological and behavioural effects of dementia (Cameron et al 2003, Walsh 1997b). It is used less often for these non-analgesic actions.

Surveys show that TENS is one of the most frequently used electrotherapies for pain relief and that it is available throughout the world (Johnson 1997, Pope et al 1995, Reeve et al 1996, Robertson & Spurritt 1998). TENS is popular because it is cheap, non-invasive, easy to administer, has few side effects and has no drug interactions. There is no potential for toxicity or overdose. TENS is commonly prescribed by doctors, physiotherapists, nurses and midwives; patients in the UK can also buy a TENS device for their own use. It is preferable for patients to administer TENS for themselves, following appropriate instruction by a healthcare professional. TENS effects are rapid in onset for most patients, so benefit can be achieved almost immediately.

During TENS, pulsed electrical currents are generated by a portable pulse generator and delivered across the intact surface of the skin via conducting pads called electrodes (Fig. 16.1). The conventional way of administering TENS is to use electrical characteristics that selectively activate large-diameter non-noxious afferents (Aβ) without activating smaller-diameter nociceptive fibres (Aδ and C). Evidence suggests that this will produce pain relief in a similar way to 'rubbing the pain better'. In practice, conventional TENS is delivered to generate a strong but comfortable paraesthesia within, or close to, the site of pain using frequencies anywhere between 1 and 200 pulses per second (pps) and pulse durations anywhere between 50 and 500 µs.

Box 16.1 Common medical conditions for which TENS has been used

Analgesic effects of TENS
Relief of acute pain
- Postoperative pain
- Labour pain
- Dysmenorrhoea
- Angina pectoris
- Orofacial pain, including dental procedures
- Physical trauma, including fractured ribs and minor medical procedures

Relief of chronic pain
- Low back pain
- Arthritic pain, including osteoarthritis, rheumatoid arthritis
- Muscle pain, including myofascial pain, muscle tension, post-exercise soreness
- Neuropathic pain, including post amputation, post-herpetic, trigeminal neuralgia
- Cancer pain, including metastatic bone pain
- Complex regional pain syndrome

Non-analgesic effects of TENS
Neuropsychological and behavioural effects
- Reducing symptoms of Alzheimer's dementia

Neuromuscular stimulating effects
- Faecal and urinary incontinence

Antiemetic effects
- Nausea from pregnancy, travelling, chemotherapy, postoperative opioid medication
- Improving blood flow
- Raynaud's disease
- Wound healing
- Ischaemia due to reconstructive surgery

HISTORY

The use of electricity to relieve pain is an age-old technique. The ancient Egyptians used electrogenic fish to treat ailments in 2500 BC, although the Roman

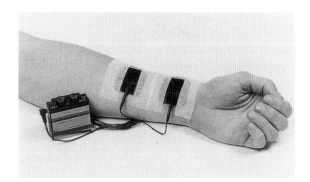

Figure 16.1 A standard device delivering TENS to the arm. There is increasing use of self-adhesive electrodes rather than black carbon-rubber electrodes that require conductive gel and tape as shown in the diagram.

physician Scribonius Largus is credited with the first written report of the use of electrogenic fish in medicine in AD 46 (Kane & Taub 1975). The development of electrostatic generators in the eighteenth century increased the use of medical electricity, although popularity declined in the nineteenth and early twentieth centuries owing to variable clinical results and the development of pharmacological treatments (Stillings 1975). Interest in the use of electricity to relieve pain was re-awakened in 1965 by Melzack and Wall, who provided a physiological rationale for electroanalgesic effects. They proposed that transmission of noxious information could be inhibited by activity in large-diameter peripheral afferents or by activity in pain inhibitory pathways descending from the brain (Fig. 16.2). Wall and Sweet (1967) used high-frequency percutaneous electrical stimulation to artificially activate large-diameter peripheral afferents and found that this relieved chronic pain in patients. Pain relief was also demonstrated when electrical currents were used to stimulate the periaqueductal grey (PAG) region of the midbrain (Reynolds 1969), which is part of the descending pain inhibitory pathway. Shealy et al (1967) found that electrical stimulation of the dorsal columns, which form the central

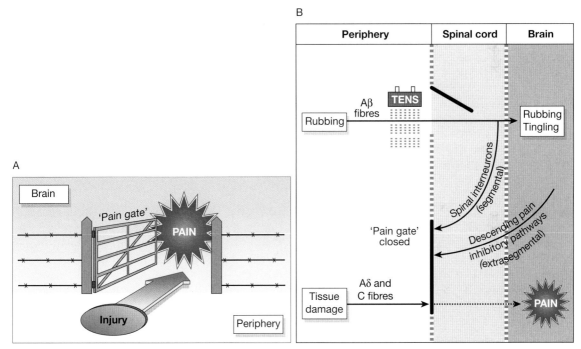

Figure 16.2 The 'pain gate'. Under normal physiological circumstances, the brain generates pain sensations by processing incoming noxious information arising from stimuli such as tissue damage. If noxious information is to reach the brain it must pass through a metaphorical 'pain gate', which is located in lower levels of the central nervous system. In physiological terms, the gate is formed by excitatory and inhibitory synapses regulating the flow of neural information through the central nervous system. This 'pain gate' is opened by noxious events in the periphery; it can be closed by activation of mechanoreceptors through 'rubbing the skin'. This generates activity in large-diameter Aβ afferents, which inhibits the onward transmission of noxious information. This closing of the 'pain gate' results in less noxious information reaching the brain, which results in a reduction in the sensation of pain. The neuronal circuitry involved is segmental in its organization. The aim of conventional TENS is to activate Aβ fibres using electrical currents. The 'pain gate' can also be closed by the activation of pain inhibitory pathways, which originate in the brain and descend to the spinal cord through the brain stem (extrasegmental circuitry). These pathways become active during psychological activities, such as motivation, and when small-diameter peripheral fibres are excited physiologically. The aim of AL-TENS is to excite small-diameter peripheral fibres to activate the descending pain inhibitory pathways.

transmission pathway of large-diameter peripheral afferents, also produced pain relief. TENS was used to predict the success of dorsal column stimulation implants until it was realised that TENS could be used as a successful modality on its own (Long 1973, 1974).

DEFINITION

By strict definition, TENS is anything that delivers electricity across the intact surface of the skin to activate underlying nerves. Healthcare professionals use the term 'TENS' to describe a 'standard TENS device' (see Fig. 16.1), although literature about TENS uses ambiguous and inconsistent nomenclature. This has resulted in inappropriate clinical practice.

THE STANDARD TENS DEVICE

Standard TENS devices are characterized by their technical output characteristics, and in the UK they retail at between £30 and £150 (Table 16.1). Standard TENS devices vary between manufacturers but these variations are minor and have a limited impact on the physiological effects produced. Standard TENS devices usually deliver biphasic pulsed currents in a repetitive manner using pulse durations of between 50 and 500 μs and pulse frequencies of between 1 and 200 pulses per second (pps) [American Physical Therapy Association (APTA) 1990, Barlas & Lundeberg 2006, Mannheimer & Lampe 1987, Sjölund et al 1990, Walsh 1997a, Woolf & Thompson 1994]. Pulses are usually delivered in a continuous pattern, although most modern devices have other patterns available, such as burst, modulated amplitude, modulated frequency, and modulated pulse duration (Fig. 16.3).

TENS-LIKE DEVICES

Developments in electronic technology have flooded the market with a variety of TENS-like devices (Table 16.2). TENS-like devices have been defined as any stimulating device that delivers electrical currents across the intact surface of the skin and whose technical output specifications

Table 16.1 Typical features on TENS devices

Feature	Examples
Weight	50–250 g
Dimensions	6 × 5 × 2 cm (small device)
	12 × 9 × 4 cm (large device)
Cost	£30–150
Pulse waveform (fixed)	Monophasic
	Symmetrical biphasic
	Asymmetrical biphasic
Pulse amplitude (adjustable)	1–50 mA into a 1 kΩ load
Pulse duration (often fixed)	50–500 μs
Pulse frequency (adjustable)	1–200 pps
Pulse pattern	Continuous, burst (random frequency, modulated amplitude, modulated frequency, modulated pulse duration)
Channels	1 or 2
Batteries	PP3 (9 V), rechargeable
Additional features	Timer
	Most devices deliver constant current output

and generic name differ from those of TENS (Johnson 2003). This includes interferential current therapy (IFT), microcurrent electrical therapy (MET), high-voltage pulsed (galvanic) current (HVPC), transcutaneous spinal electroanalgesia (TSE), action potential simulation (APS), H-wave therapy (HWT), Pain®Gone and transcranial electrical stimulation (TCES), to name but a few. TENS-like devices often have design features that are unique to a particular device and this makes categorization difficult. For example, some MET devices deliver currents at the site of pain using standard TENS electrodes; others deliver MET transcranially (e.g. as a type of TCES), and others deliver MET using a pen-like electrode. Claims about the relative effectiveness of TENS-like devices are overambitious and practitioners should use a standard TENS device in the first instance (Johnson 2003). The remainder of this chapter will focus on TENS administered using a standard TENS device.

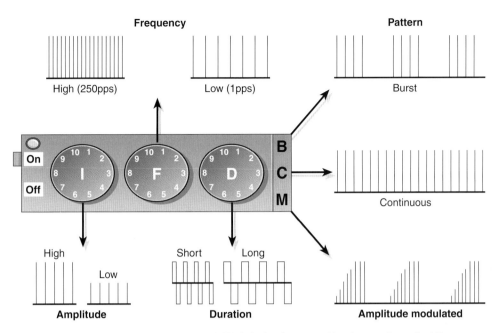

Figure 16.3 The output characteristics of a standard TENS device (topographic view, each vertical line represents one pulse). The intensity control dial (I) regulates the current amplitude of individual pulses; the frequency control dial (F) regulates the rate of pulse delivery (pulses per second; pps) and the pulse duration control dial (D) regulates the time duration of each pulse. Most TENS devices offer patterns of pulse delivery such as burst, continuous and amplitude modulated.

PHYSICAL PRINCIPLES

TENS is a technique-based intervention. Hence, outcome is dependent on the appropriateness of the TENS procedure, which is determined by the user. Users need to select the appropriate location to stimulate, type and number of electrodes, electrical characteristics of currents (i.e. pulse amplitude, frequency, pattern and duration) and dosing regimens (i.e. how often and for how long). To do this the TENS user needs to consider the physiological intention of the TENS treatment.

The physiological intention of TENS when used for pain relief is to selectively activate different populations of nerve fibres to initiate antinociceptive mechanisms that produce clinically meaningful pain relief. The electrical characteristics of TENS determines which population of nerve fibres is activated, so it is important that the TENS user is familiar with the basic principles of nerve fibre activation and how this relates to TENS technique (this is described in Chapter 13).

PRINCIPLES OF NERVE FIBRE ACTIVATION

When the pulse amplitude (intensity) of TENS is increased, non-nociceptive nerve fibres are activated first and the user experiences a non-painful tingling under the electrodes. This is because large-diameter, non-nociceptive (touch) nerve fibres (Aα and Aβ fibres) have lower thresholds of activation to electrical stimuli than their small-diameter nociceptive counterparts (Aδ and C fibres; see Chapters 5 and 6). If the pulse amplitude (intensity) of TENS is increased further, nociceptive nerve fibres are activated and the user experiences a painful tingling under the electrodes.

Pulse durations between 50 and 500 μs enable the user titrate pulse amplitude with greater precision (Howson 1978). Pulsed currents with small amplitudes (i.e. low intensity) and durations between 50 and 500 μs would be best to activate large-diameter fibres (Aβ) without activating small-diameter nociceptive fibres (Aδ and C) (Fig. 16.4). Increasing the pulse duration above 500 μs will lead to the activation of small-diameter fibres at

Table 16.2 Characteristics of some of the commercially available TENS-like devices

Device	Experimental work	Manufacturers claim	Typical Stimulating Characteristics
Action potential simulation (APS)	Odendaal & Joubert (1999)	Pain relief Improve mobility Improve circulation Reduce inflammation	Monophasic square pulse with exponential decay Delivered by two electrodes Pulse amplitude low (<25 mA), duration long (800 μs–6.6 ms), frequency fixed at 150 pps
Codetron	Pomeranz & Niznick (1987) Fargas-Babjak et al (1989; 1992)	Pain relief Reduce habituation	Square wave Delivered randomly to one of 6 electrodes Pulse amplitude low, duration long (1 ms), frequency low (2 pps)
H-wave stimulation	McDowell et al (1995; 1999)	Pain relief Improve mobility Improve circulation Reduce inflammation Promote wound healing	'Unique' biphasic wave with exponential decay Delivered by 2 electrodes Pulse amplitude low (<10 mA), duration long (fixed at 16 ms), frequency low (2–60 pps)
Interferential therapy (interference currents)	See Chapter 17	Pain relief Improve mobility Improve circulation Reduce inflammation Promote wound healing Muscle re-education	Two out of phase currents which interfere with each other to produce an amplitude modulated wave Traditionally, delivered by 4 electrodes; some devices have amplitude modulated waves that are premodulated within the device (two electrodes) Pulse amplitude low, amplitude modulated frequency 1–200 Hz, (carrier wave frequencies approximately 2–4 KHz)
Microcurrent, including transcranial stimulation and 'acupens'	Johannsen et al (1993) Johnson et al (1997)	Promote wound healing Pain relief Other indications often claimed	Modified square direct current with monophasic or biphasic pulses changing polarity at regular intervals (0.4s) Delivered by 2 electrodes Pulse amplitude low (1–600 μA with no paraesthesia), frequency depends on manufacturer (1–5000 pps) Many variants exist (e.g. transcranial stimulation for migraine and insomnia; acupens for pain)
Transcutaneous Spinal Electroanalgesia (TSE)	Macdonald and Coates (1995)	Pain relief, especially allodynia and hyperalgesia due to central sensitisation	Differentiated wave Delivered by two electrodes positioned on spinal cord at T1 and T12 or straddling C3–C5. Pulse amplitude high (although no paraesthesia), duration very short (1.5–4 μs), frequency high (600–10 000 pps)
Pain®Gone	Asbjorn (2000) Ivanova-Stoilova & Howells (2002)	Pain relief Could be non-invasive acupuncture	Hand-held pen device using piezoelectric elements Low-ampere high-voltage (e.g. 6 μA/15 000 V) single monophasic spiked pulse Delivered by giving 30–40 individual shocks at the site of pain or on acupuncture points to generate non-noxious to mild noxious pin-prick sensation; repeated whenever pain returns

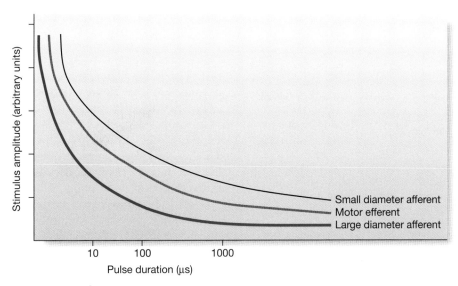

Figure 16.4 Strength–duration curve for fibre activation. As pulse duration increases, less current amplitude is needed to excite an axon to generate an action potential. Small pulse durations are unable to excite nerve axons even at high current amplitudes. Large-diameter axons require lower current amplitudes than small-diameter fibres. Thus, passing pulsed currents across the surface of the skin excites large-diameter non-noxious sensory nerves first (paraesthesia), followed by motor efferents (muscle contraction) and small-diameter noxious afferents (pain). Alteration of pulse duration is one means to help in the selective recruitment of different types of nerve fibre. For example, intense TENS should use long pulse durations (>500 μs) as they activate small-diameter afferents more readily. During conventional TENS pulse durations ~100–200 μs are used as there is a large separation (difference) in the amplitude needed to recruit different types of fibre. This enables greater precision when using the Intensity (amplitude) dial so that a strong but comfortable paraesthesia can be achieved without muscle contraction or pain.

lower pulse amplitudes. The number of nerve impulses generated by TENS will increase according to the frequency of the pulsed currents, although this is limited by the absolute and relative refractory periods for the axon. Theoretically, delivering TENS at high pulse frequencies (up to ~200 pps) should be optimum (for a discussion, see Howson 1978, Walsh 1997e, Woolf & Thompson 1994).

The type of pulsed current waveform used in TENS devices varies between manufacturers. Generally, these can be divided into monophasic or biphasic waveforms (Fig. 16.5). If the TENS device delivers a monophasic pulsed wave, the cathode should be placed proximal to the anode. This is because the cathode activates the axonal membrane, leading to an action potential, and placing the anode proximal could block nerve transmission due to hyperpolarization (Fig. 16.6, and see Chapter 13). The cathode is usually, but not

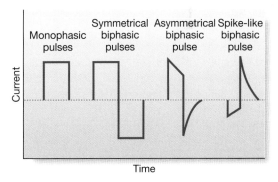

Figure 16.5 Common pulse waveforms used in TENS.

always, the black lead. Many TENS devices use biphasic waveforms whereby the cathode and anode alternate between the two electrodes during stimulation. Biphasic waveforms, which result in zero net current flow, may prevent the build-up

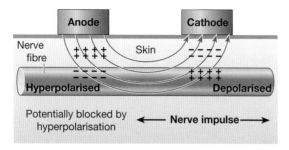

Figure 16.6 Fibre activation by TENS. When devices use waveforms that produce net DC outputs that are not zero, the cathode excites (depolarization) the axon and the nerve impulse will travel in both directions down the axon. The anode tends to inhibit the axon (hyperpolarization), which could extinguish the nerve impulse. Thus, during conventional TENS the cathode should be positioned proximal to the anode so that the nerve impulse is transmitted to the central nervous system unimpeded. However, during AL-TENS the cathode should be placed distally or over the motor point, as the purpose of AL-TENS currents is to activate a motor efferent.

of ion concentrations beneath electrodes and reduce adverse skin reactions due to polar concentrations (Kantor et al 1994, Walsh 1997e). Electrode positioning with these biphasic waveforms is less critical given the zero net DC element and therefore orientation of positive/negative is not thought to make any significant clinical difference.

The theoretical relationship between output characteristics of electrical stimuli delivered and nerve fibre activation can break down in clinical practice. It has been shown that the exact nature and distribution of currents is difficult to predict when they are passed across the intact surface of the skin, due to the complex and non-homogeneous impedance of the tissue underlying electrodes (Demmink 1993). Furthermore, the skin offers high impedance at pulse frequencies used by TENS, so it is likely that currents will remain superficial, stimulating cutaneous nerve fibres rather than the more deep-seated visceral and muscle nerve fibres. Interestingly, however, recent evidence from animal studies suggests that activity in deeper afferents may be responsible for the antinociceptive effects of TENS (Radhakrishnan & Sluka 2005).

PRINCIPLES UNDERPINNING TYPES OF TENS TECHNIQUE

The most common types of TENS technique described in the literature are conventional TENS, acupuncture-like TENS (AL-TENS) and intense TENS (Table 16.3; Barlas & Lundeberg 2006, Mannheimer & Lampe 1987, Sjölund et al 1990, Walsh 1997a, Woolf & Thompson 1994). These TENS techniques suggest the electrical characteristics of the currents that are necessary to activate different types of nerve fibre, although the emphasis on electrical characteristics has resulted in the use of inflexible 'prescriptive protocols' in clinical practice and research. In addition, the emphasis on the electrical characteristics of TENS has driven the development of TENS devices with novel output characteristics (Fig. 16.7), which are based more on technological advances in electronics than on proven physiological effect. In clinical practice in the UK, conventional TENS is most commonly used by patients whereas AL-TENS and intense TENS tend to be used only in specific situations. It is important to establish the physiological intention of each TENS technique to appreciate their relative merits.

CONVENTIONAL TENS

The physiological intention of conventional TENS is to selectively activate large-diameter Aβ fibres (touch related) without concurrently activating small-diameter Aδ and C fibres (pain-related) or muscle efferents (Fig. 16.8). Theoretically, high-frequency (~10–200 pps), low-intensity (non-painful) currents with pulse duration between 50 and 500 μs would be most efficient in selectively activating Aβ fibres (see Table 16.3). As large-diameter fibres have short refractory periods, they can generate nerve impulses at high frequencies. This means that they are more able to generate high-frequency volleys of nerve impulses when high-frequency currents are delivered, resulting in a greater afferent barrage into the central nervous system.

Large-diameter afferent activity is occurring when the user reports 'strong but comfortable' non-painful electrical paraesthesia beneath the electrodes. Animal studies have demonstrated that

Table 16.3 The characteristics of different types of TENS

	Purpose of TENS	Physiological intention of TENS (fibre type responsible for hypoalgesic effects)	Desired outcome/ patient experience	Optimal electrical characteristics	Electrode position	Analgesic profile	Duration of treatment	Main mechanism of analgesic action
Conventional TENS	Selective activation of large-diameter non-noxious afferents	Generate nerve impulses in large-diameter non-noxious afferents (Aβ) arising from mechanoreceptors	Strong, comfortable electrical paraesthesia with minimal muscle activity	High frequency/ low intensity Amplitude = low Duration = usually 100–200 μs Frequency = 10–200 pps Pattern = continuous	Over site of pain Dermatomal	Rapid onset <30 minutes after switch-on Rapid offset <30 minutes after switch-off	Continuously when in pain	Segmental
AL-TENS	Selective activation of motor efferents to produce phasic muscle twitch (cause GIII (Aδ) afferent activity)	Generate nerve impulses in small-diameter non-noxious muscle afferents GIII (Aδ) arising from ergoreceptors	Strong comfortable phasic muscle contraction	Low frequency/ high intensity Amplitude = high Duration = 100–200 μs Frequency = ~100 pps within burst Pattern = burst	Over motor point/ muscle at site of pain Myotomal	Delayed onset >30 minutes after switch-on Delayed offset >1 hour after switch-off	~30 minutes/ session	Extrasegmental Segmental
Intense TENS	Activation of small-diameter noxious afferents	Generate nerve impulses in small-diameter noxious afferents (Aδ) arising from nociceptors	Painful electrical paraesthesia that is tolerable and with minimal muscle contraction	High frequency/ high intensity Amplitude = high but tolerable Duration >500 μs Frequency = ~50–200 pps Pattern = continuous	Over site of pain or proximal over main nerve bundle	Rapid onset <30 minutes after switch-on Delayed offset >1 hour after switch-off May experience hypoaesthesia	~15 minutes/ session	Peripheral Extrasegmental Segmental

AL-TENS, Acupuncture-like TENS; GIII, Group III afferents.

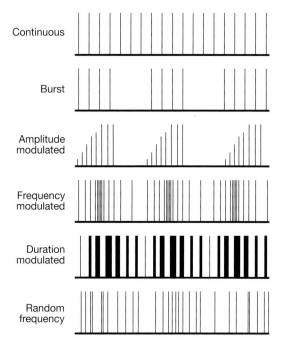

Figure 16.7 Novel pulse patterns available on TENS devices. Modulated patterns fluctuate between upper and lower limits over a fixed period of time; this is usually preset in the design of the TENS device.

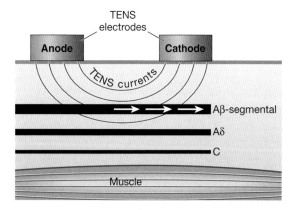

Figure 16.8 The aim of conventional TENS is to selectively activate Aβ afferents producing segmental analgesia.

TENS-induced large-diameter afferent activity inhibits ongoing transmission of nociceptive information in the spinal cord and reduces central sensitization (Garrison & Foreman 1994, 1996, Ma & Sluka 2001, Sandkuhler 2000). This effect is often rapid in onset and offset. Studies on healthy human participants exposed to experimentally induced pain in laboratory settings demonstrate that TENS applied at a strong but comfortable level produces hypoalgesic effects over and above those seen with sham TENS (Johnson & Tabasam 1999, 2003, Walsh 1997d). Hence users should be trained to titrate pulse amplitude so that it is strong enough to generate a non-noxious paraesthesia (Aβ activity) without frank pain (Aδ or C fibre activity). It is claimed that the magnitude of analgesia achieved during conventional TENS depends in part on the pulse frequency. This is supported by studies in animals, which demonstrate that high- and low-frequency TENS may generate differential antihyperalgesic effects, which use different neurochemicals (Radhakrishnan & Sluka 2003, Radhakrishnan et al 2003, Sjölund 1985, Sluka et al 2000, 2005). However, the results of experimental studies in healthy human subjects and patients are inconsistent, with some demonstrating frequency-dependent effects (De Tommaso et al 2003, Johnson et al 1989, Walsh et al 1995) and others not (Barr et al 1986, Cramp et al 2000, Foster et al 1996, Walsh et al 2000).

ACUPUNCTURE-LIKE TENS (AL-TENS)

AL-TENS is often described – in vague terms – to be the delivery of low-frequency (e.g. <10 pps), high-intensity TENS. This has led to confusion about its physiological intention (Johnson 1998). Most, but not all, opinion leaders define AL-TENS as the induction of forceful but non-painful phasic muscle contractions at myotomes related to the origin of the pain (Eriksson & Sjölund 1976, Johnson 1998, Meyerson 1983, Sjölund et al 1990, Walsh 1997a). However, most research reports articulate AL-TENS as low-frequency, high-intensity TENS without any reference to the presence or absence of muscle contractions. Some commentators describe AL-TENS as the delivery of TENS over acupuncture points irrespective of muscle activity (Lewers et al 1989, Lewis et al 1990, Longobardi et al 1989, Rieb & Pomeranz 1992). It is possible that there are differences in physiological action when TENS is applied over acupuncture points in this way (see reviews by Johnson 1998, Walsh 1996).

The physiological intention of AL-TENS, as described by the opinion leaders who developed it, is to generate activity in small-diameter muscle afferents (Aδ or group III) that arise from ergoreceptors and respond to muscle contraction (Eriksson & Sjölund 1976, Sjölund et al 1990). This is achieved indirectly by activating Aα efferents to produce a forceful but non-painful phasic muscle twitch (Anderson et al 1973, Eriksson & Sjölund 1976, Eriksson et al 1979; Fig. 16.9). AL-TENS is administered over muscles or motor points at high but non-painful intensities using low-frequency pulses (~1–10 pps) or low-frequency bursts of pulses (~2–5 bursts per second of 100 pps). Burst patterns of pulse delivery were originally incorporated on TENS devices as they were found to be more comfortable than low-frequency single pulses in producing muscle twitches (Eriksson & Sjölund, 1976). The impulses generated in small-diameter muscle afferents initiate extrasegmental antinociceptive mechanisms and the release of endogenous opioid peptides in a manner similar to that suggested for acupuncture (Meyerson 1983, Sjölund et al 1977). It should be remembered that currents delivered during AL-TENS will also activate Aβ fibres during their passage through the skin leading to segmental analgesia (see Table 16.3).

INTENSE TENS

The physiological intention of intense TENS is to activate small-diameter Aδ afferents by delivering TENS over peripheral nerves arising form the site of pain at an intensity that is just tolerable to the patient (Jeans 1979, Melzack et al 1983; Fig. 16.10). Currents are administered at high frequencies (up to 200 pps) to prevent phasic muscle twitches that would be too forceful for the patient to tolerate (see Table 16.3). Cutaneous Aδ afferent activity has been shown to block transmission of nociceptive information in peripheral nerves and to activate extrasegmental antinociceptive mechanisms (Chung et al 1984a, 1984b, Ignelzi & Nyquist 1976, 1979, Woolf et al 1980). Intense TENS will also activate Aβ fibres, producing segmental antinociceptive effects. As intense TENS acts in part as a counterirritant, it can be delivered for only a short time; however, it may prove useful for minor surgical procedures such as wound dressing and

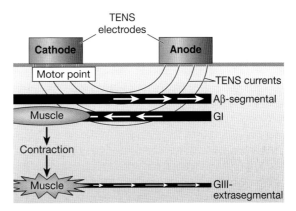

Figure 16.9 The aim of AL-TENS is to selectively activate group I (GI/Aδ) efferents, producing a muscle contraction that results in activity in ergoreceptors and group III (GIII) afferents. GIII afferents are small in diameter and have been shown to produce extrasegmental analgesia through the activation of descending pain inhibitory pathways. Aβ afferents will also be activated during AL-TENS producing segmental analgesia. Note the position of the cathode.

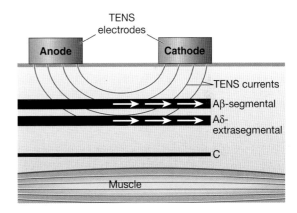

Figure 16.10 The aim of intense-TENS is to selectively activate Aδ afferents leading to extrasegmental analgesia. Aβ afferents will also be activated, producing segmental analgesia.

suture removal (Mannheimer & Lampe 1987). Despite a large published literature on TENS there is a lack of good-quality and systematic experimental work that has directly compared the clinical effectiveness and analgesic profiles of these types of TENS.

PRINCIPLES UNDERLYING APPLICATION

The patient's report of the sensation produced by TENS is the easiest means of assessing the type of fibre activity. A strong, non-painful electrical paraesthesia is mediated by large-diameter cutaneous afferents, as intended with conventional TENS; a painful electrical paraesthesia is mediated by small-diameter cutaneous afferents, as intended by intense TENS; a strong, non-painful phasic muscle contraction is likely to excite muscle ergoreceptors, as intended by AL-TENS. Patients should be trained to titrate the amplitude, frequency and duration of pulsed currents to produce the appropriate outcome. Before patients use TENS for the first time it is important to assess their pain and to instruct them on the safe use of TENS (Box 16.1).

CONTRAINDICATIONS AND PRECAUTIONS

There are very few reported cases of adverse events associated with TENS in the literature. Nevertheless, patients need to be informed of potential hazards so that they can give valid consent to treatment. Decisions on whether to prescribe TENS to a patient are taken according to the professional judgement of the healthcare professional. In difficult cases it is always wise to seek the views of medical and allied health profession colleagues.

Contraindications

In clinical practice, healthcare practitioners have to assess the risk of using TENS against the risk associated with using other available treatments, including drug medication. TENS usually evaluates favourably. Contraindications to TENS are few and mostly hypothetical (Table 16.4). TENS manufacturers list cardiac pacemakers, pregnancy and epilepsy as contraindications. From a legal perspective it may be difficult to exclude TENS as a potential cause of a problem in these patient groups. However, it is possible to use TENS in these patients providing TENS is not applied locally and the patient's progress is carefully monitored throughout (Watson 2006). Most importantly, the situation must been discussed with the patients physician.

Box 16.2 Protocol for the safe application of TENS

- Check contraindications with patient
- Test skin for normal sensation using blunt/ sharp test
- TENS device should be switched off and electrode leads disconnected
- Set electrical characteristics of TENS while device is switched off (see Tables 16.6 and 16.7)
- Connect electrodes to pins on lead wire and position electrodes on patient's skin
- Ensure TENS device is still switched off and connect the electrode wire to the TENS device
- Switch the TENS device on
- Gradually (slowly) increase the intensity until the patient experiences the first 'tingling' sensation from the stimulator
- Gradually (slowly) increase the intensity further until the patient experiences a 'strong but comfortable' tingling sensation
- This intensity should not be painful or cause muscle contraction (unless intense TENS or AL-TENS are being used)

Protocol for the safe termination of TENS
- Gradually (slowly) decrease the intensity until the patient experiences no tingling sensation
- Switch the TENS device off
- Disconnect the electrode wire from the TENS device
- Disconnect electrodes from the pins on lead wire
- Remove the electrodes from the patient's skin

Cardiac pacemakers Patients with cardiac pacemakers should not use TENS unless this has been discussed with their cardiologist. This is because the electrical field generated by TENS could interfere with implanted electrical devices. Rasmussen et al (1988) found that TENS did not interfere with pacemaker performance in 51 patients. However, Pyatt et al (2003) reported that TENS did interfere with pacemaker function in a patient who had received a biventricular ICD for malignant ventricular arrhythmias and medically refractory cardiac failure. The patient experienced bradycardia and dizziness. TENS has been reported to induce artefacts on monitoring equipment (Hauptman & Raza 1992, Sliwa & Marinko 1996). Chen et al

Table 16.4

Contraindication	Advice
'Undiagnosed pain'	Ensure patient has undergone assessment by a healthcare professional
Cardiac pacemakers	Seek approval from patient's cardiologist
	Apply over chest with extreme caution; cardiologist should monitor progress frequently
Pregnancy	Seek approval from patient's cardiologist, obstetrician and midwife
	Do not apply over anywhere over abdomen/pelvic region
Epilepsy	Seek approval from patient's neurologist
	Do not apply on neck or head
Non-adherent patients	Assess patient for competency
	If necessary, seek approval from patient's psychiatrist
Malignancy	Seek approval from patient's palliative care specialist
	In general, do not apply over active malignancy
Cardiovascular problems	Seek approval from patient's cardiologist
	Apply over chest with extreme caution; cardiologist should monitor progress frequently
Dermatological conditions or frail skin	Apply electrodes to healthy skin at appropriate dermatomes
Inappropriate electrode sites	Do not apply on anterior neck, around the eyes, over testes, through the chest (i.e. anterior and posterior electrode positions) or over damaged skin or open wounds

Precaution	Advice
Dysaesthesia/hypoaesthesia	Assess skin sensation using sharp/blunt test prior to first TENS treatment. Apply TENS on skin with normal sensation so that patient reports presence of TENS paraesthesia. Carefully monitor to ensure TENS does not aggravate dysaesthesia
Allodynia/hyperalgesia	Test skin sensation prior to first TENS treatment. Apply TENS on skin with normal sensation in first instance as TENS may, but not always, exacerbate the pain
Contact dermatitis	Change type of electrodes – use hypoallergenic electrodes
Autonomic reactions to TENS	Supervise first TENS treatment and assess severity of symptoms with a view to withdrawing TENS
Operating hazardous equipment	Advise patients never to use TENS when driving or when using hazardous equipment

(1990) reported two cases of a Holter monitor detecting interference with a cardiac pacemaker by TENS; in both instances the sensitivity of the pacemaker was reprogrammed to resolve the problem. Careful evaluation and extended cardiac monitoring should be performed when using TENS with pacemakers.

Pregnancy There is much debate about whether TENS should be contraindicated in pregnancy and a recent review of the subject found no reports of deleterious effects of TENS on pregnancy (Crothers 2003). TENS should not be administered over the abdomen or pelvis during pregnancy because the effects of TENS on fetal development are still unknown. TENS should not be administered over a pregnant uterus because currents could inadvertently cause uterine contractions and induce premature labour. Potential hazards when using TENS away from these sites seem minimal, although it would be wise to regularly monitor progress. It is known that obstetric TENS interferes with fetal monitoring equipment (Bundsen & Ericson 1982).

Epilepsy Practitioners should be cautious when giving TENS to patients with epilepsy as it may be difficult to exclude TENS as a potential cause of a seizure. Rosted (2001) reported a case of repetitive epileptic seizures in a post-stroke patient using TENS. Patients are more prone to epileptic seizures following a stroke, although in this case TENS seemed to trigger the repetitive seizures. TENS should be used with caution for post-stroke pain. Scherder et al (1999) reported increased frequency of seizures when TENS was used to improve memory and behaviour in a child with a severe psychomotor disorder and epilepsy. For these reasons, TENS should not be applied on the neck or head in patients with epilepsy.

Non-adherent patients Patients who refuse TENS treatment, do not cooperate with instructions or do not comprehend instructions should not be given TENS. This may include patients with learning difficulties, mental illness or phobias about electricity. TENS can be used on children providing they understand what to expect during TENS.

Malignancy TENS should not be applied directly over an area where there is active malignancy, except in palliative care and under the supervision of a palliative care specialist. This is because electrical currents are known to promote cell growth in vitro, although there are no known reports of TENS increasing malignancy in clinical practice.

Cardiovascular problems Therapists wishing to administer TENS to a patient with a history of cardiac disturbances, such as dysrhythmias, should always discuss the situation with a cardiologist. It is likely that TENS can be used in most cases provided it is to be applied away from the chest area. TENS is often used over the chest for angina, with much success (see the section Known efficacy: the clinical effectiveness of TENS). However, Mann (1996) reported a case of a patient who had inappropriately applied TENS electrodes on the anterior and posterior areas of the chest for unstable angina and severely compromised pulmonary ventilation owing to excessive stimulation of the intercostal muscles. The situation was resolved as soon as TENS was switched off. TENS should not be delivered through the chest using anterior and posterior electrode positions. In addition, TENS should not be applied over areas where there has been recent haemorrhage because the currents may cause further bleeding. TENS should never be applied over areas where there is ischaemic tissue and/or thrombosis, as there may be a potential for an embolism.

Dermatological conditions or frail skin TENS electrodes should not be applied on areas of broken or damaged skin, such as open wounds, although they can be placed over healthy skin surrounding a wound. Electrodes should not be applied on frail skin (e.g. some elderly patients) or on conditions such as eczema, because they may cause skin damage on removal. TENS can be placed over healthy skin around, or proximal to, an area of eczema. TENS has been used successfully for pruritus (Hettrick et al 2004, Tang et al 1999, Tinegate & McLelland 2002, Ward et al 1996).

Inappropriate electrode sites TENS should not be delivered over the anterior neck because currents may stimulate the carotid sinus leading to an acute hypotensive response via a vasovagal reflex. TENS at this site may also stimulate laryngeal nerves leading to a laryngeal spasm. TENS should not be delivered over the eyes because it may cause an increase in intraocular pressure. TENS should not be delivered through the chest using anterior and posterior electrode positions as it may affect the electrical conductivity of the heart and compromise breathing. TENS should not be administered internally except in specific circumstances and using TENS devices designed for dental, vaginal and anal stimulation. There are no known adverse effects of administering TENS on skin over or close to metal implants.

Precautions

Dysaesthesia (hyperaesthesia and hypoaesthesia) If TENS is applied to skin with diminished sensation it is likely that it will be less effective because of the presence of nerve damage. Furthermore, the patient may be unaware that high-intensity currents are being administered, and this may result in skin irritation. If TENS is applied to skin with heightened sensation (e.g. allodynia and/or hyperalgesia) it may aggravate the pain, although this is not always the case. In both cases, electrodes should be positioned on healthy skin proximal to the site of pain, and for this reason practitioners should ensure that a patient has normal skin sensation prior to using TENS.

Contact dermatitis Patients may experience minor skin irritation with TENS, such as reddening beneath or around the electrodes. This is often due to dermatitis at the site of contact with the electrodes resulting from the constituents of electrodes, electrode gel or adhesive tape (Corazza et al 1999, Meuleman et al 1996). The development of hypoallergenic electrodes has markedly reduced the incidence of contact dermatitis. Patients should be encouraged to wash the skin (and electrodes when indicated by the manufacturer) after TENS and to apply electrodes to fresh skin on a daily basis. Occasionally, patients may manifest severe contact dermatitis. There are anecdotal reports (not written up in the literature) of cases where TENS has caused an allergic response, with severe redness, blotching and irritation at local and distant sites to TENS. It is difficult to confirm the validity of such reports and whether symptoms are a direct result of TENS.

Autonomic reactions to TENS There are anecdotal reports of cases in which TENS has caused nausea, light-headedness and fainting. Caution should be taken if the patient has a history of autonomic reactions to tactile allodynia such as syncope.

Operating hazardous equipment Patients should be informed that they should not use TENS when operating vehicles or potentially hazardous equipment. In particular, drivers of motor vehicles should never use TENS while driving as a sudden surge of current could cause an accident. From a legal perspective, it would be wise for TENS users to place their TENS device in a glove compartment whenever driving as the cause of an accident may be attributed to TENS if it were attached to a driver's belt (even if it was switched off).

ELECTRODE POSITIONS

Normal skin sensation

TENS electrodes must be positioned on healthy innervated skin where sensation is intact, so it is important to check skin sensation prior to application. For most types of pain, TENS electrodes are placed around the site of pain so that paraesthesia can be directed into the painful area (Fig. 16.11). This is because conventional TENS is operating via a segmental mechanism so electrodes are placed to stimulate Aβ fibres, which enter the same spinal segment as the nociceptive fibres associated with the origin of the pain.

Heightened skin sensation (allodynia)

TENS may aggravate the pain when skin sensation has been heightened and allodynia and/or hyperalgesia exist, as may be the case when there is mechanical (tactile) allodynia. In these situations, electrodes should be positioned along the main nerves well proximal to the site of pain in the first instance. Interestingly, TENS does not always exacerbate pain in the presence of mechanical allodynia.

Diminished skin sensation (hypoaesthesia)

TENS is likely to be ineffective when applied over skin that has diminished sensation and is numb and insensitive to touch, as may be the case in chronic neuropathic wounds. In these situations, TENS electrodes should be positioned along the main nerves well proximal to the site of pain in the first instance.

Other situations

Electrodes should be positioned along the main nerves proximal to the site of pain when it is not possible to deliver currents within the site of pain, due to absence of a body part following amputation or a skin lesion. Alternatively, electrodes can be applied paravertebrally at spinal segments related to origin of pain or at contralateral dermatomes in conditions such as phantom limb pain and trigeminal neuralgia where the affected side of the face may be sensitive to touch.

DUAL CHANNEL DEVICES

Dual channel devices using four electrodes or large electrodes should be used for pain covering large areas. However, if the pain is generalized and widespread over a number of body parts it may be more appropriate to use AL-TENS at the relevant myotome, as this may produce a more generalized analgesic effect (Johnson 1998). Dual channel stimulators are useful for patients with multiple pains such as low back pain and sciatica, or for pains

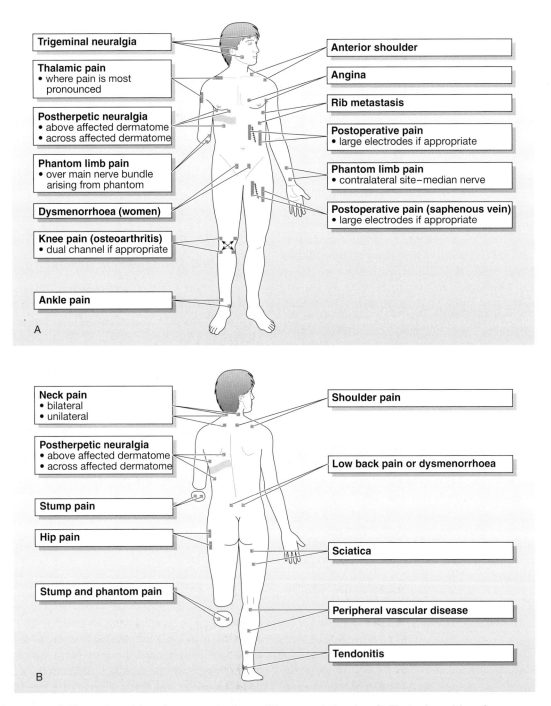

Figure 16.11 A, Electrode positions for common pain conditions – anterior view. B, Electrode positions for common pain conditions – posterior view.

which change in their location and quality over a short time period, e.g. during childbirth.

ACCURATE PLACEMENT OF PADS

Accurate placement of pads can be time-consuming. Berlant (1984) has described a useful method of determining optimal electrode sites for TENS. The therapist applies one TENS electrode to the patient at a potential placement site, holds the second electrode and uses his or her index finger to probe the patient's skin to locate the best site to place it. When the TENS device is switched on and the amplitude slowly increased, the patient and/or therapist will feel TENS paraesthesia when the circuit is made by touching the patient's skin. As the therapist probes the patient's skin, the intensity of TENS paraesthesia will increase whenever nerves on the patient's skin run superficially. This will help to target an effective electrode site.

ELECTRICAL CHARACTERISTICS OF TENS

The potential number of combinations of electrical characteristics of TENS is vast. The relationship between electrical characteristics of TENS and selective activation of nerve fibres was discussed earlier. For conventional TENS, patients are instructed to titrate the intensity of currents to achieve a strong but comfortable electrical paraesthesia without muscle contraction. No relationships have been found between pulse frequency and pattern used by patients and the magnitude of analgesia or their medical diagnosis (Johnson et al 1991b, c). In practice, patients have individual preferences for their selection of electrical characteristics of TENS and these seem to be based on the comfort of the electrical paraesthesia (Johnson et al 1991b, c). Encouraging patients to experiment with TENS settings will produce the most effective outcome.

TIMING AND DOSAGE

Experimental research suggests that maximum pain relief occurs when the TENS device is switched on and that analgesic effect usually disappears quickly once the device is switched off (Johnson & Tabasam 1999, 2003, Johnson et al 1989, 1991a, 1992b). Dosing regimens of 20 minutes at daily, weekly or monthly intervals is likely to be ineffective for conventional TENS. Thus, patients should keep the device switched on whenever the pain is present to achieve pain relief. For ongoing chronic pain this may mean that patients use TENS over the entire day. In a study of long-term users of TENS, Johnson et al (1991c) reported that 75% used TENS on a daily basis and 30% reported using TENS for more than 49 hours a week. Patients can leave electrodes in situ and administer TENS intermittently throughout the day providing they attend to skin care underneath the electrodes, as minor skin irritation may occur. Patients should take regular (although short) breaks from stimulation, should wash their skin after TENS and should apply electrodes to adjacent fresh skin on a regular basis.

Some patients report poststimulation analgesia, although the duration of this effect varies widely, lasting anywhere between 18 hours (Augustinsson et al 1976a, b) to 2 hours (Johnson et al 1991c). This may reflect natural fluctuations in symptoms and the patients' expectation of treatment duration rather than specific TENS-induced effects. It is believed that post-TENS analgesia is longer for AL-TENS than conventional TENS; this is supported by initial findings in experimental studies (Johnson et al 1992b). However, more work is needed to establish the time course of analgesic effects of different types of TENS.

GIVING A PATIENT A TRIAL OF TENS FOR THE FIRST TIME

All new TENS patients should be given a supervised trial of TENS in the first instance. This is to ensure that TENS does not aggravate pain and to give careful instruction on equipment use and expected therapeutic outcome. Patients should be allowed to familiarize themselves with the use of TENS and therapists should use the session to check that the patient can apply TENS appropriately. The initial trial can help to determine whether the patient is likely to respond to TENS and should also be seen as an opportunity to troubleshoot problems arising from poor response. Ideally, the trial should last a minimum of 30–60 minutes as it may take this long for a patient to respond (Table 16.5).

Table 16.5 Suggested characteristics to use for a patient trying TENS for the first time

	Conventional TENS	AL-TENS	Intense TENS
Electrode placement	Straddling site of pain or over main nerve bundle proximal to pain	Over muscle or motor point myotomally related to the site of pain	Straddling site of pain or over main nerve bundle proximal to pain
Pulse pattern	Continuous	Burst	Continuous
Pulse frequency	80–100 pps	80–100 pps	200 pps
Pulse duration	200 μs	200 μs	1000 μs
Pulse amplitude (intensity)	Increase intensity to produce a strong but comfortable tingling	Increase intensity to produce a strong but comfortable muscle twitch	Increase intensity to produce an uncomfortable tingling that is just bearable
Duration of stimulation in first instance	At least 30 minutes	No more than 20 minutes	No more than 5 minutes

When using TENS on a new patient for the first time it is advisable to deliver conventional TENS, as it is commonly used by long-term TENS patients (Johnson et al 1991c). A set of audio speakers (or headphones) can be plugged into the output sockets of some TENS devices to demonstrate the sound of pulses and improve patient understanding of TENS output characteristics. Following the initial trial, patients should be instructed to administer TENS in 30-minute sessions for the first few times, although once they have familiarized themselves with the equipment they should be encouraged to use TENS as much as they like. Patients should also be encouraged to experiment with all stimulator settings so that they achieve the most comfortable pulse frequency, pattern and duration (Table 16.6).

An early review of progress, ideally within a few weeks, can serve to ensure correct application, provide further instruction and to recall TENS devices which are no longer required. Most non-responders return borrowed devices at the next clinic visit (Johnson et al 1992a). Assessing TENS effectiveness at regular intervals is vital for tracking the location and continued use of devices. Some clinics and manufacturers allow patients to borrow TENS devices for a limited period with a view to purchasing the device. A point of contact should always be made available for patients who encounter problems.

APPROPRIATE EDUCATION

It is crucial that patients are educated on the appropriate administration of TENS. For example, patients (and therapists) should be encouraged to follow set safety procedures when applying and removing TENS to reduce the chance of a mild electric shock (see Box 16.2). Patients should be warned not to use TENS in the shower or bath and to keep TENS appliances out of the reach of children. TENS can be used at bedtime provided the device has a timer so that it switches off automatically.

KNOWN BIOLOGICAL EFFECTS

TENS effects can be subdivided into analgesic and non-analgesic effects (see Table 16.1). In clinical practice, TENS is predominantly used for its symptomatic relief of pain. However, there is increasing use of TENS for non-analgesic effects and there is some evidence suggesting possible effect as an antiemetic when given at acupuncture points (Dundee et al 1991, Habib et al 2006), for faecal incontinence (Hosker et al 2000), restoration of blood flow to ischaemic tissue and wounds (Burssens et al 2005, Debreceni et al 1995, Wikstrom et al 1999) and some behavioural aspects of dementia (Cameron et al 2003). There is, however, less published research on the non-analgesic effects of TENS and some of the

Table 16.6 Suggested advice following the initial trial

	Conventional TENS	AL–TENS	Intense TENS
Electrode positions	Straddle site of pain but if not successful try main nerve bundle, across spinal cord or contralateral positions; dermatomal	Over muscle belly at site of pain but if not successful try motor point at site of pain, contralateral positions; myotomal	Straddle site of pain but if not successful try over main nerve bundle
Pulse pattern	Patient preference	Burst but if not successful or uncomfortable try amplitude modulated	Continuous but if not successful or uncomfortable try frequency or duration modulated
Pulse frequency	Patient preference usually 10–200 pps	Above fusion frequency of muscle 80–100 pps within the burst	High, e.g. 200 pps
Pulse duration	Patient preference usually 50–200 µs	Patient preference 200 µs	Highest possible but if uncomfortable gradually reduce duration
Pulse amplitude (intensity)	Strong but comfortable sensation without visible muscle contraction	Strong but comfortable sensation with visible muscle contraction	Highest tolerable sensation with limited muscle contraction
Dosage	As much and as often as is required; have a break every hour or so	About 30 minutes at a time as fatigue may develop with ongoing muscle contractions	15 minutes at a time as the stimulation may be uncomfortable
Analgesic effects	Occur when stimulator on	Occur when stimulator on and for a while once the stimulator has been switched off May exacerbate pain	Occur when stimulator on and for a while once the stimulator has been switched off May exacerbate pain
General advice	Experiment with settings to maintain strong comfortable sensation	Experiment with settings (except burst) to maintain a phasic twitch	Experiment with settings to maintain highest tolerable sensation

experimental work in the field is contradictory (Walsh 1997b).

MECHANISM OF ACTION FOR ANALGESIC EFFECTS

The mechanism by which TENS produces pain relief has received much attention and can be categorized according to the anatomical site of action into peripheral, segmental and extrasegmental. The main action of conventional TENS is segmental analgesia mediated by activity in large-diameter non-noxious afferents. The main action of AL-TENS is extrasegmental analgesia mediated by ergoreceptor activity; the main action of intense TENS is extrasegmental analgesia via activity in small-diameter afferents. Conventional and intense TENS are also likely to produce peripheral blockade of afferent information in the fibre type that they activate.

PERIPHERAL MECHANISMS

The delivery of electrical currents over a nerve fibre will elicit nerve impulses that travel in both directions along the nerve axon, e.g. antidromic activation (Fig. 16.12). TENS-induced nerve impulses travelling away from the central nervous system

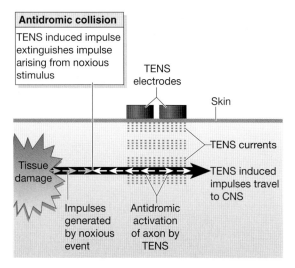

Antidromic collision

TENS induced impulse extinguishes impulse arising from noxious stimulus

TENS electrodes

Skin

Tissue damage

TENS currents

TENS induced impulses travel to CNS

Impulses generated by noxious event

Antidromic activation of axon by TENS

Figure 16.12 TENS-induced blockade of peripheral transmission. Impulses generated by TENS will travel in both directions down an axon (antidromic activation) leading to a collision with noxious impulses travelling toward the central nervous system (CNS).

will collide and extinguish afferent impulses arising from tissue damage. For conventional TENS, antidromic activation is likely to occur in large-diameter fibres but not small-diameter fibres. Tissue damage may produce activity in large-diameter fibres, so conventional TENS may mediate some of its analgesic effect by peripheral blockade in large-diameter fibres. This has been demonstrated by Walsh et al (1998), who found that TENS delivered at 110 pps significantly increased the negative peak latency of the compound action potential in healthy human subjects, suggesting a slowing of transmission in the peripheral nerve. Nardone and Schieppati (1989) have also reported that the latency of early somatosensory evoked potentials (SEPs) was increased during TENS in healthy subjects and concluded that conventional TENS could produce a 'busy line-effect' on large afferent fibres.

The contribution of peripheral blockade on analgesia is likely to be greater during intense TENS. Impulses travelling in $A\delta$ fibres induced by intense TENS will collide with nociceptive impulses, also travelling in $A\delta$ fibres. Ignelzi and Nyquist (1976) demonstrated that electrical stimulation (at intensities likely to recruit $A\delta$ fibres) can

reduce the conduction velocity and amplitude of $A\alpha$, $A\beta$ and $A\delta$ components of the compound action potential recorded from isolated nerves in the cat; the greatest change was seen in the $A\delta$ component. However, Levin and Hui-Chan (1993) have shown that healthy subjects cannot tolerate direct activation of $A\delta$ afferents by TENS, and therefore intense TENS is administered only for brief periods of time in clinical practice.

SEGMENTAL MECHANISMS

Conventional TENS produces analgesia predominantly by a segmental mechanism whereby activity generated in large-diameter fibres inhibits ongoing activity in second-order nociceptive (pain-related) neurons in the dorsal horn of the spinal cord (Fig. 16.13). Workers have shown that activity in large-diameter afferents will inhibit nociceptive reflexes in animals when the influence of pain inhibitory pathways descending from the brain has been removed by spinal transection (Sjölund 1985, Woolf et al 1980, 1988). Garrison and Foreman (1994) showed that TENS could significantly reduce ongoing nociceptor cell activity in the dorsal horn cell when it was applied to somatic receptive fields. Follow-up work after transection of the spinal cord at T12 demonstrated that spontaneously and noxiously evoked cell activities were still reduced during TENS. This demonstrates that the neuronal circuitry for conventional TENS analgesia is located in the spinal cord and it is likely that a combination of pre- and postsynaptic inhibition takes place (Garrison & Foreman 1996). Similar findings have been reported more recently by Ma and Sluka (2001), who showed a reduction in inflammation-induced sensitization of dorsal horn neurons by TENS in anaesthetized rats.

The clinical observation that conventional TENS produces analgesia that is short lasting and rapid in onset is consistent with synaptic inhibition at a segmental level. A number of workers have shown that TENS-induced activity in $A\delta$ fibres during intense TENS can lead to long-term depression (LTD) of central nociceptor cell activity for up to 2 hours (Sandkühler 2000, Sandkühler et al 1997). Latency and amplitude changes in SEPs after high-frequency (200 pps) electrical stimulation of the digital nerves in healthy subjects supports the concept

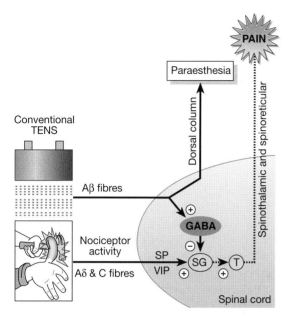

Figure 16.13 Neurophysiology of conventional TENS analgesia. Activity in Aδ and C fibres from nociceptors leads to excitation (+) of interneurons in the substantia gelatinosa (SG) of the spinal cord via neurotransmitter-like substance P (SP, cutaneous nociceptors) or vasoactive intestinal peptide (VIP, visceral nociceptors). Central nociceptor transmission neurons (T) project to the brain via spinoreticular and spinothalamic tracts to produce a sensory experience of pain. TENS-induced activity in Aβ afferents leads to the inhibition (−) of SG and T cells (dotted line) via the release of gamma amino butyric acid (GABA, black interneuron). Paraesthesia associated with TENS is generated by information travelling to the brain via the dorsal columns.

that TENS can produce LTD of central nociceptive cells (Macefield & Burke 1991). One practical outcome of this work may be introduction of 'sequential TENS', whereby conventional TENS is administered at a strong but comfortable level in the first instance, followed by a brief period of intense TENS leading to longer poststimulation analgesia (Sandkühler 2000, Sandkühler et al 1997).

EXTRASEGMENTAL MECHANISMS

TENS-induced activity in small-diameter afferents has also been shown to produce extrasegmental analgesia through the activation of structures forming the descending pain inhibitory pathways: the periaqueductal grey (PAG), nucleus raphe magnus and nucleus raphe gigantocellularis. Antinociception in animals produced by stimulation of cutaneous Aδ fibres is reduced by spinal transection, suggesting a role for extrasegmental structures (Chung et al 1984a, b, Woolf et al 1980). Phasic muscle contractions produced during AL-TENS generate activity in small-diameter muscle afferents (ergoreceptors) leading to activation of the descending pain inhibitory pathways (Fig. 16.14). The importance of muscle afferent activity in this effect has been shown in animal studies by Sjölund, (1988) who found that greater antinociception occurred when muscle rather than skin afferents were activated by low-frequency (two bursts per second) TENS. Duranti et al (1988) confirmed this in humans by demonstrating that there was no difference in analgesia produced by currents delivered through the skin (e.g. AL-TENS) compared to currents that bypassed the skin (e.g. intramuscular electrical nerve stimulation; IENS).

NEUROPHARMACOLOGY OF TENS

Many neurotransmitters and neuromodulators have been implicated in the mechanism of action of TENS, which is not surprising considering that TENS acts at multiple sites in the nervous system. Much attention has focused on the role of opioids. Originally, it was suggested AL-TENS – but not conventional TENS – is mediated by endorphins. Sjölund et al (1977) reported that AL-TENS increased cerebrospinal (CSF) endorphin levels in nine patients suffering chronic pain and that AL-TENS analgesia was naloxone reversible (Sjölund & Eriksson 1979). However, naloxone failed to reverse analgesia produced by conventional TENS in pain patients (Abram et al 1981, Hansson et al 1986, Woolf et al 1978; for a review, see Thompson 1989). Claims that conventional TENS can elevate plasma β-endorphin and β-lipotrophin in healthy subjects (Facchinetti et al 1986) have not been confirmed (Johnson et al 1992c) and it seems unlikely that β-endorphin would be able to cross the blood–brain barrier because of its large size.

More recently, research using experimental models of hyperalgesia in animal studies suggests that the antinociceptive action of low-frequency

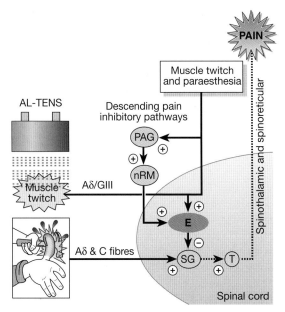

Figure 16.14 Neurophysiology of AL-TENS analgesia. Activity in Aδ and C fibres from nociceptors leads to excitation (+) of central nociceptor transmission neurons (T), which project to the brain to produce a sensory experience of pain. TENS-induced activity in small-diameter muscle afferents (Aδ, GIII) leads to the activation of brain-stem nuclei such as the periaqueductal grey (PAG) and nucleus raphe magnus (nRM). These nuclei form the descending pain inhibitory pathways, which excite interneurons that inhibit (−) SG and T cells (dotted line) via the release of met-enkephalin (E, black interneuron). It is likely that paraesthesia and sensations related to the muscle twitch are relayed to the brain via the dorsal columns.

TENS is mediated via μ opioid receptors and that antinociceptive action of high-frequency TENS medicated by δ opioid receptors, with κ receptors having no involvement (Kalra et al 2001, Sluka et al 1998, 1999). Follow-up work suggested that the anti-hyperalgesic effects of low-frequency TENS were diminished in morphine-tolerant rats but that the antihyperalgesic effects of high-frequency TENS were not affected (Sluka et al 2000). Evidence suggests that TENS-induced opioid release occurs at sites in the spinal cord and in the brainstem (Ainsworth et al 2006, Kalra et al 2001) and that opioid tolerance may develop with repeated TENS administration (Chandran & Sluka 2003).

There is also evidence to suggest the involvement of non-opioid transmitters. Studies by Duggan and Foong (1985) – using anaesthetized cats – suggest that the inhibitory neurotransmitter γ-aminobutyric acid (GABA) may have a role in pain relief by conventional TENS. Interestingly, low-frequency stimulation of Aδ fibres (1 pps, 0.1 ms), which has been shown to produce LTD in animals, is not influenced by the GABA receptor antagonist bicuculline but is abolished by D-2-amino-5-phosphonovaleric acid, a NMDA receptor antagonist (Sandkühler 2000, Sandkühler et al 1997). This suggests that glutamate rather than GABA may be involved in LTD induced by intense TENS. More recently, it has been suggested that 5-HT_2 and 5-HT_3 receptors may be involved in anti-hyperalgesia produced by low-frequency, but not high-frequency, TENS (Radakrishnan et al 2003) and that high-frequency, but not low-frequency, TENS reduces aspartate and glutamate release in the spinal cord dorsal horn. These neurotransmitters are pivotal in the central transmission of nociceptive information (Sluka et al 2005). Both low- and high-frequency TENS activate spinal muscarinic receptors (Radakrishnan & Sluka 2003) and peripheral α_{2A} adrenergic receptors (King et al 2005), and combining clonidine, a centrally acting α_2 adrenoceptor agonist, appears to augment TENS-induced antihyperalgesia (Sluka & Chandran 2002).

TIME COURSE OF ANALGESIC EFFECTS

As different mechanisms contribute to analgesia produced by different TENS techniques, it is plausible that they will have different analgesic profiles. In fact, this is the rationale for the use of different types of TENS. Evidence from laboratory and clinical studies shows that TENS analgesia is maximal when the stimulator is switched on, irrespective of the type of TENS used (for reviews, see Johnson 2003, Walsh 1997e, Woolf & Thompson 1994). This explains the finding that long-term users of TENS administer conventional TENS continuously throughout the day to achieve adequate analgesia (Chabal et al 1998, Johnson et al 1991c, Nash et al 1990). Poststimulation analgesia has been reported to occur in some patients and may be due to LTD and activation of descending pain inhibitory pathways. Reports of the duration of these poststimulation effects vary widely, from 18 hours (Augustinsson et al 1976b) to 2 hours

(Johnson et al 1991c). It is possible that natural fluctuations in symptoms and the patient's expectation of treatment duration may have contributed to these observations to some extent.

MAIN DETERMINANTS OF OUTCOME

It is becoming clear that the effectiveness of TENS is dose dependent and that the choice of electrical characteristics of TENS is important. Much has been written about the appropriate settings of TENS to use in different circumstances, although many of the claims are unfounded. Remarkably few studies have systematically investigated the analgesic profiles of TENS pulse frequencies, pulse durations and pulse patterns when all other stimulating characteristics are fixed. Existing research is conflicting, confusing and generally of very poor quality (see the tables in Walsh 1997c, d). This has opened the way for clinical practice based on ritual and mystique. Most research attention has focused on the role of pulse frequency, although in clinical practice it is likely that pulse amplitude will be the key electrical characteristic because of its relationship to fibre recruitment. Simple titration of pulse amplitude coupled with the user's report of TENS intensity enables selective activation of nerve fibres in line with the principles discussed earlier.

PULSE FREQUENCY

A great many studies have compared the analgesic effects of two pulse frequencies (usually high ~100 pps and low ~2 pps) in animals, healthy humans and patients in pain. However, it is difficult to compare the outcome of these studies because other TENS parameters such as intensity, pattern and electrode location often differ between studies. Sjölund (1985) delivered seven different stimulation frequencies (10, 40, 60, 80, 100, 120, 160 pps) to a dissected skin nerve in the lightly anaesthetized rat and reported that a stimulation frequency of 80 pps gave the most profound inhibition of the C-fibre-evoked flexion reflex. In a follow-up study, they reported that a pulse-train repetition rate of around 1 Hz was most effective in inhibition of the C-fibre-evoked flexion reflex. Gopalkrishnan and Sluka (2000) examined the effect of varying frequency, intensity and pulse duration

of TENS on primary hyperalgesia induced by carrageenan paw inflammation in rats and found that high-frequency TENS, but not low-frequency TENS, reduced primary hyperalgesia. Follow-up work in the same laboratory by King and Sluka (2001) examined the effect of frequency and intensity of TENS on secondary mechanical hyperalgesia induced by acute joint inflammation. They found that high- or low-frequency TENS was equally effective in reducing secondary mechanical hyperalgesia and that this was not influenced by intensity (for a review, see Sluka & Walsh 2003). Johnson et al (1989) assessed the analgesic effects of five stimulating frequencies (10, 20, 40, 80 and 160 pps) on cold-induced pain in healthy subjects and suggested that TENS frequencies between 20 and 80 pps produced the greatest analgesia when delivered at a strong but comfortable intensity. However, the findings of studies using healthy subjects exposed to experimental pain are variable and definitive conclusions about the most appropriate pulse frequency to use cannot be made. Nevertheless, when trying out conventional TENS on a patient for the first time it seems sensible to start with frequencies around 80 pps.

PULSE PATTERN

Johnson et al (1991a) systematically investigated the analgesic effects of burst, amplitude modulation, random (frequency of pulse delivery) and continuous TENS delivered at a strong but comfortable level on cold-induced pain in healthy subjects. All pulse patterns elevated the ice pain threshold but there were no significant differences between the groups when all other stimulating characteristics were fixed. Tulgar et al (1991a, b) demonstrated that various patterns of pulse delivery were as effective as each other in managing patients' pain. However, patients preferred modulated patterns of TENS, such as frequency modulation and burst, to continuous (Tulgar et al 1991a). This seems to contrast with Johnson et al (1991c), who found that the majority of long-term users of TENS preferred continuous rather than burst mode. More systematic investigations comparing the analgesic effects of a range (more than two) of stimulating characteristics when all other variables are fixed are clearly needed.

The variability in the findings of research into TENS settings is likely to be due to large intersubject variance in reporting pain and pain relief, even under well-controlled laboratory conditions. Nevertheless, existing evidence suggests that the 'magic bullet' for conventional TENS is a strong but comfortable electrical paraesthesia below the electrodes, as this signifies selective activation of large-diameter afferents.

DECLINING RESPONSE TO TENS

Some TENS users claim that the effectiveness of TENS declines over time, although the exact proportion of patients is not known (see Table 92-1 in Sjölund et al (1990) for a summary of studies). Eriksson et al (1979) found that effective pain relieve was achieved by 55% of chronic pain patients at 2 months, 41% at 1 year and 30% at 2 years. Loeser et al (1975) reported that only 12% of 200 chronic-pain patients obtained long-term benefits with TENS, despite 68% of patients achieving initial pain relief. Woolf and Thompson (1994) suggest that the magnitude of pain relief from TENS may decline by up to 40% for many patients over a period of 1 year.

There may be many reasons for the decline in TENS effects with time, including dead batteries, perished leads or a worsening pain problem. However, there is evidence that some patients habituate to TENS currents owing to a progressive failure of the nervous system to respond to monotonous stimuli. Pomeranz and Niznick (1987) have shown that repetitive delivery of TENS pulses at 2 pps produces habituation of late peaks (>50 ms) of SEPs. This implies that, for some people, the nervous system filters out monotonous stimuli associated with TENS. However, they found that delivering currents randomly to six different points on the body using a TENS-like device called a Codetron markedly reduced the habituation response (see Table 16.3). Fargas-Babjak et al (1989, 1992) performed a 6-week, double-blind, randomized, placebo-controlled pilot trial of the effectiveness of Codetron on osteoarthritis of the hip/knee and reported beneficial effects. Some TENS manufacturers have tried to overcome the problem of habituation by including random pulse delivery or frequency modulated pulse delivery

settings to their standard TENS devices. However, these devices have met with varied success.

If a patient reports that they are responding less well to TENS over time it may be worth experimenting with the electrical characteristics of TENS or with electrode placements to try and improve analgesia. It may also be worth considering temporarily withdrawing TENS treatment so that an objective assessment of the contribution of TENS to pain relief can be made. When this is done patients may report that their pain worsens in the absence of TENS, demonstrating that TENS was in fact beneficial.

KNOWN EFFICACY: THE CLINICAL EFFECTIVENESS OF TENS

EVIDENCE-BASED PRACTICE

There is an extensive literature on the clinical effectiveness of TENS, although the majority of reports are anecdotal or of clinical trials lacking control groups or valid sample sizes. These reports are of limited use because they cannot account for normal fluctuations in patients' symptoms, the treatment effects of concurrent interventions or patients' expectation of treatment success. Randomized, placebo-controlled clinical trials are needed to determine effects due to the active ingredient of TENS (e.g. the electrical currents) from the act of receiving TENS. In 2006, a cursory search in PubMed using the medical subject heading (MeSH) term 'transcutaneous electric nerve stimulation' resulted in over 10 000 hits, 450 clinical trials, 250 randomized controlled clinical trials (RCTs) and 10 meta-analyses. This demonstrates the wealth of information facing the practitioner. A summary of this information is provided below.

TENS and acute pain

TENS is used extensively for acute nociceptive or inflammatory pain, although opinion is divided about whether it is effective. Only one systematic review has been conducted on TENS for a variety of acute pain conditions and found that TENS was more effective than the control group in 22/39 RCTs suggesting that available evidence was inconclusive (Reeve et al 1996; Table 16.7). RCTs

Table 16.7 Outcomes of systematic reviews on acute pain

Reference and context	Condition	Data set (RCTs/patient numbers)	Outcome (trial vote count)	Outcome (meta–analysis)	Review authors' conclusion	This author's judgement	Comment on review process
Mixed populations							
Reeve et al 1996	Acute pain Mixed conditions (postoperative pain, labour pain, dysmenorrhoea, dental, back, cervical, orofacial)	39 RCTs: 34 rated as suitable quality (grade 1)	TENS > comparison group in 22/39 RCTs for pain relief and/or mobility TENS > comparison group in 19/34 grade 1 RCTs for pain relief and/or mobility	Not performed	Evidence inconclusive: poor RCT methodology	Evidence inconclusive	Comparison groups consisted of active and inactive interventions
Postoperative pain							
Reeve et al 1996 (subgroup analysis performed post hoc by Johnson)	Postoperative pain	20 RCTs	TENS > comparison group in 12/20 RCTs for pain relief and/or functional outcomes such as ventilation	Not performed	Evidence inconclusive: poor RCT methodology	Evidence inconclusive	Comparison groups consisted of active and inactive interventions. Patients allowed free access to analgesic medication in some RCTs
Carroll et al 1996	Postoperative pain	17RCTs (786 patients)	TENS > comparison groups in 2/17 RCTs for pain relief and/or analgesic sparing TENS > sham in 0/14 RCTs for pain relief and/or analgesic sparing	Not performed	Evidence of no effect	Evidence inconclusive: potential shortcomings in RCTs and review process	Comparison groups consisted of active and inactive interventions. Patients allowed free access to analgesic medication in some RCTs

(Continued)

Table 16.7 (Continued)

Reference and context	Condition	Data set (RCTs/patient numbers)	Outcome (trial vote count)	Outcome (meta-analysis)	Review authors' conclusion	This author's judgement	Comment on review process
Bjordal et al 2003	Postoperative analgesic consumption with subgroup analysis on appropriateness of TENS intervention	21 RCTs (964 patients)	11/21 RCTs met criteria for 'adequate TENS'	TENS > sham for reducing analgesic consumption (MWD = 35.5%) TENS given appropriately significantly better than TENS given inappropriately	Evidence of effect: analgesic sparing	Evidence of effect: analgesic sparing	Demonstrates many RCTs apply TENS inappropriately
Labour pain Reeve et al 1996	Labour pain	13 RCTs; nine were of suitable quality (grade 1)	TENS > comparison groups in 3/9 grade 1 RCTs for pain relief, analgesic sparing, and/or mobility	Not performed	Evidence inconclusive: poor RCT methodology	Evidence inconclusive	Comparison groups consisted of active and inactive interventions. Patients allowed free access to analgesic medication in some RCTs
Carroll et al 1997a	Labour pain	8 RCTs (712 women)	TENS > comparison groups in 1/8 RCTs for pain relief TENS > comparison groups in 3/8 RCTs for analgesic sparing TENS > sham in 2/5RCTs for analgesic sparing	Odds ratio for analgesic sparing effects of TENS vs sham = 0.57; NNT = 14 (4 RCTs) Odds ratio for pain relief	Evidence of no effect	Evidence inconclusive: potential shortcomings in RCTs and review process	Comparison groups consisted of active and inactive interventions. Patients allowed free access to analgesic medication in some RCTs

Study	Condition	Number of trials	Findings	Effect size	Conclusion	Evidence	Comments
Carroll et al 1997b (update of Carroll et al 1997a)	Labour pain	10 RCTs (877 women)	TENS > comparison groups in 0/10 RCTs for pain relief; TENS > comparison groups in 3/10 RCTs for additional analgesics	Relative risk for analgesic sparing effects of TENS vs sham = 0.88; effects of TENS vs sham = 1.89 (1 RCT)	Evidence of no effect	Evidence inconclusive: potential shortcomings in RCTs and review process	Two additional reports strengthen the argument for lack of TENS effect; One positive outcome sham controlled trial used cranial TENS
Proctor et al 2002	Primary dysmenorrhoea	7 RCTs (213 patients)		HF TENS > sham for pain relief (odds ratio = 7.2 from 2 RCTs using dichotomous data; WMD = 45 from 1 RCT using VAS) LF TENS = sham for pain relief (odds ratio = 1.3 from 2 RCTs using dichotomous data; WMD = 24.1 from 1 RCT using VAS)	Evidence of effect – pain relief for HF TENS only	Evidence inconclusive	Comparisons made on small numbers of patients and RCTs,

HF TENS, high frequency TENS; LF TENS, low frequency TENS; MWD, mean weighted difference; NNT, number needed to treat; RCT, randomized controlled trial; VAS, visual analogue scale; WMD, weighted mean difference.

and meta-analyses are available for TENS and specific acute pain conditions such as postoperative pain, labour pain, dysmenorrhoea, angina and orofacial pain.

TENS and postoperative pain

Early reports suggested that TENS reduced postoperative pain and opioid consumption (Ali et al 1981, Hymes et al 1974, Schuster & Infante 1980). However, systematic reviews performed in the mid-1990s were less favourable. Reeve et al (1996) reported that TENS demonstrated benefit against a control group in 12/20 RCTs on postoperative pain. Carroll et al (1996) reported that TENS did not produce significant postoperative pain relief in 15/17 RCTs. However, the use of pain relief as the primary outcome measure may have been compromised because patients in some of the included trials had access to additional analgesic drugs, enabling patients in sham and active TENS groups to titrate analgesic consumption to achieve similar levels of pain relief. Other potential shortcomings included inconsistencies between reviewers and trial authors because of the use of multiple outcome measures in RCTs, and insufficient statistical power to detect potential differences due to small sample sizes. A subsequent meta-analysis of 21 RCTs that accounted for these issues found that the mean reduction in analgesic consumption after TENS was 26.5% (range −6 to +51%) better than placebo (Bjordal et al 2003).

Importantly, a subgroup analysis of 11 trials (964 patients) that met criteria for optimal TENS dosage (i.e. a strong, subnoxious electrical stimulation at the site of pain) reported a mean weighted reduction in analgesic consumption of 35.5% (range 14–51%) better than placebo. In the trials without explicit confirmation of optimal TENS dosage, the mean weighted analgesic consumption was 4.1% (range −10 to +29%) in favour of active TENS. The difference in favour of adequate stimulation was highly significant ($P = 0.0002$). This review demonstrated the importance of using appropriate outcome measures and adequate TENS technique in RCTs and meta-analyses of TENS. At present, evidence suggests that TENS will reduce analgesic consumption but is inconclusive for relieving postoperative pain.

TENS and labour pain

Augustinsson et al (1976a) pioneered the use of TENS in obstetrics by applying TENS to areas of the spinal cord that correspond to the input of nociceptive afferents associated with the first and second stages of labour (T10–L1 and S2–S4, respectively; Fig. 16.15). They reported that 88% of 147 women obtained pain relief using this method, although the study failed to include a placebo control group (Augustinsson et al 1977). A series of positive outcome trials followed, which led to increased popularity and specially designed obstetric TENS devices with dual channels and a 'boost' control button for

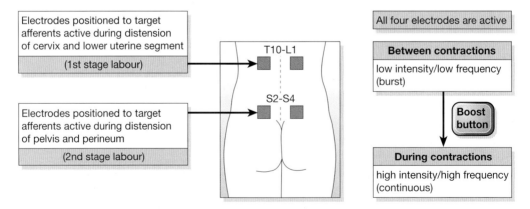

Figure 16.15 The position of electrodes and the electrical characteristics of TENS when used to manage pain during labour.

contraction pain (Augustinsson et al 1977, Bundsen et al 1978, Grim & Morey 1985, Kubista et al 1978, Miller-Jones 1980, Stewart, 1979, Vincenti et al 1982).

Systematic reviews on TENS and labour pain concluded that evidence for TENS analgesia during labour was weak, although patients in some RCTs had access to additional analgesic drugs that would compromise pain relief scores in much the same way as seen for postoperative pain trials (Carroll et al 1997a, b, Reeve et al 1996; see Table 16.7). Reeve et al (1996) reported that seven of nine RCTs showed no differences between TENS and sham TENS or conventional pain management. Carroll et al (1997a) reported that five of eight RCTs showed no benefits from TENS and this was confirmed in an updated review that included two additional RCTs (Carroll et al 1997b). Interestingly, Carroll et al (1997a) reported that the odds ratio for trials recording additional analgesic intervention was 0.57, suggesting that analgesic intervention may be less likely with TENS, although number-needed-to-treat was high (14, 95% CI 7.3 to 11.9). RCTs with high methodological scores tended to report no differences between active and sham TENS users for pain relief or additional analgesic intervention (Harrison et al 1986, Thomas et al 1988, Van der Ploeg et al 1996).

The findings of clinical research suggesting that TENS might not relieve pain conflict with the clinical experience of midwives and with patient satisfaction with the use of TENS (Johnson 1997). One reason for this difference is the difficulty of taking self-reports of pain when women are experiencing fluctuating physical and emotional conditions during childbirth. Interestingly, two RCTs with high methodological scores found that women favoured active TENS compared to sham TENS when response was taken at the end of childbirth, when women are relaxed yet still under double-blind conditions (Harrison et al 1986, Thomas et al 1988). Moreover, some RCTs included in the systematic reviews used transcranial (Limoge) TENS administered via electrodes placed on the temple and using electrical currents which have markedly different characteristics to those of conventional obstetric TENS (Champagne et al 1984, Wattrisse et al 1993; see Table 16.2). It could be argued that these studies should not have been included in the review, although both demonstrated beneficial effects. At present, the evidence is not strong for TENS and labour pain, although it would be unreasonable to dismiss the use of TENS until the discrepancy between clinical experience and clinical evidence is resolved.

TENS and dysmenorrhoea

Various types of TENS have been reported to be successful in the management of dysmenorrhoea (Dawood and Ramos 1990, Kaplan et al 1994, Lewers et al 1989, Milsom et al 1994, Neighbors et al 1987). Most often, electrodes are applied over the lower thoracic spine and sometimes on acupuncture points (see Fig. 16.11). A Cochrane review that included seven RCTs, (213 patients) reported that high-frequency, but not low-frequency, TENS was superior to sham at reducing pain associated with primary dysmenorrhoea (Proctor et al 2002). At present, there is weak evidence to suggest that may TENS be beneficial in dysmenorrhoea.

TENS and angina pectoris

There is increasing use of conventional TENS for angina with electrodes placed directly over the painful area of the chest (Börjesson et al 1997, Mannheimer et al 1982, Murray et al 2004; see Fig. 16.11). It has been demonstrated that TENS increases work capacity, decreases ST segment depression and reduces the frequency of angina attacks and nitroglycerin consumption compared to control groups (Börjesson et al 1997, Mannheimer et al 1985, 1990). At present, there is insufficient good quality evidence to determine whether TENS is beneficial for angina.

TENS and other acute pain conditions

RCTs have also shown TENS to be potentially effective for acute orofacial pain (Hansson & Ekblom 1983, Hansson et al 1986), painful dental procedures (Meechan et al 1998, Schafer et al 2000), fractured ribs (Myers et al 1977, Sloan et al 1986) and acute lower back pain (Bertalanffy et al 2005). However, there is insufficient good quality evidence to make definitive conclusions.

TENS and chronic pain

The widespread use of TENS for chronic pain is supported by a large number of clinical trials that suggest that TENS is useful for a wide range of chronic pain conditions of nociceptive, neuropathic and musculoskeletal origin. To date, three systematic reviews have examined TENS effectiveness on mixed populations of chronic pain patients (Table 16.8). Reeve et al (1996) reported that TENS was more effective than sham (7 RCTs) or no treatment (2 RCTs) in 9/20 RCTs. McQuay and Moore (1998a) reported that TENS was better than sham TENS, placebo pills or inappropriate electrode placements in 10/24 RCTs. Carroll et al (2001) reported that TENS provided better pain relief than sham or no treatment in 10/15 RCTs. All reviewers concluded that the evidence for TENS in chronic pain was inconclusive. Reviews on specific populations of chronic pain patients are also inconclusive.

TENS and low back pain

Perhaps the most common use for TENS is in the management of low back pain. The clinical practice guideline developed by the Philadelphia Panel reported that evidence to support the use of TENS for chronic low back pain (LBP) is poor and inconclusive (Philadelphia Panel 2001). This is because the findings of systematic reviews have been contradictory (see Table 16.8). A Cochrane review of five RCTs and 321 patients with LBP reported no statistically significant differences between active and sham TENS for pain relief (Brosseau et al 2002, Milne et al 2001). An update of the review by the same investigators included only two RCTs and 175 patients; one of the RCTs demonstrated significantly greater pain relief for TENS over placebo control (Khadilkar et al 2005a, b). A meta-analysis of 288 patients with LBP reported that TENS reduced pain and improved range of motion (Flowerdew & Gadsby 1997, Gadsby & Flowerdew 1997, 2000). The review included six RCTs, with 62 trials being excluded because they were either non-randomized or failed to compare active TENS with a credible placebo. The meta-analysis showed that more patients improved with acupuncture-like TENS (AL-TENS; 86.7%) than conventional TENS (45.8%) or placebo

(36.4%), with an overall odds ratio for improvement against placebo of 2.11 for any type of TENS, 7.22 for AL-TENS and 1.52 for conventional. However, the odds ratio for AL-TENS was based on the findings of only two studies, neither of which applied AL-TENS to produce muscle contractions (Gemignani et al 1991, Melzack et al 1983; for a critical review, see Johnson 1998).

Similarly, contradictory findings are found in RCTs published in prestigious journals. Marchand et al (1993) concluded that conventional TENS was significantly more efficient than placebo-TENS in reducing pain intensity, but not pain unpleasantness, in 42 patients with back pain. In contrast, an RCT by Deyo et al (1990a) concluded that treatment with TENS was no more effective than treatment with a placebo in 145 patients with chronic low back pain. At present the evidence for TENS effectiveness for LBP is inconclusive.

TENS for arthritic pain

A Cochrane review of 294 patients with knee osteoarthritis reported that TENS produced significantly better pain relief and reductions in knee stiffness than placebo (Osiri et al 2002; see Table 16.8). A Cochrane review of three RCTs, involving 78 people, concluded that evidence on the effectiveness of TENS in the treatment of pain associated with rheumatoid arthritis of the hand were conflicting (Brosseau et al 2003). Interestingly, 15 minutes of AL-TENS a week, for 3 weeks did appear to reduce rest pain but not grip pain compared to placebo, although this dosage regimen seems very low. Pelland et al (2002) conducted a Cochrane review on the effectiveness of electrical stimulation for improving muscle strength and function in patients with rheumatoid arthritis of the hand and concluded that existing evidence was inconclusive. At present, the evidence for TENS effectiveness for arthritic pain is inconclusive.

TENS and muscle pain

To date, there are no systematic reviews on TENS and muscle pain because of a lack of RCTs. Nevertheless, TENS is used for reducing localized muscle pain in the neck and shoulder arising from

Table 16.8 Outcomes of systematic reviews on chronic pain

Reference and context	Condition	Data set (RCTs/patient numbers)	Outcome (trial vote count)	Outcome (meta-analysis)	Review authors' conclusion	This author's judgement	Comment on review process
Mixed populations							
Reeve et al 1996	Mixed conditions (low back, pancreatitis, arthritis, angina)	29 RCTs; 20 were of suitable quality (grade 1)	TENS > comparison group in 16/29 RCTs for pain relief and/or mobility TENS > comparison group in 11/20 grade 1 RCTs for pain relief and/or mobility	Not performed	Evidence inconclusive: poor RCT methodology	Evidence inconclusive	Wide variation in comparison groups, outcome measures and patient groups between RCTs
McQuay & Moore 1998a	Mixed conditions (low back, pancreatitis, osteoarthritis, dysmenorrhoea)	38 RCTs	TENS > sham or no treatment control in 10/24 comparisons for pain relief and/or mobility TENS > active treatment in 3/15 comparisons for pain relief and/or mobility	Not performed	Evidence inconclusive: inadequate TENS doses	Evidence inconclusive: inadequate TENS doses	Wide variation in comparison groups, outcome measures and patient groups between RCTs
Carroll et al 2001; update of McQuay & Moore 1998a	Mixed conditions (low back, pancreatitis, osteoarthritis, dysmenorrhoea)	19 RCTs (652 patients)	TENS > sham or no treatment control in 10/15 comparisons for pain relief and/or mobility	Not performed	Evidence inconclusive: inadequate TENS doses	Evidence inconclusive: inadequate TENS doses	Wide variation in comparison groups, outcome measures and patient groups between RCTs
Low back pain							
Gadsby & Flowerdew 1997, 2000/ Flowerdew & Gadsby 1997	Chronic low back pain	6 RCTs (288 patients)	2 RCTs on AL-TENS,	Odds ratio for pain relief effects of AL-TENS/TENS vs sham = 2.1 (6 RCTs) Odds ratio for pain	Evidence of effect: poor RCT methodology	Evidence inconclusive	Definitions used to distinguish AL-TENS and conventional TENS imprecise (i.e. low

(Continued)

Table 16.8 (Continued)

Reference and context	Condition	Data set (RCTs/ patient numbers)	Outcome (trial vote count)	Outcome (meta-analysis)	Review authors' conclusion	This author's judgement	Comment on review process
				relief effects of AL-TENS vs sham = 7.2 (2 RCTs) Odds ratio for pain relief effects of cTENS vs sham = 1.5 (4 RCTs) Odds ratio for improvement of range of movement with AL-TENS vs sham = 6.6 (2 RCTs)			frequency, high intensity and high frequency, low intensity, respectively). Wide variation in comparison groups, outcome measures and TENS interventions between RCTs
Milne et al 2001/Brosseau et al 2002	Chronic low back pain	5 RCTs (421 patients)		TENS = sham for pain relief (SMD = −0.207)	Evidence of no effect	Evidence of no effect	Wide variation in TENS interventions between RCTs
Khadilkar et al 2005a, 2005b; update of Milne et al 2001/Brosseau et al 2002	Low back pain	2 RCTs (175 patients)	TENS > placebo in 1/2 RCT for pain relief	Not possible	Evidence inconclusive	Evidence inconclusive: insufficient evidence	More stringent eligibility criteria reduced the number of trials included compared to Milne et al 2001/Brosseau et al 2002
Arthritis Osiri et al 2000	Knee osteoarthritis	7 RCTs (294 patients)	TENS > sham 2/7 RCTs	TENS > sham for pain relief (SMD = −0.448 VAS) TENS > sham for knee stiffness	Evidence of effect: pain relief	Evidence inconclusive: influence of one trial may have biased meta analysis	One positive outcome RCT had major impact on outcome of analysis but used

			(WMD = −5.9cm)				Codetron, which delivered current to 13 acupuncture points, rather than standard TENS
Pelland et al 2002	Rheumatoid arthritis affecting the hand	1 RCT (15 patients)	ES > no treatment control on pinch strength and muscle endurance	Calculated ES for a variety of functional measures for each RCT; each calculation based on less than 15 participants	Evidence inconclusive	Evidence inconclusive: insufficient evidence	Review outcome based on one 15-patient RCT
Brosseau et al 2003	Rheumatoid arthritis	3 RCTs (78 patients)	TENS > sham 3/3 RCTs	Calculated ES for each RCT with a mixture of positive and negative outcomes for a range of different outcome measures. Each RCT reported at least one outcome in which TENS > sham	Evidence of effect: pain relief	Evidence inconclusive	3 RCTs predate 1985 TENS dosage very low: 15 minutes of AL-TENS per week for 3 weeks
Other conditions							
Price & Pandyan 2000, 2001	Poststroke shoulder pain	4 RCTs (170 patients)	ES = sham for pain relief; SMD = 0.13 (4 RCTs) ES > sham for pain-free range of motion shows WMD = 9.17 (4 RCTs)		Evidence inconclusive	Evidence inconclusive: insufficient evidence	Variation in ES interventions 2 RCTs used TENS to produce muscle contractions
Kroeling et al 2005a, 2005b	Neck disorders (whiplash-associated disorders and mechanical neck disorders)	11 trials (525 patients)	Fourteen comparisons made TENS > sham 1/2 RCTs for pain	Not performed	Evidence inconclusive	Evidence inconclusive: insufficient evidence	TENS effects could be isolated in 1 RCT but a microcurrent device was used rather than a

(Continued)

Table 16.8 (Continued)

Reference and context	Condition	Data set (RCTs/patient numbers)	Outcome (trial vote count)	Outcome (meta-analysis)	Review authors' conclusion	This author's judgement	Comment on review process
							standard TENS device. Two RCTs used TENS in multimodal care framework and isolation of effects was not possible
Bronfort et al 2004	Chronic recurrent headache (migraine, tension-type headache)	22 RCTs (2628 patients) Non-invasive physical agents		Cranial electrotherapy > sham for pain relief (Effect size 0.4; 95% CI 0.0 to 0.8,1 RCT on 112 patients) Biofeedback > TENS and electrical neurotransmitter modulation > relaxation for pain relief (Effect size not calculated, 1 RCT, 392 patients) Combination of automassage, TENS, stretching > acupuncture for pain relief (Effect size 0.7; 95% CI 0.1 to 1.3, 1 RCT, 48 patients)	Evidence of effect, but weak	Evidence inconclusive: insufficient evidence electrotherapy	Most studies in review on spinal manipulation therapy. Cranial not delivered by a standard TENS device. Other studies used TENS as combination therapy

CI, confidence interval; CTENS, conventional TENS; non-invasive ES, electrical stimulation; RCT, randomized controlled trial; SMD, standardized mean difference; VAS, visual analogue scale; WMD, weighted mean difference.

muscle tension and has been used to treat muscle pain resulting from minor accidents and sports injuries including post-exertion muscle pain (i.e. delayed onset muscle soreness). Kroeling et al (2005a, b) conducted a Cochrane review of any surface electrical stimulation (ES) on whiplash-associated disorders and mechanical neck disorders, which included 11 trials and 525 patients. Three TENS trials were included, although one of them had used microcurrent rather than TENS. In the remaining two trials, TENS was reported to be superior to sham for pain relief in 1/2 RCTs. TENS may be helpful for myofascial pain syndrome (Graff-Radford 1989, Hou 2002) and localized pain in fibromyalgia (Offenbacher 2000), although TENS may aggravate pain in some patients. It is unlikely that TENS will be helpful in widespread pain in fibromyalgia because it is difficult to direct TENS currents into the painful area.

TENS and neuropathic pain

Clinical experience suggests that TENS may be useful for neuropathic pain whether or not there is a sympathetic component. TENS is likely to be more effective for neuropathic pains of peripheral rather than central origin and has been reported to be beneficial for peripheral neuropathic pain due to postherpetic neuralgia (Nathan & Wall 1974), trigeminal neuralgia (Bates & Nathan 1980), phantom limb and stump pain (Finsen et al 1988, Katz & Melzack 1991, Thorsteinsson 1987). TENS may also be useful for diabetes and entrapment neuropathies such as carpal tunnel syndrome, radiculopathies (cervical, thoracic and lumbar), complex regional pain syndromes type I (reflex sympathetic dystrophy) and type II (causalgia). There are few good-quality randomized controlled clinical trials. A Cochrane review on any form of surface electrical stimulation (ES) on 170 patients with poststroke shoulder pain found no significant change in pain incidence (odds ratio = 0.64) or pain intensity [standardized mean difference (SMD) = 0.13] after ES compared with control (Price & Pandyan 2000, 2001). However, ES improved pain-free range of passive humeral lateral rotation (weighted mean difference = 9.17) and reduced the severity of glenohumeral subluxation (SMD = −1.13). At present, the evidence for the effectiveness of TENS in neuropathic pain is inconclusive.

TENS and cancer pain

Success with TENS has also been reported in the palliative care setting in both adults (Avellanosa & West 1982, Hoskin & Hanks 1988) and children (Stevens et al 1994). TENS can be used for metastatic bone disease, for pains caused by secondary deposits and for pains due to nerve compression by a neoplasm (for reviews, see Berkovitch & Waller 2005, Stannard 2002, Thompson & Filshie 1993). In these circumstances, electrodes should be placed on healthy skin near to the painful area or metastatic deposit provided sensory function is preserved, or alternatively the affected dermatome. TENS has been used for neuropathic cancer pain caused by nerve compression by a neoplasm or infiltration by a tumor, and for iatrogenic neuralgias such as postmastectomy and post-thoracotomy pains. At present the evidence for TENS effectiveness for cancer pain is inconclusive.

TENS and chronic headache

It has been suggested that TENS may be useful for the treatment of headache (Soloman & Gulielmo 1985). Bronfort et al (2004) performed a Cochrane review on the effect of non-invasive physical agents on chronic recurrent headache, including migraine and tension-type headache. Twenty-two RCTs with 2628 patients were included in the review; three RCTs examined the effectiveness of electrical stimulation. One of these reported that cranial electrotherapy was superior to sham electrotherapy for pain relief; another that TENS and electrical neurotransmitter modulation were superior to relaxation, but not biofeedback, for pain relief. One study reported that a combination of automassage, TENS and stretching was superior to acupuncture for pain relief (see Table 16.8). None of these studies enabled a definitive conclusion about the effectiveness of TENS.

TENS and children

TENS has been shown to be useful in the management of a variety of pains in children, including

Table 16.9 Outcomes of systematic reviews on non painful conditions

Reference and context	Condition	Data set (RCTs/ patient numbers)	Outcome (trial vote count)	Outcome [Meta-analysis]	Review authors' conclusion	This author's judgement	Comment on review process
Hosker et al 2000	Faecal incontinence	1 RCT (40 patients) Intra-anal electrical stimulation		Intra-anal electrical stimulation + anal EMG biofeedback + home exercises > vaginal pelvic floor manometric pressure biofeedback + home exercises for improved incontinence status (odds ratio = 0.08 95% CI 0.02 to 0.37)	Insufficient evidence	Insufficient evidence	Cannot attribute the treatment effect solely to ES
Cameron et al 2003	Dementia	8 RCTs		3 RCTs eligible for analysis TENS > sham in delayed recall of 8 words (effect size 1.06, 1 RCT), face recognition (effect size 2.77, 2 RCTs) and motivation (effect size 0.85, 1 RCT)	Evidence of effect: short lived improvements in some neuropsychological and behavioural aspects of dementia	Evidence inconclusive: insufficient evidence	TENS applied to T1 and T5 of spine to produce visible muscle contractions in 5 RCTs Microcurrent at earlobes in 1 RCT and on forehead in 1 RCT. 1 RCT did not provide sufficient detail of intervention
Say et al 1996	Promotion of fetal growth in suspected placental insufficiency	No studies were included		Not performed	Insufficient evidence	Insufficient evidence	

dental pain (Harvey & Elliott 1995, Oztas et al 1997, teDuits et al 1993), minor procedures such as wound dressing (Merkel et al 1999) and venepuncture (Lander & Fowler-Kerry 1993). Children as young as four years of age appear to be able to understand and tolerate TENS treatment (Merkel et al 1999).

TENS and non–pain conditions

Three Cochrane reviews have evaluated the evidence for the use of TENS for non-painful conditions (Table 16.11). Cameron et al (2003) claim that TENS produces some short-lived improvements in cognitive aspects of dementia based on the findings of three RCTs. A Cochrane review on the effectiveness of TENS for promoting growth in suspected placental insufficiency found no RCTs in the literature (Say et al 1996). A Cochrane review of the use of intra-anal TENS for faecal incontinence also found insufficient evidence to make a definitive conclusion (Hosker et al 2000).

SHORTCOMINGS OF SYSTEMATIC REVIEWS AND CLINICAL TRIALS

The uncertainty about the clinical effectiveness of TENS for pain relief has led to questions about TENS as a viable treatment option. Nearly all systematic reviewers conclude that the methodological quality of TENS trials is poor. The importance of using appropriate outcome measures and adequate TENS technique in reviews of TENS was demonstrated earlier for postoperative pain (Bjordal et al 2003). Nevertheless, many TENS trials lack appropriate randomization, placebo and blinding procedures, and this may seriously affect outcome. For example, an analysis of trials of TENS and postoperative pain found that 17 of 19 non-randomized controlled trials (non-RCTs) reported that TENS relieved pain, whereas 15 of 17 RCTs reported that TENS did not. Schulz et al (1995) estimates that non-RCTs overestimate treatment effects by up to 40%. Operationalizing sham TENS interventions is also difficult and often achieved by preventing TENS currents reaching the patient, for example by cutting wires within the device. Blinding is often compromised

because patients in the TENS group feel paraesthesia and those in the sham do not. This may bias the participants' report of treatment outcome and will lower methodological quality scores (Bjordal & Greve 1998, Deyo et al 1990b, McQuay & Moore 1998b, Thorsteinsson 1990). Under-dosing of TENS has been recognized as a shortcoming in some TENS trials, with outcomes often measured after a single TENS intervention or following a course of infrequent intermittent TENS treatments (Carroll et al 2001). This approach to administering TENS differs markedly from clinical practice, where long-term users of TENS administer TENS over long periods of time (Johnson et al 1991c). In addition, investigators often measure effects before and after TENS but not during TENS. If TENS effects are maximal when the TENS device is switched on, then it is possible that investigators are missing potential benefits.

SUMMARY

TENS is used extensively in health care for pain relief because it is cheap, safe, and can be administered by the patients themselves. Success with TENS depends on appropriate application, and therefore patients and therapists need an understanding of the principles of application. When used in its conventional form TENS is delivered to selectively activate Aβ afferents leading to inhibition of nociceptive transmission in the spinal cord. It is claimed that the mechanism of action and analgesic profile of AL-TENS and intense TENS differ from those of conventional TENS and they may prove useful when conventional TENS is providing limited benefit. Systematic reviews of RCTs are compromised by poor-quality RCTs and this has led to review conclusions that are inconsistent and which contrast with clinical experience. It would be inappropriate to dismiss the use of TENS until the reasons for the discrepancy in experience and published evidence are fully explored. Better-quality trials are required to determine differences in the effectiveness of different types of TENS and to compare the cost-effectiveness of TENS with other analgesic interventions, including other electrotherapies.

References

Abram SE, Reynolds AC, Cusick JF (1981) Failure of naloxone to reverse analgesia from transcutaneous electrical stimulation in patients with chronic pain. *Anesth Analg* **60**: 81–84.

Ainsworth L, Budelier K, Clinesmith M et al (2006) Transcutaneous electrical nerve stimulation (TENS) reduces chronic hyperalgesia induced by muscle inflammation. *Pain* **120**: 182–187.

Ali J, Yaffe C, Serrette C (1981) The effect of transcutaneous electric nerve stimulation on postoperative pain and pulmonary function. *Surgery* **89**: 507–512.

American Physical Therapy Association (APTA) (1990) *Electrotherapeutic Terminology in Physical Therapy, Report by the Electrotherapy Standards Committee of the Section on Clinical Electrophysiology of the American Physical Therapy Association (APTA)*. Alexandria VA, APTA.

Andersson S, Ericson T, Holmgren E, Lindqvist G (1973) Electroacupuncture. Effect of pain threshold measured with electrical stimulation of teeth. *Brain Res* **63**: 393–396.

Asbjorn O (2000) Treatment of tennis elbow with transcutaneous nerve stimulation (TNS) Online. Available: http://www.paingone.com [accessed 1 July 2002].

Augustinsson L, Bohlin P, Bundsen P et al (1976a) Analgesia during delivery by transcutaneous electrical nerve stimulation. *Lakartidningen* **73**: 4205–4208.

Augustinsson L, Carlsson C, Pellettieri L (1976b) Transcutaneous electrical stimulation for pain and itch control. *Acta Neurochir* **33**: 342.

Augustinsson L, Bohlin P, Bundsen P et al (1977) Pain relief during delivery by transcutaneous electrical nerve stimulation. *Pain* **4**: 59–65.

Avellanosa AM, West CR (1982) Experience with transcutaneous electrical nerve stimulation for relief of intractable pain in cancer patients. *J Med* **13**: 203–213.

Barlas P, Lundeberg T (2005) Transcutaneous electrical nerve stimulation and acupuncture. In McMahaon SB, Koltzenburg M (eds) *Melzack and Wall's Textbook of Pain*. Philadelphia, Elsevier: 583–590.

Barr JO, Nielsen DH, Soderberg GL (1986) Transcutaneous electrical nerve stimulation characteristics for altering pain perception. *Phys Ther* **66**: 1515–1521.

Bates J, Nathan P (1980) Transcutaneous electrical nerve stimulation for chronic pain. *Anaesthesia* **35**: 817–822.

Berkovitch M, Waller A (2005) Treating pain with transcutaneous electrical nerve stimulation (TENS). In Doyle D, Hanks G, Cherny NI, Calman K (eds) *Oxford Textbook of Palliative Medicine*. Oxford, Oxford University Press: 405–410.

Berlant S (1984) Method of determining optimal stimulation sites for transcutaneous electrical nerve stimulation. *Phys Ther* **64**: 924–928.

Bertalanffy A, Kober A, Bertalanffy P et al (2005) Transcutaneous electrical nerve stimulation reduces acute low back pain during emergency transport. *Acc Emerg Med* **12**(7): 607–611.

Bjordal J, Greve G (1998) What may alter the conclusions of systematic reviews? *Phys Ther Rev* **3**: 121–132.

Bjordal JM, Johnson MI, Ljunggren AE (2003) Transcutaneous electrical nerve stimulation (TENS) can reduce postoperative analgesic consumption by one-third. A meta-analysis with assessment of optimal treatment parameters. *Eur J Pain* **7**: 181–188.

Börjesson M, Eriksson P, Dellborg M et al (1997) Transcutaneous electrical nerve stimulation in unstable angina pectoris. *Coron Art Dis* **8**: 543–550.

Bronfort G, Nilsson N, Haas M et al (2004) Non-invasive physical treatments for chronic/recurrent headache. Cochrane Database Systematic Reviews Issue 3: CD001878.

Brosseau L, Milne S, Robinson V et al (2002) Efficacy of the transcutaneous electrical nerve stimulation for the treatment of chronic low back pain: a meta-analysis. *Spine* **27**(6): 596–603.

Brosseau L, Judd MG, Marchand S et al (2003) Transcutaneous electrical nerve stimulation (TENS) for the treatment of rheumatoid arthritis in the hand. Cochrane Database Systematic Reviews Issue 3: CD004377.

Bundsen P, Ericson, K (1982) Pain relief in labor by transcutaneous electrical nerve stimulation. Safety aspects. *Acta Obstet Gynecol Scand* **61**: 1–5.

Bundsen P, Carlsson C, Forssman L, Tyreman N (1978) Pain relief during delivery by transcutaneous electrical nerve stimulation. *Prakt Anaesth* **13**: 20–28.

Burssens P, Forsyth R, Steyaert A et al (2005) Influence of burst TENS stimulation on collagen formation after Achilles tendon suture in man. A histological evaluation with Movat's pentachrome stain. *Acta Orthop Belg* **71**(3): 342–346.

Cameron M, Lonergan E, Lee H (2003) Transcutaneous electrical nerve stimulation (TENS) for dementia. Cochrane Database Systematic Reviews Issue 3: CD004032.

Carroll D, Tramer M, McQuay H et al (1996) Randomization is important in studies with pain outcomes: systematic review of transcutaneous electrical nerve stimulation in acute postoperative pain. *Br J Anaesth* **77**: 798–803.

Carroll D, Tramer M, McQuay H et al (1997a) Transcutaneous electrical nerve stimulation in labour pain: a systematic review. *Br J Obstet Gynaecol* **104**: 169–175.

Carroll D, Moore A, Tramer M, McQuay H (1997b) Transcutaneous electrical nerve stimulation does not relieve in labour pain: updated systematic review. *Contemp Rev Obstet Gynecol* **September**: 195–205.

Carroll D, Moore RA, McQuay HJ et al (2001) Transcutaneous electrical nerve stimulation (TENS) for chronic pain. Cochrane Database Systematic Reviews. Issue 3: CD003222.

Chabal C, Fishbain DA, Weaver M, Heine LW (1998) Long-term transcutaneous electrical nerve stimulation (TENS) use: impact on medication utilization and physical therapy costs. *Clin J Pain* **14**: 66–73.

Champagne C, Papiernik E, Thierry J, Nooviant Y (1984) Electrostimulation cerebrale transutanee par les courants de Limoge au cors de l'accouchement. *Ann Franç Anesth Reeanim* **3**: 405–413.

Chandran P, Sluka KA (2003) Development of opioid tolerance with repeated transcutaneous electrical nerve stimulation administration. *Pain* **102**: 195–201.

Chen D, Philip M, Philip PA, Monga TN (1990) Cardiac pacemaker inhibition by transcutaneous electrical nerve stimulation. *Arch Phys Med Rehab* **71**: 27–30.

Chung JM, Fang ZR, Hori Y et al (1984a) Prolonged inhibition of primate spinothalamic tract cells by peripheral nerve stimulation. *Pain* **19**: 259–275.

Chung JM, Lee KH, Hori Y et al (1984b) Factors influencing peripheral nerve stimulation produced inhibition of primate spinothalamic tract cells. *Pain* **19**: 277–293.

Corazza M, Maranini C, Bacilieri S, Virgili A (1999) Accelerated allergic contact dermatitis to a transcutaneous electrical nerve stimulation device. *Dermatology* **199**: 281.

Cramp FL, Noble G, Lowe AS et al (2000) A controlled study on the effects of transcutaneous electrical nerve stimulation and interferential therapy upon the RIII nociceptive and H-reflexes in humans. *Arch Phys Med Rehab* **81**: 324–333.

Crothers E (2003) Margie Polden Memorial Lecture. The use of transcutaneous electrical nerve stimulation during pregnancy: the evidence so far. *J Assoc Chartered Physiother Women's Health* **92**: 4–14.

Dawood M, Ramos J (1990) Transcutaneous electrical nerve stimulation (TENS) for the treatment of primary dysmenorrhea: a randomized crossover comparison with placebo TENS and ibuprofen. *Obstet Gynecol* **75**: 656–660.

de Tommaso M, Fiore P, Camporeale A et al (2003) High and low frequency transcutaneous electrical nerve stimulation inhibits nociceptive responses induced by CO_2 laser stimulation in humans. *Neurosci Lett* **342**(1–2): 17–20.

Debreceni L, Gyulai M, Debreceni A, Szabo K (1995) Results of transcutaneous electrical stimulation (TES) in cure of lower extremity arterial disease. *Angiology* **46**(7): 613–618.

Demmink J (1993) *The Degree of Modulation in Interferential Current Stimulation as Used in Physiotherapy. The Effect of a Biological Conducting Medium on the Pattern of Modulation in a Two-circuit Static Interferential Field.* MSc Thesis: University of Bergen, Norway.

Deyo R, Walsh N, Martin D et al (1990a) A controlled trial of transcutaneous electrical nerve stimulation (TENS) and exercise for chronic low back pain. *N Engl J Med* **322**: 1627–1634.

Deyo R, Walsh N, Schoenfeld L, Ramamurthy S (1990b) Can trials of physical treatments be blinded? The example of transcutaneous electrical nerve stimulation for chronic pain. *Am J Phys Med Rehab* **69**: 6–10.

Duggan AW, Foong FW (1985) Bicuculline and spinal inhibition produced by dorsal column stimulation in the cat. *Pain* **22**: 249–259.

Dundee JW, Yang J, McMillan C (1991) Non-invasive stimulation of the P6 (Neiguan) antiemetic acupuncture point in cancer chemotherapy. *J Roy Soc Med* **84**(4): 210–212.

Duranti R, Pantaleo T, Bellini F (1988) Increase in muscular pain threshold following low frequency-high intensity peripheral conditioning stimulation in humans. *Brain Res* **452**: 66–72.

Eriksson M, Sjölund B (1976) Acupuncture-like electroanalgesia in TNS resistant chronic pain. In Zotterman Y (ed) *Sensory Functions of the Skin.* New York, Pergamon Press: 575–581.

Eriksson MB, Sjölund BH, Nielzen S (1979) Long term results of peripheral conditioning stimulation as an analgesic measure in chronic pain. *Pain* **6**: 335–347.

Facchinetti F, Sforza G, Amidei M et al (1986) Central and peripheral beta-endorphin response to transcutaneous electrical nerve stimulation. *NIDA Res Monogr* **75**: 555–558.

Fargas-Babjak A, Rooney P, Gerecz E (1989) Randomised control trial of Codetron for pain control in osteoarthritis of the hip/knee. *Clin J Pain* **5**: 137–141.

Fargas-Babjak A, Pomeranz B, Rooney P (1992) Acupuncture-like stimulation with codetron for rehabilitation of patients with chronic pain syndrome and osteoarthritis. *Acupunct Electrother Res* **17**: 95–105.

Finsen V, Persen L, Lovlien M et al (1988) Transcutaneous electrical nerve stimulation after major amputation. *J Bone Joint Surg* **70**: 109–112.

Flowerdew M, Gadsby G (1997) A review of the treatment of chronic low back pain with acupuncture-like transcutaneous electrical nerve stimulation and transcutaneous electrical nerve stimulation. *Compl Ther Med* **5**: 193–201.

Foster NE, Baxter F, Walsh DM et al (1996) Manipulation of transcutaneous electrical nerve stimulation variables has no effect on two models of experimental pain in humans. *Clin J Pain* **12**(4): 301–310.

Gadsby G, Flowerdew M (1997) Nerve stimulation for low back pain – a review. *Nurs Stand* **11**(43): 32–33.

Gadsby JG, Flowerdew MW (2000) Transcutaneous electrical nerve stimulation and acupuncture-like transcutaneous electrical nerve stimulation for chronic low back pain. Cochrane Database Systematic Reviews. Issue (2: CD000210.

Garrison D, Foreman R (1994) Decreased activity of spontaneous and noxiously evoked dorsal horn cells during transcutaneous electrical nerve stimulation (TENS). *Pain* **58**: 309–315.

Garrison D, Foreman R (1996) Effects of transcutaneous electrical nerve stimulation (TENS) on spontaneous and noxiously evoked dorsal horn cell activity in cats with transected spinal cords. *Neurosci Lett* **216**: 125–128.

Gemignani G, Olivieri I, Ruju G, Pasero G (1991) Transcutaneous electrical nerve stimulation in ankylosing spondylitis: a double-blind study. *Arth Rheumatol* **34**: 788–789.

Gopalkrishnan P, Sluka KA (2000) Effect of varying frequency, intensity, and pulse duration of transcutaneous electrical nerve stimulation on primary hyperalgesia in inflamed rats. *Arch Phys Med Rehab* **81**(7): 984–990.

Graff-Radford SB, Reeves JL, Baker RL, Chiu D (1989) Effects of transcutaneous electrical nerve stimulation on myofascial pain and trigger point sensitivity. *Pain* **37**(1): 1–5.

Grim L, Morey S (1985) Transcutaneous electrical nerve stimulation for relief of parturition pain. A clinical report. *Phys Ther* **65**: 337–340.

Habib AS, Itchon-Ramos N, Phillips-Bute BG, Gan TJ (2006) Transcutaneous acupoint electrical stimulation with the relief band for the prevention of nausea and vomiting during and after cesarean delivery under spinal anesthesia. *Anesth Analg* **102**(2): 581–584.

Hansson P, Ekblom A (1983) Transcutaneous electrical nerve stimulation (TENS) as compared to placebo TENS for the relief of acute oro-facial pain. *Pain* **15**(2):157–165.

Hansson P, Ekblom A, Thomsson M, Fjellner B (1986 Influence of naloxone on relief of acute oro-facial pain by transcutaneous electrical nerve stimulation (TENS) or vibration. *Pain* **24**: 323–329.

Harrison R, Woods T, Shore M et al (1986) Pain relief in labour using transcutaneous electrical nerve stimulation (TENS). A TENS/TENS placebo controlled study in two parity groups. *Br J Obstet Gynaecol* **93**: 739–746.

Harvey M, Elliott M (1995) Transcutaneous electrical nerve stimulation (TENS) for pain management during cavity preparations in pediatric patients. *J Dent Child* **62**: 49–51.

Hauptman P, Raza M (1992) Electrocardiographic artifact with a transcutaneous electrical nerve stimulation unit. *Int J Cardiol* **34**: 110–112.

Hettrick HH, O'Brien K, Laznick H et al (2004) Effect of transcutaneous electrical nerve stimulation for the management of burn pruritus: a pilot study. *J Burn Care Rehab* **25**: 236–240.

Hosker G, Norton C, Brazzelli M (2000) Electrical stimulation for faecal incontinence in adults. Cochrane Database Systematic Reviews. Issue 2: CD001310.

Hoskin PJ, Hanks GW (1988) The management of symptoms in advanced cancer: experience in a hospital-based continuing care unit. *J Roy Soc Med* **81**: 341–344.

Hou CR, Tsai LC, Cheng KF et al (2002) Immediate effects of various physical therapeutic modalities on cervical myofascial pain and trigger-point sensitivity. *Arch Phys Med Rehab* **83**(10): 1406–1414.

Howson D (1978) Peripheral neural excitability. Implications for transcutaneous electrical nerve stimulation. *Phys Ther* **58**: 1467–1473.

Hymes A, Raab D, Yonchiro E et al (1974) Electrical surface stimulation for control of post operative pain and prevention of ileus. *Surg Forum* **65**: 1517–1520.

Ignelzi RJ, Nyquist JK (1976) Direct effect of electrical stimulation on peripheral nerve evoked activity: implications in pain relief. *J Neurosurg* **45**: 159–165.

Ignelzi RJ, Nyquist JK (1979) Excitability changes in peripheral nerve fibers after repetitive electrical stimulation. Implications in pain modulation. *J Neurosurg* **51**: 824–833.

Ivanova-Stoilova T, Howells D (2002) The usefulness of PainGone pain killing pen for self-treatment of chronic musculoskeletal pain – a pilot study. The Pain Society of Great Britain Annual Scientific Meeting Abstracts, April 9–12 Bournemouth, UK, Abstract 104.

Jeans M (1979) Relief of chronic pain by brief, intense transcutaneous electrical stimulation – a double blind study.

In Bonica JJ, Leibeskind J, Albe-fessard D (eds) *Advances in Pain Research and Therapy*, Vol 3. New York: Raven Press: 601–606.

Johannsen F, Gam A, Hauschild B et al (1993) Rebox: an adjunct in physical medicine? *Arch Phys Med Rehab* **74**: 438–440.

Johnson MI (1997) Transcutaneous electrical nerve stimulation (TENS) in the management of labour pain: the experience of over ten thousand women. *Br J Midwifery* **5**: 400–405.

Johnson MI (1998) The analgesic effects and clinical use of Acupuncture-like TENS (AL-TENS). *Phys Ther Rev* **3**: 73–93.

Johnson MI (2003) TENS and TENS-like devices. Do they provide pain relief? *Pain Rev* **8**: 121–158.

Johnson MI, Tabasam G (1999) A double blind placebo controlled investigation into the analgesic effects of interferential currents (IFC) and transcutaneous electrical nerve stimulation (TENS) on cold induced pain in healthy subjects. *Physiother Theory Pract* **15**: 217–233.

Johnson MI, Tabasam G (2003) A single-blind placebo controlled investigation into the analgesic effects of interferential currents (IFC) and transcutaneous electrical nerve stimulation (TENS) on ischaemic pain in healthy subjects. *Phys Ther* **83**(3): 208–223.

Johnson MI, Ashton CH, Bousfield DR, Thompson JW (1989) Analgesic effects of different frequencies of transcutaneous electrical nerve stimulation on cold-induced pain in normal subjects. *Pain* **39**: 231–236.

Johnson MI, Ashton CH, Bousfield DR, Thompson JW (1991a) Analgesic effects of different pulse patterns of transcutaneous electrical nerve stimulation on cold-induced pain in normal subjects. *J Psychosom Res* **35**: 313–321.

Johnson MI, Ashton CH, Thompson JW (1991b) The consistency of pulse frequencies and pulse patterns of transcutaneous electrical nerve stimulation (TENS) used by chronic pain patients. *Pain* **44**: 231–234.

Johnson MI, Ashton CH, Thompson JW (1991c) An in-depth study of long-term users of transcutaneous electrical nerve stimulation (TENS). Implications for clinical use of TENS. *Pain* **44**: 221–229.

Johnson MI, Ashton CH, Thompson J (1992a) Long term use of transcutaneous electrical nerve stimulation at Newcastle Pain Relief Clinic. *J Roy Soc Med* **85**: 267–268.

Johnson MI, Ashton CH, Thompson JW (1992b) Analgesic effects of Acupuncture Like TENS on cold pressor pain in normal subjects. *Eur J Pain* **13**: 101–108.

Johnson MI, Ashton CH, Thompson JW et al (1992c) The effect of transcutaneous electrical nerve stimulation (TENS) and acupuncture on concentrations of beta endorphin, met enkephalin and 5 hydroxytryptamine in the peripheral circulation. *Eur J Pain* **13**: 44–51.

Johnson MI, Penny P, Sajawal MA (1997) An examination of the analgesic effects of microcurrent stimulation (MES) on cold-induced pain in healthy subjects. *Physiother Theory Pract* **13**: 293–301.

Kalra A, Urban MO, Sluka KA (2001) Blockade of opioid receptors in rostral ventral medulla prevents antihyperalgesia produced by transcutaneous electrical nerve stimulation (TENS). *J Pharmacol Exp Ther* **298**(1): 257–263.

Kane K, Taub A (1975) A history of local electrical analgesia. *Pain* **1**: 125–138.

Kantor G, Alon G, Ho H (1994) The effects of selected stimulus waveforms on pulse and phase characteristics at sensory and motor thresholds. *Phys Ther* **74**: 951–962.

Kaplan B, Peled Y, Pardo J et al (1994) Transcutaneous electrical nerve stimulation (TENS) as a relief for dysmenorrhea. *Clin Exp Obstet Gynecol* **21**: 87–90.

Katz J, Melzack R (1991) Auricular transcutaneous electrical nerve stimulation (TENS) reduces phantom limb pain. *J Pain Sympt Manage* **6**: 73–83.

Khadilkar A, Milne S, Brosseau L et al (2005a) Transcutaneous electrical nerve stimulation (TENS) for chronic low-back pain. Cochrane Database of Systematic Reviews. Issue 3: CD003008.

Khadilkar A, Milne S, Brosseau L et al (2005b) Transcutaneous electrical nerve stimulation for the treatment of chronic low back pain: a systematic review. *Spine* **30**(23): 2657–2666.

King EW, Sluka KA (2001) The effect of varying frequency and intensity of transcutaneous electrical nerve stimulation on secondary mechanical hyperalgesia in an animal model of inflammation. *J Pain* **2**(2): 128–133.

King EW, Audette K, Athman GA et al (2005) Transcutaneous electrical nerve stimulation activates peripherally located alpha-2A adrenergic receptors. *Pain* **115**(3): 364–373.

Kroeling P, Gross A, Houghton PE (2005a) Electrotherapy for neck disorders. Cochrane Database of Systematic Reviews. Issue 2: CD004251.

Kroeling P, Gross AR, Goldsmith CH (2005b) Cervical Overview Group. A Cochrane review of electrotherapy for mechanical neck disorders. *Spine* **30**(21): 641–648.

Kubista E, Kucera H, Riss P (1978) The effect of transcutaneous nerve stimulation on labour pain. *Geburtschilfe Frauenheilkd* **38**: 1079–1084.

Lander J, Fowler-Kerry S (1993) TENS for children's procedural pain. *Pain* **52**: 209–216.

Levin M, Hui-Chan C (1993) Conventional and acupuncture-like transcutaneous electrical nerve stimulation excite similar afferent fibers. *Arch Phys Med Rehab* **74**: 54–60.

Lewers D, Clelland J, Jackson J et al (1989) Transcutaneous electrical nerve stimulation in the relief of primary dysmenorrhoea. *Phys Ther* **69**: 3–9.

Lewis SM, Clelland JA, Knowles CJ et al (1990) Effects of auricular acupuncture-like transcutaneous electric nerve stimulation on pain levels following wound care in patients with burns: a pilot study. *J Burn Care Rehab* **11**: 322–329.

Loeser J, Black R, Christman A (1975) Relief of pain by transcutaneous electrical nerve stimulation. *J Neurosurg* **42**: 308–314.

Long DM (1973) Electrical stimulation for relief of pain from chronic nerve injury. *J Neurosurg* **39**: 718–722.

Long DM (1974) External electrical stimulation as a treatment of chronic pain. *Minnesota Med* **57**: 195–198.

Longobardi A, Clelland J, Knowles C, Jackson J (1989) Effects of auricular transcutaneous electrical nerve stimulation on distal extremity pain: a pilot study. *Phys Ther* **69**: 10–17.

Ma YT, Sluka KA (2001) Reduction in inflammation-induced sensitization of dorsal horn neurons by transcutaneous electrical nerve stimulation in anesthetized rats. *Exp Brain Res* **137**(1): 94–102.

Macdonald ARJ, Coates TW (1995) The discovery of transcutaneous spinal electroanalgesia and its relief of chronic pain. *Physiotherapy* **81**: 653–660.

Macefield G, Burke D (1991) Long-lasting depression of central synaptic transmission following prolonged high-frequency stimulation of cutaneous afferents: a mechanism for post-vibratory hypaesthesia. *Electroencephal Clin Neurophysiol* **78**: 150–158.

Mann CJ (1996) Respiratory compromise: a rare complication of transcutaneous electrical nerve stimulation for angina pectoris. *J Acc Emerg Med* **13**: 68–69.

Mannheimer JS, Lampe GN (1987) *Clinical Transcutaneous Electrical Nerve Stimulation*. Philadelphia, FA Davis.

Mannheimer C, Carlsson C, Ericson K et al (1982) Transcutaneous electrical nerve stimulation in severe angina pectoris. *Eur Heart J* **3**: 297–302.

Mannheimer C, Carlsson C, Emanuelsson H et al (1985) The effects of transcutaneous electrical nerve stimulation in patients with severe angina pectoris. *Circulation* **71**: 308–316.

Mannheimer C, Emanuelsson H, Waagstein F (1990) The effect of transcutaneous electrical nerve stimulation (TENS) on catecholamine metabolism during pacing-induced angina pectoris and the influence of naloxone. *Pain* **41**: 27–34.

Marchand S, Charest J, Li J et al (1993) Is TENS purely a placebo effect? A controlled study on chronic low back pain. *Pain* **54**: 99–106.

McDowell BC, Lowe AS, Walsh DM et al (1995) The lack of hypoalgesic efficacy of H-wave therapy on experimental ischaemic pain. *Pain* **61**: 27–32.

McDowell BC, McCormack K, Walsh DM et al (1999) Comparative analgesic effects of H-wave therapy and transcutaneous electrical nerve stimulation on pain threshold in humans. *Arch Phys Med Rehab* **80**: 1001–1004.

McQuay HJ, Moore RA (1998a) TENS in chronic pain. In McQuay HJ, Moore RA (eds) *An Evidence-Based Resource for Pain Relief*. Oxford, Oxford University Press: 207–211.

McQuay HJ, Moore RA (1998b) Judging the quality of trials. In McQuay HJ, Moore RA (eds) *An Evidence-Based Resource for Pain Relief*. Oxford, Oxford University Press: 10–13.

Meechan JG, Gowans AJ, Welbury RR (1998) The use of patient-controlled transcutaneous electronic nerve stimulation (TENS) to decrease the discomfort of regional anaesthesia in dentistry: a randomised controlled clinical trial. *J Dentistry* **26**(5–6): 417–420.

Melzack R, Wall P (1965) Pain mechanisms: A new theory. *Science* **150**: 971–979.

Melzack R, Vetere P, Finch L (1983) Transcutaneous electrical nerve stimulation for low back pain. A comparison of TENS and massage for pain and range of motion. *Phys Ther* **63**: 489–493.

Merkel SI, Gutstein HB, Malviya S (1999) Use of transcutaneous electrical nerve stimulation in a young child with pain from open perineal lesions. *J Pain Symptom Manage* **18**: 376–381.

Meuleman V, Busschots A, Dooms-Goossens A (1996) Contact allergy to a device for transcutaneous electrical neural stimulation (TENS). *Contact Dermatitis* **35**: 53–54.

Meyerson B (1983) Electrostimulation procedures: effects presumed rationale, and possible mechanisms. In Bonica JJ Lindblom U, Iggo A (eds) *Advances in Pain Research and Therapy*, Vol 5. New York, Raven Press: 495–534.

Miller-Jones C (1980) Transcutaneous nerve stimulation in labour. *Anaesthesia* **35**: 372–375.

Milne S, Welch V, Brosseau L et al (2001) Transcutaneous electrical nerve stimulation (TENS) for chronic low back pain. Cochrane Database of Systematic Reviews. Issue 2: CD003008.

Milsom I, Hedner N, Mannheimer C (1994) A comparative study of the effect of high-intensity transcutaneous nerve stimulation and oral naproxen on intrauterine pressure and menstrual pain in patients with primary dysmenorrhea. *Am J Obstet Gynecol* **170**: 123–129.

Murray S, Collins PD, James MA (2004) An investigation into the 'carry over' effect of neurostimulation in the treatment of angina pectoris. *Int J Clin Pract* **58**(7): 669–674.

Myers RA, Woolf CJ, Mitchell D (1977) Management of acute traumatic pain by peripheral transcutaneous electrical stimulation. *S Afr Med J* **52**: 309–312.

Nardone A, Schieppati M (1989) Influences of transcutaneous electrical stimulation of cutaneous and mixed nerves on subcortical and cortical somatosensory evoked potentials. *Electroencephal Clin Neurophysiol* **74**: 24–35.

Nash T, Williams J, Machin D (1990) TENS: does the type of stimulus really matter? *Pain Clin* **3**: 161–168.

Nathan PW, Wall PD (1974) Treatment of post-herpetic neuralgia by prolonged electric stimulation. *Br Med J* **3**: 645–647.

Neighbors L, Clelland J, Jackson J et al (1987). Transcutaneous electrical nerve stimulation for pain relief in primary dysmenorrhea. *Clin J Pain* **3**: 17–22.

Odendaal CL, Joubert G (1999) APS therapy – a new way of treating chronic backache – a pilot study. *S Afr J Anaesthesiol Analg* **5**: 1–5.

Offenbacher M, Stucki G (2000) Physical therapy in the treatment of fibromyalgia. *Scand J Rheumatol* (suppl) **113**: 78–85.

Osiri M, Welch V, Brosseau L et al (2002) Transcutaneous electrical nerve stimulation for knee osteoarthritis. Cochrane Database of Systematic Reviews. Issue 4: CD002823.

Oztas N, Olmez A, Yel B (1997) Clinical evaluation of transcutaneous electronic nerve stimulation for pain control during tooth preparation. *Quint Int* **28**: 603–608.

Pelland L, Brosseau L, Casimiro L et al (2002 Electrical stimulation for the treatment of rheumatoid arthritis. The Cochrane Database of Systematic Reviews Issue 2: CD003687.

Philadelphia Panel (2001) Philadelphia Panel evidence-based clinical practice guidelines on selected rehabilitation interventions for low back pain. *Phys Ther* **81**(10): 1641–1674.

Pomeranz B, Niznick G (1987) Codetron, a new electrotherapy device overcomes the habituation problems of conventional TENS devices. *Am J Electromed* **First quarter**: 22–26.

Pope G, Mockett S, Wright J (1995) A survey of electrotherapeutic modalities: ownership and use in the NHS in England. *Physiotherapy* **81**: 82–91.

Price CI, Pandyan AD (2000) Electrical stimulation for preventing and treating post-stroke shoulder pain. Cochrane Database of Systematic Reviews. Issue 4: CD001698.

Price CI, Pandyan AD (2001) Electrical stimulation for preventing and treating post-stroke shoulder pain: a systematic Cochrane review. *Clin Rehab* **15**(1): 5–19.

Proctor ML, Smith CA, Farquhar CM, Stones RW (2002) Transcutaneous electrical nerve stimulation and acupuncture for primary dysmenorrhoea. Cochrane Database of Systematic Reviews. Issue (1: CD002123.

Pyatt JR, Trenbath D, Chester M, Connelly DT (2003) The simultaneous use of a biventricular implantable cardioverter defibrillator (ICD) and transcutaneous electrical nerve stimulation (TENS) unit: implications for device interaction. *Europace* **5**(1): 91–93.

Radhakrishnan R, Sluka KA (2003) Spinal muscarinic receptors are activated during low or high frequency TENS-induced antihyperalgesia in rats. *Neuropharmacology* **45**(8): 1111–1119.

Radhakrishnan R, Sluka KA (2005) Deep tissue afferents, but not cutaneous afferents, mediate transcutaneous electrical nerve stimulation-Induced antihyperalgesia. *J Pain* **6**(10): 673–680.

Radhakrishnan R, King EW, Dickman JK et al (2003) Spinal 5-HT(2) and 5-HT(3) receptors mediate low, but not high, frequency TENS-induced antihyperalgesia in rats. *Pain* **105**(1–2): 205–213 [erratum in: *Pain* 2004 **107**(1–2): 197].

Rasmussen M, Hayes D, Vlietstra R, Thorsteinsson G (1988) Can transcutaneous electrical nerve stimulation be safely used in patients with permanent cardiac pacemakers? *Mayo Clin Proc* **63**: 443–445.

Reeve J, Menon D, Corabian P (1996) Transcutaneous electrical nerve stimulation (TENS): a technology assessment. *Int J Technol Ass Health Care* **12**: 299–324.

Reynolds DV (1969) Surgery in the rat during electrical analgesia induced by focal brain stimulation. *Science* **164**: 444–445.

Rieb L, Pomeranz B (1992) Alterations in electrical pain thresholds by use of acupuncture-like transcutaneous electrical nerve stimulation in pain-free subjects. *Phys Ther* **72**: 658–667.

Robertson V, Spurritt D (1998) Electrophysical agents: Implications of their availability and use in undergraduate clinical placements. *Physiotherapy* **84**: 335–344.

Rosted P (2001) Repetitive epileptic fits – a possible adverse effect after transcutaneous electrical nerve stimulation (TENS) in a post-stroke patient. *Acupuncture Med* **19**: 46–49.

Sandkühler J (2000) Long-lasting analgesia following TENS and acupuncture: Spinal mechanisms beyond gate control. In: Devor M, Rowbotham MC, Wiesenfeld-Hallin Z (eds) *Progress in Pain Research and Management*, Vol 16. Seattle, WA, IASP Press: 359–369.

Sandkühler J, Chen JG, Cheng G, Randic M (1997) Low-frequency stimulation of afferent Adelta-fibers induces long-term depression at primary afferent synapses with substantia gelatinosa neurons in the rat. *J Neurosci* **17**: 6483–6491.

Say L, Gülmezoglu AM, Hofmeyr GJ (1996) Transcutaneous electrostimulation for suspected placental insufficiency (diagnosed by Doppler studies). Cochrane Database of Systematic Reviews Issue (1: CD000079).

Schafer E, Finkensiep H, Kaup M (2000) Effect of transcutaneous electrical nerve stimulation on pain perception threshold of human teeth: a double-blind, placebo-controlled study. *Clin Oral Invest* **4**(2): 81–86.

Scherder E, Van Someren E, Swaab D (1999) Epilepsy: a possible contraindication for transcutaneous electrical nerve stimulation. *J Pain Symptom Manage* **17**: 152–153.

Schulz KF, Chalmers I, Hayes RJ, Altman DG (1995) Empirical evidence of bias. Dimensions of methodological quality associated with estimates of treatment effects in controlled trials. *J Am Med Assoc* **273**: 408–412.

Schuster G, Infante M (1980) Pain relief after low back surgery: the efficacy of transcutaneous electrical nerve stimulation. *Pain* **8**: 299–302.

Shealy CN, Mortimer JT, Reswick JB (1967) Electrical inhibition of pain by stimulation of the dorsal columns: preliminary clinical report. *Anesth Analg* **46**: 489–491.

Sjölund B (1985) Peripheral nerve stimulation suppression of C-fiber-evoked flexion reflex in rats. Part 1: parameters of continuous stimulation. *J Neurosurg* **63**: 612–616.

Sjölund B (1988) Peripheral nerve stimulation suppression of C-fiber-evoked flexion reflex in rats. Part 2: parameters of low-rate train stimulation of skin and muscle afferent nerves. *J Neurosurg* **68**: 279–283.

Sjölund BH, Eriksson MB (1979) The influence of naloxone on analgesia produced by peripheral conditioning stimulation. *Brain Res* **173**: 295–301.

Sjölund B, Terenius L, Eriksson M (1977) Increased cerebrospinal fluid levels of endorphins after electroacupuncture. *Acta Physiol Scand* **100**: 382–384.

Sjölund B, Eriksson M, Loeser J (1990) Transcutaneous and implanted electric stimulation of peripheral nerves. In Bonica JJ (ed) *The Management of Pain* Vol 2. Philadelphia, Lea and Febiger: 1852–1861.

Sliwa J, Marinko M (1996) Transcutaneous electrical nerve stimulator-induced electrocardiogram artifact. A brief report. *Am J Phys Med Rehab* **75**: 307–309.

Sloan J, Muwanga C, Waters E et al (1986) Multiple rib fractures: transcutaneous nerve stimulation versus conventional analgesia. *J Trauma* **26**: 1120–1122.

Sluka KA, Chandran P (2002) Enhanced reduction in hyperalgesia by combined administration of clonidine and TENS. *Pain* **100**(1–2): 183–190.

Sluka KA, Walsh D (2003) Transcutaneous electrical nerve stimulation: basic science mechanisms and clinical effectiveness. *J Pain* **4**(3): 109–121.

Sluka KA, Bailey K, Bogush J et al (1998) Treatment with either high or low frequency TENS reduces the secondary hyperalgesia observed after injection of kaolin and carrageenan into the knee joint. *Pain* **77**(1): 97–102.

Sluka KA, Deacon M, Stibal A et al (1999) Spinal blockade of opioid receptors prevents the analgesia produced by TENS in arthritic rats. *J Pharmacol Exp Ther* **289**(2): 840–846.

Sluka KA, Judge MA, McColley MM et al (2000) Low frequency TENS is less effective than high frequency TENS at reducing inflammation-induced hyperalgesia in morphine-tolerant rats. *Eur J Pain* **4**(2):185–193.

Sluka KA, Vance CG, Lisi TL (2005) High-frequency, but not low-frequency, transcutaneous electrical nerve stimulation reduces aspartate and glutamate release in the spinal cord dorsal horn. *J Neurochem* **95**(6): 1794–1801.

Solomon S, Guglielmo KM (1985) Treatment of headache by transcutaneous electrical stimulation. *Headache* **25**(1): 12–15.

Stannard C (2002) Simulation-induced analgesia in cancer pain management. In Sykes N, Fallon MT, Patt RB (eds) *Textbook of Clinical Pain Management*. London, Edward Arnold: 245–252.

Stevens M, Dalla Pozza L, Cavalletto B et al (1994) Pain and symptom control in paediatric palliative care. *Cancer Surv* **21**: 211–231.

Stewart P (1979) Transcutaneous electrical nerve stimulation as a method of analgesia in labour. *Anaesthesia* **34**: 361–364.

Stillings D (1975) A survey of the history of electrical stimulation for pain to 1900. *Med Instrument* **9**: 255–259.

Tang WY, Chan LY, Lo KK, Wong TW (1999) Evaluation on the antipruritic role of transcutaneous electrical nerve stimulation in the treatment of pruritic dermatoses. *Dermatology* **199**(3): 237–241.

teDuits E, Goepferd S, Donly K et al (1993) The effectiveness of electronic dental anesthesia in children. *Pediatr Dent* **15**: 191–196.

Thomas I, Tyle V, Webster J, Neilson A (1988) An evaluation of transcutaneous electrical nerve stimulation for pain relief in labour. *Aust NZ J Obstet Gynaecol* **28**: 182–189.

Thompson J (1989) The pharmacology of transcutaneous electrical nerve stimulation (TENS). *Intract Pain Soc Forum* **7**: 33–39.

Thompson J, Filshie J (1993) Transcutaneous electrical nerve stimulation (TENS) and acupuncture. In Doyle D, Hanks G, Cherny NI, Calman K (eds) *Oxford Textbook of Palliative Medicine*. Oxford, Oxford University Press: 229–244.

Thorsteinsson G (1987) Chronic pain: use of TENS in the elderly. *Geriatrics* **42**: 75–77, 81–82.

Thorsteinsson G (1990) Can trials of physical treatments be blinded? The example of transcutaneous electrical nerve stimulation for chronic pain. *Am J Phys Med Rehab* **69**: 219–220.

Tinegate H, McLelland J (2002) Transcutaneous electrical nerve stimulation may improve pruritus associated with haematological disorders. *Clin Lab Haematol* **24**(6): 389–390.

Tulgar M, McGlone F, Bowsher D, Miles J (1991a) Comparative effectiveness of different stimulation modes in relieving pain. Part I. A pilot study. *Pain* **47**: 151–155.

Tulgar M, McGlone F, Bowsher D, Miles J (1991b) Comparative effectiveness of different stimulation modes in relieving pain. Part II. A double-blind controlled long-term clinical trial. *Pain* **47**: 157–162.

van der Ploeg J, Vervest H, Liem A et al (1996) Transcutaneous nerve stimulation (TENS) during the first stage of labour: a randomized clinical trial. *Pain* **68**: 75–78.

Vincenti E, Cervellin A, Mega M (1982) Comparative study between patients treated with transcutaneous electric stimulation and controls during labour. *Clin Exp Obstet Gynaecol* **9**: 95–97.

Wall PD, Sweet WH (1967) Temporary abolition of pain in man. *Science* **155**: 108–109.

Walsh DM (1996) Transcutaneous electrical nerve stimulation and acupuncture points. *Compl Ther Med* **4**: 133–137.

Walsh DM (1997a) *TENS. Clinical Applications and Related Theory.* New York, Churchill Livingstone.

Walsh DM (1997b) Non-analgesic effects of TENS. In Walsh DM (ed) *TENS. Clinical Applications and Related Theory.* New York, Churchill Livingstone: 125–138.

Walsh DM (1997c) Review of clinical studies on TENS. In Walsh DM (ed) *TENS. Clinical Applications and Related Theory.* New York, Churchill Livingstone: 83–124.

Walsh DM (1997d) Review of experimental studies on TENS. In Walsh DM (ed) *TENS. Clinical Applications and Related Theory.* New York, Churchill Livingstone: 63–81.

Walsh DM (1997e) TENS: Physiological principles and stimulation parameters. In Walsh DM (ed) *TENS. Clinical Applications and Related Theory.* New York, Churchill Livingstone: 25–40.

Walsh DM, Liggett C, Baxter D, Allen JM (1995) A double-blind investigation of the hypoalgesic effects of transcutaneous electrical nerve stimulation upon experimentally induced ischaemic pain. *Pain* **61**(1): 39–45.

Walsh DM, Lowe AS, McCormack K et al (1998) Transcutaneous electrical nerve stimulation: effect on peripheral nerve conduction, mechanical pain threshold, and tactile threshold in humans. *Arch Phys Med Rehab* **79**: 1051–1058.

Walsh DM, Noble G, Baxter GD, Allen JM (2000) Study of the effects of various transcutaneous electrical nerve stimulation (TENS) parameters upon the RIII nociceptive and H-reflexes in humans. *Clin Physiol* **20**(3):191–199.

Ward L, Wright E, McMahon SB (1996) A comparison of the effects of noxious and innocuous counter stimuli on experimentally induced itch and pain. *Pain* **64**(1): 129–138.

Watson T (2006) Transcutaneous electrical nerve stimulation (TENS). Online. Available: http://www.electrotherapy. org [accessed 24 May 2006].

Wattrisse G, Leroy B, Dufossez F, Tai RBH (1993) Electrostimulation cerebrale transcutanee: etude comparative des effets de son association a l'anesthesie peridurale par bupivacaine-fentanyl au cours de l'analgesie obstetricale [Transcutaneous electric stimulation of the brain: a comparative study of the effects of its combination with peridural anaesthesia using bupivacaine-fentanyl during obstetric analgesia]. *Cahiers anesthésiol* **41**: 489–495.

Wikstrom SO, Svedman P, Svensson H, Tanweer AS (1999) Effect of transcutaneous nerve stimulation on microcirculation in intact skin and blister wounds in healthy volunteers. *Scand J Plast Reconstr Surg Hand Surg* **33**(2): 195–201.

Woolf C, Thompson JW (1994) Segmental afferent fibre-induced analgesia: Transcutaneous electrical nerve stimulation (TENS) and vibration. In Wall PD, Melzack R (eds) *Textbook of Pain.* Edinburgh, Churchill Livingstone: 1191–1208.

Woolf C, Mitchell D, Myers RA, Barrett GD (1978) Failure of naloxone to reverse peripheral transcutaneous electro-analgesia in patients suffering from acute trauma. *S Afr Med J* **53**: 179–180.

Woolf C, Mitchell D, Barrett GD (1980) Antinociceptive effect of peripheral segmental electrical stimulation in the rat. *Pain* **8**: 237–252.

Woolf C, Thompson S, King A (1988) Prolonged primary afferent induced alterations in dorsal horn neurones, an intracellular analysis in vivo and in vitro. *J Physiol* **83**: 255–266.

Chapter 17

Interferential current

Shea Palmer and Denis Martin

CHAPTER CONTENTS

INTRODUCTION

Interferential current (IFC) was developed in the 1950s and became increasingly popular in the UK during the 1970s (Ganne 1976). Although the actual definition of IFC has not been standardized in the literature, it can be described as the transcutaneous application of medium-frequency alternating currents, the amplitude of which is modulated at low frequency for therapeutic purposes. From this definition it can be seen that IFC is a form of transcutaneous electrical nerve stimulation (TENS).

IFC has been reported to reduce the skin resistance (and thus the discomfort) incurred by traditional low-frequency currents, while still producing low-frequency effects within the tissues (De Domenico & Strauss 1985, Low & Reed 2000). It has also been claimed to permit the treatment of deep tissues (De Domenico & Strauss 1985, Goats 1990, Hansjuergens 1986, Low & Reed 2000, Nikolova 1987, Willie 1969). Both of the above claims, which are unique to IFC, are largely unsubstantiated and have been challenged (Alon 1987, Palmer et al 1999a).

IFC has been reported to be available in between 77 and 98% of physiotherapy departments in Australia (Lindsay et al 1990, Robertson & Spurritt 1998), England (Pope et al 1995) and the Republic of Ireland (Cooney et al 2000). A strong relationship between the availability of IFC and its use has been established (Cooney et al 2000, Lindsay et al 1990, Robinson & Snyder-Mackler 1988), with 90% of physiotherapy clinicians with access to IFC reported to use it at least once per day (Lindsay et al 1990). Turner and Whitfield (1997) found that IFC was used by 43% of physiotherapists working in all clinical specialties in England. In terms of the conditions treated with IFC, 91% of respondents to one survey (Johnson & Tabasam 1998) used IFC to relieve pain. In a follow-up study (Tabasam & Johnson 2000), 26% of treatments were found to be for acute pain, 50% for chronic pain, and 16% for reduction of swelling. In another survey 88% of clinicians in the UK and Ireland reported using IFC to treat non-specific low back pain (Foster et al 1999). In addition to the treatment of pain IFC has also been used for other clinical conditions, including asthma (Emberson 1996), fractures (Fourie & Bowerbank 1997), incontinence (Laycock & Green 1988), psoriasis (Philipp et al 2000) and swelling (Christie & Willoughby 1990); and for accelerating tissue healing (Nikolova 1987), enhancing blood flow (Lamb & Mani 1994) and muscle strengthening (Bircan et al 2002).

These studies illustrate both a high rate of access to and use of IFC, at least in the UK, Ireland and Australia. It is interesting to note the prevalence of its usage for pain, indicating a perceived benefit to patients in terms of IFC-mediated effects on pain. Clinical trials of the effects of IFC on pain and other conditions, however, still remain scarce and largely inconclusive. Reports of the effectiveness of IFC have traditionally been scholarly statements in electrotherapy textbooks (De Domenico 1987, Kahn 1987, Nikolova 1987, Savage 1984) or largely descriptive journal articles (Belcher 1974, De Domenico 1982, Ganne 1976, Goats 1990, Willie

1969). The current emphasis on evidence-based practice, however, demands a more critical approach to clinical reasoning and treatment choices. This chapter will concentrate primarily on the literature related to IFC in the management of pain due to the prevalence of this use. Other claimed effects of IFC, such as on bone and tissue healing and muscle stimulation will be addressed in less detail.

A fundamental issue in the chapter is whether IFC is a singular, distinctive form of treatment, or simply another type of TENS. This is an important consideration because, if not the former, then the need for IFC is undermined.

PHYSICAL PRINCIPLES OF INTERFERENTIAL CURRENT

IFC describes a current applied at approximately 4000 Hz (usually referred to in physiotherapy as medium frequency) that rhythmically increases and decreases in amplitude at low frequency (adjustable between 0 and 200–250 Hz). IFC is produced by mixing two slightly out-of-phase medium-frequency currents, either by applying them so that they 'interfere' within the tissues or, alternatively, by mixing them within the stimulator prior to application ('premodulated' current). One current is normally of fixed frequency, for example at 4000 Hz, the other is adjustable, for example between 4000 and 4200 Hz. Theoretically, the two currents summate or cancel each other out in a predictable manner, producing the resultant amplitude modulated 'interferential current'. The

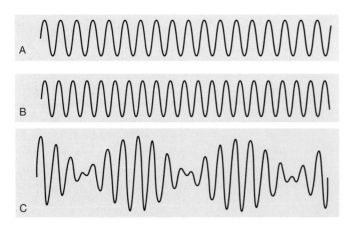

Figure 17.1 Interference between two medium-frequency currents (A, 4000 Hz and B, 4100 Hz) produces a resultant 'interferential current' (C) 4050 Hz and an amplitude modulated frequency of 100 Hz.

frequency of the resultant current will be equal to the mean of the two original currents and will vary in amplitude at a frequency equal to the difference between these two currents. This latter frequency is known as the 'amplitude modulated frequency' (AMF) or 'beat frequency'. Figure 17.1 illustrates the production of IFC: two currents of 4000 and 4100 Hz are mixed, resulting in a medium-frequency current of 4050 Hz, which is amplitude modulated at a frequency of 100 Hz.

TREATMENT PARAMETERS AND METHODS OF APPLICATION

Amplitude modulated frequency

The AMF is traditionally considered to be the effective component of IFC, mimicking low-frequency currents and creating differential stimulation of nerve and tissue types (De Domenico 1982, Ganne 1976, Goats 1990, Low & Reed 2000, Nikolova 1987, Szehi & David 1980, Willie 1969). The theory of IFC is that the medium-frequency components simply act as 'carrier' currents, bringing the low-frequency AMF into the tissues (De Domenico 1982), where the body must be able to demodulate it.

The mechanisms of this demodulation have not been established (Johnson 1999) and claims for the AMF to be the effective component of IFC have been challenged (Johnson 1999, Kinnunen & Alasaarela 2004, Martin 1996, Martin & Palmer 1995a, Palmer et al 1999a). It has been demonstrated that alteration of the AMF has little effect on the threshold activation of sensory, motor and pain responses (Kinnunen & Alasaarela 2004, Martin & Palmer 1995a, Palmer et al 1999a). IFC certainly did not follow the very clear frequency-dependent effects displayed by TENS, suggesting that the AMF does not, in fact, mimic low-frequency stimulation. In addition, the omission of an AMF (pure 4000 Hz current) displayed similar effects to when an AMF was used. It was concluded from this latter observation that the medium-frequency component of IFC, and not the AMF, was the dominant stimulating parameter (Palmer et al 1999a).

To illustrate this point, the mean sensory thresholds (the point at which the current was first reported as being perceived) from Palmer et al

(1999a) are presented in Figure 17.2. These results can be explained by consideration of Table 17.1, which illustrates the effect of altering the AMF on the other components of IFC. This highlights that the resultant current frequency, and thus phase duration, change little. If the medium frequency is the main stimulating parameter then it is perhaps not surprising that the effect of the AMF might prove not to be as important as traditionally thought. However, it is obvious that the responses induced by IFC stimulation change with different AMF settings. Low AMFs, for example, elicit a 'beating' or 'tapping' sensation and muscle twitch responses, whereas higher AMFs elicit a 'buzzing'

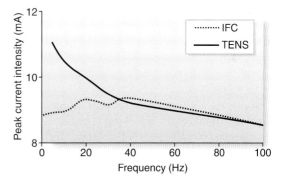

Figure 17.2 Mean sensory thresholds for IFC and TENS (from Palmer et al 1999a). Frequency has little effect on sensory thresholds with IFC, whereas clear frequency-dependent effects are demonstrated with TENS.

Table 17.1 Interferential current characteristics with a range of amplitude modulated frequencies (4000 Hz carrier frequency)

Amplitude modulated frequency (AMF)	Resultant medium frequency (Hz)	Resultant medium-frequency phase duration (µs)
100	4050	123.5
40	4020	124.4
30	4015	124.5
20	4010	124.7
15	4007.5	124.8
10	4005	124.9
5	4002.5	124.9
0	4000	125

or 'tingling' sensation and a tetanic muscle contraction. This proposes some ability of the body to distinguish between high and low AMF settings. It has been found that participants experienced a 5 Hz AMF setting as being significantly more uncomfortable than either 50 or 100 Hz, with no significant difference between the level of discomfort at 50 and 100 Hz (Martin & Palmer 1996). In fact, at frequencies above approximately 40 Hz there seems to be little difference in the effects of IFC and TENS on somatosensory and motor thresholds (Palmer et al 1999a), with the comfort associated with muscle stimulation at 80 Hz also being demonstrated to be similar (Bircan et al 2002).

The AMF, at least in the lower frequency range (up to approximately 40 Hz) might therefore have a role in altering perceived comfort (Martin & Palmer 1996), but the main component of stimulation seems to be the medium frequency (Kinnunen & Alasaarela 2004, Martin & Palmer 1995a, Palmer et al 1999a). The AMF may be a synergistic partner, along with the medium frequency, but its role may be minor. As AMF selection has traditionally been a major component of clinical decision making with IFC, these observations have important significance.

AMF settings across a wide range between 1 and 130 Hz have been recommended in the literature for the treatment of pain, with little consensus. Clinically, however, the most popular (38% of replies) AMF used for pain relief was 130 Hz in the South West of Scotland (Scott & Purves 1991), although a 'great range' of AMF settings were used. In another survey of the AMFs used to treat a range of clinical conditions (Tabasam & Johnson 2000), it was reported that the mean was 85 Hz (range 1–150 Hz) when IFC was applied at a fixed frequency. In Northern Ireland, 70% of therapists used 80–120 Hz for the treatment of low back pain (Gracey et al 2001).

In conclusion, recent evidence has questioned the importance of the AMF. Most participants appear to prefer higher (50–100 Hz) to lower AMF settings (5 Hz) and the most commonly used frequencies clinically are also in this higher band. It is therefore difficult, and perhaps unnecessary, to recommended specific AMF settings. Initially, it may prove beneficial to use one that is most comfortable for the patient and carefully evaluate the effects of treatment.

Frequency sweep

A frequency sweep is available on most IFC stimulators, where the AMF is altered over time. A sweep may be set between two prefixed AMFs, for example between 50 and 100 Hz. The pattern of change in frequency can also be adjusted on most machines. For example, it may be set to slowly increase and decrease over a period of 6 seconds (normally depicted by 6∧6), or to give 1 second of stimulation at one frequency and then to automatically switch to the other frequency (1|1). It has been reported that 96% of treatments by physiotherapists that employed a frequency sweep used a 6∧6 pattern (Tabasam & Johnson 2000).

A frequency sweep has been claimed to reduce adaptation (Low & Reed 2000, Nikolova 1987, Savage 1984), although evidence for the importance of this feature is, at best, only weak (Johnson 1999). One study, albeit small, demonstrated that the inclusion of a frequency sweep had no effect on the amount of adaptation experienced by participants (Martin & Palmer 1995b). This study requires replication, but empirical evidence for a frequency sweep reducing adaptation is certainly lacking.

A frequency sweep has also been claimed to allow stimulation of a greater range of excitable tissues (Low & Reed 2000, Savage 1984), thereby extending the scope of potential treatment effects. It has been found that cold pain threshold increased with a 6∧6 sweep pattern compared to a 1|1 pattern or sham stimulation (Johnson & Wilson 1997). Although the results of this study were not subjected to statistical analysis, it suggested a possible effect of frequency sweep. A later, larger study contradicted these results, however, finding no effect of frequency sweep (1|1, 6|6, 6^6, or burst) on cold-induced pain threshold, intensity and unpleasantness (Johnson & Tabasam 2003b).

Because of a lack of experimental evidence, and the argument in the previous section that the AMF may be of limited importance, it is again difficult, and perhaps unnecessary, to recommend the inclusion or selection of specific frequency sweeps. The value of the sweep depends largely on the value attached to the AMF. If used clinically, the effectiveness of frequency sweep may be monitored by careful assessment.

FOUR-ELECTRODE AND TWO-ELECTRODE APPLICATION

IFC may be produced either by applying the two medium-frequency currents via four electrodes so that they intersect in the tissues (sometimes called 'quadripolar' or '4 pole' IFC), or alternatively by mixing the two currents in the stimulator prior to application via two electrodes (premodulated 'bipolar' or '2 pole' method). It is claimed that a four-electrode application of IFC produces modulated current in a 'clover-leaf' pattern, as depicted in Figure 17.3, with the 'leaves' set up at right-angles to the two medium-frequency currents (Kahn 1987, Low & Reed 2000, Savage 1984).

It has been claimed that premodulated IFC displays a different distribution within tissues compared with four-electrode application (Hansjuergens 1986, Savage 1984). Whereas four-electrode IFC is claimed to be created deep within the tissues, premodulated IFC will be distributed similarly to conventional electrical stimulation (Savage 1984), with maximal current intensities underneath the electrodes, progressively decreasing with distance (Hansjuergens 1986). It has also been suggested that the wide dispersal of the area of interference with premodulated IFC might also reduce the effectiveness of treatment (Goats 1990). Such claims have been challenged.

Treffene (1983) found that there was a good correlation between the expected and the actual pattern of IFC fields in a homogeneous water medium. The amplitude modulated current was set up not only in the central area between electrodes, however, but also underneath the electrodes. Lambert et al (1993), using computer models of a non-homogeneous medium and a human thigh, demonstrated that destructive interference (where the positive and negative charges of the two medium-frequency currents cancel each other out) was impossible with four-electrode IFC. Although some interference was evident, this varied at different positions in the thigh and there was no point at which there was zero resultant current. It was concluded that four-electrode application of IFC was fundamentally different from a two-electrode application, and that 100% modulation can only be obtained using two electrodes. Demmink (1995) directly measured the distribution of four-electrode IFC fields within pork tissue, discovering the current pattern and degree of modulation to be unreliable and haphazard. Additionally, the current did not follow a straight line between electrodes in each circuit. It must be concluded, therefore, that the pattern of IFC depicted in traditional textbooks is unrepresentative of that produced in biological tissue.

A haphazard distribution of modulated current, with modulation also occurring underneath the electrodes, seems to invalidate claims of the supremacy of four-electrode application. A premodulated application ensures that modulation is always

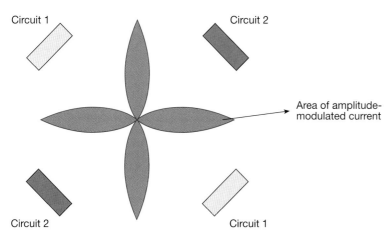

Circuit 1   Circuit 2

Area of amplitude-modulated current

Circuit 2   Circuit 1

Figure 17.3 'Clover-leaf' pattern with four-electrode IFC, where 'interferential current' is theoretically created at right-angles to the two medium-frequency currents. Research evidence has demonstrated that this theoretical pattern is impossible in biological tissue.

100% (Lambert et al 1993, Low & Reed 2000), although, as discussed, previously the AMF may not prove to be critical in any case. Ozcan et al (2004) found that four-electrode IFC was similar to two-electrode premodulated IFC in terms of the ratio between motor and sensory thresholds. Two-electrode IFC produced higher muscle torque values and less discomfort, however, suggesting that the two-electrode current was superior. A premodulated application has been found to be most commonly used by physiotherapists (79% of treatments) (Tabasam & Johnson 2000), although 80% of therapists have reported using four electrodes for the treatment of low back pain (Gracey et al 2001).

The use of two-electrode (premodulated) IFC is the only way to ensure 100% modulation and there is evidence that it may be more effective and comfortable in muscle stimulation. It also provides the easier alternative in a practical sense (De Domenico & Strauss 1985, Martin 1996). Evidence for differences in the effectiveness of two- and four-electrode IFC is embryonic, however. A four-electrode application can treat a larger area and, given that complete modulation may be relatively unimportant, this may present a valid treatment choice.

SUCTION AND PLATE ELECTRODES

IFC is often applied via electrodes that are held in place using an intermittent suction unit (with damp sponge inserts to ensure effective skin contact). Alternatively, flat carbon–rubber electrodes in damp sponge covers may be used. No literature has investigated the relative merits of either technique, although Tabasam and Johnson (2000) revealed that 90% of IFC treatments in their survey used carbon–rubber electrodes. Suction electrodes have been reported to have the advantage of allowing application to large flat areas or to patients who are relatively immobile (Savage 1984). The suction itself has also been claimed to stimulate cutaneous nerves and cause vasodilation (Low & Reed 2000). Such claims remain to be validated.

In recommendations for selection, ease of application should probably guide the choice of method. Flat carbon–rubber electrodes may be easier to apply to peripheral limbs, when they may be held in position by bandages or elasticated Velcro® straps. On the other hand there may be

anatomical areas that are less accessible, and in these cases the suction option may be advantageous.

ELECTRODE PLACEMENT

For muscle stimulation, it has been recommended that a large electrode can be placed on the nerve supplying the muscle to be stimulated and another smaller electrode over the relevant motor point. Alternatively, two electrodes of equal size may be placed at the proximal and distal ends of the muscle (De Domenico & Strauss 1985). A process of trial and error may be used to find the placement that produces the strongest and most comfortable contraction. For pain relief, electrode placements may be used as for TENS (see Chapter 16). There is some preliminary evidence in people with low back pain (Hurley et al 2001) that application of IFC via electrodes placed over the spinal nerve root demonstrated better improvement in functional disability than when applied to the painful area (both were administered in combination with an evidence-based information booklet). There were no differences, however, between groups in terms of pain severity or overall health scores. For the treatment of low back pain, 80% of therapists have reported using electrode placements over the painful area and 50% over the spinal nerve root (Gracey et al 2001).

There is not yet any definitive evidence for the superiority of different electrode placements and therefore clinicians and patients should be encouraged to use a process of trial and error to find the most comfortable and effective application.

CURRENT INTENSITY

For pain relief, most authors advocate a current intensity that produces a 'strong but comfortable' sensation (Goats 1990, Nikolova 1987, Savage 1984, Wadsworth & Chanmugam 1980). In an unpublished study, however, it was observed that the peak current intensity producing 'strong but comfortable' sensation in the forearm varied significantly between individuals and over time (Palmer 2002). Factors such as the area treated and the size and placement of electrodes will also determine the sensation induced by specific current intensities.

By definition, 'strong but comfortable' stimulation should be determined by participant report rather than peak current intensity settings. Intensity should be slowly increased until the patient signals that the required sensation has been reached. If used for muscle stimulation, the aim should be to use an intensity that produces a comfortable muscle contraction. Periodic adjustment of the intensity is recommended to compensate for any adaptation (Goats 1990, Robinson & Snyder-Mackler 1995, Savage 1984).

TREATMENT DURATION

Recommendations for treatment time have included 10–15 minutes with no longer than 20 minutes to one area (Savage 1984) or 10 minutes for most painful conditions (Wadsworth & Chanmugam 1980). Clinicians have reported actual treatment time to be between 11 and 15 minutes in the majority (61–72%) of cases (Tabasam & Johnson 2000, Gracey et al 2001, respectively). These treatment durations have no theoretical basis, however, and are more likely to be the result of practical constraints as opposed to scientific rationale (Johnson 1999). There is some evidence that IFC has short-lived effects, with raised experimentally induced cold pain thresholds returning to baseline levels within 10–20 minutes (Johnson & Tabasam 1999a, Johnson & Wilson 1997, Tabasam et al 1998). The applicability of such observations to the clinical situation continues to stimulate debate. However, if the reader accepts a fair degree of validity, then it may temper any expectancy of lasting pain relief following such short treatment sessions. This has yet to be specifically investigated clinically, however. The advent of small, portable IFC stimulators, as opposed to the traditional application via large, expensive and bulky stimulators in outpatient departments, is to be welcomed. These smaller stimulators will allow IFC to be used for longer periods, as recommended for TENS (McQuay et al 1997).

On existing knowledge, recommendation of specific treatment durations is potentially misleading. Logically, the same guidelines as for TENS should be used. However, in the absence of portable machines, time constraints in the clinical setting often limit the use of IFC to 10–20 minutes.

USE AS A TREATMENT ADJUNCT

It has been reported that IFC was used as an adjunct to other treatments in 73% of cases (Tabasam & Johnson 2000). Treatment combinations reported for low back pain have included exercise (90% of respondents), mobilization (80%) and manipulation (40%) (Gracey et al 2001). This suggests that IFC might not be seen as an effective treatment in its own right but rather as part of a comprehensive treatment programme. Turner and Whitfield (1997), in their multivariate analysis of techniques used by English physiotherapists, found that those who often used passive manipulation techniques were also high users of IFC and ultrasound. (Exercise therapy was commonly used by all therapists). Physiotherapy for painful conditions should incorporate a biopsychosocial approach (Martin & Palmer 2005) and, as such, it is important to elucidate the effects of IFC when combined with other treatments. Some of the investigations that have attempted to do so will be outlined later.

HAZARDS

A number of adverse effects have been reported with IFC treatment, including burns, increased pain, general malaise, nausea, vomiting, dizziness/faintness, migraine/headache and neurological effects (Kitchen 2000a, b, Partridge & Kitchen 1999). Very high current densities can produce a burn with any type of electrical current. This may occur where the effective size of the electrode is reduced by poor contact with the skin, and care must therefore be taken to ensure an even current density through equally damp electrode covers and good skin–electrode contact (CSP 1995). IFC should be incapable of producing chemical changes (and thus a chemical burn) as it is an evenly alternating current. Stimulation of the autonomic nervous system may account for some of the more general effects reported. At present, there are no adequate screening tools to identify patients who may experience undesirable reactions to IFC but close attention to equipment safety and servicing is of the utmost importance (CSP 1991). When applied to intact skin, decontamination of sponge electrode covers using hot water and detergent is recommended as an adequate infection control measure (Mercier & Haig 1993), although many centres use an antiseptic solution.

Participants should be tested for pain sensitivity before the first application and, if indicated, on other occasions. Contraindications should include application to patients where disturbance of a thrombus, spread of infection or cancerous cells, or haemorrhage might result; pacemakers; and application across the abdomen during pregnancy, across the chest wall in patients with cardiac problems, or where there is skin damage. These recommendations are based on prudence as opposed to scientific evidence, however.

CONCLUSIONS

It is clear from this overview that there is a wide array of possible application methods of IFC, with little rationale or evidence for many of them. In some cases, such as for the claimed importance of the AMF, the available evidence actually contradicts traditional theory. The wide choice of parameters with IFC makes the investigation of its efficacy all the more difficult and makes their selection for clinical use confusing. On the other hand, if the reader accepts their limited importance, then comparison of different applications is eased and clinical choice is simplified.

THEORETICAL MECHANISMS OF INTERFERENTIAL CURRENT

A number of mechanisms have been quoted to support the claimed effects of IFC, although conclusive evidence for those mechanisms is elusive. Some of the literature equates IFC with TENS (Johnson 1999, Kloth 1991), carrying with it an assumption that the stimulus characteristics of the two modalities are comparable. This has been demonstrated not to be the case (Palmer et al 1999a). The use of literature on claimed frequency-specific effects of TENS to explain the mechanisms of action of IFC may therefore be inappropriate, particularly below approximately 40 Hz. Johnson (1999) has observed a multiplicity of claims of the actions of specific AMFs. Given the evidence for the relative lack of importance of the AMF (Palmer

et al 1999a), claims of such specificity will not be detailed in this chapter. Each theoretical mechanism will now be addressed in turn.

NEURAL EFFECTS

Some authors have explained the effects of IFC on pain in terms of the classic pain gate theory (Melzack & Wall 1965), where impulses in large-diameter sensory nerves (Aβ-fibres) inhibit dorsal horn neurons normally responsive to nociceptive afferent nerves (C and Aδ fibres) (De Domenico 1982, Goats 1990, Rennie 1988, Shafshak et al 1991). This effectively 'closes the gate' to nociceptive impulses (Wall 1999). IFC can stimulate large-diameter peripheral nerves, as evidenced by the sensation produced. It is logical, therefore, to suggest that this mechanism may be activated, although specific experimental evidence is unavailable.

It has also been proposed that IFC may elicit descending pain suppression through stimulation of afferent Aδ and C fibres (De Domenico 1982, Goats 1990, Low & Reed 2000, Rennie 1988). This increases activity in fibres descending from the raphe nuclei, releasing inhibitory neurotransmitters at spinal level (Goats 1990, Rennie 1988). Resulting analgesia may be long lasting but pain may initially increase due to stimulation of nociceptive Aδ and C fibres (Goats 1990). Unfortunately, no direct evidence for the effectiveness of IFC in eliciting these mechanisms has been found in the literature.

IFC stimulation of peripheral nociceptive fibres at rates above their maximum conduction frequency may cause cessation of action potential propagation (De Domenico 1982, Goats 1990, Low & Reed 2000, Rennie 1988, Shafshak et al 1991) through increased thresholds and synaptic fatigue (Goats 1990). Authors have been careful to point out that physiological block of nerve fibres has not been demonstrated with IFC stimulation (De Domenico 1982, Ganne 1986, Noble et al 2000a). An interesting review by Ganne (1986) of the literature on conduction block with electrical stimulation concluded that there was no evidence for this phenomenon. Howson (1978) also stated that published evidence suggested insufficient blockage of small fibre activity to account for substantial pain reduction with electrical stimulation. Both authors concluded, therefore, that pain relief with electrical stimulation most likely depended upon maximizing normal responses of nerve fibres rather than blocking them. It has been observed that IFC did not significantly alter conduction velocity in the ulnar and median nerves (Belcher 1974), or affect RIII or H-reflexes in the sural nerve (Cramp et al 2000). These results question the claims of conduction block with IFC.

BLOOD FLOW AND SWELLING

IFC has been claimed to improve the circulation of blood and swelling, which may wash away the chemicals that stimulate nociceptive nerve endings (De Domenico 1982, Goats 1990, Rennie 1988, Shafshak et al 1991). Reduced swelling may concomitantly reduce tissue pressure. These phenomena are reportedly due to mild muscle contraction or action on the autonomic nervous system, decreasing blood vessel tone (Low & Reed 2000, Rennie 1988).

PLACEBO

Placebo responses have been identified as a potential factor with IFC stimulation (De Domenico 1982, Goats 1990, Low & Reed 2000, Rennie 1988, Taylor et al 1987), as with the majority of medical interventions. Taylor et al (1987) concluded that IFC treatment involved a large placebo component, as some 65% of participants in their placebo group reported an improvement in pain. Other authors have suggested, however, that in the context of their specific experiments placebo was unlikely to be a major factor (Shafshak et al 1991, Stephenson & Johnson 1995). Like the other claimed mechanisms, therefore, the extent of placebo responses with IFC stimulation remains unclear.

MUSCLE STIMULATION

As with other forms of electrical stimulation, as IFC intensity is increased, there is a progressive recruitment of sensory and motor responses (Palmer et al 1999a). This is readily observable and IFC has, therefore, been recommended as a method of re-educating muscle activity (De Domenico 1987, De Domenico & Strauss 1985). It has been particularly advocated in the treatment of incontinence (Laycock & Green 1988).

BONE AND TISSUE HEALING

The reader is referred to Chapter 4 for a detailed discussion of the healing process. It has been claimed that IFC offers similar benefits in fracture healing to low-frequency stimulation due to demodulation of the AMF from the medium frequency current, although, as already discussed, any mechanism of demodulation is not established (Johnson & Tabasam 2003a). Nikolova (1987) claimed that IFC may alter activity of the autonomic nervous system and cells, and alter production of important chemical mediators. Such claims are difficult to assess as they are evidenced by poorly conducted, often uncontrolled trials open to bias. Important work by Sontag and colleagues has suggested some effects of IFC on cells in vitro and this evidence will be described later.

BRONCHODILATION

IFC has been reported to have a bronchodilation effect (Emberson 1996, Nikolova 1987, Savage 1984) and thus to relieve symptoms associated with asthma. Appropriate research evidence for such effects is lacking.

CONCLUSIONS

IFC is thus associated with an impressive range of claimed physiological effects, many of which lack empirical evidence owing to a lack of appropriate investigation. Whereas a mechanism involving the stimulation of peripheral nerves in line with the gate theory is likely to be related to IFC, the more radical explanation of blocking of nerve conduction is unlikely to contribute to pain relief with this modality. Other mechanisms, such as descending pain suppression, increased circulation and placebo, cannot be easily discounted, although they do require verification. Similarly, the ability of IFC to stimulate muscle is clearly evident, although evidence for mechanisms related to bone and tissue healing and bronchodilation is more elusive. The following sections will address the laboratory and clinical evidence in more depth.

EVIDENCE FOR THE EFFECTS OF INTERFERENTIAL CURRENT

LABORATORY INVESTIGATIONS

A number of laboratory studies of the effects of IFC have been undertaken. The value of these studies is that they can indicate the presence of effects in a controlled environment, which if also found in the clinical environment could be associated with patient benefit. Noble et al (2001) provide an excellent review of the effects of IFC on experimental pain models and neurophysiological indices.

Ischaemic pain

There is some evidence that IFC is more effective than either control or placebo stimulation in reducing experimental ischaemic pain intensity and unpleasantness (Johnson & Tabasam 1999, 2002, 2003c, Tabasam & Johnson 1999b). This finding is not consistent within the literature, however (Scott & Purves 1991). Johnson and Tabasam (2003c) demonstrated that IFC reduced ischaemic pain intensity when compared with sham stimulation. When compared to TENS, however, there was no significant difference.

Cold-induced pain

Cold pain is interesting because it is mediated by both C- and Aδ-fibre nerve pathways (Verdugo & Ochoa 1992, Yarnitsky & Ochoa 1990). Any change in the experience of cold pain may, therefore, indicate more global effects on the perception of activity within peripheral nociceptive pathways. A number of studies have demonstrated that IFC reduces reported pain perception using the cold pressor test (Johnson & Wilson 1997, Johnson & Tabasam 1999a, b, Stephenson & Johnson 1995, Tabasam & Johnson 1999a), although the results are often dependent on the outcome measure used. Johnson and Tabasam (2003a) found no effect of IFC on cold pain threshold, intensity or unpleasantness. There was also no effect of altering IFC frequency (20, 60, 100, 140, 180, 220 Hz). Stephenson and Walker (2003) similarly found no effects of different frequencies (30 or 100 Hz) or placements (ipsilateral or contralateral) of IFC on cold pain threshold, when compared with sham stimulation or control.

Johnson and Tabasam (2003b) did find significant changes in cold-induced pain threshold, intensity and unpleasantness over time, however, suggesting analgesic effects of IFC. Different swing patterns (1|1, 6|6, 6^6 or burst) had no effect. Together, these studies suggest that modulation of specific elements of the experience of cold-induced pain may be possible with IFC treatment.

Thermal quantitative sensory testing

Quantitative sensory testing (QST) allows the assessment of, and differentiation between, the perception of activity within C- and Aδ-fibre nerve pathways (Palmer et al 2000, Price 1996, Verdugo & Ochoa 1992). Assessment of specific thermal thresholds (the very first perception of a thermal sensation) gives information on the perception of activity within these neural pathways. Warm sensation (WS), for example, is mediated by C fibres (Morin & Bushnell 1998, Verdugo & Ochoa 1992, Yarnitsky & Ochoa 1990, 1991), cold sensation (CS) by Aδ fibres (Verdugo & Ochoa 1992, Yarnitsky & Ochoa 1991), heat pain (HP) by C fibres (Morin & Bushnell 1998, Verdugo & Ochoa 1992, Yarnitsky & Ochoa 1991) and cold pain (CP) by a mixture of C and Aδ fibres (Verdugo & Ochoa 1992, Yarnitsky & Ochoa 1990). Effects of modalities on specific sensations may, therefore, indicate effects on specific nerve fibre types. QST has previously been shown to be sensitive to TENS (Eriksson et al 1985, Marchand et al 1991) and vibration (Yarnitsky et al 1997).

Despite initial reports of an effect of 100 Hz IFC on the perception of CP and CS (Palmer et al 1999b), a much larger follow-up study found no significant effect of a range of IFC AMFs (0, 5 and 100 Hz) in altering the perception of activity in these peripheral pathways compared to controls, TENS (5 Hz and 100 Hz), or placebo stimulation (Palmer et al 2004).

Mechanical pain

Alves-Guerreiro et al (2001) found no significant differences between the effects of IFC, TENS, action potential stimulation (APS) and a control condition on mechanical pain threshold, concluding that no modality displayed hypoalgesic effects.

Delayed-onset muscle soreness (DOMS)

Schmitz et al (1997) found that both 10 Hz and 100 Hz IFC ($n = 5$ in each group) significantly reduced the pain associated with DOMS in the elbow flexors but there was no difference between groups. Serum cortisol levels (used as a marker of β-endorphin release) were unchanged, suggesting that the mechanism of pain relief was not endorphin mediated. The authors concluded that both forms of IFC were effective but suggested that their results were limited by not including a placebo group. Minder et al (2002) found no significant effects of low- or high-frequency IFC (10–20 Hz or 80–100 Hz, respectively) when compared with sham stimulation. The evidence for effects on DOMS therefore remains equivocal.

Blood flow

Two experimental studies have found no evidence of increased tissue perfusion with IFC stimulation (Indergand & Morgan 1995, Nussbaum et al 1990). Another found that IFC significantly increased blood flow but that this effect was no greater than with placebo or TENS (Olson et al 1999). One study, which observed increased arterial circulation and skin perfusion during and after IFC (Lamb & Mani 1994), was unable to determine whether these effects were caused by muscle stimulation or effects on the sympathetic nervous system. Noble et al (2000b) found no overall effects of a range of IFC settings (10–20 Hz, 10–100 Hz, 80–100 Hz, placebo and control) on cutaneous blood flow, although there was a short-lived increase in the 10–20 Hz group after 12 minutes. The evidence to date, therefore, is contradictory as to the effect of IFC on circulation.

Cell activity

Sontag and colleagues have demonstrated that specific combinations of IFC parameters can alter cell activity in vitro, whereas others do not. Complex interactions were demonstrated between IFC parameters and a wide range of inflammatory mediators, including prostaglandin E_2, leukotriene B4, interleukines 1b and 8, adenosine 3′:5′-cyclic monophosphate (cAMP), guanosine 3′:5′-cyclic monophosphate (cGMP) and tumour necrosis factor α (TNFα) (Sontag 2000, 2001, 2004, Sontag & Dertinger 1998). These changes were particularly marked when cells were in the presence of a chemical stimulant. Effects were shown to be dependent on specific combinations of IFC exposure time, current intensity and stimulation frequency, in addition to the concentration of the chemical stimulus. This complex interaction between parameters demonstrated either a suppression or enhancement of activity in different combinations. Such 'window' effects illustrate the possible interaction between different IFC parameters but also support possible effects on the healing process. No changes were observed in cell respiration or energy levels (Sontag 1998), intracellular calcium (Sontag & Dertinger 1998) or interleukin 6 (Sontag 2000), or thromboxane B2 (Sontag 2001), suggesting some specificity in terms of IFC-mediated effects. Such evidence supports the theoretical basis of IFC in tissue healing but these results have yet to be replicated in clinical conditions.

Muscle stimulation

During muscle stimulation, Baker et al (1988) found that a symmetrical, biphasic square wave was more comfortable than either IFC or a monophasic, paired, spike waveform. The authors did state, however, that a subgroup found IFC to be most comfortable and recommended that it should be used for patients who could not tolerate other current types. Bennie et al (2002) found that IFC was unable to produce a sustained muscle contraction at 10% of the maximum voluntary contraction and that a sine waveform was preferable (in terms of the mean peak current intensity and comfort). Bircan et al (2002) investigated the effectiveness of premodulated two-electrode IFC (2500 Hz carrier frequency, 80 Hz AMF) and low-frequency stimulation (symmetrical biphasic, 100 μs, 80 Hz) in enhancing quadriceps muscle strength in healthy participants. Isokinetic strength increased significantly with both forms of stimulation relative to a control group, although there was no statistically significant difference between them. The perceived discomfort associated with stimulation was also similar between IFC and low-frequency stimulation. The available evidence suggests, therefore, that IFC may not be the best method of producing effective and comfortable muscle stimulation.

IFC compared with TENS

At the beginning of the chapter we proposed that a key issue is whether IFC is superior to or even different from TENS, a question that has been highlighted by other authors in the field (Alon 1987, Johnson 1999). The controlled environment of a laboratory is a suitable arena for comparing IFC and TENS on fundamental effects.

In the laboratory setting it has been observed that IFC and TENS had different effects on cold-induced pain, with TENS increasing threshold but not altering pain intensity ratings, whereas IFC decreased intensity ratings but had no effect on threshold (Salisbury & Johnson 1995). Another study, however, discovered no significant differences between the effects of IFC and TENS on cold-induced pain (Johnson & Tabasam 1999a) or ischaemic pain (Johnson & Tabasam 2003c). Using quantitative sensory testing methods, IFC and TENS were equally ineffective in altering the perception of activity within peripheral nerve pathways (Palmer et al 2004). There have also been no differences observed in the effects of IFC and TENS on RIII and H-reflexes (Cramp et al 2000), mechanical pain threshold (Alves-Guerreiro et al 2001), blood flow (Olson et al 1999), or muscle strengthening in healthy subjects (Bircan et al 2002). Baker et al (1988) reported, however, that TENS pulses elicited more comfortable muscle stimulation.

The laboratory evidence suggests, therefore, that there are no conclusive differences in the degree or nature of the effects of IFC and TENS.

Conclusions

This overview proposes some evidence that IFC stimulation may alter some but not all elements of ischaemic and cold-induced pain, DOMS and cell activity. This is consistent with IFC having a clinical use, although its effects may not be different from those of TENS.

CLINICAL INVESTIGATIONS

The research evidence for the effects of IFC on clinical conditions is maturing and will be detailed in this section.

'Musculoskeletal' conditions

Rush and Shore (1994) surveyed 100 rheumatologists and 100 rehabilitation specialists on the perceived benefits (their subjective opinions) of 11 physical modalities in treating seven different musculoskeletal problems. The rehabilitation specialists reported a greater perceived effectiveness of all modalities on all conditions compared with rheumatologists, suggesting differences in the exposure to and knowledge of the modalities. TENS was consistently perceived to be more effective than IFC for all conditions when all 200 specialists were analysed together. The results, however, did not distinguish between the effects that the modalities may have on specific symptoms associated with the conditions. The survey does, however, give an interesting insight into clinical experience and opinion.

Knee osteoarthritis

Knee osteoarthritis (OA) has most commonly been the target of clinical trials of IFC. Quirk et al (1985) compared IFC coupled with an exercise programme with shortwave diathermy (SWD) and exercise, and exercise alone. There were no significant differences between groups, although all exhibited significant improvements in pain, range of knee movement (ROM) and overall clinical condition. The results did not, therefore, suggest an additive effect of IFC over exercise alone. Young et al (1991) found that both IFC and placebo stimulation significantly reduced knee OA pain but that there were no significant differences between groups. Adedoyin et al (2002), however, compared the effects of IFC and placebo stimulation (both combined with supervised exercise and dietary advice). Pain significantly improved in both groups, with the IFC group being significantly better than placebo at the end of the 4-week trial. Defrin et al (2005) also found that IFC significantly improved pain intensity, morning stiffness, and ROM in patients with knee OA. Both noxious and innocuous stimulation (30% above and below pain threshold respectively) were effective, although noxious stimulation was more effective in reducing pain intensity and pain threshold. Sham and control groups were included, adding credibility to these results.

Ní Chiosoig et al (1994) assessed the effects of two-electrode and four-electrode IFC on eight patients with bilateral knee OA. The authors reported statistically significant improvements in pain, ROM and muscle strength but no differences between groups. It was suggested that two-electrode IFC produced faster improvements (based on pain reduction after six treatments) although after 12 treatments the groups were very similar. The small sample size and lack of a control group limit definitive conclusions, but the results suggest a potential difference in the effectiveness of IFC applied by the two methods. Interestingly, six out of eight participants preferred two-electrode IFC. Another OA knee pain study (Shafshak et al 1991) classified 44% of patients as 'responders' to IFC treatment (50% or more relief for at least 5 days after treatment). The study aimed to establish whether personality was associated with 'responders' and 'non-responders' (25% or less relief for at least 5 days after treatment), finding no differences in personality types between these rather arbitrary classifications. The authors offered the conclusion that because personality did not affect the response to IFC treatment, placebo responses may be a minor factor in IFC treatment, although this supposition relies on an as yet unfounded premise, personality characteristics are a major factor in the placebo response.

In conclusion, with regard to pain associated with knee OA, there is some evidence to suggest positive effects of IFC. The research evidence is equivocal, however, and is generally of poor quality.

Jaw pain

Taylor et al (1987) found that both IFC and placebo stimulation improved jaw pain over the three treatments administered but differences between groups were not significant, leading the authors to conclude that IFC treatment displayed a high placebo component. There were also no changes in a functional measure (vertical jaw opening).

Fracture pain

In patients with proximal humerus fractures, Martin et al (2000) found no significant differences in pain and ROM following treatment with IFC, placebo stimulation (in conjunction with both exercise and passive mobilization) and exercise and mobilization alone. All outcome measures improved over time but it was concluded that IFC did not provide any additional benefit over exercises and mobilization alone. Incomplete randomization and small participant numbers in this study, however, prevent definitive conclusions.

Low back pain

Werners et al (1999) compared IFC with mechanical traction and massage on patients with low back pain. Significant improvements in pain and disability were observed at 3 months but there were no significant differences between groups. The lack of control or placebo groups in this study makes it impossible to gauge the clinical significance of the results, which may be due to natural progression, equal effectiveness (or ineffectiveness) of the two modalities, equivalent placebo responses, or a combination of these situations. Hurley et al (2001) also studied the effects of IFC applied to either the painful area or spinal nerve root (both also received an evidence-based information booklet) or the booklet in isolation. All groups improved significantly in terms of pain intensity, disability and quality of life, with those receiving the booklet and IFC to the spinal nerve improving to a greater degree than the other groups. The authors concluded that IFC electrode placement was an important consideration. Hurley et al (2004) also demonstrated that both IFC and manipulation, whether used in combination or isolation, significantly improved pain, functional disability and quality of life. The improvements were similar for all groups and were maintained at 6 and 12 months. Taken together, these results suggest some effect of IFC in the treatment of low back pain.

Shoulder disorders

Van Der Heijden et al (1999) investigated the effects of IFC and ultrasound (US) on patients with shoulder pain and/or reduced shoulder movement. Patients received one of a combination of active and dummy US and IFC (both applied together), or no additional treatment. All groups also received exercise therapy, individualized to each patient. There were no differences between groups in recovery, function, main complaint, pain and ROM (statistical analysis was not performed). This suggested that active or dummy IFC and US did not provide additional treatment effects to those achieved by exercise alone. Further appreciation of the results is difficult owing to the limited and ambiguous analysis methods employed.

Palmar psoriasis

Philipp et al (2000) demonstrated significant effects of a 12-week period of IFC treatment (twice per day) on erythema, fissures, induration, pustules and scaling associated with palmar psoriasis. Twelve patients who had previously been resistant to change by traditional therapy were included in this quasi-controlled study, with 11 displaying significant or complete improvement. The results are encouraging and merit further investigation in a more tightly controlled experimental study.

Fibromyalgia

Almeida et al (2003) found that IFC, when used in conjunction with ultrasound (so-called combined therapy), improved multiple indices of pain and sleep in patients with fibromyalgia. The relative contribution of each of the treatment components is, however, unclear.

Knee surgery

Jarit et al (2003) investigated the effects of IFC on pain, ROM, and swelling in patients who had anterior cruciate ligament (ACL) reconstruction, meniscectomy or knee chondroplasty. Patients received a portable IFC device to use at home which was either active (treatment group) or inactive (placebo group). The active IFC group reported greater improvements in pain and ROM at all time points. ACL and meniscectomy patients also had reduced swelling at all time points, and chondroplasty patients demonstrated reduced swelling for up to 4 weeks. Treatment was applied three times per day for 28 minutes during each session and continued for 7–9 weeks. This mode of treatment is very different from traditional IFC applications, involving home treatment with a portable device, and is thus more akin to TENS treatment. It would be interesting to investigate such applications further, particularly given the positive results of this study. The small portable

IFC devices now commercially available would provide a suitable comparison with TENS.

Swelling

Conclusive published evidence for the influence of IFC in reducing swelling is elusive. Quirk et al (1985) found no effects of IFC and exercise on the girth of OA knees, and Christie and Willoughby (1990) found no significant effect of IFC on swelling post open reduction and internal fixation of the ankle. As described above, however, Jarit et al (2003) did find significant effects of a comprehensive home IFC regimen on swelling associated with a range of knee surgery procedures.

Muscle stimulation and treatment of incontinence

A survey of therapists involved in treating stress urinary incontinence found that 144 of 189 (76%) of respondents used IFC in treatment (Mantle & Versi 1991). The CSP guidelines on the treatment of stress urinary incontinence contain several evidence statements about the usefulness of electrical stimulation in the treatment of this condition, although some concerns are noted about using IFC due to possible effects on cellular activity in the pelvic and abdominal organs (Laycock et al 2001).

Wilson et al (1987) found that women with genuine stress incontinence (GSI) significantly improved with a regimen of supervised pelvic floor exercises (PFE), whether or not they were combined with IFC or faradic stimulation, when compared with home PFE. Dumoulin et al (1995) investigated the effects of IFC and PFE in eight women with postpartum GSI. Frequency of incontinence, volume of urine loss and maximal pelvic floor muscle pressure all improved with treatment. No control group was included, however, and the effectiveness of the programme and the relative effectiveness of each component cannot, therefore, be clearly ascertained. Laycock and Jerwood (1993) reported two separate trials of the effectiveness of IFC in the treatment of GSI. The first trial found both IFC and PFE to be equally effective, although the second study demonstrated active IFC to be significantly better than placebo stimulation on a range of outcome measures. IFC may therefore be effective, but no more so than active exercises. In another uncontrolled study

(Dougall 1985) descriptive analysis found that there was a reduction in frequency of voiding, nocturia and incontinence following treatment with IFC alone. Vahtera et al (1997) used a regimen of IFC stimulation and PFE in patients with lower urinary tract dysfunction due to multiple sclerosis and included a control group. Power and endurance of the pelvic floor increased and symptoms associated with dysfunction were significantly better in the treatment group. Again, the relative effectiveness of the two interventions cannot be determined, but the combination of IFC stimulation and PFE seems to be effective in this population. A small, uncontrolled pilot study investigating the effectiveness of IFC in anorectal incontinence found no evidence of long-term improvement in symptoms (Sylvester & Keilty 1987). Overall, therefore, evidence for the effectiveness of IFC in the treatment of incontinence is not clear.

Bone healing

Ganne et al (1979) found that treatment with IFC of nine patients predisposed to non-union of mandibular fractures (out of 150 consecutive fractures) reduced the incidence to zero. This compared with a retrospective study of a further 150 subjects who did not receive IFC, where three (2%) fractures resulted in non-union. Ganne (1988) also demonstrated that treatment of acute tibial shaft fractures with IFC significantly reduced time to union compared with matched controls. In a large randomized placebo-controlled trial, Fourie and Bowerbank (1997) found no statistically significant difference in time to union of tibial shaft fractures between IFC, control and placebo groups. The evidence for the effects of IFC on bone healing is thus equivocal and further research is required.

Conclusions

In summary, there seems to be some clinical evidence for the effectiveness of IFC in the management of a range of conditions, although rigorous scientific scrutiny of this modality is still in its relative infancy. The number and standard of clinical trials of IFC is gradually increasing, however, and this is very encouraging.

OVERALL CONCLUSIONS

This chapter has introduced the characteristics of IFC, the theoretical mechanisms of action of this method of electrical stimulation, and the evidence for these mechanisms. An overview has also been made of the relevant laboratory and clinical investigations.

Although there are inherent problems with existing systematic reviews of TENS (Johnson 2000), the best evidence suggests that it may be ineffective for the relief of acute pain (McQuay et al 1997). In the management of chronic pain, McQuay et al (1997) report that much larger trials are needed and that it needs to be applied for long periods of time, rather than in short-duration treatment packages. This latter view is shared by Johnson (1999), who stated that analgesic effects have been demonstrated to mainly occur during the time that TENS is switched on. Taking the lead from the TENS evidence, therefore, there is little to suggest that the traditional application of IFC in short treatment sessions provides optimal conditions for efficacy.

Many fundamental questions remain. It is still not clear whether IFC is, indeed, efficacious or which aspects of clinical conditions are affected. There is also the key question of whether IFC is any more effective than other, more accessible, forms of electrical stimulation such as TENS. Initial work would suggest that it may not be, but this requires further clarification if IFC is to remain as a singular, distinctive treatment modality deserving of its own niche in the field of electrotherapy.

References

Adedoyin RA, Olaogun MOB, Fabeja OO (2002) Effect of interferential current stimulation in management of osteo-arthritic knee pain. *Physiotherapy* **88**(8): 493–499.

Almeida TF, Roizenblatt S, Benedito-Silva AA et al (2003) The effect of combined therapy (ultrasound and interferential current) on pain and sleep in fibromyalgia. *Pain* **104**: 665–672.

Alon G (1987) Interferential current news. *Phys Ther* **67**(2): 280–281.

Alves-Guerreiro J, Noble JG, Lowe AS et al (2001) The effect of three electrotherapeutic modalities upon peripheral nerve conduction and mechanical pain threshold. *Clin Physiol* **21**(6): 704–711.

Baker LL, Bowman BR, McNeal DR (1988) Effects of waveform on comfort during neuromuscular electrical stimulation. *Clin Orthop Rel Res* **233**: 75–85.

Belcher JF 1974 Interferential therapy. *NZ J Physiother* **6**:29–34.

Bennie SD, Petrofsky JS, Nisperos J et al (2002) Toward the optimal waveform for electrical stimulation of human muscle. *Eur J Appl Physiol* **88**: 13–19.

Bircan C, Senocak O, Peker O et al (2002) Efficacy of two forms of electrical stimulation in increasing quadriceps strength: a randomized controlled trial. *Clin Rehab* **16**(2): 194–199.

Chartered Society of Physiotherapy (CSP) (1991) *Standards for the Use of Electrophysical Modalities*. London, CSP.

Chartered Society of Physiotherapy (CSP) (1995) *Factsheet PA22: Burns and Interferential Therapy*. London, CSP.

Christie AD, Willoughby GL (1990) The effect of interferential therapy on swelling following open reduction and internal fixation of ankle fractures. *Physiother Theory Pract* **6**:3–7.

Cooney M, Gallen C, Mullins G (2000) A survey of ownership and use of electrotherapeutic modalities in public out-patient departments and private practice in the Republic of Ireland. *Physiother Ireland* **21**(2): 3–8.

Cramp FL, Noble G, Lowe AS et al (2000) A controlled study of the effects of transcutaneous electrical nerve stimulation and interferential therapy upon the RIII nociceptive and H-reflexes in humans. *Arch Phys Med Rehab* **81**: 324–333.

De Domenico G (1982) Pain relief with interferential therapy. *Aust J Physiother* **28**(3): 14–18.

De Domenico G (1987) *New Dimensions in Interferential Therapy. A Theoretical and Clinical Guide*. Lindfield, New South Wales, Australia, Reid Medical Books.

De Domenico G, Strauss GR (1985) Motor stimulation with interferential currents. *Aust J Physiother* **31**(6): 225–230.

Defrin R, Ariel E, Peretz C (2005) Segmental noxious versus innocuous electrical stimulation for chronic pain relief and the effect of fading sensation during treatment. *Pain* **115**: 152–160.

Demmink JH (1995) The effect of a biological conducting medium on the pattern of modulation and distribution in a two-circuit static interferential field. In *Proceedings of the 12th International Conference of the World Confederation for Physical Therapy*, Washington DC: 583.

Dougall DS (1985) The effects of interferential therapy on incontinence and frequency of micturition. *Physiotherapy* **71**(3): 135–136.

Dumoulin C, Seaborne DE, Quiron-DeGirardi C et al (1995) Pelvic-floor rehabilitation, part 2: pelvic-floor reeducation with interferential currents and exercise in the treatment of genuine stress incontinence in postpartum women – a cohort study. *Phys Ther* **75**(12): 1075–081.

Emberson W (1996) Asthma and interferential therapy (IFT). *In Touch* **79**: 2–8.

Eriksson MBE, Rosén I, Sjölund B (1985) Thermal sensitivity in healthy subjects is decreased by a central mechanism after TENS. *Pain* **22**: 235–242.

Foster NE, Thompson KA, Baxter GD et al (1999) Management of non-specific low back pain by physiotherapists in Great Britain and Ireland. A descriptive questionnaire of current clinical practice. *Spine* **24**(13): 1332–1342.

Fourie JA, Bowerbank P (1997) Stimulation of bone healing in new fractures of the tibial shaft using interferential currents. *Physiother Res Int* **2**(4): 255–268.

Ganne JM (1976) Interferential therapy. *Aust J Physiother* **22**(3): 101–110.

Ganne JM (1986) Interferential therapy. *Aust J Physiother* **32**(1): 63–65.

Ganne JM (1988) Stimulation of bone healing with interferential therapy. *Aust J Physiother* **34**(1): 9–20.

Ganne JM, Speculand B, Mayne LH et al (1979) Interferential therapy to promote union of mandibular fractures. *Aust NZ J Surg* **49**(1): 81–83.

Goats GC (1990) Interferential current therapy. *Br J Sports Med* **24**(2): 87–92.

Gracey JH, Noble WH, Noble JG (2001) *Clinical use of interferential therapy in the management of low back pain. A survey of current practice in Northern Ireland*. The Physiotherapy Research Society, University of Ulster.

Hansjuergens A (1986) Interferential current clarification. *Phys Ther* **66**(6): 1002.

Howson DC (1978) Peripheral neural excitability – implications for transcutaneous electrical nerve stimulation. *Phys Ther* **58**(12): 1467–1473.

Hurley DA, Minder PM, McDonough SM et al (2001) Interferential therapy electrode placement in acute low back pain: a preliminary investigation. *Arch Phys Med Rehab* **82**: 485–493.

Hurley DA, McDonough SM, Dempster M et al (2004) A randomized clinical trial of manipulative therapy and interferential therapy for acute low back pain. *Spine* **29**(20): 2207–2216.

Indergand HJ, Morgan BJ (1995) Effect of interference current on forearm vascular resistance in asymptomatic humans. *Phys Ther* **75**(4): 306–312.

Jarit GJ, Mohr KJ, Waller R et al (2003) The effects of home interferential therapy on post-operative pain, edema, and range of motion of the knee. *Clin J Sport Med* **13**(1): 16–20.

Johnson MI (1999) The mystique of interferential currents when used to manage pain. *Physiotherapy* **85**(6): 294–297

Johnson MI (2000) The clinical effectiveness of TENS in pain management. *Crit Rev Phys Rehab Med* **12**: 131–149.

Johnson MI, Tabasam G (1998) *A Questionnaire Survey on the Clinical Use of Interferential Currents (IFC) by Physiotherapists*. Leicester University, The Pain Society Annual Scientific Meeting, 22–24 April 1998.

Johnson MI, Tabasam G (1999a) A double blind placebo controlled investigation into the analgesic effects of interferential currents (IFC) and transcutaneous electrical nerve stimulation (TENS) on cold-induced pain in healthy subjects. *Physiother Theory Pract* **15**: 217–233.

Johnson MI, Tabasam G (1999b) *Differential Analgesic Effects of Amplitude Modulated Frequencies of Interferential Currents*

(IFC) on Cold-induced Pain in Normal Subjects. Vienna, 9th World Congress on Pain: 453.

Johnson MI, Tabasam G (2002) A single-blind placebo-controlled investigation into the analgesic effects of interferential currents on experimentally induced ischaemic pain in healthy subjects. *Clin Physiol Funct Imag* **22**: 187–196.

Johnson MI, Tabasam G (2003a) An investigation into the analgesic effects of different frequencies of the amplitude-modulated wave of interferential current therapy on cold-induced pain in normal subjects. *Arch Phys Med Rehab* **84**: 1387–1394.

Johnson MI, Tabasam G (2003b) A single-blind investigation into the hypoalgesic effects of different swing patterns of interferential currents on cold-induced pain in healthy volunteers. *Arch Phys Med Rehab* **84**: 350–357.

Johnson MI, Tabasam G (2003c) An investigation into the analgesic effects of interferential currents and transcutaneous electrical nerve stimulation on experimentally induced ischemic pain in otherwise pain-free volunteers. *Phys Ther* **83**: 208–223.

Johnson MI, Wilson H (1997) The analgesic effects of different swing patterns of interferential currents on cold-induced pain. *Physiotherapy* **83**(9): 461–467.

Kahn J (1987) Principles and practice of electrotherapy. New York, Churchill Livingstone.

Kinnunen M, Alasaarela E (2004) Registering the response of tissues exposed to an interferential electric current stimulation. *Acupuncture Electrother Res* **29**(3–4): 213–226.

Kitchen S (2000a) Audit of the unexpected effects of electrophysical agents. Interim report: responses to December 1999. *Physiotherapy* **86**(3): 152–155.

Kitchen S (2000b) Audit of the unexpected effects of electrophysical agents. Interim report: responses January to June, 2000. *Physiotherapy* **86**(10): 509–511.

Kloth LC (1991) Interference current. In Nelson RM, Currier DP. *Clinical Electrotherapy*. Norwalk, Connecticut: Appleton & Lange: 221–260.

Lamb S, Mani R (1994) Does interferential therapy affect blood flow? *Clin Rehab* **8**: 213–218.

Lambert HL, Vanderstraeten GG, De Cuyper HJ et al (1993) Electric current distribution during interferential therapy. *Eur J Phys Med Rehab* **3**(1): 6–10.

Laycock J, Green RJ (1988) Interferential therapy in the treatment of incontinence. *Physiotherapy* **74**(4): 161–168.

Laycock J, Jerwood D (1993) Does pre-modulated interferential therapy cure genuine stress incontinence? *Physiotherapy* **79**(8): 553–560.

Laycock J, Standley A, Crothers E et al (2001) Clinical guidelines for the physiotherapy management of females aged 16–65 with stress urinary incontinence. London, Chartered Society of Physiotherapy.

Lindsay D, Dearness J, Richardson C et al (1990) A survey of electromodality usage in private physiotherapy practices. *Aust J Physiother* **36**(4): 249–256.

Low J, Reed A (2000) *Electrotherapy Explained. Principles and Practice*, 3rd edn. Oxford, Butterworth–Heinemann.

Mantle J, Versi E (1991) Physiotherapy for stress urinary incontinence: a national survey. *Br Med J* **302**: 753–755.

Marchand S, Bushnell MC, Duncan GH (1991) Modulation of heat pain perception by high frequency TENS. *Clin J Pain* **7**: 122–129.

Martin DJ (1996) Interferential current. In Kitchen S, Bazin S (eds) *Clayton's Electrotherapy*, 10th edn. London, WB Saunders.

Martin DJ, Palmer S (1995a) *Amplitude Modulation of 4 KHz Alternating Current (Interferential Current) Does Not Permit Selective Stimulation of Nerve Types*. Biological Engineering Society Symposium on Electrical Stimulation – Clinical Systems, Glasgow: 37–38.

Martin DJ, Palmer S (1995b) *Sensory Adaptation to Interferential Current is Not Affected by Modulation of the Stimulus*. Proceedings of the 12th International Conference of the World Confederation for Physical Therapy, Washington DC: 584.

Martin DJ, Palmer S (1996) The effect of beat frequency on perceived comfort during stimulation of healthy subjects with interferential current. *Physiotherapy* **82**(11): 639.

Martin DJ, Palmer S (2005) Soft tissue pain and physical therapy. *Anaesth Intens Care Med* **6**(1): 23–25.

Martin DJ, Palmer S, Heath C (2000) Interferential current as an adjunct to exercise and mobilisation in the treatment of proximal humerus fracture pain: lack of evidence of an additional effect. *Physiotherapy* **86**(3): 147.

McQuay HJ, Moore RA, Eccleston C et al (1997) Systematic review of outpatient services for chronic pain control. *Health Technol Assess* **1**(6): 1–135.

Melzack R, Wall P (1965) Pain mechanisms: a new theory. *Science* **150**(3699): 971–979.

Mercier C, Haig L (1993) Infection control in physiotherapy. *Physiotherapy* **79**(6): 385–387.

Minder PM, Noble JG, Alves-Guerreiro J et al (2002) Interferential therapy: lack of effect upon experimentally induced delayed onset muscle soreness *Clin Physiol Funct Imag* **22**: 339–347.

Morin C, Bushnell MC (1998) Temporal and qualitative properties of cold pain and heat pain: a psychophysical study. *Pain* **74**: 67–73.

Ní Chiosoig F, Hendriks O, Malone J (1994) A pilot study of the therapeutic effects of bipolar and quadripolar interferential therapy, using bilateral osteoarthritis as a model. *Physiother Ireland* **15**(1): 3–7.

Nikolova L (1987) *Treatment with Interferential Current*. Singapore, Churchill Livingstone.

Noble JG, Henderson G, Cramp AF et al (2000b) The effect of interferential therapy upon cutaneous blood flow in humans. *Clin Physiol* **20**(1): 2–7.

Noble JG, Lowe AS, Walsh DM (2000a) Interferential therapy review. Part 1. Mechanism of analgesic action and clinical usage. *Phys Ther Rev* **5**: 239–245.

Noble JG, Lowe AS, Walsh DM (2001) Interferential therapy review part 2: experimental pain models and neurophysiological effects of electrical stimulation. *Phys Ther Rev* **6**(1): 17–37.

Nussbaum E, Rush P, Disenhaus L (1990) The effects of interferential therapy on peripheral blood flow. *Physiotherapy* **76**(12): 803–807.

Olson SL, Perez JV, Stacks LN et al (1999) The effects of TENS and interferential current on cutaneous blood flow in healthy subjects. *Physiother Canada* **51**(1): 27–31.

Ozcan J, Ward AR, Robertson VJ (2004) A comparison of true and premodulated interferential currents. *Arch Phys Med Rehab* **85**: 409–415.

Palmer S (2002) *The Effects of Interferential Current on C- and Aδ-mediated thermal perception. A comparison with Transcutaneous Electrical Nerve Stimulation.* PhD Thesis. Open University/Queen Margaret University College, Edinburgh.

Palmer S, Martin D, Steedman W et al (1999a) Interferential current and transcutaneous electrical nerve stimulation frequency: effects on nerve excitation. *Arch Phys Med Rehab* **80**: 1065–1071.

Palmer S, Martin D, Steedman W et al (1999b) *The Effects of Interferential Current on Thermal Sensation and Thermal Pain in Healthy Female Volunteers.* The Pain Society Annual Scientific Meeting, Edinburgh, 14–16 April 1999: 11.

Palmer S, Martin D, Steedman W et al (2000) C and Aδ-fibre mediated thermal perception: response to the rate of temperature change using method of limits. *Somatosens Motor Res* **17**(4): 325–333.

Palmer S, Martin D, Steedman W et al (2004) Effects of electric stimulation on C and A delta fiber-mediated thermal perception thresholds. *Arch Phys Med Rehab* **85**(1): 119–128.

Partridge CJ, Kitchen SS (1999) Adverse effects of electrotherapy used by physiotherapists. *Physiotherapy* **85**(6): 298–303.

Philipp A, Wolf GK, Rzany B et al (2000) Interferential current is effective in palmar psoriasis: an open prospective trial. *Eur J Dermatol* **10**(3): 195–198.

Pope GD, Mockett SP, Wright JP (1995) A survey of electrotherapeutic modalities: ownership and use in the NHS in England. *Physiotherapy* **81**(2): 82–91.

Price DD (1996) Selective activation of A-delta and C nociceptive afferents by different parameters of nociceptive heat stimulation: a tool for analysis of central mechanisms of pain. *Pain* **68**: 1–3.

Quirk A, Newman RJ, Newman KJ (1985) An evaluation of interferential therapy, shortwave diathermy and exercise in the treatment of osteoarthrosis of the knee. *Physiotherapy* **71**(2): 55–57.

Rennie S (1988) Interferential current therapy. In Peat M (ed) *Current Physical Therapy.* Philadelphia, BC Decker: 196–206.

Robertson VJ, Spurritt D (1998) Electrophysical agents: implications of their availability and use in undergraduate clinical placements. *Physiotherapy* **84**(7): 335–344.

Robinson AJ, Snyder-Mackler L (1988) Clinical application of electrotherapeutic modalities. *Phys Ther* **68**(8): 1235–1238.

Robinson AJ, Snyder-Mackler L (1995) *Clinical Electrophysiology: Electrotherapy and Electrophysiologic Testing*, 2nd edn. Baltimore, MD, Williams & Wilkins.

Rush PJ, Shore A (1994) Physician perceptions of the value of physical modalities in the treatment of musculoskeletal disease. *Br J Rheumatol* **33**(6): 566–568.

Salisbury L, Johnson M (1995) The analgesic effects of interferential therapy compared with TENS on experimental cold induced pain in normal subjects. *Physiotherapy* **81**: 741.

Savage B (1984) *Interferential Therapy.* London, Faber & Faber.

Schmitz RJ, Martin DE, Perrin DH et al (1997) Effect of interferential current on perceived pain and serum cortisol associated with delayed onset muscle soreness. *J Sport Rehab* **6**(1): 30–37.

Scott S, Purves C (1991) *The Effect of Interferential Therapy in the Relief of Experimentally Induced Pain: A Pilot Study.* Proceedings of the 11th International Congress of the World Confederation for Physical Therapy, Book II: 743–745.

Shafshak T, El-Sheshai AM, Soltan HE (1991) Personality traits in the mechanisms of interferential therapy for osteoarthritic knee pain. *Arch Phys Med Rehab* **72**: 579–581.

Sontag W (1998) Treatment of zymosan-activated HL-60 cells with low frequencies electric fields does not change cellular ATP and ADP levels and reactive oxygen species. *Bioelectrochem Bioenerg* **46**: 255–261.

Sontag W (2000) Modulation of cytokine production by interferential current in differentiated HL-60 cells. *Bioelectromagnetics* **21**: 238–244.

Sontag W (2001) Release of mediators by DMSO-differentiated HL-60 cells exposed to electric interferential current and the requirement of biochemical prestimulation. *Int J Radiation Biol* **77**(6): 723–734.

Sontag W (2004) Response of cyclic AMP by DMSO differentiated HL-60 cells exposed to electric interferential current after prestimulation. *Bioelectromagnetics* **25**: 176–184.

Sontag W, Dertinger H (1998) Response of cytosolic calcium, cyclic AMP, and cyclic GMP in dimethylsulfoxide-differentiated HL-60 cells to modulated low frequency electric currents. *Bioelectromagnetics* **19**: 452–458.

Stephenson R, Johnson M (1995) The analgesic effects of interferential therapy on cold-induced pain in healthy subjects: a preliminary report. *Physiother Theory Pract* **11**: 89–95.

Stephenson R, Walker EM (2003) The analgesic effects of interferential (IF) current on cold-pressor pain in healthy subjects: A single blind trial of three IF currents against sham IF and control. *Physiother Theory Pract* **19**(2): 99–107.

Sylvester KL, Keilty SEJ (1987) A pilot study to investigate the use of interferential in the treatment of ano-rectal incontinence. *Physiotherapy* **73**(4): 207–208.

Szehi E, David E (1980) The stereodynamic interferential current – a new electrotherapeutic technique. *Electromedica* **38**: 13–17.

Tabasam G, Johnson MI (1999a) *The Analgesic Effects of Different Swing Patterns of Interferential Currents (IFC) on Cold-induced Pain in Healthy Subjects.* The Pain Society Annual Scientific Meeting, Edinburgh, 14–16 April 1999: 12.

Tabasam G, Johnson MI (1999b) *The Analgesic Effects of Interferential Currents (IFC) and Transcutaneous Electrical Nerve Stimulation (TENS) on Ischaemic Pain in Healthy Subjects.* 9th World Congress on Pain, Vienna: 81.

Tabasam G, Johnson MI (2000) *A Survey of the Procedures Used to Administer Interferential Currents (IFC) by Physiotherapists.* Pain Society Annual Scientific Meeting, Warwick, 3–5 April 2000: 90.

Tabasam G, Johnson MI, Turja J (1998) *A Double Blind Placebo Controlled Investigation into the Analgesic Effects of Interferential Currents (IFC) and Transcutaneous Electrical Nerve Stimulation (TENS) on Cold-induced Pain in Normal Subjects*. Pain Society Annual Scientific Meeting, Leicester University, 22–24 April 1998.

Taylor K, Newton R, Personius W et al (1987) Effects of interferential current stimulation for treatment of subjects with recurrent jaw pain. *Phys Ther* **67**(3): 346–350.

Treffene RJ (1983) Interferential fields in a fluid medium. *Aust J Physiother* **29**(6): 209–216.

Turner PA, Whitfield TWA (1997) A multidimensional scaling analysis of the techniques that physiotherapists use. *Physiother Res Int* **2**(4): 237–254.

Vahtera T, Haaranen M, Viramo-Koskela AL et al (1997) Pelvic floor rehabilitation is effective in patients with multiple sclerosis. *Clin Rehab* **11**: 211–219.

Van Der Heijden GJ, Leffers P, Wolters PJ et al (1999) No effect of bipolar interferential electrotherapy and pulsed ultrasound for soft tissue shoulder disorders: a randomised controlled trial. *Ann Rheum Dis* **58**(9): 530–540.

Verdugo R, Ochoa JL (1992) Quantitative somatosensory thermotest: a key method for functional evaluation of small calibre afferent channels. *Brain* **115**: 893–913.

Wadsworth H, Chanmugam APP (1980) *Electrophysical Agents in Physiotherapy. Therapeutic and Diagnostic Use*. Marrickville, Australia: Science Press.

Wall P (1999) *Pain: The Science of Suffering*. London. Weidenfield & Nicolson.

Werners R, Pynsent PB, Bulstrode CJK (1999) Randomised trial comparing interferential therapy with motorised lumbar traction and massage in the management of low back pain in a primary care setting. *Spine* **24**(15): 1579–1584.

Willie CD (1969) Interferential therapy. *Physiotherapy* **55**(12): 503–505.

Wilson PD, Al Samarrai T, Deakin M et al (1987) An objective assessment of physiotherapy for female genuine stress incontinence. *Br J Obstet Gynaecol* **94**: 575–582.

Yarnitsky D, Ochoa JL (1990) Release of cold-induced burning pain by block of cold-specific afferent input. *Brain* **113**: 893–902.

Yarnitsky D, Ochoa JL (1991) Warm and cold specific somatosensory systems: psychophysical thresholds, reaction times and peripheral conduction velocities. *Brain* **114**: 1819–1826.

Yarnitsky D, Kunin M, Brik R et al (1997) Vibration reduces thermal pain in adjacent dermatomes. *Pain* **69**(1–2): 75–77.

Young SL, Woodbury MG, Fryday-Field K et al (1991) Efficacy of interferential current stimulation alone for pain reduction in patients with osteoarthritis of the knee: a randomized placebo control clinical trial. *Phys Ther* **71**(6): S52.

Chapter 18

Functional electrical stimulation

David Ewins and Sally Durham

INTRODUCTION

Functional electrical stimulation (FES) can be considered to be the application of electrical impulses to the body, to restore lost or impaired function. Many practitioners would consider that FES implies that the functional benefit should be immediate (or direct), e.g. reduction of foot-drop following stroke, resulting in the use of terms such as electrical orthoses or neural prostheses. However, for some, a less immediate (or indirect) benefit (e.g. muscle strengthening with stimulation) that, in time, leads to improvements in function, would also be considered to be FES. In both cases, the muscle contraction is usually very clear.

Strengthening through electrical stimulation is sometimes called therapeutic electrical stimulation (TES). For added confusion, the abbreviation 'TES' has also been used for threshold electrical stimulation, in which extended periods (e.g. night-time) of very low-level intensity stimulation have been used to improve motor skills. The results from such stimulation are mixed (Dali et al 2002) and this technique will not be discussed further. The terms 'neuromuscular electrical stimulation' (NMES) and 'functional neuromuscular stimulation' (FNS) are also used in the literature to cover direct and indirect functional applications of electrical stimulation.

In most reported applications of FES, electrical impulses are applied to innervated muscles such that impulses result in nerve depolarization and then subsequent muscle contraction. The basic theory behind this has already been reviewed in Chapters 13–15, but typical stimulation parameters for FES are pulse widths of 100–1000 μs and frequencies of 10–100 Hz. The amplitude varies with the application and the impedance characteristics of the patient; however, for surface stimulation, values of up to 120 mA (assuming a 1 kΩ load) are not uncommon. In some cases, electrical impulses have been used to recruit denervated muscle by direct depolarization of muscle fibres. However, the electrical impulses have a pulse width that is usually 100–1000 times greater than those used for innervated muscle stimulation, so necessitating the development of a different range of stimulation equipment. Nonetheless, work in this area has the potential to restore function, and some success has been reported, e.g. maintenance of standing posture following spinal cord injury (SCI) (Kern et al 2005). Although this is a very relevant and interesting area of work, for the remainder of this chapter, innervated muscle will be assumed.

The electrical impulses may be applied using skin surface electrodes, percutaneous electrodes (e.g. through the skin and into the muscle belly, near the motor point), or totally implanted electrodes (e.g. peripheral nerve cuffs or spinal roots, receiving power and control through an RF link from an external unit), with skin electrodes being the most common in routine clinical practice.

Skin-surface electrodes are often used in pairs, such that one (called the active or negative) electrode is usually placed over the motor point and the other (indifferent) electrode is placed at the proximal or distal end to complete the circuit and minimize recruitment of other muscles (Fig. 18.1). In some cases, rather than direct stimulation of the motor nerve, stimulation may be used to target a reflex action. The classic example is that of stimulation of the common peroneal nerve withdrawal reflex, which, if successful, can lead to a combination of hip and knee flexion, and ankle dorsiflexion (Fig. 18.2). It should not be forgotten that surface stimulation has a sensory component that, in some patients, can lead to disuse and make stimulation of less superficial muscles problematic. In addition, in some cases, particularly with finger/hand stimulation, it can be difficult to achieve or maintain the necessary specificity for clinical use. Percutaneous and implanted systems can address some of these

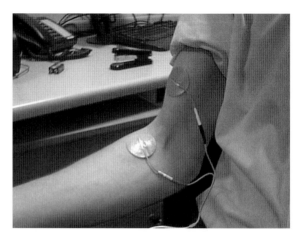

Figure 18.1 Typical electrode position for stimulation of biceps brachii. Active (negative) electrode placed over motor point, inactive (positive) electrode placed distally.

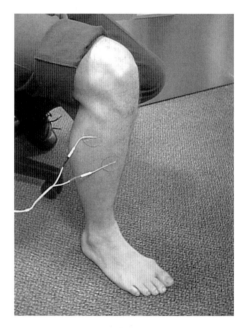

Figure 18.2 Typical electrode position for flexion withdrawal response. Active electrode placed over the common peroneal nerve (just below head of fibula), indifferent electrode placed over motor point of tibialis anterior.

problems, but the benefits have to be balanced against cost and clinical convenience.

In the following sections, a number of common applications of FES for upper and lower limb applications will be discussed and practical examples presented, however, it is a dynamic field and the review is indicative only. The reader is also encouraged to review other areas, for example restoration of bladder and bowel function, phrenic nerve stimulation, the use of stimulation to encourage fibre type conversion, and the general area of neuromodulation. Further recommended reading and information sources are given at the end of the chapter. For specific guidance on surface electrode positions the work by Baker et al (2000) and the information available from Odstock Medical Ltd (Salisbury District Hospital, Salisbury, UK) will be of particular interest.

LOWER LIMB STIMULATION

For some time, there has been considerable interest in the application of FES following SCI. Much of the earlier work used surface systems, and benefits in muscle bulk and blood flow through regular use of surface electrical stimulation have been reported (Taylor et al 1993). The use of surface systems to provide standing and walking has also been investigated (Fig. 18.3). The type of work reported ranges from stimulation-only-based systems (Ewins et al 1988) to hybrid approaches in which FES and mechanical (orthotic) systems are combined, for example Davis et al (1999) combined stimulation with a specially designed ankle–foot orthosis (AFO), and Sykes et al (1996) evaluated the benefits of combining FES with a reciprocating gait orthosis (RGO). The benefits of stimulation only systems are the lack of encumbrance of external mechanical aids and therefore reliance on and use of the subject's own musculature. The downside includes fatigue, resulting from synchronous recruitment of motor units (with a potentially greater proportion of type II muscle fibre following SCI), which can lead to short standing durations, and the issues surrounding control of a complex biomechanical system with a limited number of stimulation channels.

Routine clinical take-up of surface systems (standalone and otherwise) has been limited because of a combination of factors, including system complexity, cosmesis, time to attach/remove components and relative functional gain provided when compared to, for example, advances in

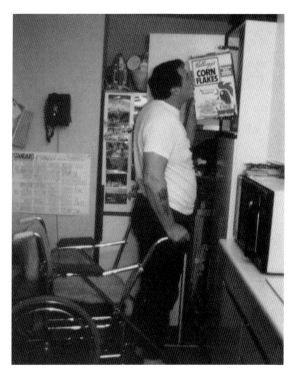

Figure 18.3 Surface FES assisted standing. Standing is supported through stimulation of the quadriceps muscle group. The stimulation parameters are controlled through measurement of knee ankle. The frame is used to provide support in the standing up and sitting down process, but balance only once standing.

wheelchair technology. Some of these problems have been addressed through the development of percutaneous and implanted stimulators, but further work in, for example, implantable sensor technology and system modelling, is required before routine daily use becomes practicable. This has led to a refocusing of interest in the use of FES for SCI, certainly in the UK, with growing emphasis on areas such as FES to assist fitness through its application in cycling (Fig. 18.4) and rowing (Hunt et al 2006, Wheeler et al 2002). In such systems, stimulation of large muscles groups, e.g. quadriceps and hamstring muscles, have the potential to provide overall performance and health benefits, doing so as part of regular recreational activities, which should encourage transfer of the technology to more routine use.

One of the earliest published examples of FES was as a gait assist for patients who present with a

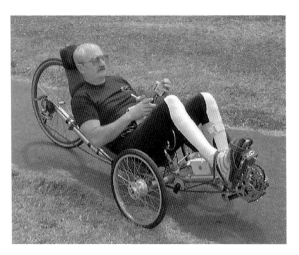

Figure 18.4 FES-assisted cycling using surface stimulation of quadriceps, hamstrings and gluteal muscles. Stimulation timing is controlled by measurement of the pedal (crank) angle. Courtesy of the Implanted Devices Group, University College London, UK.

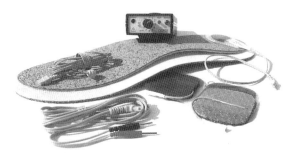

Figure 18.5 Salisbury ODFS111 stimulator, innersoles, footswitch, electrode pads and leads. The stimulator is a single-channel device designed primarily for gait assist. Courtesy of the Department of Clinical Science and Engineering, Salisbury District Hospital, UK.

flaccid foot drop (Liberson et al 1961). In the simplest case, the FES system consists of a single-channel device stimulating the peroneal nerve to induce ankle dorsiflexion and hip and knee flexion during the swing phase of the gait cycle. A sensible starting point for the electrode positions would be as shown in Figure 18.2; however, a number of electrode positions may have to be evaluated before an optimal response is found. The system employs a sensor that controls the timing of the stimulation. This is often a footswitch placed under the heel. In most cases, stimulation starts once the heel of the affected leg rises off the ground and ends when the heel makes contact with the ground during the swing to stance transition. The stimulator is usually worn either in a pocket or attached to a belt. Figure 18.5 shows a modern version of the stimulation equipment. Other physical sensors, e.g. tilt sensors, goniometers and electromyographic signals, have been investigated with varying levels of success, although the tilt sensor based WalkAide system (Innovative Neurotronics, Maryland, USA) is now marketed in the USA.

The dropped-foot stimulation system is now perhaps the most widespread clinical application of FES. The technology has advanced such that the equipment, particularly the foot switch, is more reliable and the stimulation timing is more subtle. The use of two-channel devices is also more common, with the second channel being used to assist with, for example, knee extension during stance (stimulation of quadriceps), 'push off' in late stance (calf stimulation), or for cases of bilateral foot drop.

The most commonly cited patient groups for dropped-foot stimulation are stroke and multiple sclerosis. For example, Taylor et al (1999a) reported a significant increase in walking speed and decreased energy consumption in a stroke patient group, and reported similar orthotic benefits in patients with multiple sclerosis. They also found smaller but still significant 'carry-over' benefits when the stimulation was not used. Kottink et al (2004) concluded that their review suggested a positive orthotic effect of FES on walking speed following stroke.

The authors' experience is that a very wide range of responses is shown to stimulation in stroke and MS patient groups, from quite dramatic improvements (Fig. 18.6) to no visible change. Despite a lack of observable improvement, some patients in the latter group report the FES to be helpful in assisting walking. This could be as a result of the sensory cue delivered by stimulation. Some preliminary work in patients with Parkinson's disease (Mann et al 2004) supports this observation.

When reviewing the evidence for the application of FES in improving motor control, the Royal College of Physicians' (2004) *National Clinical*

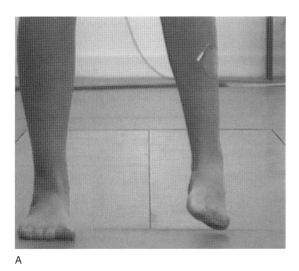 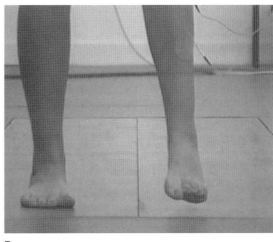

A   B

Figure 18.6 A, without and B, with stimulation, illustrating the improvement in foot positioning during swing. Stimulation was controlled by a hand switch controlled by a therapist.

Guidelines for Stroke concludes that 'FES should not be used on a routine basis and that individual patients should be considered for FES as an orthosis in certain circumstances, such as improving arm movement, ankle dorsiflexion and gait performance.' The guidelines go onto say that 'when considering the use of FES as an orthosis, local teams may wish to specify which patients are considered suitable; and how its benefit is to be judged for any patient trying it.' The need for further research in this patient group was also identified in the review by Pomeroy et al (2006), who found that questions such as the most effective type of stimulation, dose and time after stroke require further investigation.

Surface FES has also been investigated to assist in the gait of children with cerebral palsy (CP). One example is for those children who present with an equinus gait. There are two apparently opposing approaches, with some studies reporting positive results from stimulating the anterior tibial muscles (Durham et al 2004, Hazlewood et al 1994, Pape et al 1993), whereas others support stimulation of the calf or triceps surae muscle group. The rationale for electrical stimulation to the anterior tibial muscle is to produce active dorsiflexion at the ankle during the swing phase of gait, which at the same time reciprocally inhibits the antagonist, triceps surae (Hazelwood et al 1994).

By contrast, stimulating the triceps surae is thought to favourably modify altered muscle activation patterns with a reduction in spasticity (Rose 1998). In a study of four children (Carmick 1993, 1995), gait was improved through the application of electrical stimulation to triceps surae. In this study there was good evidence of a carry-over effect with improvements remaining when stimulation was not used in two of the four children. In a further study (Comeaux et al 1997), electrical stimulation of the gastrocnemius alone and then the gastrocnemius and tibialis anterior resulted in a trend towards increased dorsiflexion at initial toe contact. It made no difference whether gastrocnemius alone was stimulated or gastrocnemius and tibialis anterior alternately; both produced significant and similar results. This improvement was small but followed only short periods of limited use. Whereas both approaches have shown some encouraging results, they fail to produce conclusive evidence as to which is the treatment method of choice, or to provide prescription guidelines for appropriate patient selection. With this uncertainty, and as indicated by the work of Postans and Granat (2005), use of formal assessment techniques such as gait analysis might lead to more effective use of FES by allowing the clinical team to develop a greater understanding of the underlying reasons for the presenting problem.

The use of electrical stimulation for the treatment of congenital talipes equinovarus (CTEV) was suggested by Kirsch and Pape (1992). Their treatment involved two children aged 7 and 11 and a 44-year-old patient who suffered from persistent residual problems of CTEV. The results showed an increase in the active range of motion of the ankle and foot, an increased muscle bulk of the thigh and calf, and an improvement in the number of steps per 6 m and the distance travelled in a 6-minute walk. They suggested that the outcome of CTEV may improve by including treatment of the muscle atrophy with electrical stimulation and that younger children might demonstrate a greater benefit. Studies into the effect of stimulation on children with CTEV are being conducted at Queen Mary's Hospital, Roehampton, using surface electrodes following treatment by the Ponseti method. Figure 18.7 shows typical electrode positions used in this work to improve muscle strength of the weaker dorsiflexors and evertors. The preliminary results showed an improvement in foot position in both standing and walking and emphasized the need for further research in this area.

Apart from the sensory effects, which can be a major problem for some patients, a limitation of surface-electrode FES systems is electrode placement. In a review of use of the Odstock dropped-foot stimulator, Taylor et al (1999b) noted that one of the principal reasons for discontinuing with the FES system was electrode positioning difficulties; the other was changes (both improvements and deterioration) in mobility. Developments in percutaneous and fully implantable systems may address this problem. The use of percutaneous stimulation in the work by Johnston et al (2004) and Pierce et al (2004) in children with CP does demonstrate that this technique can be applied successfully. However, when much longer-term use is required, fully implanted systems may well be preferred. Recent commercial products that partly address this problem for patients with foot drop include the STIMuSTEP system (Finetech Medical Limited, Welwyn Garden City, UK), and the ActiGait system (Neurodan A/S, Aalborg SV, Denmark). These systems use an external control and power unit that transmits to an implanted receiver, with stimulation timed through an external foot switch mounted in the shoe.

As with the standing and walking in complete SCI discussed above, the use of hybrid approaches following, for example, stroke and CP have also been investigated. For example, a dropped-foot stimulation system can be combined with a hinged AFO to provide foot lift during swing (FES) and ankle/foot stability (orthosis) during stance. Others have investigated the simultaneous use of botulinum toxin with electrical stimulation (e.g. Detrembleur et al 2002, Johnson et al 2004). The results have been mixed, with some investigators reporting increased benefit with the hybrid approach and others reporting no change, suggesting that further work is required.

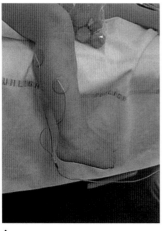

A

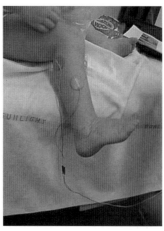

B

Figure 18.7 Stimulation being used to strengthen muscles in a child presenting with CTEV. A, without stimulation; B, with stimulation.

UPPER LIMB ASSIST

There has been considerable interest in the use of FES for upper limb assistance. Three areas that will be introduced here are shoulder subluxation and pain, muscle strength, and direct restoration of upper limb function.

SHOULDER SUBLUXATION AND SHOULDER PAIN

Shoulder subluxation and pain are common after stroke, with shoulder pain arising in approximately 30% of patients following stroke (Royal College of Physicians 2004), with the guidelines concluding that pain is not related to subluxation of the shoulder, and its relationship to handling and positioning remains uncertain. Figure 18.8 shows electrode positions that have been used to reduce shoulder subluxation through stimulation, in this case through stimulation of supraspinatus

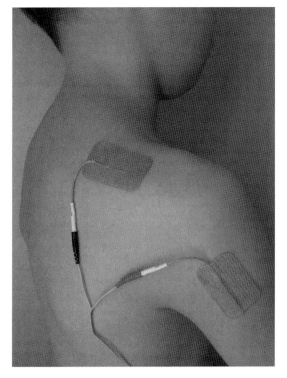

Figure 18.8 Use of stimulation to reduce shoulder subluxation after stroke. The electrodes are positioned for supraspinatus and deltoid muscles.

and deltoid muscles. In one particular case, stimulation was increased from 5 minutes to 30 minutes a day over the course of a week. Regular physiotherapy was maintained, but in the view of the treating therapist the patient's condition had stabilized prior to the FES sessions. X-rays were taken at assessment, and then without and with stimulation at 6 weeks (Fig. 18.9). Accepting the limitations of body positioning in the collection of the images, they do suggest that after 6 weeks the level of subluxation has decreased through stimulation, and that there is a further decrease when stimulation is actually applied.

The result discussed above is typical of that reported in the literature (for a review, see Price & Pandyan 2001). However, although Price and Pandyan accept that there appear to be benefits for passive humeral lateral rotation, possibly through reduction of glenohumeral subluxation, they believe that it is not conclusive that electrical stimulation (in a variety of formats) around the shoulder influences reports of pain. The effectiveness of FES in the motor recovery has also been reported to be affected by time since injury (Wang et al 2002) and, as for gait assist, the sensory component associated with stimulation can lead to disuse. Advances in implanted techniques, such as the BION stimulator (AMI, University of Southern California, Los Angeles, USA; reported by Leob et al 2006), offers potential for future development of the technique.

MUSCLE STRENGTH

There is growing interest in the use of FES to facilitate upper limb mobility and function through increases in muscle strength and reduction in antagonist muscle activity. Figure 18.10 illustrates the electrode positioning used with a single-channel stimulator to activate wrist and finger extensors in a chronic stroke patient. The change with stimulation is apparent. However, given the dynamics of conditions such as CP and stroke, and the complexity of the anatomy of the forearm, achieving a suitable response using surface electrodes can be very time consuming, with small changes in arm position and stimulation intensity resulting in quite dramatic changes in response in some patients, which can lead to disuse (Mangold et al 2005). Nonetheless, in clinical studies, the use of upper

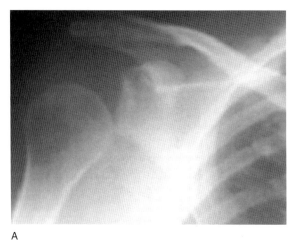

A

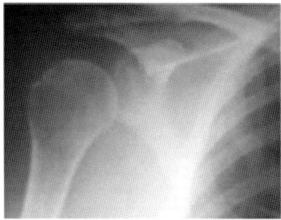

B

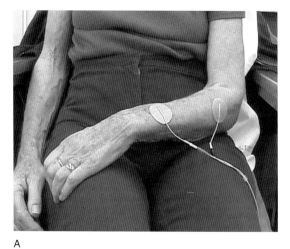

C

Figure 18.9 X-rays taken at the start and after 6 weeks of stimulation of supraspinatus and deltoid muscles to decrease shoulder subluxation in a post-stroke patient. A, at assessment; B, at 6 weeks and stimulation OFF; C, at 6 weeks and stimulation ON.

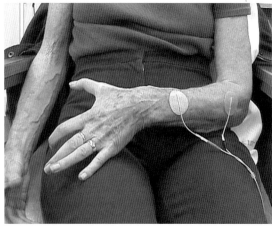

A

B

Figure 18.10 Stimulation being used to provide general wrist and hand extension. A, without stimulation; B, with stimulation.

limb stimulation in CP (Wright & Granat 2000), spinal cord injury (Mangold et al 2005) and post stroke (Gritsenko & Prochazka 2004, Ring & Rosenthal 2005) has been shown to provide some benefit to mobility and function. Odstock Medical Limited and NESS (Ra'anana, Israel) are two suppliers of FES equipment for upper limb strengthening.

As with gait assist, benefits have been shown when electrical stimulation has been combined with other interventions, e.g. dynamic splinting (Ozer et al 2006) and botulinum toxin injections (Hesse et al 2001). However, although the work is promising, further studies are required as results are not conclusive. For example, Carda and Molteni (2005) found taping following botulinum toxin injections to be more effective in reducing wrist and finger hypertonia than postinjection use of electrical stimulation and splinting.

DIRECT RESTORATION OF UPPER LIMB FUNCTION

As indicated above, it is relatively easy to use surface stimulation to recruit upper limb muscles but it is more difficult to do this in such a way that

leads to a system that can restore fine motor control on a practical basis. A number of systems have been investigated, e.g. the Bionic Glove, evaluated for C5–C7 spinal cord injured patients by Popovic et al (1999), and although laboratory success has often been demonstrated, these have yet to become available routinely.

To date, perhaps the most widely reported system for restoring hand function following spinal cord injury is the implanted Freehand system (previously available from Neurocontrol, USA). Illustrated in Figure 18.11, this system involves transfer of tendons together with the implantation of electrodes in the muscles of the forearm and hand of patients with tetraplegia. The electrode wires go up the arm to a control box located under the skin in the pectoral region. A movement detector is placed externally on the opposite shoulder. When the patient elevates and depresses, or protracts and retracts, this shoulder the movement is relayed to the control box, which is programmed to coordinate the activity in the electrodes and cause the hand to open and close. Taylor et al (2002) and Mulcahey et al (2004), among others, have concluded that the Freehand system does provide substantive functional benefits.

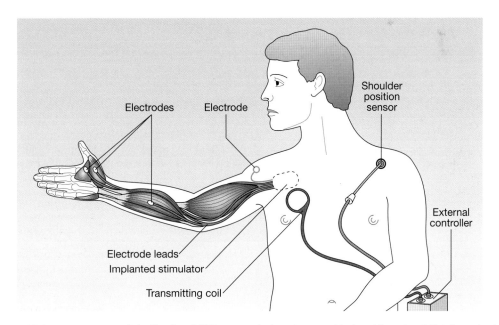

Figure 18.11 Major components of the Freehand FES system designed to provide hand function following spinal cord injury.

CONCLUSIONS

Published work makes a case for suggesting that FES has a part to play in current clinical practice. However, in many applications, uncertainty remains on issues such as selection criteria, protocols for use and appropriate outcome measures. In addition, FES is often only one of a range of options that could be explored at any given time and so its cost effectiveness also requires further investigation. At present, the use of FES is probably best undertaken following a multidisciplinary team review, which should include the patient and/or parent/carer as appropriate. The review would normally benefit from conventional assessments, such as joint range of motion and functional assessment tests to, as in the case of lower limb applications, a full three-dimensional movement analysis, to establish how stimulation can be best applied.

A very wide range of FES equipment has been developed, but in most cases the practicalities of routine clinical work will necessitate the use of surface systems with a limited number of output channels. With developments in electrode array technologies and integrated sensors that can lead to intelligent garments, the (non-sensory) limitations of multichannel surface electrode systems may be overcome.

Electrical stimulation equipment is not without risk, e.g. its use during pregnancy or with a cardiac pacemaker is often contraindicated. It is therefore important that healthcare professionals receive appropriate education and training in the use of electrical stimulation technologies. It is also important to ensure that the patient and/or parent/carer demonstrate their competence in the use of the equipment before it is used at home and that they are aware of any limitations when the stimulation is used to directly restore function. Regular reviews are often required to ensure effective use, and these may need to be more frequent during initial use. Care should also be taken to ensure that the patient's local therapy team are involved in the process, as this can improve compliance and the chances of success of the intervention.

In the longer term, more complex implantable systems will become available, such as those based on the BION stimulators referred to earlier. These will make use not only of technological developments but also of advances in (closed-loop) control techniques. Current sensing systems based on physical sensors, e.g. foot switches, goniometers, gyroscopes, accelerometers and load cells, will be supplemented by the use of natural sensors, for example, from the recording and processing of (afferent) nerve signals (Hansen et al 2004). These developments will offer exciting opportunities for more widespread use of FES.

References

Baker LL, Wederich CL, McNeal DR et al (2000) *Neuromuscular Electrical Stimulation – A Practical Guide*, 4th edn. Rancho Los Amigos Medical Centre, Downey, CA, Rancho Rehabilitation Engineering Program.

Carda S, Molteni F (2005) Taping versus electrical stimulation after botulinum toxin type A injection for wrist and finger spasticity. A case controlled study. *Clin Rehab* **19**(6): 621–626.

Carmick J (1993) Clinical use of neuromuscular electrical stimulation for children with cerebral palsy, part 1: Lower extremity. *Phys Ther* **73**(8): 505–513.

Carmick J (1995) Managing equinus in children with cerebral palsy: Electrical stimulation to strengthen the triceps surae muscle. *Dev Med Child Neurol* **37**: 965–975.

Comeaux P, Patterson N, Rubin M, Meiner R (1997) Effect of neuromuscular electrical stimulation during gait in children with cerebral palsy. *Pediatr Phys Ther* **9**: 103–109.

Dali C, Hansen FJ, Pedersen SA et al (2002) Threshold electrical stimulation (TES) in ambulant children with CP: a randomized double-blind placebo-controlled clinical trial. *Dev Med Child Neurol* **44**(6): 364–369.

Davis R, Houdayer T, Andrews B, Barriskill A (1999) Paraplegia: prolonged standing using closed loop functional electrical stimulation and Andrews ankle–foot orthosis. *Artif Organs* **23**(5): 418–420.

Detrembleur C, Lejeune TM, Renders A, Van den Bergh PYK (2002) Botulinum toxin and short-term electrical stimulation in the treatment of equinus in cerebral palsy. *Move Dis* **17**(1): 162–169.

Durham S, Eve L, Stevens C, Ewins D (2004) Effect of functional electrical stimulation on asymmetries in gait of children with hemiplegic cerebral palsy. *Physiotherapy* **90**: 82–90.

Ewins DJ, Taylor PN, Crook SE et al (1988) Practical low cost stand/sit system for mid thoracic paraplegics. *J Biomed Eng* **10**(2): 184–188.

Gritsenko V, Prochazka A (2004) A functional electrical stimulation-assisted exercise therapy system for hemiplegic hand function. *Arch Phys Med Rehab* **85**(6): 881–885.

Hansen M, Haugland MK, Sinkjaer T (2004) Evaluating robustness of gait event detection based on machine learning and natural sensors. *IEEE Trans Neural Syst Rehab Eng* **12**(1): 81–88.

Hazlewood ME, Brown JK, Rowe PJ, Salter PM (1994). The use of therapeutic electrical stimulation in the treatment of hemiplegic cerebral palsy. *Dev Med Child Neurol* **36**: 661–673.

Hesse S, Brandi-Hesse B, Bardeleben A et al (2001) Botulinum toxin A treatment of adult upper and lower limb spasticity. *Drugs Aging* **18**(4): 255–262.

Hunt KJ, Ferrario C, Grant S et al (2006) Comparison of stimulation patterns for FES-cycling using measures of oxygen cost and stimulation cost. *Med Eng Phys* **28**(7): 710–718.

Johnson CA, Burridge JH, Strike PW et al (2004) The effect of combined use of botulinum toxin type A and functional electrical stimulation in the treatment of spastic drop foot after stroke: a preliminary investigation. *Arch Phys Med Rehabil* **85**(6): 902–909.

Johnston TE, Finson RL, McCarthy JJ et al (2004) Use of functional electrical stimulation to augment traditional orthopaedic surgery in children with cerebral palsy. *J Pediatr Orthop* **24**(3): 283–291.

Kern H, Salmons S, Mayr W et al (2005) Recovery of long term denervated human muscles induced by electrical stimulation. *Muscle Nerve* **31**(1): 98–101.

Kirsch SE, Pape KE (1992) Changes in unilateral congenital talipes equinovarus in a 44 year old man following transcutaneous electrical stimulation. *Am Acad Pediatr* [orthopedics section].

Kottink AI, Oostendorp LJ, Buurke JH et al (2004) The orthotic effect of functional electrical stimulation on the improvement of walking in stroke patients with a dropped foot: a systematic review. *Artif Organs* **28**(6): 577–586.

Leob GE, Richmond FJ, Baker LL (2006) The BION devices: Injectable interfaces with peripheral nerves and muscle. *Neurosurg Focus* **20**(5): E2.

Liberson WT, Holmquest HJ, Scot D, Margot D (1961) Functional electrotherapy: stimulation of the peroneal nerve synchronised with the swing phase of gait of hemiplegic subjects. *Arch Phys Med Rehab* **42**: 101–105.

Mangold S, Keller T, Curt A, Dietz V (2005) Transcutaneous functional electrical stimulation for grasping in subjects with cervical spinal cord injury. *Spinal Cord* **43**(1): 1–13.

Mann GE, Finn SM, Taylor PN (2004) *A Pilot Study to Investigate the Effects of Functional Electrical Stimulation on Gait in Parkinson's Disease*. 9th Annual Conference of the International FES Society and 2nd FESnet Conference: 62–64.

Mulcahey MJ, Betz RR, Kozin SH et al (2004) Implantation of the freehand system during initial rehabilitation using minimally invasive techniques. *Spinal Cord* **42**(3): 146–155.

Ozer K, Chesher SP, Scheker LR (2006) Neuromuscular electrical stimulation and dynamic bracing for the management of upper extremity spasticity in children with cerebral palsy. *Dev Med Child Neurol* **48**(7): 559–563.

Pape K, Kirsch S, Galil A et al (1993) Neuromuscular approach to the deficits of cerebral palsy: A pilot study. *J Pediatr Orthop* **13**: 628–633.

Pierce S, Orlin MN, Lauer RT et al (2004) Comparison of percutaneous and surface functional electrical stimulation during gait in a child with hemiplegic cerebral palsy. *Am J Phys Med Rehab* **83**: 798–805.

Pomeroy VM, King L, Pollock A et al (2006) Electrostimulation for promoting recovery of movement or functional ability after stroke (review). Cochrane Library, Issue 2.

Popovic D, Stojanovic A, Pjanovic A et al (1999) Clinical evaluation of the bionic glove. *Arch Phys Med Rehab* **80**(3): 299–304.

Postans NJ, Granat MH (2005) Effect of functional electrical stimulation, applied during walking, on gait in spastic cerebral palsy. *Dev Med Child Neurol* **47**(1): 46–52.

Price CI, Pandyan AD (2001) Electrical stimulation for preventing and treating post stroke shoulder pain: a systematic Cochrane review. *Clin Rehab* **15**(1): 5–19.

Ring H, Rosenthal N (2005) Controlled study of neuroprosthetic functional electrical stimulation in sub-acute post stroke rehabilitation. *J Rehab Med* **37**(1): 32–36.

Rose J (1998) The motor unit in cerebral palsy. *Dev Med Child Neurol* **40**: 270–277.

Royal College of Physicians (2004) *National Clinical Guidelines for Stroke*, 2nd edn. London, Royal College of Physicians.

Sykes L, Campbell IG, Powell ES et al (1996) Energy expenditure of walking with spinal cord lesions using the reciprocating gait orthosis and functional electrical stimulation. *Spinal Cord* **34**(11): 659–665.

Taylor PN, Ewins DJ, Fox BA et al (1993) Limb blood flow, cardiac output and quadriceps muscle bulk following spinal cord lesion and the effect of training for the Odstock functional electrical stimulation standing system. *Paraplegia* **31**: 303–310.

Taylor PN, Burridge JH, Dunkerley AL et al (1999a) Clinical use of the Odstock dropped foot stimulator: its effect on the speed and effort of walking. *Arch Phys Med Rehab* **80**(12): 1577–1583.

Taylor P, Burridge J, Dunkerley A et al (1999b) Clinical audit of 5 years provision of the Odstock dropped foot stimulator. *Artif Organs* **23**(5): 440–442.

Taylor P, Esnouf J, Hobby J (2002) The functional impact of the Freehand system on tetraplegic hand function: clinical results. *Spinal Cord* **40**(11): 560–566.

Wang RY, Yang YR, Tsai MW et al (2002) Effects of functional electrical stimulation on upper limb motor function and shoulder range of motion in hemiplegic patients. *Am J Phys Med Rehab* **81**(4): 283–290.

Wheeler GD, Andrews B, Lederer R et al (2002) Functional electrical stimulation-assisted rowing: Increasing cardiovascular fitness through functional electric stimulation rowing training in persons with spinal cord injury. *Arch Phys Med Rehab* **83**(8): 1093–1099.

Wright PA, Granat MH (2000) Therapeutic effects of functional electrical stimulation of the upper limb of eight children with cerebral palsy. *Dev Med Child Neurol* **42**(11): 724–727.

Further reading and information sources

Agnew WF, McCreery DB (eds) (1990) *Neural Prostheses: Fundamental Studies*. London, Prentice Hall.

Baker LL, Wederich CL, McNeal DR et al (2000) *Neuromuscular Electrical Stimulation – A Practical Guide,* 4th edn. Rancho Los Amigos Medical Centre, Downey, CA, Rancho Rehabilitation Engineering Program.

Brindley GS, Rushton DN (eds) (1995) *Neuroprostheses. Clinical Neurology Series.* Vol 4, No 1, London, Baillière Tindall.

FESnet (UK network for Rehabilitation using Functional Electrical Stimulation). Online. Available: http://fesnet.eng.gla.ac.uk/

Hambrecht FT, Reswick JB (eds) (1977) *Functional Electrical Stimulation: Applications in Neural Prostheses* New York, Marcel Dekker.

IFESS (International Functional Electrical Stimulation Society). Online. Available: http://www.ifess.org/

Institute of Physics in Engineering and Medicine (2004) The clinical use of functional electrical stimulation in neurological rehabilitation. In *Horizons in Medicine 16: Updates on Major Clinical Advances*. London, Royal College of Physicians.

Kralj A, Bajd T (1989) *Functional Electrical Stimulation: Standing and Walking after Spinal Cord Injury*. Boca Raton, FL, CRC Press.

Web address for examples of suppliers of FES equipment cited in the text

Alfred Mann Institute (BION stimulators): http://ami.usc.edu/

Finetech Medical Limited (STIMuSTEP): http://www.finetech-medical.co.uk/

Innovative Neurotronics (WalkAide System): http://www.walkaide.com/

NESS (Neuromuscular Electrical Stimulation Systems Ltd): http://www.nessltd.com/

Neurodan A/S (ActiGait): http://www.neurodan.com/

Odstock Medical Limited: http://www.odstockmedical.com/

Chapter 19

Electrical stimulation for enhanced wound healing

Tim Watson

INTRODUCTION

Chronic wounds are a continuing problem within the healthcare sector: the costs of care are high, thus effective care is of great importance. Such wounds are treated in a wide variety of ways, one of which is electrical stimulation based on the observed differences in electrical potential resulting from wounding and persisting through the stages of healing. This chapter considers the current evidence for the efficacy of treatment using electrical stimulation linked with the endogenous bioelectric evidence summarized in Chapter 3. The use of electrical stimulation as a means of enhancing wound healing is not new. Reports dating back to the seventeenth century record the use of gold-leaf applications to cutaneous lesions associated with smallpox. Although there have been many publications in this research area, especially in more recent years, there appears to be a reluctance to use the therapy in the clinical environment. Given the drive towards evidence-based practice, this appears to be a strange phenomenon.

A chronic wound is any interruption in the continuity of the body's surface that requires a prolonged time to heal, does not heal or recurs (Ojingwa & Isseroff 2002, Wysocki 1996). In a recent Cochrane review, Kranke et al (2004) concluded that chronic wounds are common and constitute a significant health problem. The true incidence and impact are difficult to assess accurately because of the wide range of disease, the fact that much care is delivered at home, and also because many wound-care products are purchased directly from a variety of sources. Evidence is cited to suggest that 1% of the population of industrialized countries will experience a leg ulcer at some time (Baker et al 1991).

Healthcare costs for chronic wound vary depending on the method of calculation adopted by the authors, but McGuckin et al (2001) suggest that, in the UK, the financial cost of venous disease has been estimated between £294 and £650 million per year; more recently, Kranke et al (2004) suggested that wound care in the UK costs in excess of £1 billion per year. In the United States, costs are estimated between $2.5 and $3 billion, with a loss of 2 million work days per year.

Many forms of electrotherapy have been used in relation to wound healing, including laser therapy, ultrasound and pulsed shortwave and magnetic therapies. While acknowledging these other interventions, this chapter focuses exclusively on electrical stimulation; previous chapters have identified key issues in relation to other modalities.

PROBLEMS ASSOCIATED WITH CHRONIC WOUNDS

A relatively small proportion of wounds present with healing problems and many will heal spontaneously without major therapeutic intervention. However, some wound types are notoriously slow to heal, for example chronic venous ulcers and pressure sores. These tend to be lesions of long duration and are often resistant to many forms of treatment. The most commonly encountered wounds in Western medical practice are a consequence of diabetes, arterial and/or venous disease, sustained pressure or as a result of radiotherapy (Kranke et al 2004). They can result in significant medical, social and economic problems for patients, their relatives and the medical professionals involved.

The factors responsible for poor wound healing are legion and beyond the scope of this chapter, but they remain central to the philosophy of the use of electrical stimulation as a modality to enhance healing. Interference with one or more levels of the cascade of events associated with any healing process can lead to inadequate healing and repair responses. Frank and Szeto (1983) summarized the possible general factors as follows:

- inability to form a blood clot or mount an adequate inflammatory reaction

- inability to produce new cells or scar components in adequate quantity or quality

- inability to organize the scar into an appropriate functional or cosmetic unit.

These factors can be considered on both a local and a systemic level. The local factors include infection, inadequate blood flow and inadequate nutrition, resulting in low oxygen levels and a poor inflammatory response. Repeated wound stresses or sustained pressure can also make a significant contribution. Systemic effects that might be detrimental include age-related changes, concurrent disease states and hormonal disturbance. Clearly, one could add to these lists with ever more detailed categories, but in principle a large number of factors might be responsible for the interruption of a component of the healing process, and thus in achieving a major healing dysfunction by interfering with the cascade nature of the normal healing events and the complex interactions between components of the processes.

Chronic wounds behave differently from acute wounds and some authorities have suggested that they are different in a more fundamental way than just their duration. Cutting (2006) suggests that the overall picture found within chronic wound tissue is not simply one of decreased cellular activity but rather disorder, where unregulated cellular functions can be identified. It is argued that to achieve resolution to these chronic problems, a reaction needs to be initiated, then order established before closure can be achieved. The process of wound healing was reviewed in Chapter 4, which together with the bioelectric background information from Chapter 3 provides a platform for this chapter on electrical stimulation for enhancement of wound healing.

REVIEWS

There have been several detailed reviews relating to the use of electrical stimulation in relation to wound healing and wound management. Gardner et al (1999), for example, reported the outcome of a meta-analysis that aimed to quantify the effect of electrical stimulation on chronic wound healing. Fifteen studies were analysed and the average rate of healing per week was calculated for the electrical stimulation and control samples, giving 22% for electrical stimulation samples and 9% for control samples. Further analysis by type of electrical stimulation failed to demonstrate a clear differential between stimulation modes and it was concluded that although electrical stimulation produces a substantial improvement in the healing of chronic wounds, further research is needed to identify which electrical stimulation devices are most effective and which wounds respond best to this treatment.

A very comprehensive and detailed review by Kloth (2005) did not attempt meta-analysis but did consider a raft of evidence from cellular, animal and clinical studies, with a focus on lower limb wounds. Rather than divide the available research up in terms of stimulation mode, Kloth took a clinical problem focused approach which evaluated over 150 papers. Ojingwa and Isseroff (2002) provide a more traditional review considering the various modalities on the basis of their mode of intervention which acts as a useful complement to the Kloth paper.

VARIETY OF APPROACHES

Although numerous studies have looked at the basic and clinical science of wound electrical stimulation, one of the key issues, commented on by nearly all reviewers in the field, is the inhomogeneity of the research. Very few of the cellular, animal or clinical studies have employed the 'same' form of stimulation, and thus identifying the essential and common threads in the research remains problematic. Almost every review identifies the need for further research and larger-scale randomized controlled trials (RCTs) in particular (e.g. Cutting 2006, Kloth 2005, Ojingwa & Isseroff 2002).

For the purposes of this chapter, the use of electrical stimulation to enhance or stimulate wound healing has been divided into three main approaches. Each approach described has reported beneficial clinical effects and, at present, the available evidence does not appear to identify a distinct advantage of one approach over another. This chapter sets out to consider the effects of electrical stimulation on chronic skin wounds, particularly chronic venous ulcers, pressure sores and allied lesions. The substantial and growing body of literature concerning electrical stimulation for promoting bone healing and other soft-tissue repair is not discussed in any detail in this chapter; reviews of this additional material can be found in Albert and Wong (1991), Black (1987), Childs (2003), Gardner et al (1999), Rodriguez-Merchan and Forriol (2004) and Watson (2006). At the end of the chapter, a summary of the proposed mechanisms by which stimulation is able to bring about the positive clinical effects is considered.

ELECTRICAL ACTIVITY IN THE SKIN RELATED TO WOUNDS AND HEALING

The key issues associated with tissue batteries, endogenous bioelectric activity and the relationship between these phenomena and tissue injury and repair were considered in some detail in Chapter 3. An unreferenced summary will be provided here for continuity.

Tissue, in its non-injured state, exhibits bioelectric activity that is actively maintained. These endogenous bioelectric signals are derived from a variety of sources at both the cellular and tissue level, possibly supplemented by organism-wide electrical energy systems. When insult, injury or pathology affects the tissues, there is both a local and an organism-wide change in this electrical activity (generally referred to as the 'current of injury'), and these changes have been associated with effective tissue repair. If this electrical activity is at too low a level, or indeed is absent in the damaged tissue, the 'normal' process of healing is either significantly inhibited or effectively absent.

It is argued that the use of exogenous (i.e. from outside the body) electric stimulation can supplement the naturally occurring bioelectric activity and, by this mechanism, facilitate the process of tissue repair.

CELLULAR STUDIES

A substantial volume of work has been published concerning the effects of electrical stimulation on cell cultures and in-vivo animal experiments. Numerous studies have demonstrated cellular responses to direct current, often at magnitudes comparable to those found physiologically (see Chapter 3). Whereas it can be argued that laboratory-based cell studies are not directly clinically relevant, it is important to establish that cells of various types are electrically sensitive, demonstrate a change in metabolic activity, and also change their direction and rate of movement in response to electric fields (Cutting 2006, Kloth 2005). The key findings are summarized here.

Fibroblasts

Fibroblasts have been investigated by numerous groups, although not all studies have used human cultures. Using an applied direct current (DC) stimulation, Dunn (1988) demonstrated fibroblast invasion of a collagen matrix placed in a skin wound in the guinea pig. The fibroblast ingrowth and collagen fibre alignment were significantly increased compared to controls. Goldman and Pollack (1996) studied the effect of electrical stimulation on human fibroblasts in vitro. Various current intensities and frequencies were evaluated and a field strength of between 31 and 50 mV/mm was found to be effective at 10 Hz, but not at 100 Hz. The concept of frequency and amplitude windows appears to be supported by this work, and the effective parameters match those identified in the endogenous bioelectric state [see Chapter 1 and Watson (2000)].

Erickson and Nuccitelli (1984) demonstrated fibroblast migration towards the cathode when the cells were exposed to a DC field. The threshold field strength was found to be between 1 and 10 mV/mm. In addition to cell migration, they demonstrated changes in cell orientation, the fibroblasts realigning with their long axes perpendicular to the field direction. Field strengths of up to 10 times greater than those necessary to induce fibroblast responses have been measured in vivo. Ross et al (1989) also demonstrated (human) fibroblast alignment when exposed to an electric field with field strengths of 0.1–1.5 V/mm (100–1500 mV/mm). Further studies that have demonstrated significant beneficial effects on fibroblast motility, proliferation and protein synthesis include Bourguignon and Bourguignon (1987),

Canseven and Atalay (1996), Goldman and Pollack (1996) and Thawer and Houghton (2001).

Fibroblasts are crucial in terms of tissue repair and the published literature would support the overall finding that fibroblasts are both sensitive and responsive to electrical fields.

Epidermal cells

When considering wound healing and closure, epidermal cells are of the utmost importance. Epidermal cell orientation and migration have been demonstrated in DC fields (Cooper & Schliwa 1985). The threshold for these effects was in the region of 0.5 V/cm (50 mV/mm), which represents some 1–4 mV per cell diameter. The demonstration by Winter (1964) that epithelial cells migrating from the periphery of an ulcer move in response to the voltage gradient is also pertinent to the discussion on the effects of electrical stimulation for wound healing (Kloth 1995, 2005).

In addition to fibroblasts and epidermal cells, several other cell types have been shown to respond to electrical stimuli; some of the key papers for each main cell type are included in Table 19.1.

There has been considerable interest, over the last few years, in the role of angiogenesis in tissue repair (see Chapter 4) and a recent paper by Bai et al (2004) demonstrated a significant beneficial effect of DC stimulation on the angiogenic response in human-derived cells. Furthermore, Zhao et al (2004) demonstrated a similar effect, and identified vascular endothelial growth factor (VEGF) as the mediator of the response, whereas Goldman et al (2004) demonstrated an increase in capillary bed density with electrical stimulation.

Antibacterial effects

The delay of wound healing due to local infection is not doubted (Bowler et al 2001) and healing will inevitably be delayed while the infection persists. Electrical stimulation has been shown to have both bacteriostatic and bacteriocidal effects. It is also suggested that even wounds that do not demonstrate overt signs of infection are very often 'colonized' (Hansson 1995), which will almost certainly have an inhibitory effect. It is a well-demonstrated clinical principle that dealing with the contaminated wound is an essential early phase of wound management

Table 19.1 Key papers relating to cell reactivity in response to electrical stimulation

Cell type	References
Fibroblasts	Bourguinon & Bourguinon 1987, Canseven & Atalay 1996, Cheng & Goldman 1998, Goldman & Pollack 1996, Reger et al 1999, Thawer & Houghton 2001
Neutrophils	Fukushima et al 1953, Gentzkow & Miller 1991
Macrophages	Cho et al 2000, Orida & Feldman 1982
Mast cells	Gentzkow 1993, Reich et al 1991, Taskan et al 1997
Endothelial cells	Chang et al 1996, Goldman et al 2004, Li et al 2002, Nissen et al 1998, Zhao et al 2004
Myofibroblasts	Brown & Gogia 1987, Gabbiani 2003
Epidermal cells	Farbould et al 2000, Nishimura et al 1996, Nuccitelli 2003, Pullar et al 2001, Sheridan et al 1996, Zhao et al 1999

(Schultz et al 2003) and successful wound closure cannot expected if the infection cannot be managed.

There is considerable evidence that electrical stimulation has a marked inhibitory effect on several common pathogens. On balance, the DC stimulation modes appear to be more effective than their alternating current (AC) counterparts.

Kincaid and Lavoie (1989) published a series of results highlighting the effects of high-voltage pulsed current (HVPC) on cultured bacterial species in a series of in-vitro experiments. Three commonly isolated bacterial strains were exposed to positive and negative HVPC. All three strains were affected equally by 2 hours of HVPC above 250 V. Cathodal (−ve) exposure resulted in bacterial death, whereas at the anode (+ve), toxic electrochemical end-products appeared to be responsible for the bacterial demise. The authors suggested that HVPC could have significant antibacterial effects in the clinical environment. Szuminsky et al (1994) have also identified a definite antimicrobial effect of high-voltage stimulation (monophasic twin peak).

Merriman et al (2004) compared the efficacy of various electrical stimulation modes on bacterial growth in vitro. Microamp stimulation (DC, pulsed DC monophasic and biphasic) and HPVC were compared in their effect on culture plates containing *Staphylococcus aureus*. The zone of inhibition surrounding each electrode was measured following stimulation and a significant inhibitory effect was shown for continuous DC and HVPC but not for the pulsed monophasic and biphasic modes.

There appears to be evidence of benefit from various forms of electrical stimulation in relation to antibacterial effect and the clinical application of this therapy, intended to stimulate wound healing, might have part of its beneficial action attributed to bacteriocidal effects.

ANIMAL STUDIES

Before considering the effects of electrical stimulation for wound healing in the clinical environment, it is pertinent to summarize the evidence generated from numerous animal experiments. It is difficult to extrapolate directly from this animal work as the wound-healing process is not the same as in humans and, although there are similarities between species, there are no directly equivalent animal-healing models. The experimentation does, nevertheless, provide useful background material for the principles supporting clinical intervention. A more comprehensive review of animal research is found in Kloth (2005) and Ojingwa and Isseroff (2002). The key issues will be identified below to provide a foundation for the clinical studies. In addition, a substantial number of studies have considered the electrical correlates of healing and regeneration in amphibian and vertebrate species, reviewed in a series of papers by Borgens and colleagues (Borgens 1981, 1982, Borgens & McCaig 1989, Borgens et al 1977, 1989). Research evidence will be briefly considered under three themes: collagen content and tensile strength, wound closure and tissue necrosis.

Collagen content and increased wound tensile strength

Several animal wound models include tensile strength measures as a key outcome, although this is not a commonly reported clinical outcome (for obvious reasons). Some doubt has been raised as to the validity of measuring wound healing in terms of tensile strength alone (Forrest 1983) and strength changes combined with collagen content analysis appear to be preferable.

Thawer and Houghton (2001) demonstrated an increase in collagen deposition in diabetic mice wounds. Skin incision work in rabbits is reported by Konikoff (1976), who used bilateral, full-thickness paravertebral incisions with one side receiving DC stimulation and a sham treatment to the contralateral wound. A DC current (20 mA) was used and the wounds were tested at 1 week for tensile strength, at which time the treated lesions demonstrated an average 53% increase in tensile strength compared to the sham-treated wounds.

Bach et al (1991) used a rat-skin wound model to compare the effects of DC, AC and sham treatments on wound strength. Neither type of electrical stimulation had a significant effect on wound strength when compared with controls, but both electrical stimulation groups showed significant increases in collagen content in and around the wound compared with the sham group.

The effects of electrical stimulation (through a metallic suture) in abdominal muscle lesions were investigated by Wu et al (1967). Two suture materials were compared for effects: stainless steel and platinum. DC stimulation at 40–400 mA was used and it was found that the rabbits with steel sutures gained greater wound strength than those with platinum sutures. The increases in wound strength did not appear to be related to stimulation polarity or intensity, and it was therefore suggested that the benefits of stimulation might be due to electrode products (Fe) rather than the stimulation itself.

There are many animal experiments in this field, and Ojingwa and Isseroff (2002) provide a useful summary, concluding that several forms of stimulation have shown an increase in wound strength, but on balance, the DC stimulation modes appear to have generated the stronger results.

Wound closure

The widely cited experimental work of Alvarez et al (1983) used a pig model to compare the effects of DC stimulation, sham stimulation and no treatment on skin wounds that were evaluated for re-epithelialization and collagen synthesis. It was found that collagen content increased in the DC stimulation group and the epithelial covering was more rapid than in the sham and no-treatment groups.

Taskan et al (1997) compared the effect of ultrasound and electrical stimulation in a rat wound model. Four groups were compared: real and sham electrostimulation (ES), and real and sham ultrasound (US). Both real ES and US have beneficial effects but the ES results were found to be superior to those attributed to the US.

Stromberg (1988) reported the results of different electrical stimulation protocols on skin wounds in pigs, measuring wound contraction rates and the open wound area. The stimulation groups received either DC stimulation (35 mA unipolar square-wave stimulation for 30 minutes twice a day with the negative electrode at the wound) or an identical electrical stimulation but with the wound electrode polarity reversed every 3 days. The first group, with the consistently negative wound electrode, appeared to gain no benefit from the treatment, with a trend towards a retarded healing process. By contrast, in the group where the stimulating polarity was reversed the wound size decreased to 18% of the original size in 2 weeks, and down to 5% of the original size by the end of 3 weeks of treatment.

Reger et al (1999) compared the efficacy of DC and AC stimulation with a control condition on experimental skin ulcers in a pig model. Interestingly, both the AC and DC stimulation resulted in reduced healing time compared with the control condition, but the DC group showed the most rapid reduction in the wound area and the AC stimulation showed the most rapid reduction in wound volume.

Tissue necrosis

Using a full-thickness skin excision and replacement model in rats, Politis et al (1989) used a necrotic area of skin that resulted under control conditions following this procedure. After 1 week, the size of the necrotic area was compared in a control group and two treatment groups who had received DC stimulation with opposite-polarity currents. The group with the anode to the skin surface and the cathode implanted deep to the wound showed least necrosis (50%), whereas the reverse polarity stimulation group and the sham treatment group both had 80–90% necrosis after the same time period.

Wound healing in pig skin has been extensively studied as it provides an animal model that more closely resembles human skin. Im et al (1990) raised bilateral bipedicle skin flaps, the central portion of which is known to become ischaemic without intervention. This central zone was treated with electrical stimulation (pulsed DC) at 35 mA, 128 Hz, for 30 minutes twice a day over 9 days. The treatment protocol involved negative stimulation on days 1–3, positive stimulation on days 4–6 and negative stimulation again for days 7–9. The necrotic area in the treated animals was significantly smaller than in the control group.

CLINICAL TRIALS

One of the problems with reviewing the literature on electrical stimulation for wound healing is that there are multiple approaches, several variations with each area and a lack of controlled trials with large sample sizes. Almost all those who have seriously reviewed the literature in recent years have made the same comments (Cutting 2006, Kloth 2005, Ojingwa & Isseroff 2002). Additionally, there is some confusion (or ambiguity) concerning the terms employed to describe the stimulation, with a complexity of terminology, some of which relates to machine-specific features, and with several authors using similar terms in quite different ways. It is suggested that a description of the essential features of the stimulation mode in terms of stimulus amplitude, frequency and duration are the essential features and that, additionally, pulse 'shape' could be usefully added. Whether the delivered current is monophasic or biphasic certainly appears to have an impact in the context of wound healing; if biphasic, whether the pulses are symmetrical or asymmetrical is also important. Given, then, what is supposed to be a 'short' list of features, it is still not a simple task to compare stimulation modes.

The mechanisms by which electrical stimulation achieves its results are still poorly understood and, although there are clearly links that can be established between the hypothetical effects of the treatment and the outcome of the intervention, the theoretical basis for the treatment remains tenuous

in places. Nevertheless, the general trend of the clinical research reports is for beneficial effects to dominate, with only a minority of trials reporting zero or negative effects.

The various clinical interventions are divided as follows for the purpose of this review:

- direct currents (DC)
- pulsed direct currents (pulsed DC), which are further divided into high and low intensity
- alternating currents (AC).

Any classification is prone to failure at some point and this change in categorization, although different from that employed previously, is probably the most appropriate at the current time. The direct currents would include a range of modalities that are often referred to as 'microcurrent' stimulation or low-intensity direct current (LIDC). Other terms that have been used as 'categories' – such as high-voltage pulsed galvanic stimulation (HVPGS) – would be incorporated into the pulsed DC group, under the high-intensity section. The classification is capable of further refinement (in that subgroups can be added) and should be sufficiently flexible to enable 'new' stimulation modes to be fully incorporated without the need for adjusting the main groupings. It remains to be seen whether this hierarchy will become more widely employed. A basic representation of commonly employed current/pulse forms is identified in Figure 19.1.

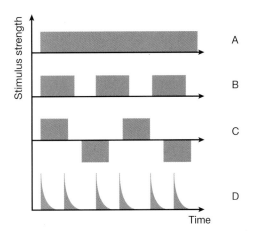

Figure 19.1 Representation of basic stimulating current forms. A, direct current; B, monophasic pulsed DC; C, symmetric biphasic pulsed; D, twin peak monophasic.

In an interesting novel development, Lee et al (2004) have used a combination of electrical stimulation and gene therapy to derive a combined beneficial effect of both interventions. The process of electroporation – a form of electrical stimulation used to enhance the permeability of the cell membrane to allow penetration of macromolecules – is already employed in several areas of gene- and electrically enhanced chemotherapy. In the experimental work reported by Lee et al, the combination of electrical stimulation and gene intervention [related to transforming growth factor (TGF-β1)] was significantly better than either therapy alone, and therefore opens up new areas of combined intervention. Whether such combined intervention fits the existing framework, or whether an additional category needs to be added, remains to be seen.

Direct current (including microcurrent)

The measurement of small DC potentials associated with injury and the repair processes following musculoskeletal lesions (reviewed in Chapter 3) has resulted in a number of research groups using low-intensity DC as a therapeutic tool in the management of non-healing or delayed-healing wounds. Recent developments, both in wound management research and other areas involving soft-tissue injury, have involved the delivery of small-magnitude DCs, which are of similar magnitude to the endogenous currents identified as being part of normal tissue healing. Given that these (endogenous) currents have been shown to be of low microamp magnitude and DC in nature, the term 'microcurrent' has been coined by some researchers, manufacturers and other authorities in the field. It is a perfectly acceptable term, although, strictly, it does not refer to a specific modality – it relates to the magnitude or intensity of the applied stimulation.

DC stimulation was one of the first forms of electrical stimulation to be used clinically, with reports as early as the seventeenth century concerning the application of charged gold leaf to smallpox lesions (see Dayton & Palladino 1989). Many of the animal studies outlined in the previous section used DC stimulation with encouraging results. The philosophy for the use of DC exogenous

stimulation is that it can supplement or enhance the naturally occurring DC potentials associated with repair, and thereby stimulate the healing process, particularly in cases where the process is slow or appears to have stopped, as might be the case with chronic venous ulcers and chronic pressure sores.

The use of low-intensity DC in this field has been through numerous phases of popularity and one of the first of the more recent research reports was by Assimacopoulos (1968), who treated chronic leg ulcers that had been resistant to all previous forms of therapy with DC stimulation. The ulcers were treated with negative polarity stimulation with direct currents up to 0.1 mA intensity. Complete healing was reported in 6 weeks. The main problem with this study was the very small sample ($n = 53$) and lack of any control group, thus limiting the strength of the results.

Soon after this, Wolcott et al (1969) published the results of a more extensive study in which 83 ischaemic ulcers were investigated. The DC stimulation involved three sessions a day, each of which lasted for 2 hours using current intensities of between 0.2 and 0.8 mA. One electrode was placed in the wound and the other on the skin surface, proximally. The intensity of the stimulation was determined empirically as it was found that stimulation with too great an intensity resulted in a bloody exudate from the ulcer, whereas stimulation with too low an intensity resulted in a serous exudate. The applied intensity fell between these two limits, being determined for each patient individually. The wound electrode was made negative initially, and maintained so for at least 3 days. If the ulcer was not infected at this stage, the electrode polarity was then reversed such that the wound electrode was made positive. Infected ulcers were stimulated with a negative wound electrode until the infection had cleared, and then for three further days; only then was the wound electrode made positive. All patients had the polarity of the wound electrode reversed each time a plateau was reached in the healing process.

The results from the 75 patients with a single ulcer were encouraging: 34 (45%) achieved 100% healing over 9.6 weeks, with an average healing rate of 18.4% per week; of the remaining 41 ulcers, the mean healing rate was 9.3% per week and these patients achieved an average 64.7% healing over 7.2 weeks. Additional data were derived from a group of patients who presented with bilateral ulcers of comparable size and aetiology; these patients received electrical stimulation to only one of the ulcers, the other acting as a control lesion. The results from these patients showed that six of the eight treated ulcers healed completely and that the remaining two achieved 70% healing. The control ulcers from the same patients healed less well, with three of the eight showing no healing, a further three healing less than 50% and the remaining two healing by 75%. The average healing rate for the treated ulcers was 27% per week and for the control ulcers was 5% per week. Although these trial results are more convincing because of the increased sample size and the fact that there was a control group for part of the work, there are nevertheless pertinent issues that need to be highlighted. First, the control ulcers did also show signs of healing, and this might be due either to natural processes at work or to the effects of the electrical stimulation to one ulcer causing the release of a systemic mediator substance, which in turn stimulated the contralateral ulcer. It is not possible with this experimental design to differentiate between the possibilities. Second, a placebo effect cannot be discounted.

The work of Wolcott et al (1969) is one of the most frequently cited in the field of electrical stimulation for wound healing and, although there have been criticisms of the design and protocol (e.g. Vodovnik & Karba 1992) it remains an important paper. It is of interest that, although in principle the treatment was based on supplementing or enhancing the naturally occurring currents associated with healing, the polarity reversal on reaching a growth plateau does not appear to be based on a recognized physiological phenomenon. The published works that have measured rather than manipulated the potentials occurring with repair do not report multiple polarity reversals during the healing process (in non-regenerating species) and, although in this study the effects were beneficial, the rationale for the approach is questioned.

A trial, similar in design that of Wolcott et al, was conducted by Gault and Gatens (1976) involving 76 patients with a total of 106 ischaemic ulcers of differing aetiologies and locations. Six patients presented with bilateral ulcers, providing a small control group. For patients with a single ulcer, the mean healing rate was 28.4% per week (an improvement over the unilateral ulcer result from Wolcott's study). For the patients with bilateral ulcers, where one was treated with electrical stimulation and one acted as a control, the mean healing rate of the control ulcers was 14.7% per week, and that of the treated ulcers was 30% per week.

The third widely cited trial involving LIDC was a more rigorously controlled study by Carley and Wainapel (1985), using a similar but not identical protocol to Wolcott et al (1969) and Gault and Gatens (1976). Thirty hospital inpatients were involved in the study, divided equally into a treatment and a control group by random selection. In addition to the equal size of groups, the patients were matched (paired) on the basis of age, diagnosis and wound aetiology, location and size.

The patients in the control group received conventional conservative therapy. The LIDC group received 2 hours of LIDC twice a day, 5 days a week in addition to the conventional therapy. The two stimulation sessions were separated by a 2–4-hour rest period when the machine gave no output but remained in situ. One electrode was placed at the wound site and a dispersive electrode was placed on the skin proximal to the wound. The wound electrode had negative polarity for the first 3 days of the trial, after which time the polarities were reversed. The wound-positive arrangement was maintained until the wound healed or until there was a healing plateau, in which case the wound electrode was made negative again for a further 3 days and then reverted to positive. The current intensity was between 300 and 700 mA, determined empirically in the same manner as Wolcott et al (1969). Wounds were measured and photographed on a weekly basis, and the programme continued for 5 weeks or until the ulcer had healed.

The results of the study showed that the patients in the LIDC group showed healing rates that were 1.5–2.5 times faster than those of their paired controls and the overall healing rate was two times greater. There was no significant difference between the wounds in the two groups at the commencement of the study and the difference did not become apparent until week 3 of the study, after which it became progressively more significant.

In addition to the increased rate of healing, the scar tissue from the treatment group appeared to be stronger and there were fewer problems with wound infection. In the control group the healed tissue appeared thin and fragile and reopened in some patients. No patients in the treatment group required wound debridement during the trial period, whereas in the control group patients typically required repeated debridement. Patients in the LIDC group also reported decreased pain and discomfort compared with those in the control group.

The rationale for alternating the wound electrode polarity appears to be derived from the animal experimentation identified in the previous section concerning the effects of opposite polarities on rabbit wound healing. It was suggested that a negative-polarity wound electrode appears to encourage the resolution of infection but does not stimulate healing, whereas the wound-positive electrode stimulates both infection and healing. Therefore, the suggestion that the wound electrode should be made negative until the infection cleared, then positive to promote the repair, has a rational basis. The alternating wound electrode polarity on reaching a healing plateau cannot be traced to the published literature.

A new development in the DC stimulation group involves a wound dressing that incorporates a small DC stimulator that is permanently 'on'. This approach would be entirely consistent with the background research literature (see Chapter 3) in that the endogenous currents are normally present 24 hours a day rather than for short duration 'treatment' periods and, additionally, it has been shown that maintaining a moist wound environment is distinctly advantageous in terms of facilitating wound healing and promoting endogenous current flow (Jaffe & Vanable 1984, Cheng et al 1995).

The stimulator (Posifect®) has been developed on the back of this research literature and there has, as yet, been a limited range of studies involving its use in the clinical environment (Fig. 19.2). Feldman et al (2005) conducted a small scale study with two active and two control patients over a 16-week period, with 8-week treatment and 8-week control blocks. The main aim of the work was to try and establish effective stimulation protocols for maximally beneficial effect, and the results were incorporated into a subsequent trial by Hampton and King (2005), which was a report of a case study utilizing the new protocol with a 4-month treatment period looking at wound closure in what appears to be a somewhat 'difficult case', and further case material in Hampton and Collins (2006). These are clearly not the large-scale RCT-type designs that are needed for convincing evidence, but rather the early-stage investigations of a low-intensity 'always on' stimulator incorporated into the wound dressing; they appear to fit the existing evidence. It is anticipated that this approach (whether with the Posifect® or other devices) will gain ground in the clinical field and hopefully add to the research literature in the DC stimulation group.

Pulsed direct current

Low–intensity pulsed DC Several research reports related to the use of pulsed DC stimulation in wound-healing studies appeared in the early 1990s. Mulder (1991) and Feedar et al (1991) both reported the results from a randomized, double-blind, multicentre study with results presented from 47 patients with a total of 50 wounds. These wounds were of several different pathologies, covering nine different sites and at stages II–IV, which is a somewhat heterogeneous group. Of the 50 wounds, 24 were allocated (randomly) to the control group and 26 to the treatment group. Patients in both groups were treated twice daily (with real or sham stimulation) using a small, battery-powered device. Each session was for 30 minutes with a rest period of 4–8 hours between sessions. Treatment was thus applied 7 days a week for the first 4 weeks. The stimulation protocol was varied according to wound state (infected or non-infected) and wound stage (II–IV).

Infected wounds were treated at 128 pulses per second (pps) at a nominal current of 35 mA with a negative wound electrode. This stimulation was continued until the wound was infection free, and then continued for a further 3 days. Following this initial phase, the polarity of the wound electrode was alternated every 3 days until the wound reached stage II. After this time, the pulse repetition rate was reduced to 64 pps and the wound electrode polarity was reversed daily. The initial part of the trial was conducted on a double-blind

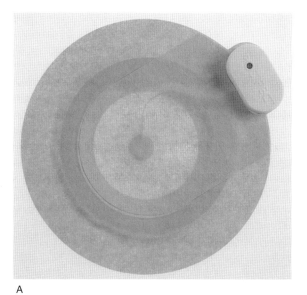

A

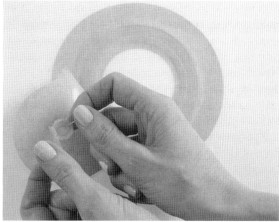

B

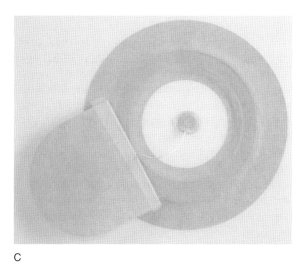

C

Figure 19.2 Posifect® microcurrent stimulation device incorporated into wound dressing.

basis and, after completion of this phase, patients from the sham treatment (control) group were allowed to join the full-treatment programme along with any patient from the treatment group who had not achieved full healing.

The results were presented for the initial 4-week period and, additionally, for the follow-up study, with wound size reported as a percentage of the original size. Following the 4-week blind element, the treatment group wounds were 44% of their original size on average, whereas the control wounds averaged 67% of their initial size. The mean healing rate of the treated lesions was 14%

per week compared with the control group healing rate of 8.25% per week. No wounds in the treatment group increased in size, compared to five wounds in the control group.

In the second phase, 14 wounds were crossed-over to the stimulation protocol. The mean reduction in wound size during the sham treatment had been 11.3% at an average rate of 2.9% per week. After 4 weeks of active electrical stimulation, these wounds had reduced to 49% of their size at crossover and had demonstrated a mean healing rate of 12.8% per week. The authors concluded that the results support the use of pulsed LIDC in the management of chronic dermal wounds at stages II, III and IV; the strength of the results is enhanced by the improvements in the cross-over group.

Weiss et al (1989) compared scar thickness and hypertrophic scar formation at the skin-graft donor site in a small study of four patients. Each patient had bilateral split skin grafts taken from the anterior thigh. One site was given electrical stimulation whereas the other acted as a control. The electrical stimulation started on the day of surgery and consisted of two sessions daily, each of 30 minutes' duration, which were continued for 7 days. The stimulation was delivered by a small unit as a pulsed DC stimulation at 128 pps, the pulses being of 150 ms duration, at a peak current of 35 mA. The wound electrode was maintained at a positive polarity throughout the study. A combination of evaluation by three independent physicians and donor site punch biopsies at 2–3 months postsurgery provided data for the analysis.

The subjective findings strongly suggested that the scars at the donor sites that had been subjected to electrical stimulation were softer, flatter and more cosmetically acceptable than the untreated scars. These differences were apparent by 1 month post-surgery and were persistent, but less marked, at 6 months. The biopsy data support the subjective (blinded) findings, the treated scars being on average 46% of the thickness of the untreated scars. Biopsies also showed fewer mast cells in the stimulated scars. The effect of electrical stimulation under these conditions suggests that it can decrease fibrosis, possibly by reducing the number of mast cells.

High–intensity pulsed DC A further development in the use of electrical stimulation for wound healing utilizes a pulsed DC current applied at a high voltage, known either as HVPGS or HVPC. The pulses are commonly monophasic 'twin pulses' of short duration and high intensity (100–500 V; see Fig. 19.1D).

A trial looking at the effects of HVPGS was reported by Kloth and Feedar (1988). A group of 16 patients with stage IV decubitus ulcers were recruited for the trial; all had lesions that had been unresponsive to previous treatment. Patients were allocated randomly to a treatment group ($n = 59$) or sham treatment group ($n = 57$). The electrical stimulation consisted of monophasic twin-pulse stimulation at 105 pps delivered at a voltage just below that required to achieve visible muscle contraction (typically 100–175 V). These stimulation parameters are reported as being arbitrarily set. Electrical stimulation was given for one 45-minute session a day for 5 days a week. Sham group patients had electrodes placed in the same way, but the machine output was set to zero. Electrode polarity was set initially for the wound electrode to be positive, with the negative electrode placed on the skin surface proximally. If a healing plateau was reached during the trial, the wound electrode was made negative and the treatment continued. If a second plateau was reached, the electrode polarity was reversed daily thereafter. Whichever electrode was placed at the wound site, the relative arrangement was maintained in that the positive electrode was always placed cephalad in relation to the negative electrode.

All patients in the treatment group achieved complete healing of their ulcers (on average over 7.3 weeks at a mean healing rate of 44.8% per week). The control-group patients did less well, with an increase in mean wound size of almost 29% between the first and last treatments. A sub-group of three patients who were in the control group went on to complete a course of electrical stimulation following the main trial; all three achieved full healing of their ulcers over 8.3 weeks, with an average healing rate of 38% per week.

Griffin et al (1991) assessed the effects of HVPC on pressure-sore healing in a group of patients with spinal cord injury. Seventeen patients were assigned randomly to either a treatment or a control (sham treatment) group. Electrical stimulation treatments were carried out for 1 hour a day for 20 consecutive days with repeated wound assessments during this period. HVPC was delivered by means of a negative wound electrode with the stimulator delivering 100 pps at an intensity of 200 V using similar twin pulses to the previous study. The percentage change (decrease) in ulcer size for the treatment group was significantly greater at days 5, 15 and 20 and the average change for all ulcers in the treatment group was an 80% size reduction compared with a 52% decrease for the control group.

A more recent study by Houghton et al (2003) involved 27 patients with a total of 42 chronic

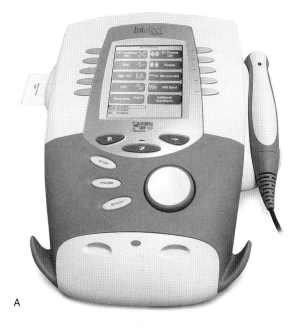

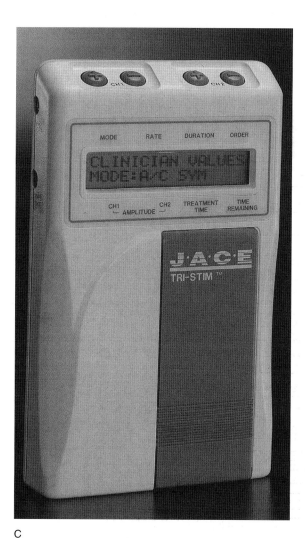

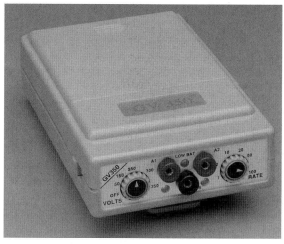

A

B

C

Figure 19.3 Examples of machines delivering high-voltage pulsed current (HVPC).

leg ulcers of varying aetiologies (diabetic, arterial, venous) and employed a placebo-controlled RCT design. Following initial assessment, there was a stable (baseline) period during which only 'conventional' therapy was employed, followed by a 4-week treatment phase with the patients divided into treatment or sham groups. The high-voltage pulses were delivered at 150 V, 100 pps and 100 μs duration, using 45-minute treatment periods, three times a week for the 4 weeks. The wound electrode was made negative throughout the treatment period, i.e. no polarity reversal. Assessment included a 1-month follow-up period. The treatment group wounds significantly reduced in size (mean 44% of original) compared to the sham group (mean 16%). The significant differences were not maintained at the 1-month follow-up assessment, although there was a clear trend seen in the results.

Goldman et al (2002) aimed to evaluate the ability of HVPC to increase microcirculation in critically ischaemic wounds and, as a result, to improve wound healing. The diabetic patients presented with ischaemic malleolar lesions and serial measures were made of wound parameters, including oxygen tension. The results indicated that the use of electrical stimulation in these patients objectively improved tissue oxygenation and improved the anticipated wound healing profile.

Alternating current

Stefanovska et al (1993) conducted a comparative study involving three patient groups (DC stimulation, AC stimulation and a control group) with 250 patients, 170 of whom were spine-injured patients with 'pressure wounds'. The electrical stimulation groups received conventional therapy in addition to the stimulation (DC stimulation utilized a 600-mA current for 2 hours daily; the AC group patients were treated with low-frequency pulsed currents for 2 hours daily; further details of parameters are provided in the report.) The results suggested that the AC-stimulation group achieved better results than the DC and control groups.

A study reported by Baker et al (1997) compared the effect of asymmetric biphasic and symmetric biphasic square-wave pulsed stimulation with a control group. Eighty patients with open ulcers were involved in the study, the results of which demonstrated a significant increase in the healing rate: almost 60% in the group given the asymmetric stimulation. Symmetric pulse stimulation, by contrast, showed no significant advantage over the control condition. To some extent at least, this would be consistent with the endogenous bioelectric background and the DC group results in that if the bioelectric currents influencing repair are DC in nature, then an asymmetric AC current form has a net polarization (which is effectively a DC component incorporated into the AC stimulation) whereas the symmetric stimulation will provide a zero net DC current [similar to transcutaneous electrical nerve stimulation (TENS) and interferential], which lacks the DC element and is therefore less likely to be effective in this context.

A report by Adunsky and Ohry (2005) uses a device that delivers an unspecified mixture of alternating and direct currents. This multicentre trial, involving 63 patients in a placebo and a treatment group, achieved some interesting and potentially useful results but the overt non-disclosure of the machine stimulation parameters makes it difficult to place the stimulation mode into the existing framework.

Lundberg et al (1992) carried out a controlled study of the effects of electrical nerve stimulation in conjunction with a standard treatment for healing chronic diabetic ulcers in 64 patients divided into two groups. All patients received standard treatment plus stimulation or sham stimulation, which was an alternating current (80 Hz frequency, 1 ms pulse duration at sufficient intensity to bring about a strong paraesthesia), which was delivered for 20 minutes twice daily for 12 weeks. The results demonstrated significant differences in the wound area in the treated compared with the placebo group (42% reduction for stimulation group compared with 15% for the sham group).

Few other trials have directly involved AC type stimulation devices, although trials involving TENS-type applications (e.g. Kaada 1983, 1988, Westerhof & Bos 1983) have provided some interesting and encouraging results.

POSSIBLE MECHANISMS

The exact mechanism by which electrical stimulation appears to enhance wound healing remains unidentified, even with hundreds of research papers (cell and tissue studies, animal studies and clinical trials, case studies and RCTs) available. Much of the background physiology and biophysics has been reasonably well established, and the clinical outcome work appears to support the intervention. The critical area for further research (apart from the ever-needed large-scale RCTs) is to fully establish the link between the physiological events associated with endogenous bioelectric phenomena, tissue injury and repair, and the exogenous electrical stimulation of apparently non responding (and therefore 'chronic') wounds. The clinical evidence reviewed in this chapter would support the use of electrical stimulation in a variety of forms as a method that contributes to the management of chronic skin ulceration.

In terms of the explanations offered and supported – to some extent at least – by the evidence, several potential mechanisms exist, including cell-membrane-mediated effects, chemical mediator release or production modification and bioelectric enhancement.

Cutting (2006) takes the view that cellular processes in chronic wounds are not normal and appear to demonstrate greater disorganization than usual. The use of exogenous stimulation might be a mechanism that promotes organization and thereby facilitates the repair response. It has been suggested (Vodovnik et al 1992) that cellular proliferation is modified by DC stimulation. If the proliferative rate is too low, it can be increased and, conversely, if the rate is too high then downregulation occurs with a reduced proliferative rate.

Frank and Szeto (1983) suggest that electrical stimulation can affect soft-tissue healing by inhibiting negative healing factors, by speeding normal healing processes or by creating new and improved healing pathways, thus improving both the rate and the endpoint of scar formation of tissue regeneration.

Dayton & Palladino (1989) suggest that the possible effects of electrical stimulation on wounds include reduction of bacterial count, increased rate of wound healing, increased wound strength, improved scar quality and pain relief, whereas Biedebach (1989) suggests both a local tissue response and a general vasodilatory response, which might be neuronal or chemically mediated. There is also some evidence for this being a CNS-mediated mechanism, for instance the demonstration that in spinal injury patients the response to electrical stimulation is less marked than in other patients (Wolcott et al 1969).

Dodgen et al (1987), Gagnier et al (1988) and Peters et al (1998) provide evidence that electrical stimulation increases the oxygen tension in the limb, which can be associated with successful repair (see Chapter 4).

Bourguignon and Bourguignon (1987) contribute to the evidence for a chemically mediated effect demonstrating activation of fibroblasts by electrical stimulation and, in a separate study, showed the effects of electrical stimulation on T lymphocytes, with increased levels of calcium ions (Ca^{2+}) and kinase activity, receptor clustering and increased DNA synthesis. It is suggested that Ca^{2+} might act as the mediator for many of the changes in cell activation that have been observed, with the Ca^{2+} acting as a second messenger (this would be very similar to mechanisms associated with therapeutic ultrasound, laser and pulsed shortwave therapies). It is possible that increased cellular Ca^{2+} uptake not only results in increased cellular motility but is also linked to the production of cellular energy (in the form of adenosine triphosphate; ATP) via mitochondrial mechanisms. The angiogenic responses [identified previously and evidenced in the papers by Bai (2004) and Zhao et al (2004)] also contribute to the chemically mediated effect.

The galvanotactic response to electrical stimulation is evidenced by numerous authors, including Kloth (1995), Nuccitelli (1988, 2003) and Robinson (1985), with several authors also evidencing the increased collagen fibre alignment with electrical stimulation (Brown et al 1989, Cruz et al 1989, Reger et al 1999).

Dunn (1988) has proposed a wider-ranging descriptive model: that electrical stimulation might accelerate wound healing as a consequence of:

- modification of endogenous bioelectricity
- activation or attraction of inflammatory cells
- presence of products of electrode breakdown
- attraction of connective tissue cells
- enhanced cell replication
- enhanced cell biosynthesis
- inhibition of infectious microorganisms.

Lundberg et al (1988) demonstrated significant changes in capillary-filling mechanisms in tissue with venous stasis, with subsequent reduction of oedema and stasis, whereas Griffin et al (1991) suggest several attractive hypotheses. These include the attraction of connective tissue and inflammatory cells, modification of endogenous electrical potentials of tissue, stimulation of cellular biosynthesis and replication, bactericidal effects, enhanced circulation and the generation of a cellular electrophysiological effect.

There is, as yet, no universally accepted model for the mode of action through which electrical stimulation achieves clinical effectiveness. All the potential mechanisms identified above have evidence at one level or another to support them. A universal bioelectric theory that binds all the (apparently) disparate elements might emerge, or there might be new evidence to establish which of the current contending theories is most appropriate.

CONCLUSIONS AND CLINICAL IMPLICATIONS

As the biomedical, biophysical, bioelectrical and clinical evidence continues to accumulate, it is anticipated that an increased understanding of the means by which electrical stimulation is able to facilitate the process of wound healing will emerge. When further understanding of the mechanism has been gained, it is probable that the most efficient stimulation parameters will also be clarified. At the present time, DC, pulsed DC and AC stimulation modes all appear to have a measurable, beneficial effect and although differentiation between these modes of intervention is currently problematic, there is little doubt – from the evidence – that they do have a clinically significant effect.

References

Adunsky A, Ohry A (2005) Decubitus direct current treatment (DDCT) of pressure ulcers: results of a randomized double-blinded placebo controlled study. *Arch Gerontol Geriatr* **41**(3): 261–269.

Albert SF, Wong E (1991) Electrical stimulation of bone repair. *Clin Podiatr Med Surg* **8**(4): 923–935.

Alvarez OM, Mertz PM, Smerbeck RV et al (1983) The healing of superficial skin wounds is stimulated by external electrical current. *J Invest Dermatol* **81**: 144–148.

Assimacopoulos D (1968) Wound healing promotion by the use of negative electric current. *Am Surg* **34**(6): 423–431.

Bach S, Bilgrav K, Gottrup F et al (1991) The effect of electrical current on skin incision. *Eur J Surg* **157**: 171–174.

Bai H, McCaig CD, Forrester JV et al (2004) DC electric fields induce distinct preangiogenic responses in microvascular and macrovascular cells. *Arterioscler Thromb Vasc Biol* **24**(7): 1234–1239.

Baker LL, Chambers R, DeMuth SK et al (1997) Effects of electrical stimulation on wound healing in patients with diabetic ulcers. *Diabetes Care* **20**(3): 405–412.

Baker SR, Stacey MC, Jopp-McKay AG et al (1991) Epidemiology of chronic venous ulcers. *Br J Surg* **78**: 864–867.

Biedebach MC (1989) Accelerated healing of skin ulcers by electrical stimulation and the intracellular physiological mechanisms involved. *Acupunct Electrother Res* **14**(1): 43–60.

Black J (1987) *Electrical Stimulation: Its Role in Growth, Repair and Remodelling of the Musculoskeletal System*. New York, Praeger.

Borgens RB (1981) Injury, ionic currents and regeneration. In Becker R (ed) *Mechanisms of Growth Control*. Springfield, Illinois, Charles C Thomas, 107–136.

Borgens RB (1982) What is the role of naturally produced electric current in vertebrate regeneration and healing? *Int Rev Cytol* **76**: 245–298.

Borgens RB, McCaig CD (1989). Endogenous currents in nerve repair, regeneration and development. In Borgens R (ed) *Electric Fields in Vertebrate Repair*. New York, Alan Liss Inc, 77–116.

Borgens RB, Vanable JW, Jaffe LF (1977) Bioelectricity and regeneration: Large currents leave the stumps of regenerating newt limbs. *Proc Natl Acad Sci USA* **74**(10): 4528–4532.

Borgens RB, Robinson K, Vanable J et al (1989). *Electric Fields in Vertebrate Repair: Natural and Applied Voltages in Vertebrate Regeneration and Healing*. New York, Alan R Liss Inc.

Bourguignon GJ, Bourguignon LY (1987) Electric stimulation of protein and DNA synthesis in human fibroblasts. *Faseb J* **1**(5): 398–402.

Bowler PG, Duerden BI, Armstrong DG (2001) Wound microbiology and associated approaches to wound management. *Clin Microbiol Rev* **14**(2): 244–269.

Brown M, Gogia PP (1987) Effects of high voltage stimulation on cutaneous wound healing in rabbits. *Phys Ther* **67**(5): 662–667.

Brown M, McDonnell MK, Menton DN (1989) Polarity effects on wound healing using electric stimulation in rabbits. *Arch Phys Med Rehab* **70**(8): 624–627.

Canseven AG, Atalay NS (1996) Is it possible to trigger collagen synthesis by electric current in skin wounds? *Indian J Biochem Biophys* **33**(3): 223–227.

Carley PJ, Wainapel SF (1985) Electrotherapy for acceleration of wound healing: low intensity direct current. *Arch Phys Med Rehab* **66**(7): 443–446.

Chang PC, Sulik GI, Soong HK et al (1996) Galvanotropic and galvanotaxic responses of corneal endothelial cells. *J Formos Med Assoc* **95**(8): 623–627.

Cheng K, Goldman RJ (1998) Electric fields and proliferation in a dermal wound model: cell cycle kinetics. *Bioelectromagnetics* **19**(2): 68–74.

Cheng K, Tarjan P, Oliveira-Gandia M (1995) An occlusive dressing can sustain natural electrical potential of wounds. *J Invest Dermatol* **104**(4): 662–665.

Childs SG (2003) Stimulators of bone healing. Biologic and biomechanical. *Orthop Nurs* **22**(6): 421–428.

Cho MR, Thatte HS, Lee RC et al (2000) Integrin-dependent human macrophage migration induced by oscillatory electrical stimulation. *Ann Biomed Eng* **28**(3): 234–243.

Cooper MS, Schliwa M (1985) Electrical and ionic controls of tissue cell locomotion in DC electric fields. *J Neurosci Res* **13**: 223–244.

Cruz NI, Bayron FE, Suarez AJ (1989) Accelerated healing of full-thickness burns by the use of high-voltage pulsed galvanic stimulation in the pig. *Ann Plast Surg* **23**(1): 49–55.

Cutting KF (2006) Electric stimulation in the treatment of chronic wounds. *Wounds UK* **2**(1): 3–11.

Dayton PD, Palladino SJ (1989) Electrical stimulation of cutaneous ulcerations. A literature review. *J Am Podiatr Med Assoc* **79**(7): 318–321.

Dodgen PW, Johnson BW, Baker LL (1987) The effects of electrical stimulation on cutaneous oxygen supply in older adults. *Phys Ther* **67**(5): 793.

Dunn MG (1988) Wound healing using collagen matrix: Effect of DC electrical stimulation. *J Biomed Mater Res* **22**(A2 suppl): 191–206.

Erickson CA, Nuccitelli R (1984) Embryonic fibroblast motility and orientation can be influenced by physiological electric fields. *J Cell Biol* **98**(1): 296–307.

Farboud B, Nuccitelli R, Schwab IR et al (2000) DC electric fields induce rapid directional migration in cultured human corneal epithelial cells. *Exp Eye Res* **70**(5): 667–673.

Feedar JA, Kloth LC, Gentzkow GD (1991) Chronic dermal ulcer healing enhanced with monophasic pulsed electrical stimulation. *Phys Ther* **71**(9): 639–649.

Feldman D, Andino RV, Jennings JA (2005). Clinical evaluation of an electrical stimulation bandage (Posifect Dressing). *ETRS/EWMA/DFGW*. Stuttgart, Germany.

Forrest L (1983) Current concepts in soft connective tissue wound healing. *Br J Surg* **70**: 133–140.

Frank CB, Szeto AY (1983) A review of electromagnetically enhanced soft tissue healing. *IEEE Eng Med Biol* **2**: 27–32.

Fukushima K, Densa N, Inui H (1953) Studies on galvano-taxis of human neutrophilic leukocytes and methods of its measurement. *Med J Osaka Univ* **4**: 195–208.

Gabbiani G (2003) The myofibroblast in wound healing and fibrocontractive diseases. *J Pathol* **200**(4): 500–503.

Gagnier K, Manix N, Baker L (1988) The effects of electrical stimulation on cutaneous oxygen supply in paraplegics. *Phys Ther* **68**(5): 835–839.

Gardner SE, Frantz RA, Schmidt FL (1999) Effect of electrical stimulation on chronic wound healing: a meta- analysis. *Wound Repair Regen* **7**(6): 495–503.

Gault WR, Gatens PF Jr (1976) Use of low intensity direct current in management of ischemic skin ulcers. *Phys Ther* **56**(3): 265–269.

Gentzkow GD (1993) Electrical stimulation to heal dermal wounds. *J Dermatol Surg Oncol* **19**(8): 753–758.

Gentzkow GD, Miller KH (1991) Electrical stimulation for dermal wound healing. *Clin Podiatr Med Surg* **8**(4): 827–841.

Goldman R, Pollack S (1996) Electric fields and proliferation in a chronic wound model. *Bioelectromagnetics* **17**(6): 450–457.

Goldman R, Brewley BI, Golden MA (2002) Electrotherapy reoxygenates inframalleolar ischemic wounds on diabetic

patients: a case series. *Adv Skin Wound Care* **15**(3): 112–120.

Goldman R, Rosen M, Brewley B et al (2004) Electrotherapy promotes healing and microcirculation of infrapopliteal ischemic wounds: a prospective pilot study. *Adv Skin Wound Care* **17**(6): 284–294.

Griffin JW, Tooms RE, Mendius RA et al (1991) Efficacy of high voltage pulsed current for healing of pressure ulcers in patients with spinal cord injury. *Phys Ther* **71**(6): 433–442; discussion 442–444.

Hampton S, Collins F (2006) Treating a pressure ulcer with bio-electric stimulation therapy. *Br J Nurs* **15**(6): s14–s18.

Hampton S, King L (2005) Healing an intractable wound using bio-electrical stimulation therapy. *Br J Nurs* **14**(15): S30–S32.

Houghton PE, Kincaid CB, Lovell M et al (2003) Effect of electrical stimulation on chronic leg ulcer size and appearance. *Phys Ther* **83**(1): 17–28.

Im MJ, Lee WP, Hoopes JE (1990) Effect of electrical stimulation of survival of skin flaps in pigs. *Phys Ther* **70**(1): 37–40.

Jaffe LF, Vanable JW Jr (1984) Electric fields and wound healing. *Clin Dermatol* **2**(3): 34–44.

Kaada B (1983) Promoted healing of chronic ulceration by transcutaneous nerve stimulation (TNS). *Vasa* **12**: 262–269.

Kaada B, Emru M (1988) Promoted healing of leprous ulcers by transcutaneous nerve stimulation. *Acupunct Electrother Res* **13**(4): 165–176.

Kincaid CB, Lavoie KH (1989) Inhibition of bacterial growth in vitro following stimulation with high voltage, monophasic, pulsed current. *Phys Ther* **69**(8): 651–655.

Kloth LC (1995) Physical modalities in wound management: UVC, therapeutic heating and electrical stimulation. *Ostomy Wound Manage* **41**(5): 18–20, 22–24, 26–27.

Kloth LC (2005) Electrical stimulation for wound healing: a review of evidence from in vitro studies, animal experiments, and clinical trials. *Int J Low Extrem Wounds* **4**(1): 23–44.

Kloth LC, Feedar JA (1988) Acceleration of wound healing with high voltage, monophasic, pulsed current. *Phys Ther* **68**(4): 503–508.

Kloth LC, McCulloch JM (1996) Promotion of wound healing and electrical stimulation. *Adv Wound Care* **9**(5 part 1): 42–45.

Konikoff JJ (1976) Electrical promotion of soft tissue repairs. *Ann Biomed Eng* **4**(1): 1–5.

Kranke P, Bennett M, Roeckl-Wiedmann I et al (2004) Hyperbaric oxygen therapy for chronic wounds. Cochrane Database Syst Rev(2): CD004123.

Lee PY, Chesnoy S, Huang L (2004) Electroporatic delivery of TGF-beta1 gene works synergistically with electric therapy to enhance diabetic wound healing in db/db mice. *J Invest Dermatol* **123**(4): 791–798.

Li X, Kolega J (2002) Effects of direct current electric fields on cell migration and actin filament distribution in bovine vascular endothelial cells. *J Vasc Res* **39**(5): 391–404.

Lundeberg TC, Eriksson SV, Malm M (1992) Electrical nerve stimulation improves healing of diabetic ulcers. *Ann Plast Surg* **29**(4): 328–331.

Lundeberg T, Abrahamsson P, Bondesson L et al (1988) Effect of vibratory stimulation on experimental and clinical pain. *Scand J Rehab Med* **20**(4): 149–159.

McGuckin M, Williams L, Brooks J et al (2001) Guidelines in practice: the effect on healing of venous ulcers. *Adv Skin Wound Care* **14**(1): 33–36.

Merriman HL, Hegyi CA, Albright-Overton CR et al (2004) A comparison of four electrical stimulation types on *Staphylococcus aureus* growth in vitro. *J Rehab Res Dev* **41**(2): 139–146.

Mulder GD (1991) Treatment of open-skin wounds with electric stimulation. *Arch Phys Med Rehab* **72**: 375–377.

Nishimura KY, Isseroff RR, Nuccitelli R (1996) Human keratinocytes migrate to the negative pole in direct current electric fields comparable to those measured in mammalian wounds. *J Cell Sci* **109**(Pt 1)): 199–207.

Nissen NN, Polverini PJ, Koch AE et al (1998) Vascular endothelial growth factor mediates angiogenic activity during the proliferative phase of wound healing. *Am J Pathol* **152**(6): 1445–1452.

Nuccitelli R (1988) Ionic currents in morphogenesis. *Experientia* **44**(8): 657–666.

Nuccitelli R (2003) A role for endogenous electric fields in wound healing. *Curr Top Dev Biol* **58**: 1–26.

Ojingwa JC, Isseroff RR (2002) Electrical stimulation of wound healing. *Prog Dermatol* **36**(4): 1–12.

Ojingwa JC, Isseroff RR (2003) Electrical stimulation of wound healing. *J Invest Dermatol* **121**(1): 1–12.

Orida N, Feldman JD (1982) Directional protrusive pseudopodial activity and motility in macrophages induced by extracellular electric fields. *Cell Motil* **2**(3): 243–255.

Peters EJ, Armstrong DG, Wunderlich RP et al (1998) The benefit of electrical stimulation to enhance perfusion in persons with diabetes mellitus. *J Foot Ankle Surg* **37**(5): 396–400; discussion 447–448.

Politis MJ, Zanakis MF, Miller JE (1989) Enhanced survival of full-thickness skin grafts following the application of DC electrical fields. *Plast Reconstr Surg* **84**(2): 267–272.

Pullar CE, Isseroff RR, Nuccitelli R (2001) Cyclic AMP-dependent protein kinase A plays a role in the directed migration of human keratinocytes in a DC electric field. *Cell Motil Cytoskel* **50**(4): 207–217.

Reger SI, Hyodo A, Negami S et al (1999) Experimental wound healing with electrical stimulation. *Artif Organs* **23**(5): 460–462.

Reich JD, Cazzaniga AL, Mertz PM et al (1991) The effect of electrical stimulation on the number of mast cells in healing wounds. *J Am Acad Dermatol* **25**(1 Pt 1): 40–46.

Robinson KR (1985) The responses of cells to electrical fields: A review. *J Cell Biol* **101**: 2023–2027.

Rodriguez-Merchan EC, Forriol F (2004) Nonunion: general principles and experimental data. *Clin Orthop Relat Res*(419): 4–12.

Ross SM, Ferrier JM, Aubin JE (1989) Studies on the alignment of fibroblasts in uniform applied electrical fields. *Bioelectromagnetics* **10**: 371–384.

Schultz GS, Sibbald RG, Falanga V et al (2003) Wound bed preparation: a systematic approach to wound management. *Wound Repair Regen* **11**(suppl 1): S1–S28.

Sheridan DM, Isseroff RR, Nuccitelli R (1996) Imposition of a physiologic DC electric field alters the migratory response of human keratinocytes on extracellular matrix molecules. *J Invest Dermatol* **106**(4): 642–646.

Stefanovska A, Vodovnik L, Benko H et al (1993) Treatment of chronic wounds by means of electric and electromagnetic fields. Part 2. Value of FES parameters for pressure sore treatment. *Med Biol Eng Comput* **31**(3): 213–220.

Stromberg BV (1988) Effects of electrical currents on wound contraction. *Ann Plast Surg* **21**(2): 121–123.

Szuminsky NJ, Albers AC, Unger P, et al (1994) Effect of narrow, pulsed high voltages on bacterial viability. *Phys Ther* **74**(7): 660–667.

Taskan I, Ozyazgan I, Tercan M et al (1997) A comparative study of the effect of ultrasound and electrostimulation on wound healing in rats. *Plast Reconstr Surg* **100**(4): 966–972.

Thawer HA, Houghton PE (2001) Effects of electrical stimulation on the histological properties of wounds in diabetic mice. *Wound Repair Regen* **9**(2): 107–115.

Vodovnik L, Karba R (1992) Treatment of chronic wounds by means of electric and electromagnetic fields. Part 1. Literature review. *Med Biol Eng Comput* **30**(3): 257–266.

Vodovnik L, Miklavcic D, Sersa G (1992) Modified cell proliferation due to electrical currents. *MBEC* **30**: CE21–CE28.

Watson T (2000) The role of electrotherapy in contemporary physiotherapy practice. *Manual Ther* **5**(3): 132–141.

Watson T (2006) Electrotherapy and tissue repair. *Sportex Med* **29**: 7–13.

Weiss DS, Eaglstein WH, Falanga V (1989) Exogenous electric current can reduce the formation of hypertrophic scars. *J Dermatol Surg Oncol* **15**: 1272–1275.

Westerhof W, Bos JD (1983) Trigeminal trophic syndrome: a successful treatment with transcutaneous electrical stimulation. *Br J Dermatol* **108**(5): 601–604.

Winter GD (1964). Epidermal regeneration studies in the domestic pig. In Montagna W, Billingham RE (eds) *Advances in the Biology of Skin*. Oxford, Pergamon Press: 113–127.

Wolcott LE, Wheeler PC, Hardwicke HM et al (1969) Accelerated healing of skin ulcer by electrotherapy: preliminary clinical results. *South Med J* **62**(7): 795–801.

Wu KT, Go N, Dennis C et al (1967) Effects of electric currents and interfacial potentials on wound healing. *J Surg Res* **7**: 122–128.

Wysocki AB (1996) Wound fluids and the pathogenesis of chronic wounds. *J Wound Ostomy Continence Nurs* **23**(6): 283–290.

Zhao M, Bai H, Wang E et al (2004) Electrical stimulation directly induces pre-angiogenic responses in vascular endothelial cells by signaling through VEGF receptors. *J Cell Sci* **117**(Pt 3): 397–405.

Zhao M, Forrester JV, McCaig CD (1999) A small, physiological electric field orients cell division. *Proc Natl Acad Sci USA* **96**(9): 4942–4946.

SECTION 4

Ultrasound imaging

SECTION CONTENTS

Chapter **20**

Musculoskeletal ultrasound imaging

John Leddy

CHAPTER CONTENTS

INTRODUCTION

Ultrasound imaging enables the clinician to look directly at the soft tissues of the body. The dynamic, real-time, moving image that is produced is ideal for evaluating the structure and behaviour of muscles, tendons and other soft tissues. Not only can ultrasound be used to evaluate pathological changes, it is also possible to analyse muscle contractions, the movement of tendons and joints, and their effect on surrounding structures.

The relatively low cost and safety (owing to the absence of ionizing radiation) of ultrasound scanners make them a practical tool in the clinical setting and, unsurprisingly, they are no longer the preserve of radiology and maternity departments. For many clinicians, such as cardiologists, anaesthetists and surgeons, using ultrasound is now seen as a natural extension of their clinical examination in much the same way as the stethoscope.

The use of ultrasound imaging in physiotherapy is still in its infancy but has already developed applications beyond those traditionally performed in radiology. Monitoring response to treatment, along with evaluating function and the dynamic interaction between structures, is often of more relevance to the therapist. This chapter introduces the reader to ultrasound imaging and highlights those applications that might be relevant to physiotherapy practice.

HISTORY

The use of ultrasound to image the human body began shortly after the Second World War, using technology borrowed from military and metallurgy applications. Early studies required the subject to be immersed in a water bath, and produced a single, static, cross-sectional image.

By the early 1980s, a moving image could be produced. This was acquired by applying a small probe to the skin surface, which allowed quick and straightforward examinations of many of the organs of the body. At around this time CT and MRI also became available as alternative methods of producing cross-sectional images. Each modality was found to have its own strengths and weaknesses and, despite rapid developments over the past 20 years, they remain complementary, rather than rival approaches to imaging.

Musculoskeletal ultrasound applications began to emerge in the mid-1980s (Crass et al 1984) as the resolution of scanners improved. Physiotherapy researchers found ultrasound to be ideal for the direct visualization and evaluation of both muscle size and activity (Stokes & Young 1986). By the late 1990s, the development of high-frequency probes, with resolution in some respects superior to MRI, had led to renewed interest in musculoskeletal ultrasound. This continues today as falling costs and increased portability have made high-resolution ultrasound imaging feasible in the clinic and on the ward.

Ultrasound continues to evolve, with numerous recent innovations including the use of contrast agents, software that can measure the elasticity of tissue and three-dimensional (3D) and four-dimensional (4D) imaging. These will lead to new insights and applications, which will enable clinicians to further refine the accuracy and effectiveness of diagnoses and therapeutic interventions.

PRINCIPLES

GREY SCALE

When a sound wave passes through the body, a small percentage of the wave's energy (typically less than 1%) is reflected at each boundary that is encountered. The ultrasound image is acquired using a probe that generates a series of short, tightly focused pulses. These pass through the body and the sound waves reflected back to the probe by successive boundaries are recorded. Each pulse produces a single line of data, and a single image may be made up over a hundred such lines.

With each image taking as little as 1/100th of a second to construct, it can be updated continuously, giving a real time cinematic view of the body that allows even fast-moving structures such as the heart, active muscles, or even small children to be imaged.

SCANNERS

Scanners are typically made up of one or more hand-held probes attached via flexible cables to a central unit, which processes and displays the image (Fig. 20.1). The probes operate at one or more fundamental frequencies, which determine the maximum depth and resolution of the images they generate. At higher frequencies, the shorter wavelengths mean that shorter pulses can be

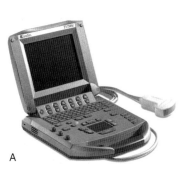

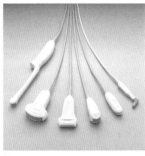

A   B

Figure 20.1 Portable ultrasound scanner (A) and probes (B) (courtesy of Sonosite).

produced, giving better resolution. At lower frequencies, the resolution is reduced but the ultrasound is absorbed less readily as it passes through the body, enabling deeper structures to be examined.

The most commonly used probes are the linear and curvilinear probes (Fig. 20.1B). Linear probes are normally designed to operate at frequencies of 7.5 MHz and above; these produce high-resolution, rectangular images to a depth of around 5 cm. Curvilinear probes generate a fan-shaped image with a wider field of view than a linear probe. They operate at lower frequencies, typically between 2 and 5 MHz, and can produce images to a depth of up to 15 cm but at the cost of lower resolution.

A detailed discussion of resolution and image generation lies beyond the scope of this chapter and the reader will find more comprehensive descriptions in dedicated ultrasound texts, in particular Hedrick et al (2005).

DOPPLER

Doppler is used to detect the flow of blood within the body by measuring the change in frequency of a sound wave that occurs when it is reflected by a moving structure. The two common display modes are colour and pulsed Doppler.

Colour Doppler

This samples the flow velocities over a wider area of the image and displays the presence of flow by adding colour to the greyscale image (Fig. 20.2A). Blue and red are typically used, although these represent flow either away or towards the ultrasound probe rather than venous and arterial flow.

Pulsed or spectral Doppler

This detects the flow of blood through a small part of the image and displays it in the form of the spectrum of velocities detected against time (Fig. 20.2B).

Power Doppler

This variation of colour Doppler utilizes only one colour, normally orange, to display the presence of flow without directional information. This modality

is more sensitive in detecting low speeds and volumes of flow.

APPEARANCES: FEATURES OF AN ULTRASOUND IMAGE

Presentation

The orientation of the screen is not fixed but for most applications the top of the image corresponds to the surface in contact with the ultrasound probe. For ultrasound applications such as abdominal scanning, the convention used in CT and MRI is generally adhered to, with the left side of a transverse section image corresponding to the right side of the patient. This is done so that the image corresponds to what the clinician sees when facing the patient, looking up from the feet. By convention, the left side of a longitudinal or coronal ultrasound image represents the cephalic direction, which corresponds with what would be seen by an observer looking from the right side of the patient. For musculoskeletal scanning these conventions are not always appropriate as the position of the patient and operator are not standardized, though ambiguous images should be adequately labelled.

The depth of the image is displayed as a scale of distance from the probe, running down the side of the picture. The maximum depth that can be displayed is determined primarily by the frequency the probe operates at, but is also dependent on the power output, and by how strongly the sound is absorbed (attenuated) by the intervening tissue.

Typical appearance of normal tissue

The normal appearance of structures varies from person to person. The frequency used and the quality of the scanner also determines the amount of detail in the image. The most significant factors affecting the image, however, are the amount and nature of tissue that the sound has to pass through to reach the structure of interest.

Figure 20.3 demonstrates some typical appearances of soft tissues:

- **Skin**: appears smooth and bright (echogenic, hyperechoic, highly reflective).

- **Fat**: can be bright or dark (hypoechoic, low echogenicity, low reflectivity), but subcutaneous fat is typically dark, with numerous fine bright septa running through it.

- **Muscle**: is also dark when viewed in cross-section. In long section, sound is reflected back by the muscle fibres and the internal structure of the muscle can be clearly visualized.

- **Fluid**: whether blood, effusion or the content of cysts, is generally black (anechoic), although thicker fluids (such as pus or those containing debris) can be bright or dark. Fluid generally absorbs less of sound than the surrounding soft tissue (translucence). This has the effect of

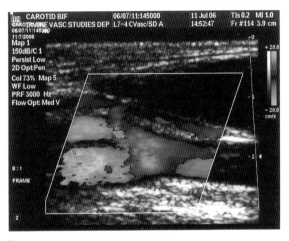

A

Figure 20.2 Colour Doppler image of the carotid bulb (A) and common carotid artery with spectral trace (B).

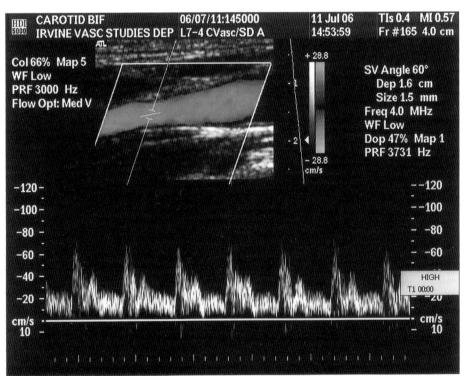

B

making the image deep to fluid-filled structures appear relatively bright (enhancement).

- **Tendons**: are typically bright, although this varies with their orientation relative to the sound waves emitted by the probe (anisotropy, see Fig. 20.7).

- **Nerves**: in the periphery also appear bright or dark depending on their orientation, and are distinguished from tendons dynamically, by

following their course through the surrounding tissues.

- **Bone**: the surface of bone appears as a particularly bright line due to the dramatic difference in acoustic impedance between bone and soft tissue. Because so much of the sound is reflected back by this boundary, very little is seen of what lies deep to the bone surface (shadowing).

IMAGING APPLICATIONS

MUSCLE

Ultrasound is often the imaging modality of choice for examining muscle. The internal structure and the interfaces between muscles are very well seen, in contrast to MRI and CT, and muscle contractions along with their effect on neighbouring structures can be observed in real time (Fig. 20.4).

Ultrasound has been particularly useful in evaluating the function of the deep muscles of the abdomen and pelvis, which are difficult to assess manually (Hides et al 1994 1995). Techniques that were developed for research are increasingly being used clinically in the treatment of low back pain and pelvic dysfunction.

Muscles such as the transverse abdominis, along with the overlying internal and external oblique, can be observed simultaneously in real time

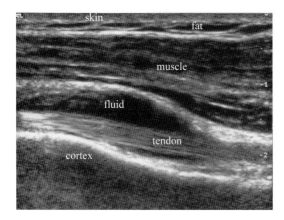

Figure 20.3 Longitudinal section of the biceps tendon surrounded by an effusion in the tendon sheath. Note the highly reflective cortex, and the subtle reduction in brightness of the tendon from left to right as the fibres change direction (anisotropy).

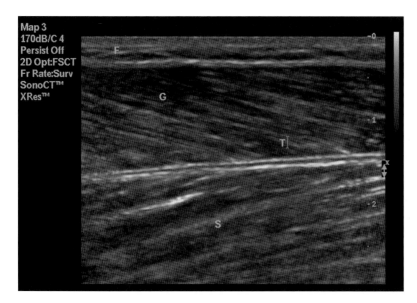

Figure 20.4 Longitudinal section through the medial head of gastrocnemius. The thin bright layer at the top of the image is the skin; immediately below is a thin layer of relatively dark subcutaneous fat (F) with fine bright septations. (G) is the muscle belly of the medial gastrocnemius with the muscle fibres seen angling down to the bright tendon (T), which separates it from the underlying soleus (S) muscle.

(Fig. 20.5), so that the extent to which individual muscles are being recruited during conscious and unconscious activation can be evaluated. This approach can be used for assessing almost any muscle group, but is particularly useful in assessing the lumbar paraspinal muscles, the diaphragm and the pelvic floor.

The pelvic floor can be scanned from the abdominal wall through the bladder, or from the perineum. Using the perineal approach, the continence mechanism can be evaluated directly by observing the effect of pelvic floor activity on the course of the urethra.

Biofeedback

Patients are becoming used to looking at ultrasound images, due mainly to its use in obstetrics. The size and mobility of modern scanners makes it feasible to scan in such a way that the patients can see the live image, allowing them to simultaneously observe the muscles they are trying to recruit and the effect this has on surrounding structures.

Objective measurement

Ultrasound can be used to accurately measure the cross-sectional area of muscle (Martinson & Stokes 1991). The increase in muscle thickness during contraction can also be measured, although the correlation with effort is multifactorial and not yet fully described (Hodges et al 2003, McMeeken et al 2004). Muscle atrophy has a characteristic appearance, with the muscle appearing relatively bright. Ultrasound techniques to quantify the degree of fatty infiltration associated with muscle atrophy are still in their infancy and MRI remains the examination of choice for this (Strobel et al 2005).

Muscle injuries

The appearance of muscle sprains and tears is highly variable. The appearances of low-grade tears are often very subtle, requiring experience to reliably evaluate. This is particularly true immediately after injury, as changes that can be detected by ultrasound may take more than a day to develop.

Larger tears are seen as a loss of continuity or a gap in the fibrous pattern, which may be highlighted by the presence of haematoma. Careful examination will also highlight muscle hernias and anatomical variations.

The appearance of a haematoma will also vary dramatically as it goes through different stages

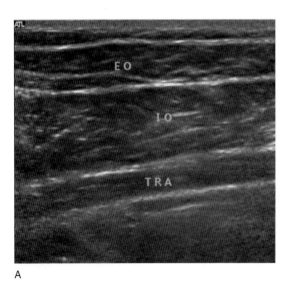
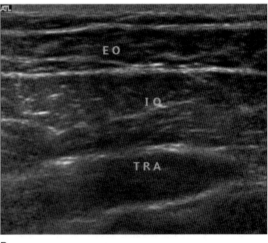

A   B

Figure 20.5 Transverse section of the lateral abdominal wall when standing at rest (A). A significant increase in the thickness of internal oblique (IO) and transverse abdominis (TRA) is noted when the subject was asked to draw in his stomach (B). EO, external oblique.

before being reabsorbed. Myositis ossificans is well seen with ultrasound as calcification has a bright appearance similar to bone and will typically cast a characteristic acoustic shadow artefact (Fig. 20.6).

TENDON

Ultrasound examination of tendons can be very rewarding. Not only can tendinopathy, tears,

calcinosis, enthesitis and tenosynovitis be visualized, but it is also possible to dynamically evaluate the movement of tendons in relation to surrounding structures. This enables adhesions and subluxations to be visualized.

Normal appearance

Normal tendon appears bright in an ultrasound image, so long as the surface of the probe is held roughly parallel with the direction of the tendon fibres. This allows incident sound to be reflected back to the probe. Once the angle changes significantly, the ultrasound no longer strikes the tendon at 90°, so much of the sound is reflected away from the probe making the tendon appear dark. This effect is known as anisotropy (Fig. 20.7).

Tendinopathy

The thickness of tendons such as the Achilles increases with tendinosis and the diameter can be compared with the unaffected side and/or normal values. The diameter and the echogenicity of the Achilles tendon return to normal as the tendon recovers (Ohberg et al 2004) and it may be that ultrasound can be used to tailor rehabilitation, although much work still needs to be done on this.

Focal tendinosis appears as dark areas within a tendon. This appearance can be mimicked by areas

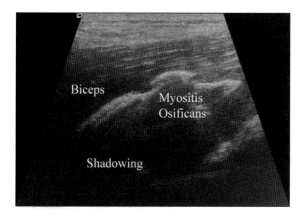

Figure 20.6 Myositis osificans in biceps femoris. Characteristic bright calcified outline seen within the muscle, with loss of image (shadowing) behind. (Supplied by Dr Gina Allen FRCR MFSEM(UK), MSK radiologist, Royal Orthopaedic and University Hospitals, Birmingham).

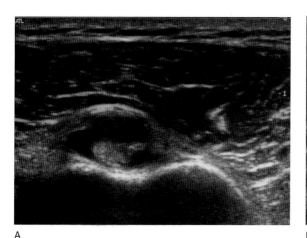

A

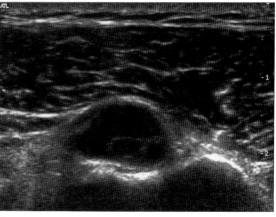

B

Figure 20.7 Transverse section through the long head of biceps tendon highlighted by an effusion within the biceps sheath. A, the image is made with the probe correctly aligned; B, in this image the probe is tilted slightly and the tendon appears dark due to anisotropy.

of normal tendon due to the anisotropy described above, and so considerable care is required in evaluating subtle tendon injuries.

The synovial sheath that is present around some tendons is not easily identified when normal. In the presence of inflammation it becomes oedematous and has an easily identified thickened hypoechoic (darkened) appearance. Ultrasound is very effective at identifying fluid within a tendon sheath, although it should be remembered that in some sheaths a small amount of fluid may be normal.

The ability to move joints and simultaneously visualize tendons also allows subluxation to be confirmed, typically with tendons such as biceps and the peroneii. Tethering can be identified when a tendon is seen to draw the surrounding soft tissue with it as it moves rather than gliding freely. Within the hand the flexor tendons can be seen moving through their pulleys, and with good high-frequency probes the pulleys themselves can be examined (Boutry et al 2005).

Tendon tears

Ultrasound is often used to confirm whether a tendon has ruptured, and the relative position of the free ends. Where tendons are superficial this is a relatively straightforward task, made easier by the ability to visualize the relative movement in real time. Partial tears can also be seen, but as with muscle tears, are more difficult to evaluate when there is not a clear gap in the fibrous pattern.

Calcific deposits

Calcification in tendons appears as a bright, rimmed (hyperechoic) mass (Fig. 20.8), often casting a characteristic acoustic shadow, which obscures the image lying behind it.

BONES

The surfaces of bones are highly reflective and are well seen with ultrasound. Fractures often appear as a clear break in the outline of the bone and ultrasound will pick up some fractures not apparent on plain-film X-ray (Herneth et al 2001, Rutten et al 2006). Despite this, ultrasound is not usually the imaging modality of choice as it is not normally

possible to examine the whole outline of the bone and in particular the intra-articular elements.

In paediatrics, where ossification of the bones is not complete, ultrasound can often complement X-rays, as the cartilaginous sections are well seen, in contrast to plain films. Ultrasound is used to assess the depth of the acetabulum in neonates, where it has been shown to facilitate the early detection of developmental dysplasia of the hip (Roovers et al 2005).

JOINTS

The margins of peripheral joints are easily identified with ultrasound and can be examined in some detail with a high frequency probe. Although the typical appearance of different joints varies greatly, with experience synovial hypertrophy, erosions, osteophytes, ligament injuries and evidence of inflammation can be discerned. Ultrasound is particularly useful for detecting and characterizing effusions (Delaunoy et al 2003, Kane et al 2003) and for directing therapeutic injections and aspiration.

The movement of joints can also be visualized along with the surrounding soft tissue, although this can be technically challenging owing to movement of the probe in contact with the body. X-ray fluoroscopy is currently the imaging method of choice for detecting subtle carpal bone subluxation;

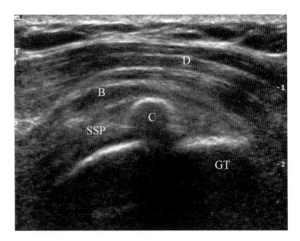

Figure 20.8 Round calcific deposit (C) in the supraspinatus tendon (SSP) just distal to its insertion into the greater tubercle (GT). Note a distended subacromial bursa (B) deep to the deltoid muscle (D).

however, with the advent of real-time three-dimensional ultrasound imaging (4D) it may be possible to evaluate movement of the carpi without the use of ionizing radiation.

Guided injections

The accuracy of blind injections has often been questioned. Ultrasound guidance enables precise placement of the needle tip within the intended structure and can be used for most of the commonly performed therapeutic orthopaedic injections (Fig. 20.9). This may lead to reductions in the required dosage and recent studies suggest that ultrasound guidance improves the efficacy of therapeutic injections (Naredo et al 2004). Ultrasound is generally the imaging modality of choice for the guided aspiration of superficial effusions and collections, as it is superior to CT at differentiating fluids and solid matter. Using ultrasound has the added benefit that structures such as blood vessels and nerves can be identified and avoided.

NERVES

Ultrasound is relatively underused in examining nerves, although improvement in the resolution available in recent years has lead to increased interest. Nerves in the periphery appear bright (similar to tendons), presumably due to their multiple fibrous septations (Fig. 20.10A). By contrast, the spinal nerves appear dark as they exit the cervical foramina before joining the brachial plexus, and so are often mistaken for blood vessels (Fig. 20.10B).

Ultrasound has been shown to have a sensitivity and specificity approaching those of nerve conduction studies (NCS) in evaluating patients with suspected carpal tunnel syndrome (CTS). Findings include increased thickness and vascularity of the nerve just proximal to the tunnel (Mallouhi et al 2006). Ultrasound has the advantage of demonstrating occult structural abnormalities and soft-tissue lesions that might be present, as well as being painless and so better tolerated than NCS.

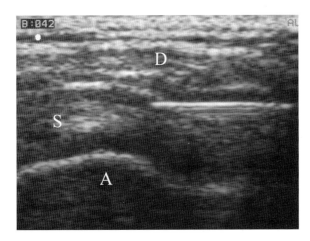

Figure 20.9 Subacromial injection. A 23-gauge needle with its tip in a mildly distended subacromial bursa. (D) Deltoid muscle, (S) supraspinatus tendon, (A) humeral head.

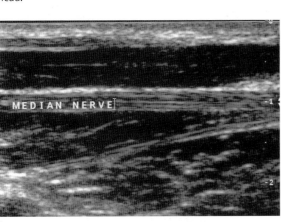
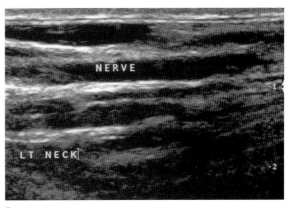

A   B

Figure 20.10 A, shows a long section of the median nerve which appears bright (echogenic) in relation to the surrounding muscle. B, shows a nerve root in the neck, which appears almost black (anechoic).

The movement of nerves can also be visualized relative to the surrounding soft tissue. When present, subluxation of the ulnar nerve can be seen at the elbow during passive flexion, and reduced transverse glide of the median nerve has been described in patients with carpal tunnel syndrome (Erel et al 2003, Nakamichi & Tachibana 1995).

Ultrasound is often used to determine the presence or absence of a Morton's neuroma, although this is a technically difficult examination, the sensitivity and specificity of which are dependent on the skill and experience of the operator.

VASCULAR

Doppler ultrasound is used in physiotherapy research to assess blood flow in the vertebral arteries (Arnold et al 2004, Mitchell et al 2004), because of concerns regarding adverse effects of cervical manipulation. The relative roles of vertebral and carotid arteries in adverse events have yet to be determined, but in the future ultrasound may have a role in premanipulation screening.

Grey-scale imaging is used to examine the structure of blood vessels, whereas Doppler is applied to evaluate the blood flow. Blood vessel walls appear as bright tubes on ultrasound, with blood appearing black (anechoic) in a grey-scale image. Arteries and veins are easily distinguished as the latter collapse with gentle probe pressure and the pulsatility of flow in arteries is unmistakable when viewed with Doppler.

Thrombus within vessels is not always visible on grey scale as it can have the same echo texture as blood; however, it can be detected in veins by dynamic testing, as the vessel will not completely collapse when compressed if there is thrombus within the lumen at that point. Within arteries, stenoses resulting from intramural thrombus cause changes in blood flow which can be detected with Doppler.

LUMPS AND BUMPS

Evaluation of palpable masses, or 'lumps and bumps' as they are commonly referred to, requires considerable experience. Ultrasound appearances are almost never entirely specific and so these always require clinical correlation, and often further imaging.

Ultrasound is very useful in detecting foreign bodies, especially those not well seen with X-ray, such as wood splinters. These will often appear bright, casting an acoustic shadow, and may be surrounded by a dark halo of reactive oedematous tissue. Ganglia, including Baker's cysts appear as fluid-filled sacks, and often a tail can be seen tracking towards the structure they arise from, giving them a C shape or 'speech bubble' appearance (Fig. 20.11).

Ultrasound does not suffer from the problems of MRI and CT in imaging prostheses. These generally have sonographic qualities similar to bone, so although their internal integrity cannot be assessed, their superficial surface, effusions, collections and the overlying soft tissues can be visualized.

LUNGS

Ultrasound is not normally associated with the examination of the lungs, however in radiology the chest wall is commonly examined to confirm the presence of pleural effusions and collections as well as to guide the placement of drains. Passing comment is often made with regard to the presence of underlying collapse or consolidation of the basal segments as these are clearly visible, although whether this information is of any clinical value is unclear.

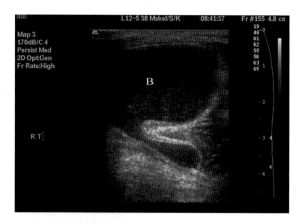

Figure 20.11 Typical speech-bubble appearance of a Baker's cyst (B). Note that the cyst does not appear black (anechoic) owing to the presence of blood products within it (haematoma).

LIMITATIONS OF ULTRASOUND

Ultrasound imaging is not without its limitations, considerable skill and experience being required to perform more complex tasks. The ability that ultrasound scanners afford – to continually change the plane being scanned – means that the operator must interpret the moving image dynamically, taking into consideration factors such as the orientation of the probe and the presence of artefacts. Indeed, the static images that are taken only reflect the operator's ability to acquire a representative image in a single plane, and so cannot be reliably re-interpreted in the same manner as MRI or CT.

With the exception of specialized Doppler studies of the circle of Willis, ultrasound cannot be used to examine tissue lying deep to calcified bone. Air also represents a barrier to ultrasound, limiting examinations of the thorax and bowel.

Other limitations include reduced image quality when examining large subjects. This can be alleviated to some extent by using lower-frequency probes, but at the cost of reduced resolution.

SAFETY

Ultrasound is perceived as a safe form of imaging and, to date, no harmful side effects have been reported from the clinical use of real-time ultrasound in the paediatric and adult populations. Developments in ultrasound technology, however, have led to ever higher power outputs, particularly with applications such as tissue harmonic imaging and Doppler, and the possibility of tissue damage cannot be discounted. The potential risks are from heating and from mechanical effects such as cavitation (outlined in Chapter 12). These effects are likely to be negligible when using standard grey-scale imaging of musculoskeletal structures; however, it is prudent to avoid scanning over a fixed point for longer than is necessary for assessment and training purposes.

Concerns about the safety of ultrasound have been focused on in-utero scanning, where ultrasound may have an effect on the rapidly developing fetus. Unnecessary scanning of the fetus should therefore be avoided (BMUS Safety Guidelines 2000) and should be carried out only by operators with the appropriate training.

The most significant risk to the patient from the use of ultrasound comes not from the ultrasound itself but from misinterpretation of ultrasound findings, and it is essential that clinicians using ultrasound can recognize the limitations imposed by equipment, image quality and their own experience and training.

CONCLUSION

Ultrasound imaging has the potential to revolutionize physiotherapy practice by allowing the clinician to directly image the structures of interest, whether the patient is on the couch or the treadmill. Muscle recruitment and its effect on other structures can be evaluated with increased accuracy. With appropriate training, focal soft-tissue lesions and pathological changes can also be evaluated and, because patients are seen regularly throughout the rehabilitation process, physiotherapists have the unique opportunity to monitor and document the healing of tendons, muscles, joints and even possibly nerve injuries. In this way, ultrasound offers physiotherapy not only a powerful adjunct to clinical assessment but also a much-needed objective tool for evaluating the effectiveness of practice, and the diverse range of treatment modalities, including those described in this text.

References

Arnold C, Bourassa R, Langer T, Stoneham G (2004) Doppler studies evaluating the effect of a physical therapy screening protocol on vertebral artery blood flow. *Man Ther* **9**:13–21.

BMUS Safety Guidelines (2000) Online. Available: http://www.bmus.org/public-info/pi-safety03.asp

Boutry N, Titecat M, Demondion X et al (2005) High-frequency ultrasonographic examination of the finger pulley system. *J Ultrasound Med* **24**(10): 1333–1339.

Crass J, Craig E, Thompson R, Feinberg S (1984) Ultrasonography of the rotator cuff: surgical correlation. *J Clin Ultrasound* **12**(8): 487–491.

Delaunoy I, Feipel V, Appelboom T, Hauzeur J (2003) Sonography detection threshold for knee effusion. *Clin Rheumatol* **22**(6): 391–392.

Erel E, Dilley A, Greening J et al (2003) Longitudinal sliding of the median nerve in patients with carpal tunnel syndrome. *J Hand Surg* **28**(5): 439–443.

Hedrick W, Hykes,D, Starchman D (2005) *Ultrasound Physics and Instrumentation*, 4th edn. St Louis, MO, Mosby.

Herneth A, Siegmeth A, Bader T et al (2001) Scaphoid fractures: evaluation with high-spatial-resolution US initial results. *Radiology* **220**(1): 231–235.

Hides J, Stokes M, Saide M et al (1994) Evidence of multifidus wasting ipsilateral to symptoms in patients with acute/subacute low back pain. *Spine* **19**(2): 165–177.

Hides J, Richardson C, Jull G (1995) Magnetic resonance imaging and Ultrasonography of the lumbar multifidus muscle. Comparison of two different modalities. *Spine* **20**(1): 54–58.

Hodges P, Pengel L, Herbert R, Gandevia S (2003) Measurement of muscle contraction with ultrasound imaging. *Muscle Nerve* **27**(6): 682–692.

Kane D, Balint P, Sturrock R (2003) Ultrasonography is superior to clinical examination in the detection and localization of knee joint effusion in rheumatoid arthritis. *J Rheumatol* **30**(5): 966–971.

Mallouhi A, Pultzl P, Trieb T et al (2006) Predictors of carpal tunnel syndrome: accuracy of grey-scale and colour Doppler sonography. *Am J Roentgenol* **186**(5): 1240–1245.

Martinson H, Stokes M (1991) Measurement of anterior tibial muscle size using real-time ultrasound imaging, *Eur J Appl Physiol Occup Physiol* **63**(3–4): 250–254.

McMeeken J, Beath I, Newham D et al (2004) The relationship between EMG and change in thickness of transverse abdominis. *Clin Biomech* **19**(4): 337–342.

Mitchell J, Keen D, Dyson C et al (2004) Is cervical spin rotation, as used in the standard vertebrobasilar insufficiency test, associated with a measurable change in intracranial vertebral artery blood flow? *Man Ther* **9**(4): 220–227.

Nakamichi K, Tachibana S (1995) Restricted motion of the median nerve in carpal tunnel syndrome. *J Hand Surg* **20**(4): 460–464.

Naredo E, Cabero F, Beneyto P et al (2004) A randomised comparative study of short term response to blind injection vs. sonographic-guided injection of local corticosteroids in patients with painful shoulder. *J Rheumatol* **31**(2): 308–314.

Ohberg L, Lorentzon R, Alfredson H (2004) Eccentric training in patients with chronic Achilles tendinosis: normalised tendon structure and decreased thickness at follow up. *Br J Sports Med* **38**(1): 8–11.

Roovers E, Boere-Boonekamp M, Castelein R et al (2005) Effectiveness of ultrasound screening for developmental dysplasia of the hip. *Arch Dis Child (Foetal Neonatal Ed)* **90**(1): F25–F30.

Rutten M, Jager G, de Waal Malefijt M et al (2006) Double line sign: a helpful sonographic sign to detect occult fractures of the proximal humerus. *Eur Radiol* **17**: 762–767

Stokes M, Young A (1986) Measurement of quadriceps cross-sectional area by ultrasonography: a description of the technique and its applications in physiotherapy. *Physiother Pract* **2**: 31–36.

Strobel K, Hodler J, Meyer D et al (2005) Fatty atrophy of supraspinatus and infraspinatus muscles: accuracy of US. *Radiology* **237**(2): 584–589.

SECTION 5

Contraindications, dangers and precautions

Chapter 21

Guidance for the clinical use of electrophysical agents 2006

Reproduced with permission of the CSP, 14 Bedford Row, London WC1R 4ED

Sarah Bazin, Sheila Kitchen, David Maskill, Ann Reed, Alison Skinner,

Deirdre Walsh and Tim Watson

CHAPTER CONTENTS

SECTION 1: INTRODUCTION

This guidance, developed by the Chartered Society of Physiotherapy, has been written to provide advice on the safe practice of electrophysical agents, where the use of such agents is indicated following assessment. Treatment parameters should be decided on the basis of the assessment, the known physiological effects of treatment, and any modifying factors, for example medication, past medical history. It would therefore be inappropriate for this document to include prescriptive protocols.

Chartered physiotherapists need to ensure that any interventions given will be clinically effective. Evidence of effectiveness can be drawn from research, expert opinion and patients' and professionals' experience. Recommendations in this document are based on a combination of the above, together with experience of the authors. A number of references are included in each section with additional suggested general literature in Section 9. Although these provide some key citations, they in no way provide a comprehensive review of the literature. The body of literature pertaining to electrophysical agents is both large and disparate. It is the responsibility of the user to keep up to date with this material.

1.1 DISCLAIMER

Although the information in this publication is relevant and accurate at the time of publication, readers and users of the material will need to take responsibility for identifying additional new information of relevance as it becomes available. It does not override the responsibility of the physiotherapist to make appropriate decisions for individual patients, in consultation with the patient and/or guardian or carer.

The authors and publisher disclaim responsibility for any adverse effects resulting directly or indirectly from the suggested procedures, from any undetected errors, or from the reader's misunderstanding of the text.

This guidance was arrived at after careful consideration of the available evidence and should be used in conjunction with the Chartered Society of Physiotherapy's (CSP) Core Standards of Physiotherapy Practice (CSP 2005), Rules of Professional Conduct (CSP 2002), Core Standards, CSP guideline paper PA47, Medical Devices Agency guidance, 1998 (see Section 4) and relevant legislation, including the Consumer Protection Act and Health and Safety at Work Act (1974). See also websites, e.g.:

● *www.doh.gov.uk/hhsexec/manrec.htm* (Managing records in NHS Trusts and Health Authorities), and

● *www.open.gov.uk/doh/coinh.htm* (Using electronic patient records in hospitals: legal requirements and good practice).

Although it is important for the profession to provide guidance, physiotherapists, when implementing the advice, will also need to take account of local regulations and policies.

SECTION 2: SCOPE OF PRACTICE, CONSENT AND MONITORING

2.1 SCOPE OF PRACTICE

● Physiotherapists should confine themselves to the use of electrophysical agents which they are able to apply safely and competently. In order to achieve this, physiotherapists should ensure that they, as individuals, follow the guidance on competence to practise contained in Section 5 of this publication, and on Safety, in Section 6. Physiotherapists who are giving advice to others with regard to electrophysical agents must ensure that they are familiar with the guidance laid down in Section 3, Relationships with and Advice to Third Parties.

● Physiotherapists should be aware of the guidance and standards that relate to each specific physiotherapeutic agent. When using a procedure which is not specifically listed, they should follow the principles laid down for other agents, and also make reference to Section 8, Novel Agents and Equipment.

● The individual physiotherapist is ultimately responsible for the assessment and treatment they deliver. This responsibility is not absolved if a prescriptive treatment programme is followed, or if the task is delegated (Section 3.2). Attention is drawn to Rule 4 of the Rules of Professional Conduct (2002), which relates to the responsibility of the physiotherapist for their intervention, regardless of what may have been prescribed by, for example, a medical practitioner, manufacturer or another physiotherapist. The physiotherapist has to decide whether the treatment is appropriate, and if in doubt, it is their responsibility to seek further professional/expert opinion before undertaking the treatment.

● Before proceeding with the proposed treatment, physiotherapists must ensure that patients receive sufficient information, including the risks, benefits and alternatives, to allow them to make an informed decision.

● Physiotherapists must maintain an adequate record of the agents they use. This should include the assessment, the tests carried out and their results, the clinical reasoning and the patient interaction that led to the decision to apply these.

● Physiotherapists should be aware of, and comply with, the maintenance issues highlighted in Section 4 of this document. Although it is not the responsibility of physiotherapists to carry out the majority of the formal safety and calibration tests, it *is* their responsibility to ensure that these have been carried out for the equipment they are using. They also have a responsibility to ensure that a safety check programme is up to date. Physiotherapists should not use a machine which does not have an 'in date' safety check.

● Attention is also drawn to Rules 7 and 8 of the Rules of Professional Conduct, which relate to the advertising and sale of equipment and services. Care should be taken to ensure that patients are given adequate information with regard to machine purchase or hire.

The professional responsibilities of physiotherapists in relation to the application of electrophysical agents should conform to the principles set out in the Rules of Professional Conduct (CSP 2002).

2.2 VALID CONSENT

Patients must have the capacity to give valid consent to treatment. They should be able to comprehend and retain material information, especially consequences, and be able to use and weigh information in decision making. Information given by the physiotherapist should enable the patient to make a balanced judgement, understand material or significant risks, and questions should be answered truthfully. The DH Consent website *www.dh.gov.uk/consent* has the full text of all DH Consent publications.

2.3 MONITORING PERFORMANCE

Clinical audit

Routine clinical audit should include procedures that measure performance.

Unexpected effects reporting

In addition, it is the responsibility of the individual physiotherapist to report all unexpected effects of electrophysical treatments both in the appropriate way locally, and to the professional body. It is an important component of professional audits that all such unexpected effects are recorded and detailed accurately and fully. Included in this booklet is the current report form (Appendix 1) which should be completed and returned to the Clinical Effectiveness Unit of the CSP electronically via *enquiries@csp.org.uk* or to the postal address quoted in the event of a patient experiencing an unexpected response to treatment.

SECTION 3: RELATIONSHIPS WITH AND ADVICE TO THIRD PARTIES

There are a number of situations where a physiotherapist may give advice on the use of electrophysical devices. In all such situations, the physiotherapist should be aware of the full implications of giving such advice.

3.1 LOAN/HIRE OF ELECTROPHYSICAL DEVICES FOR USE BY A PATIENT (e.g. home use of a TENS unit)

Patients who are loaned or hired an electrophysical device by a physiotherapist, receive instruction on its safe and effective application.

Criteria

- Equipment is checked for electrical safety, output and cleanliness prior to the loan.

- The patient is fully instructed in the safe and effective use of the apparatus.

- There is a demonstration on the patient of the application of the device.

- The patient is supervised in practising the application of the device.

- Simple written instructions detailing use, adequate care, hazards of the apparatus, and contact details for assistance, are provided.

- A copy of the written instructions to patients is placed in the patient's record.

- The loan of equipment is recorded in the patient's record.

- A record is kept of all equipment loaned/hired.

- The patient's use of the loan equipment is monitored normally on a monthly basis.

- Equipment returned by patients/third parties (e.g. another department or family member) is checked upon return, in accordance with a local protocol.

3.2 DELEGATION OF TASKS TO PHYSIOTHERAPY ASSISTANTS

The responsibility for the patient's care remains with the physiotherapist, who will undertake the initial assessment and make the decision that the application of an electrophysical agent is indicated, and prescribe the dose. The physiotherapist is responsible for the re-evaluation of the patient's condition at each attendance, and has a responsibility for monitoring the assistant's technique of application. Tasks should be delegated in accordance with the CSP's Information Paper PA 6, 'The delegation of tasks to physiotherapy assistants and other support workers'.

The physiotherapist must ensure, in every case, that the assistant has received adequate, documented training on the relevant and specific apparatus. This will include the operation of relevant devices, and information about potential dangers, risks and contraindications to treatment. Equally, the physiotherapy assistant should alert the physiotherapist if they feel their training is inadequate to allow the safe application of the agent.

Physiotherapy assistants who apply electrophysical agents to patients are responsible for satisfying themselves the task has been appropriately delegated and carried out.

Criteria

Physiotherapy assistants will:

● only use equipment for which they have received training

● apprise the delegating physiotherapist where they believe their training in the use of the specific equipment to be applied is inadequate

● ensure that all instructions are received in writing

● ensure that all instructions include body part, dose and application time

● inform the delegating physiotherapist of the progress of treatment

● notify the delegating physiotherapist immediately, whenever any unexpected reactions to treatment are observed, or where potential risks or contradictions become apparent.

3.3 ADVICE TO ANOTHER PHYSIOTHERAPIST

Regardless of any specific expertise or length of experience, physiotherapists considering giving advice to another physiotherapist are encouraged to be fully apprised of all relevant facts in the case in question, and preferably in writing. In such cases, it should be noted that the duty of care remains with the physiotherapist responsible for the treatment.

3.4 ADVICE FROM MANUFACTURERS/ SUPPLIERS/DEVELOPERS

The claims, whether in terms of effects, efficacy or safety, of manufacturers, suppliers or developers should not be accepted by the physiotherapist in isolation. Evidence from reliable studies, or advice from suitably qualified clinicians, e.g. physiotherapists or physicians who are familiar or experienced in the use of the particular apparatus (in the case of a new machine) or agent (in the case of novel treatments), should be additionally sought.

3.5 ADVICE TO MANUFACTURERS/ SUPPLIERS/DEVELOPERS

Individual physiotherapists should only undertake technical consultancy after fully considering the implications of the subsequent use of the advice provided.

Provision of written or oral testimonials should normally be avoided.

3.6 ADVICE TO OTHER RECOGNISED HEALTH CARE PRACTITIONERS

Individual physiotherapists are encouraged not to provide *informal* advice on electrophysical agents to other recognized healthcare professionals e.g. physicians, nurses, chiropractors, osteopaths, podiatrists. Where the other party can demonstrate relevant knowledge and competence, advice may be given at the discretion of the physiotherapist in line with the recommendations noted above for advice given to other physiotherapists, *i.e. in such cases, the duty of care remains with the other healthcare professionals, not the physiotherapist.*

Under some circumstances, formalized training may be provided for such professionals by suitably qualified physiotherapists; in such cases, due consideration should be given to the implications for the profession(s) concerned and their recognized competencies.

3.7 ADVICE TO UNQUALIFIED PRACTITIONERS, EXCLUDING PHYSIOTHERAPY ASSISTANTS

It is considered inadvisable for physiotherapists to provide advice to practitioners whose qualifications are not recognized by statute, regardless of the 'expertise' or length of experience of the practitioner, as there is no continuing jurisdiction over their practice, unlike the position with physiotherapy assistants.

3.8 ADVICE TO INDIVIDUALS NOT UNDER THE DIRECT CARE OF A RECOGNIZED PRACTITIONER

In some cases, members of the general public may avail themselves of opportunities to obtain electrophysical apparatus directly from the manufacturer or supplier (e.g. by mail order) and subsequently seek advice on its use.

Physiotherapists approached in such cases should encourage the individual to seek assessment from a chartered physiotherapist or other suitably qualified practitioner, who can then advise on the suitability and appropriateness of the apparatus or agent purchased. Physiotherapists are encouraged not to provide informal advice to such patients, regardless of individual circumstances e.g. patient with chronic pain, unless a full assessment has been performed and the physiotherapist is familiar with the apparatus in question and its suitability.

SECTION 4: MAINTENANCE ISSUES

The standards for the maintenance of electrophysical equipment should be read in conjunction with Section 7, as they may be modified for specific electrophysical agents.

4.1 ELECTROPHYSICAL EQUIPMENT RECEIVES ROUTINE AND APPROPRIATE MAINTENANCE, WHICH INCLUDES QUALITY ASSURANCE OF FUNCTION AND SAFETY FEATURES

Criteria

● There is a local policy for the maintenance of all electrotherapeutic equipment

● There is a contract for the maintenance and repair and quality assurance of equipment with:
  ● manufacturer/supplier and/or
  ● hospital Medical Engineers Department and/or
  ● hospital Medical Physics Department and/or
  ● a reputable third-party maintenance organization.

● The contract specifies maintenance and quality assurance to be carried out at least once per year.

● There is a written record of all maintenance, repairs and quality assurance results, which should be accurate, detailed and readily assessable. Consideration should be given to permanent preservation of records (publication HSC1999/053 refers and can be found via *www.dh.gov.uk*).

● Prior to use a visual check of all electrotherapy equipment includes:
  ● electrodes
  ● leads
  ● cables
  ● plugs
  ● power outlets
  ● switches
  ● controls
  ● dials
  ● screens
  ● indicator lights
  ● mechanical stability.

● Faults, or suspected faults, are reported immediately.

● Machines or parts with faults or suspected faults are removed from use immediately until repaired.

● Where a piece of electrophysical apparatus is loaned by a supplier, an indemnity form is signed by both supplier and a representative of the health authority or practice, prior to the start of the loan period.

● All new equipment is tested in accordance with the manufacturer's guidance to ensure that it is functioning as intended and is safe for the patient and operator.

The Medical Devices Agency, an Executive Agency of the Department of Health, has produced guidance on 'Acceptance Testing' and 'The Management of Medical Equipment and Devices' (*www.medical-devices.gov.uk*).

All new equipment sold in the European Community should be CE marked, in accordance with the Medical Devices Directive. European Standards describe the specification to which equipment should be manufactured, and are documented in the British Standards BS EN46000 series. Manufacturing and maintenance organizations should be aware of these, and the user is unlikely to need to refer to them. If the equipment gives rise to any major concerns, the user may wish to consult the documents, which are available from the British Standards Institute, or from major city or university reference libraries.

SECTION 5: COMPETENCE TO PRACTISE

Professional competence is essential to safe and effective practice. Before using the electrophysical agent, practitioners must ensure that they are knowledgeable about its physical, physiological and clinical effects and efficacy, based on the best available evidence. Contraindications, precautions and methods of safe application must also be known.

Rule 1 of the Rules of Professional Conduct of the CSP states 'Chartered physiotherapists shall only practise to the extent that they have established and maintained their ability to work safely and competently…' (CSP 2002). Physiotherapists should therefore confine themselves to the use of agents in which they have undertaken relevant pre- and/or post-qualifying programmes. Learning from manufacturer's literature alone is not adequate. Physiotherapists have a responsibility for updating themselves, as new knowledge becomes available.

Continuing professional development is described by the CSP as 'the lifelong learning that professionals need to undertake throughout their career in order to maintain, enhance and broaden professional competence'. As in other areas of the profession, competence to practise is maintained through the incorporation of information obtained from a variety of sources, including:

- participating in courses, workshops

- reviewing research, equipment evaluations and safety literature on a regular basis

- discussing the use and effects of relevant agents with other knowledgeable professionals.

SECTION 6: CONTRAINDICATIONS, PRECAUTIONS, SAFETY AND APPLICATION ISSUES

The following guidelines apply to all the equipment referred to in Section 7. Additional safety measures are also specified in Section 7 for specific agents, and these should also be adhered to.

In order to ensure safety during the application of electrophysical agents, the physiotherapist must consider the patient, the electrotherapy apparatus, the surrounding environment and other people.

6.1 CONTRAINDICATIONS FOR ALL AGENTS

During the selection and application of any electrophysical agents (EPAs), the following measures should be taken to ensure safety and good practice.

	Reference
• Those who are unable to comprehend instructions, or who are unable to co-operate	CSP Core Standards (2005)
• The application of electrophysical agents over the abdomen, lower back or pelvis is normally contraindicated during the first 35 weeks of pregnancy. Refer to specific information for each agent	Expert opinion
• In the area of a tumour where there is active or suspected malignancy, except for palliative care	001*/002*/003* 004*/005*/006* 007*/008*/009*
• Areas of recent bleeding tissue or haemorrhage	Expert opinion
• Active tuberculosis in treatment area	Expert opinion

*001 Auda SP, Hall G, Elias J et al (1979) Selective tumor heating and growth retardation by shortwave radiofrequency. *Surg Forum* 30: 154–156.

*002 Auda SP, Steinert HR, Elias EG et al (1980) Selective tumor heating by shortwave radiofrequency (RF). *Cancer* 46(9): 1962–1968.
*003 Habal MB (1980) Effect of applied dc currents on experimental tumor growth in rats. *J Biomed Mater Res* 14(6): 789–801.
*004 Jarm T, Wickramasinghe YA, Deakin M et al (1999) Blood perfusion of subcutaneous tumours in mice following the application of low-level direct electric current. *Adv Exp Med Biol* 471: 497–506.
*005 Lejbkowicz F, Zwiran M, Salzberg S et al (1993) The response of normal and malignant cells to ultrasound in vitro. *Ultrasound Med Biol* 19(1): 75–82.
*006 Marino A (1993) Electromagnetic fields, cancer and the theory of neuroendocrine related promotion. *Bioelectrochem Bioenerget* 29(3): 255–276.
*007 Miyagi N, Sato K, Rong Y et al (2000) Effects of PEMF on a murine osteosarcoma cell line: drug-resistant (P-glycoprotein-positive) and non-resistant cells. *Bioelectromagnetics* 21: 112–121.
*008 Sicard-Rosenbaum L, Lord D, Danoff JV et al (1995) Effects of continuous therapeutic ultrasound on growth and metastasis of subcutaneous murine tumors. *Phys Ther* 75(1): 3–13.
*009 Verschaeve L (1995) Can nonionising radiation induce cancer. *Cancer J* 8(5): 237–249.

6.2 PRECAUTIONS FOR ALL AGENTS

Treatment should not normally be carried out:

	Reference
• Over the anterior aspect of the neck	Expert opinion
• Where there is significant impairment in the circulation/sensory loss of the area to be treated	Expert opinion
• Where there is devitalized tissue, e.g. after recent radiotherapy	Expert opinion
• Where there are local acute skin conditions, e.g. eczema, dermatitis	Expert opinion

6.3 HEALTH AND SAFETY CONSIDERATIONS

	Reference
• Treatment is carried out in compliance with local regulations	Norm
• The surrounding environment is safe for treatment	Expert opinion
• There is a warning sign relating to patients with internal stimulators where high-frequency equipment is used	Expert opinion

6.4 QUICK REFERENCE GRID

CONTRAINDICATION/PRECAUTION — AGENT	Pregnancy (in fetal region)	Pregnancy (anywhere)	Malignancy	Specialized tissue	Active implants, inc pacemaker	Active epiphysis	Metal implants	Local circulation insufficiency	Epilepsy	Devitalized tissue	Bleeding tissue	THERMAL SKIN TEST	SHARP/BLUNT SKIN TEST
ELECTRICAL STIMULATION													
GENERIC				E,T					N			○	✓
INTERFERENTIAL				E,T					N			○	✓
LOW FREQUENCY				E,T					N			○	✓
TENS				E,T					N			○	✓
NON THERMAL													
LASER				E,T								○	○
PULSED SHORTWAVE				E,T								○	○
ULTRASOUND				E,T								○	○
THERMAL													
HOT PACK				E								✓	○
INFRARED				E								✓	○
MICROWAVE				E,T								✓	○
SHORTWAVE (CONT/PULSED)				E,T								✓	○
ULTRASOUND				E,T								✓	○
WAX				E								✓	○
OTHERS													
BIOFEEDBACK (NO STIMULATION)												○	○
COLD THERAPY				E								✓	○
ULTRAVIOLET													○

E = EYE
T = TESTIS
N = NECK

Pattern	Meaning
CONTRAINDICATION	
LOCAL CONTRAINDICATION	
PRECAUTION	
NO KNOWN ADVERSE EFFECT	
SEE SPECIFIC AGENT	
NECESSARY	✓
NOT REQUIRED	○

6.5 APPLICATION FOR ALL AGENTS

	Reference
Measures should be taken to ensure that the electrophysical equipment is applied in a manner that is conducive to safe usage	Expert opinion
The user manual for each piece of equipment is read and understood before its use	Expert opinion
Equipment and accessories are checked as appropriate prior to application	Core standard 18
Relevant technical safety checks are carried out for the specific apparatus	Core standard 18
Equipment is kept clean	Expert opinion

(Continued)

(Continued)

	Reference
Where appropriate, the intensity indicator is set at zero prior to switching on or off	Expert opinion
The equipment is switched on/off in the correct sequence	Expert opinion
Where appropriate, intensity dials are turned up or down gradually	Expert opinion
The patient should be positioned comfortably with adequate support to remain in the given position for the duration of the treatment	Expert opinion
Preparation of patient	
• an explanation of the planned treatment is given to enable valid consent	010*/011*
• the sensation of the planned treatment to be experienced is explained	010*/011*
• the patient is warned of any effects that should be reported	010*/011*
Examination and testing	
• this refers to specific examination of the part of the body to be treated for possible hazards, contraindications and precautions, plus any appropriate tests. A check should be made to ascertain whether the patient might suffer an allergic reaction to any substance being applied to the skin	010*/011*
Drug information	
• information must be obtained from the patient concerning medication that may interfere with or mask the effects of the electrophysical agent.	Expert opinion
Assembly of apparatus	
• visual checks are made of electrodes, leads, cables, plugs, power outlets, switches, controls, dials and indicator lights	010*/011*
Preparation and testing of apparatus	
• the operator(s) should minimize their own exposure to the agent	010*/011*
Preparation of the part to be treated	
• this involves any preparatory procedure, e.g. washing the area	010*/011*
Setting up	
• the apparatus should be set up to ensure optimum therapeutic effect and safety	010*/011*
• where possible the same piece of equipment is used at each visit.	Expert opinion
• the functional output of the equipment is tested on the day of use	Expert opinion
• local policies relating to infection control are adhered to, and specialist advice is sought where appropriate	Expert opinion
Application	
• the patient should be monitored appropriately to ensure that treatment is progressing satisfactorily and without unexpected effect	010*/011*
Treatment	
• if pain, discomfort or unexpected sensations are experienced by the patient treatment intensity should be modified	Expert opinion
• at the termination of treatment the part treated should be examined, and the general condition of the patient evaluated	010*/011*
For those devices that allow a hands-free application:	
• a member of staff remains within calling distance during treatment	Expert opinion
• the patient is provided with a means of calling for assistance	Expert opinion
Recording	
• an accurate record of assessment findings, machine settings, all treatment parameters and effects must be made. This is required to enable accurate treatment replication and as a legal requirement.	010*/011* Core standard 14 Core standard 18

*010 Kitchen S (ed) (2002) *Electrotherapy: Evidence-based Practice*. London, Churchill Livingstone.
*011 Low J, Reed A (2000) *Electrotherapy Explained – Principles and Practice*, 3rd edn. Oxford, Butterworth-Heinemann: 27–28.

Supplementary reading: all agents – application

Chartered Society of Physiotherapy (CSP) Safety of Electrotherapy Equipment working group (1990) Guidelines for the safe use of ultrasound therapy equipment. *Physiotherapy* **76**(11): 683–684.

Chartered Society of Physiotherapy (CSP) Safety of Electrotherapy Equipment working group (1991) Guidelines for the safe use of microwave therapy equipment. *Physiotherapy* **77**(9): 653–654.

SECTION 7: AGENTS

The information in the following sections should be read in conjunction with the generic information in Section 6.

7.1 BIOFEEDBACK

7.1.1 Introduction

A technique which enables the individual to readily determine the activity levels of a particular physiological process, and with appropriate training, learn to manipulate the same process by an internalized mechanism.

[For the purpose of this documentation, *Biofeedback* will specifically relate to the use of EMG Biofeedback, although it is acknowledged that there are many different forms of this therapy.]

The EMG Biofeedback unit allows the detection of the gross electrical signals arising from active muscle, passes them through several electronic processes and presents them to the patient in a simplified format (lights, sound).

7.1.2 Contraindications

None known.

7.1.3 Precautions

	Reference
• Ensure that the skeletal and soft tissues are capable of withstanding the enhanced forces that may be generated by the facilitated muscle.	Expert opinion

7.1.4 Hazards

Patients with epilepsy may experience an adverse response to the visual display (flashing lights/computer screen). Such patients should be treated with caution and careful monitoring, following consultation between the therapist and the appropriate medical practitioner.

7.1.5 Application and mandatory warnings

Patients should not feel any skin irritation, discomfort or pain. Any such sensations should be reported to the therapist immediately.

7.1.6 Treatment record

See 'Application for all agents' – *Recording*.

7.2 COLD THERAPY

7.2.1 Introduction

Read in conjunction with the generic information in Section 6.

Cold therapy is the application of cooling agents to the tissues to produce a reduction in body tissue temperature. The temperature changes affect a wide variety of structures including skin, muscle, nerves and blood vessels.

Little evidence is available to support the following contraindications, which are based on current clinical norms.

7.2.2 Contraindications

	Reference
• Acute febrile illness	Expert opinion
• Vasospasm (e.g. Raynaud's disease/development of white/blue fingers with cold)	Expert opinion
• Cryoglobulinaemia	Expert opinion
• Cold urticaria/allergy	Expert opinion

7.2.3 Precautions

	Reference
• Appropriate precautions should be taken in the presence of open wounds, infected tissue and skin lesions	Expert opinion
• Very large areas (e.g. bilateral lower limbs) should never be subjected to very low temperatures	Expert opinion

7.2.4 Hazards

● Cold burns.

7.2.5 Application and mandatory warnings

● The treatment can result in a cold burn.

1. Ice pack/towel

The ice pack/towel is applied directly to the area in question, ensuring appropriate contact between the cold source and the skin surface, e.g. water, oil or other medium.

A timed dosage is delivered.

The comfort and skin condition of the patient are checked at least once during the treatment period.

The skin normally becomes bright pink (possibly verging towards bright red) in colour – it should never show signs of becoming blue–red – a sign of venostasis. In the early stages blanching may occur.

2. Ice bath

The temperature of the ice bath is checked and considered to be appropriate.

The part is placed in the bath.

A timed dosage is delivered.

3. Ice massage

An ice cube may be brushed over dermatomes or myotomes to provide a stimulatory effect.

Ice cube massage can be effectively used as a replacement for ice pack therapy.

7.2.6 Treatment record

See 'Application for all agents' – *Recording.*

Supplementary reading: cold therapy

Basur R, Shephard E, Mouzos G (1976) A cooling method in the treatment of ankle sprains. *Practitioner* **216**: 708.

Curkovic B, Vitulic V, Babic-Naglic D, Durrigl T (1993) The influence of heat and cold on the pain threshold in rheumatoid arthritis. *Zeitschr für Rheumatol* **52**: 289–291.

Cuthill JA, Cuthill SC (2005) Partial thickness burn to the leg following application of a cold pack: case report and results of a questionnaire survey of Scottish physiotherapists in private practice. *Physiotherapy* **92**: 61–65.

Green GA, Zachazewski JE, Jordan SE (1989) Peroneal nerve palsy induced by cryotherapy. *Phys Sports Med* **17**(9): 63–70.

Harris ED, McCroskery PA (1974) The influence of temperature and fibril stability on degradation of cartilage collagen by rheumatoid synovial collegenase. *N Engl J Med* **290**: 1–6.

Hunter J, Kerr EH, Whillans MG (1952) The relation between joint stiffness upon exposure to cold and the characteristics of synovial fluid. *Can J Med Sci* **30**: 367–377.

Jutte LS, Merrick MA, Ingersoll CD, Edwards JE (2001) The relationship between intramuscular temperature, skin temperature and adipose thickness during cryotherapy and rewarming. *Arch Phys Med Rehab* **82**: 845–850.

Lee JM, Warren MP, Mason SM (1978) Effects of ice on nerve conduction velocity. *Physiotherapy* **64**: 2–6.

Lessard LA, Scudds RA, Amendola A, Vaz MD (1997) The effect of cryotherapy following arthroscopic knee surgery. *J Orthop Sports Phys Ther* **26**(1): 14–22.

McMaster WC, Liddle S, Waugh TR (1978) Laboratory evaluation of various cold therapy modalities. *Am J Sports Med* **6**(5): 291–294.

Melzac R, Jeans ME, Stratford JG, Monks RC (1980) Ice massage and transcutaneous electrical stimulation: comparison of treatment for low back pain. *Pain* **9**: 209–217.

Meussen R, Lievens P (1986) The use of cryotherapy in sports injuries. *Sports Med* **3**: 398–414.

Oliver RA, Johnson DJ, Wheelhouse WW et al (1979) Isometric muscle contraction response during recovery from reduced intramuscular temperature. *Arch Phys Med Rehab* **60**: 126.

Otte JW, Merrick MA, Ingersoll CD, Cordova ML (2002) Subcutaneous adipose tissue thickness alters cooling time during cryotherapy. *Arch Phys Med Rehab* **83**: 1501–1505.

Parker JT, Small NC, Davis DG (1983) Cold induced nerve palsy. *Athletic Training* **18**: 76.

Pegg SMH, Littler TR, Littler EN (1969) A trial of ice therapy and exercise in chronic arthritis. *Physiotherapy* **55**: 51–56.

Roberts D, Wallis C, Carlile J et al (1992) Relief of chronic low back pain: heat versus cold. In *Evaluation and Treatment of Chronic Pain*, Aronoff GM (ed), 2nd edn. Baltimore, MD, Urban and Schwarzenberg: 263–266.

Waylonis GW (1967) The physiological effect of ice massage. *Arch Phys Med Rehab* **48**: 37–41.

Wright V, Johns RJ (1961) Quantitative and qualitative analysis of joint stiffness in normal subjects and in patients with connective tissue disease. *Ann Rheumatol Dis* **20**: 26–36.

Yurtkurtan M, KocagilT (1999) Electroacupuncture and ice massage: a comparison of treatment for osteoarthritis of the knee. *Am J Acupuncture* **27**: 133–140.

Supplementary reading: contrast baths

Myrer JW, Draper DO, Durrant E (1994) Contrast therapy and intramuscular temperature in the human leg. *J Athletic Training* **29**(4): 318–322.

7.3 ELECTRICAL STIMULATION

7.3.1 Introduction

Read in conjunction with the generic information in Section 6.

Electrical stimulation involves the application of electrical currents to the tissues through the skin. Agents include:

- LOW FREQUENCY (typically < 250 Hz):
  - neuromuscular electrical stimulation (NMES), which is commonly used to stimulate muscle by means of the motor nerve
  - transcutaneous electrical nerve stimulation (TENS) which is commonly used for the relief of pain by means of afferent nerve stimulation.

- MEDIUM FREQUENCY
  - interferential therapy is the application of two medium-frequency currents (typically 2–6 kHz) to the skin to produce amplitude modulation at a low frequency (< 250 Hz) within the tissues
  - Russian stimulation is the application of medium frequency (2500 Hz) carrier current, interspersed with 10 ms periods when no current is flowing, producing 50 bursts per second.

There are numerous other forms of electrical stimulation not specifically identified above.

7.3.2 Contraindications.

None agent specific.

7.3.3 Precautions

	Reference
• Patients who have epilepsy, advanced cardiovascular conditions, e.g. severe angina or cardiac arrhythmias, should be treated at the discretion of the physiotherapist in consultation with the appropriate medical practitioner	012* 013*
• Transthoracic electrical stimulation should be applied with great caution	Expert opinion
• Caution should be used when applying suction electrodes where skin or tissue damage is likely, e.g. anticoagulant therapy, long-term steroid therapy	Expert opinion
• Avoid active epiphyseal regions in children	014*
• Select stimulation parameters to produce an appropriate level of muscle contraction. Inappropriate stimulation parameters may cause muscle damage, reduction in blood flow through the muscle and low-frequency muscle fatigue	Expert opinion

*012 Aldrich T, Laborde D et al (1992) A meta-analysis of the epidemiologic evidence regarding human health risk associated with exposure to electromagnetic fields. *Electro Magnetobiol* **11**(2): 127–143.

*013 Rosted P (2001) Repetitive epileptic fits-a possible adverse effect after transcutaneous electrical nerve stimulation (TENS) in a post-stroke patient. *Acupuncture Med* **19**(1): 46–49.

*014 Sato O, Akai M (1990) Effect of direct-current stimulation on the growth plate. In vivo study with rabbits. *Arch Orthop Trauma Surg* **109**(1): 9–13.

7.3.4 Hazards

- Skin burns, e.g. currents that involve a net DC component or excess current density. This can be minimized by the use of zero net DC current
- Haematomas may occur when using suction electrodes

- Electrical shock

Supplementary reading: electrical stimulation

Bomba G, Kowalski IM, Szarek J et al (2001) The effect of spinal electrostimulation on the testicular structure in rabbit. *Med Sci Monit* **7**(3): 363–368.

Broadley AJ (2000) The diagnostic dilemma of 'pseudopacemaker spikes.' *Pacing Clin Electrophysiol* **23**(2): 286–288.

Bundsen P, Ericson K (1982) Pain relief in labor by transcutaneous electrical nerve stimulation. Safety aspects. *Acta Obstet Gynecol Scand* **61**(1): 1–5.

Bundsen P, Ericson K, Peterson LE et al (1982) Pain relief in labor by transcutaneous electrical nerve stimulation. Testing of a modified stimulation technique and evaluation of the neurological and biochemical condition of the newborn infant. *Acta Obstet Gynecol Scand* **61**(2): 129–136.

Bundsen P, Peterson LE, et al (1981) Pain relief in labor by transcutaneous electrical nerve stimulation. A prospective matched study. *Acta Obstet Gynecol Scand* **60**(5): 459–468.

Burck G, Hentschel R, Wledemann D et al (1988) [Modification of cardiac pacemakers of the MCP and LCP series by electrodiagnostic and electrotherapy procedures].' *Z Gesamte Inn Med* **43**(20): 572–576.

Capelle HH, Simpson RK Jr, Kronenbuerger M et al (2005) Long-term deep brain stimulation in elderly patients with cardiac pacemakers. *J Neurosurg* **102**(1): 53–59.

Chen D, Philip M, Philip PA et al (1990) Cardiac pacemaker inhibition by transcutaneous electrical nerve stimulation. *Arch Phys Med Rehab* **71**(1): 27–30 [published erratum appears in *Arch Phys Med Rehab* 1990 **71**(6): 388].

Doyle J, Kobetic R, Marsolais EB et al (1992) 'Effect of functional neuromuscular stimulation on anterior tibial compartment pressure.' *Clin Orthop Relat Res* (284): 181–188.

Dunn PA, Rogers D, Halford K et al (1989) Transcutaneous electrical nerve stimulation at acupuncture points in the induction of uterine contractions. *Obstet Gynecol* **73**(2): 286–290.

Genbun Y (1991) [The effects of electrical stimulation on epiphyseal cartilage]. *Nippon Ika Daigaku Zasshi* **58**(4): 21–28.

Griffin DT, Dodd NJ, Moore JV et al (1994) The effects of low-level direct current therapy on a preclinical mammary carcinoma: tumour regression and systemic biochemical sequelae. *Br J Cancer* **69**(5): 875–878.

Habal MB (1980). Effect of applied dc currents on experimental tumor growth in rats. *J Biomed Mater Res* **14**(6): 789–801.

Hardell L, Holmberg B, Malker H et al (1995) Exposure to extremely low frequency electromagnetic fields and the risk of malignant diseases – an evaluation of epidemiological and experimental findings. *Eur J Cancer Prevention* **4**(S1): 3–107.

Heiberg E, Nalesnik WJ, Janney C (1991) Effects of varying potential and electrolytic dosage in direct current treatment of tumors. *Acta Radiol* **32**(2): 174–177.

Jarm T, Cemazar M, Steinberg F et al (2003) Pertubation of blood flow as a mechanism of anti-tumour action of direct current electrotherapy. *Physiol Meas* **24**: 75–90.

Jarm T, Wickramasinghe YA, Deakin M et al (1999) Blood perfusion of subcutaneous tumours in mice following the application of low-level direct electric current. *Adv Exp Med Biol* **471**: 497–506.

Kyank HR, Seidenschnur G (1988) [Intrauterine growth retardation-CTG findings in pre-partum oxygen respiration and transcutaneous nerve stimulation]. *Zentralbl Gynakol* **110**(22): 1407–1415.

Madersbacher H, Fischer J (1993) Sacral anterior root stimulation: prerequisites and indications. *Neurourol Urodyn* **12**(5): 489–494.

May AE, Elton CD (1998) The effects of pain and its management on mother and fetus. *Baillières Clin Obstet Gynaecol* **12**(3): 423–441.

O'Clock GD (1997) The effects of in vitro electrical stimulation on eukaryotic cells: suppression of malignant cell proliferation. *J Orthomol Med* **12**(3): 173–181.

Paterson DC, Lewis GN, Cass CA et al (1980) Treatment of delayed union and nonunion with an implanted direct current stimulator. *Clin Orthop Relat Res* **148**: 117–28.

Philippon J, Fohanno D, Gazengel J (1977) [Treatment of chronic pain syndromes by transcutaneous stimulation. Preliminary results. A propos of 40 cases]. *Neurochirurgie* **23**(1): 89–92.

Pyatt JR, Trenbath D, Chester M, Connelly DT (2003) The simultaneous use of a biventricular implantable cardioverter defibrillator (ICD) and transcutaneous electrical nerve stimulation (TENS) unit: implications for device interaction. *Europace* **5**(1): 91–93.

Rosen T, de Veciana M, Miller HS et al (2003) A randomized controlled trial of nerve stimulation for relief of nausea and vomiting in pregnancy. *Obstet Gynecol* **102**(1): 129–135.

Rosted P (2001) Repetitive epileptic fits-a possible adverse effect after transcutaneous electrical nerve stimulation (TENS) in a post-stroke patient. *Acupuncture Med* **19**(1), 46–49.

Sato O, Akai M (1990) Effect of direct-current stimulation on the growth plate. In vivo study with rabbits. *Arch Orthop Trauma Surg* **109**(1): 9–13.

Sauermann S, Bijak M, Schmutterer C et al (1997). Computer aided adjustment of the phrenic pacemaker: automatic functions, documentation, and quality control. *Artif Organs* **21**(3): 216–218.

Seif C, Junemann KP, Braun PM et al (2004) Deafferentation of the urinary bladder and implantation of a sacral anterior root stimulator (SARS) for treatment of the neurogenic bladder in paraplegic patients. *Biomed Tech (Berl)* **49**(4): 88–92.

Shade SK (1985) Use of transcutaneous electrical nerve stimulation for a patient with a cardiac pacemaker. A case report. *Phys Ther* **65**(2): 206–208.

Slotnick RN (2001) Safe, successful nausea suppression in early pregnancy with P-6 acustimulation. *J Reprod Med* **46**(9): 811–814.

Sluka KA, Walsh D (2003) TENS: basic science mechanisms and clinical effectiveness. *J Pain* **4**(3): 109.

Tal Z, Frankel ZN, Ballas S et al (1988) Breast electrostimulation for the induction of labor. *Obstet Gynecol* **72**(4): 671–674.

Taylor TV, Engler P, Pullan BR et al (1994) Ablation of neoplasia by direct current. *Br J Cancer* **70**(2): 342–345.

Tronnier VM, Staubert A, Hahnel S et al (1999) Magnetic resonance imaging with implanted neurostimulators: an in vitro and in vivo study. *Neurosurgery* **44**(1): 118–125; discussion 125–126.

Turler A, Schaefer H, Schaefer N et al (2000) Local treatment of hepatic metastases with low-level direct electric current: experimental results. *Scand J Gastroenterol* **35**(3): 322–328.

Turler A, Schaefer H, Schaefer N et al (2000) Experimental low-level direct current therapy in liver metastases: influence of polarity and current dose. *Bioelectromagnetics* **21**(5): 395–401.

Tuschl H, Neubauer G, Garn H et al (1999). Occupational exposure to high frequency electromagnetic fields and its effect on human immune parameters. *Int J Occup Med Environ Health* **12**(3): 239–251.

van der Ploeg JM, Vervest HA, Liem AL et al (1996) Transcutaneous nerve stimulation (TENS) during the first stage of labour: a randomized clinical trial. *Pain* **68**(1): 75–78.

Vodovnik L, Miklavcic D, Sersa G et al (1992) Modified cell proliferation due to electrical currents. *Med Biol Eng Comput* **30**(4): CE21–CE28.

Wang Y, Hassouna MM (1999) Electrical stimulation has no adverse effect on pregnant rats and fetuses. *J Urol* **162**(5): 1785–1787.

7.3.5 Application and mandatory warnings

See Section 6.

Preparation:

● The electrode covers (for rubber electrodes) or sponge inserts (for suction application) are in good condition and suitably moistened.

● Adjustable parameters (frequency, pulse width, pulse shape, ramping, duty cycle, timer) are set to those required for the treatment.

Application:

● Where appropriate the patient is advised on reducing and increasing the intensity (e.g. TENS); if the patient feels any pain stop the treatment immediately, resume using a lower intensity.

7.3.6 Treatment record

See 'Application for all agents' – *Recording.*

7.4 HIGH FREQUENCY THERAPY

Read in conjunction with the generic information in Section 6.

7.4.1 Introduction

These agents include microwave diathermy, shortwave diathermy and pulsed shortwave therapy.

Microwave diathermy (MWD) involves the use of a particular frequency of electromagnetic radiation which falls within the 300 MHz–300 GHz band.

Shortwave diathermy (SWD) is an electromagnetic radiation, coming from the high-frequency part of the electromagnetic spectrum. Therapeutic machines utilize a frequency of 27.12 MHz, and a corresponding wavelength of 11 metres.

Pulsed shortwave therapy (PSWT) involves the intermittent application of SWD at 27.12 MHz delivered in short duration pulses (20–400 μs) and with a variable number of pulses per second (20–800).

7.4.2 Contraindications

	Reference
● It is unsafe to deliver more than 5 watts mean power when there is metal in the tissue	015*
● Metal plinths/furniture are generally considered unacceptable when applied mean power is more than 5 watts	015*

*015 Chartered Society of Physiotherapy (CSP) (2001) Physios warned of diathermy danger. *Frontline* **7**: 9.

Supplementary reading

Bricknell R, Watson T (1995) The thermal effects of pulsed shortwave therapy. *Br J Ther Rehab* **2**(8): 430–434.

7.4.3 Precautions

Safety

In the interest of the physiotherapist's safety, it is recommended that once the machine has been switched on, the physiotherapist and all other personnel keep at least one metre from the operating machine, leads and electrodes. Pregnant physiotherapists or others with concerns may want to ask a colleague to turn the machine on. Almost all modern machines turn themselves off. It is recommended that physiotherapists consult the 'Safe Practice with Electrotherapy (Shortwave Therapies)' document (CSP 1997), for further information.

Supplementary reading

(1987) Evaluation report: shortwave therapy units. *J Med Eng Technol* **11**(6): 285–298.

(1988) Health Protection Branch of Health & Welfare Canada. *Physiother Canada* **40**: 205–206.

(1997) Electrotherapy and the risks. *Physiother Frontline* **3**(11): 10–11.

Aldrich T, Laborde D, et al (1992) A meta-analysis of the epidemiologic evidence regarding human health risk associated with exposure to electromagnetic fields. *Electro Magnetobiol* **11**(2): 127–143.

Bassen HI, Coakley RF Jr (1981) United States radiation safety and regulatory considerations for radiofrequency hyperthermia systems. *J Microw Power* **16**(2): 215–226.

Friend B (1997) Keep your distance. Do not stand within one metre of shortwave electrotherapy. *Physiother Frontline* **3**(1): 7.

Other electrophysical apparatus

It is recommended that other electrophysical devices, especially electrical stimulation apparatus, be kept at least two metres from the machine. The output of some machines (e.g. interferential therapy devices) can be affected by close proximity to an operating high-frequency machine. Departments/physiotherapists should establish the conflicts between their particular machine and electrical stimulation apparatus as these will not be the same for all combinations of equipment. It is considered unwise to operate two high-frequency machines simultaneously without maintaining a separation of at least 3 metres.

● Hearing aids and similar devices should removed from the field prior to commencement of the treatment.

● Avoid treatment of the abdomen and pelvic region during menstruation.

● Thermal treatments may aggravate acute inflammatory lesions.

7.4.4 Hazards

● Thermal burn	● Scald (if the skin is wet/damp after the skin sensation check)

7.4.5 Application and mandatory warnings

Safety:

There is some controversy as to the thermal nature of pulsed treatments, but in the light of recent research, it is suggested that in order to stay below the level at which thermal accumulation may occur, a mean power of less than 5 watts should be employed if tissue heating is considered inappropriate.

For thermal applications ensure there is no metal in the field adjacent to or on the patient, e.g. jewellery, chairs, treatment couch, wheelchair.

Preparation:

The skin is thoroughly dried following the thermal sensation test and prior to treatment.

Application:

● The cables are clear of the machine, the patient and the couch.

● When applying a thermal dose, the patient should feel only feel a mild warmth. Any sensation greater than mild warmth could cause a burn.

● The patient should not move during the treatment and should remain aware of the heat being produced throughout.

7.4.6 Treatment record

See 'Application for all agents' – *Recording*.

Supplementary reading

(1987) Evaluation report: shortwave therapy units. *J Med Eng Technol* **11**(6): 285–298.

(1997) Electrotherapy and the risks. *Physiother Frontline* **3**(11): 10–11.

Aldrich T, Laborde D, Griffith J et al (1992) A meta-analysis of the epidemiologic evidence regarding human health risk associated with exposure to electromagnetic fields. *Electro Magnetobiol* **11**(2): 127–143.

Auda SP, Hall G, Elias J et al (1979) Selective tumor heating and growth retardation by shortwave radiofrequency. *Surg Forum* **30**: 154–156.

Auda SP, Steinert HR, Elias EG et al (1980) Selective tumor heating by shortwave radiofrequency (RF). *Cancer* **46**(9): 1962–1968.

Bassen HI, Coakley RF Jr (1981) United States radiation safety and regulatory considerations for radiofrequency hyperthermia systems. *J Microw Power* **16**(2): 215–226.

Bocker B, Callies R, Zenner I (1992) [Pregnancy and shortwave therapy]. *Geburtshilfe Frauenheilkd* **52**(6): 378.

Bricknell R, Watson T (1995) The thermal effects of pulsed shortwave therapy. *Br J Ther Rehab* **2**(8): 430–434.

Brown-Woodman PD, Hadley JA, Waterhouse J et al (1988) Teratogenic effects of exposure to radiofrequency radiation (27.12 MHz) from a shortwave diathermy unit. *Indust Health* **26**(1): 1–10.

Brown-Woodman PD, Hadley JA, Richardson L et al (1989) Evaluation of reproductive function of female rats exposed to radiofrequency fields (27.12 MHz) near a shortwave diathermy device. *Health Phys* **56**(4): 521–525.

Chantraine A (1977) [High-frequency currents: indications and contra-indications]. *Z Unfallmed Berufskr* **70**(4): 202–208.

Chartered Society of Physiotherapy (CSP) (2001) Physios warned of diathermy danger. *Physiother Frontline* **7**: 9.

Chung MK, Kim JC, Myung SH (2004) Lack pf adverse effects in pregnant/lactating female rats and their offspring following pre- and postnatal exposure to ELF magnetic fields. *Bioelectromagnetics* **25**: 236–244.

Coppell RB (1988) Survey of stray electromagnetic emissions from microwave and shortwave diathermy equipment. *NZ J Physiother* **16**(3): 9–14.

Delpizzo V, Joyner K (1987) On the safe use of microwave and shortwave diathermy units. *Aust J Physiother* **33**(3): 152–158.

Docker M, Bazin S, Dyson M et al (1992) Guidelines for the safe use of continuous shortwave therapy equipment. *Physiotherapy* **78**(10): 755–757.

Elwood JM (2003) Epidemiological studies of radiofrequency exposures and human cancer. *Bioelectromagnetics* **Suppl 6**: S63–S73.

Friend B (1997) Keep your distance. Do not stand within one metre of shortwave electrotherapy. *Physiother Frontline* **3**(1): 7.

Goldsmith J (1996) Epidemiologic studies of radiofrequency radiation – current status and areas of concern. *Sci Total Environ* **180**(1): 3–8.

Guberan E, Campana A, Faval P et al (1994) Gender ratio of offspring and exposure to shortwave radiation amongst female physiotherapists. *Scand J Work Environ Health* **20**(5): 345–348.

Hamburger S, Logue JN, Silverman PM et al (1983) Occupational exposure to non-ionizing radiation and an association with heart disease: an exploratory study. *J Chronic Dis* **36**(11): 791–802.

Hardell L, Holmberg B, Malker H et al (1995) Exposure to extremely low frequency electromagnetic fields and the risk of malignant diseases – an evaluation of epidemiological and experimental findings. *Eur J Cancer Prev* **4**(S1): 3–107.

Heick A, Espersen T, Pedersen HL et al (1991) Is diathermy safe in women with copper-bearing IUDs? *Acta Obstet Gynecol Scand* **70**(2): 153–155.

Heynick LN, Merritt JH (2003) Radiofrequency fields and teratogenesis. *Bioelectromagnetics* **Suppl 6**: S174–S186.

Heynick LN, Johnston SA, Mason PA et al (2003) Radio frequency electromagnetic fields: cancer, mutagenesis and genotoxicity. *Bioelectromagnetics* **Suppl 6**: S74–S100.

Hocking B, Joyner K (1995) Miscarriages among female physical therapists who report using radio-frequency and microwave-frequency electromagnetic radiation. *Am J Epidemiol* **141**(3): 273–274.

Jones SL (1976) Electromagnetic field interference and cardiac pacemakers. *Phys Ther* **56**(9): 1013–1018.

Larsen A (1991) Congenital malformations and exposure to high frequency electromagnetic radiation among Danish physiotherapists. *Scand J Work Environ Health* **17**(5): 318–323.

Larsen A, Olsen J, Svane O (1991) Gender specific reproductive outcome and exposure to high frequency electromagnetic radiation among physiotherapists. *Scand J Environ Health* **17**: 324–329.

Leitgeb N (1993) Analysis of epidemiologic studies on cancer risks caused by magnetic fields. *Biomedizinische Technik* **38**(5): 111–116.

Lerman Y, Jacubovich R, Caner A et al (1996) Electromagnetic fields from shortwave diathermy equipment in physiotherapy departments. *Physiotherapy* **82**(8): 456–458.

Logue J, Hamburger S, Silverman PM et al (1985) Congenital anomalies and paternal occupational exposure to shortwave, microwave, infrared and acoustic radiation. *J Occup Med* **27**(6): 451–452.

Marino A (1993) Electromagnetic fields, cancer and the theory of neuroendocrine related promotion. *Bioelectrochem Bioenerget* **29**(3): 255–276.

Martin C, McCallum HM, Heaton B et al (1990) An evaluation of radiofrequency exposure from therapeutic diathermy equipment in the light of current recommendations. *Clin Phys Physiol Meas* **11**(1): 53–63.

Martin C, McCallum H, Strelley S et al (1991) Electromagnetic fields from therapeutic diathermy equipment: a review of hazards & precautions. *Physiotherapy* **77**(1): 3–7.

Matsui N, Ohta H, Otsoka T et al (1989) [Hyperthermia in malignant tumors of the extremities—experimental heating by a radiofrequency applicator and its clinical significance]. *Gan To Kagaku Ryoho* **16**(4 Pt 2–3): 1788–1794.

McDowell AD, Lunt MJ (1991) Electromagnetic field strength measurements on megapulse units. *Physiotherapy* **77**(12): 805–809.

Meltz ML (2003) Radiofrequency exposure and mammalian cell toxicity, genotoxicity and transformation. *Bioelectromagnetics* **Suppl 6**: S196–S213.

Miyagi N, Sato K, Rong Y et al (2000) Effects of PEMF on a murine osteosarcoma cell line: drug-resistant (P-glycoprotein-positive) and non-resistant cells. *Bioelectromagnetics* **21**: 112–121.

Osepchuk JM, Petersen RC (2003) Historical review of RF exposure standards and the International Committee on Electromagnetic Safety (ICES). *Bioelectromagnetics* **Suppl 6**: S7–S16.

Ouellet-Hellstrom R, Stewart WF (1993) Miscarriages among female physical therapists who report using radio- and microwave-frequency electromagnetic radiation [see comments]. *Am J Epidemiol* **138**(10): 775–786.

Pachocki KA, Gajewski AK (1991) Exposure to electromagnetic fields and risk of leukemia. *Rocz Panstw Zakl Hig* **42**(3): 217–221.

Pang L, Traitcheva N, Gothe G et al (2002) Elf-electromagnetic fields inhibit the proliferation of human cancer cells and induce apoptosis. *Electromagnet Biol Med* **21**(3): 243–248.

Pyrpasopoulou A, Kotoula V, Cheva A et al (2003) Bone morphogenic protein expression in newborn rat kidneys after prenatal exposure to radiofrequency radiation. *Bioelectromagnetics* **25**: 216–227.

Rongen MJ, Beets-Tan RG, Backes WH et al (2004) The effects of high field strength MRI on electrodes and pulse generator in dynamic graciloplasty. *Colorectal Dis* **6**(2): 113–116.

Savitz D (1993) Overview of epidemiologic research on electric and magnetic fields and cancer. *Am Ind Hyg Assoc J* **54**(4): 197–204.

Scherder E, Van Someren E, Swaab D et al (1999) Epilepsy: a possible contraindication for transcutaneous electrical nerve stimulation. *J Pain Symptom Manage* **17**(3): 152–153.

Scowcroft AT, Mason AH, Hayne CR (1977). Safety with microwave diathermy: Preliminary report of the CSP working party. *Physiotherapy* **63**(11): 359–361.

Shields N, Gormley J, O'Hare N (2001) Short-wave diathermy in Irish physiotherapy departments. *Br J Ther Rehab* **8**(9): 331–339.

Shields N, Gormley J, O'Hare N (2002) Contraindications to continuous and pulsed short-wave diathermy. *Phys Ther Rev* **7**: 133–143.

Shields N, O'Hare N, Gormley J (2003) Short-wave diathermy and pregnancy: what is the evidence? *Adv Physiother* **5**(1): 2–14.

Shields N, O'Hare N, Gormley N et al (2004) Contra-indications to shortwave diathermy: Survey of Irish physiotherapists. *Physiotherapy* **90**: 42–53.

Taskinen H, Kyyronen P, Hemminki K (1990) Effects of ultra-sound, shortwaves and physical exertion on pregnancy outcome in physiotherapists. *J Epidemiol Commun Health* **44**: 196–201.

Tuschl H, Neubauer G, Garn H et al (1999) Occupational exposure to high frequency electromagnetic fields and its effect on human immune parameters. *Int J Occup Med Environ Health* **12**(3): 239–51.

Valtonen EJ, Lilius HG, Tiula E (1975) Disturbances in the function of cardiac pacemaker caused by short wave and microwave diathermies and pulsed high frequency cur-rent. *Ann Chir Gynaecol Fenn* **64**(5): 284–287.

Verschaeve L (1995) Can nonionising radiation induce can-cer. *Cancer J* **8**(5): 237–249.

Wessman HC (1971) Effect of shortwave diathermy to the abdomen on peripheral circulation during pregnancy. *Phys Ther* **51**(1): 43–47.

Williams CD, Markov MS (2001) Therapeutic electromag-netic field effects on angiogenesis during tumor growth: a pilot study in mice. *Electro Magnet Biol* **20**(3): 323–329.

Yerman Y, Jacubovich R, Caner A et al (1996) Electromagnetic fields from shortwave diathermy equipment in physio-therapy departments. *Physiotherapy* **82**(8): 456–458.

7.5 HOT PACKS/BATHS

Read in conjunction with the generic information in Section 6.

7.5.1 Introduction

Hot packs and baths may be used to provide local con-tact heating (conductive heating), normally to rela-tively small areas. A tissue temperature of around 40–42°C is the accepted norm.

7.5.2 Contraindications

	Reference
None agent specific.	Expert opinion

7.5.3 Precautions

	Reference
• Never allow a patient to lie on top of a hot pack, particularly if treating the trunk	Expert opinion
• Avoid using hot packs on very overweight patients as the tissues may not dissipate the heat efficiently and thus lead to a burn	Expert opinion
• Moisture may encourage damaged or infected skin to break down	Expert opinion

7.5.4 Hazards

• Thermal burns	• Oedema
• Blistering	

7.5.5 Application and mandatory warnings

Hot packs are applied using appropriate insulation materials to prevent overheating.

The patient is checked after 5 minutes and further insulation added if there is a mottled erythema.

The patient should feel only a mild warmth. Any sensation greater than mild warmth could cause a burn.

Preparation:

The integrity and temperature of the hot pack/baths are checked.

7.5.6 Treatment record

See 'Application for all agents' – *Recording*.

Supplementary reading

Batavia M (2004) Contraindications for superficial heat and therapeutic ultrasound: do sources agree? *Arch Phys Med Rehab* **85**(6): 1006–1012.

7.6 INFRARED (IR)

Read in conjunction with the generic information in Section 6.

7.6.1 Introduction

Infrared is an electromagnetic radiation coming from the region of the electromagnetic spectrum which gives rise to heating. The radiations lie between microwaves and visible light on the spectrum and have a wavelength of between 780 and 1 000 000 nm.

That of clinical IR is normally between 700 and 1500 nm.

7.6.2 Contraindications

None agent specific.

7.6.3 Precautions

	Reference
• Never position the lamp so that it could fall onto the patient.	Norm

7.6.4 Hazards

- Thermal burns
- Oedema
- Blistering
- Permanent pigmentation (with prolonged use)

7.6.5 Application and mandatory warnings

Safety

● The patient should feel only a mild warmth. Any sensation greater than mild warmth could cause a burn.

Preparation:

● The mechanical safety of the lamp (stability, secure joints and screws) is checked.

● The lamp is placed 60–80 cm away from the body part, the final distance being governed by the patient response.

● The lamp is positioned parallel to, but not directly above, the area to be treated.

Application:

● The comfort and skin condition of the patient are checked at least once during the treatment period.

7.6.6 Treatment record

See 'Application for all agents' – *Recording*.

Supplementary reading

Batavia M (2004) Contraindications for superficial heat and therapeutic ultrasound; do sources agree? *Arch Phys Med Rehab* **85**: 1006–1012.

Kitchen S (ed) (2002) *Electrotherapy: Evidence-based Practice*. Edinburgh, Churchill Livingstone.
Lehmann J (1982) *Therapeutic Heat and Cold*. Baltimore, MD, Williams & Wilkins.
Lehmann JF, de Lateur BJ (1989) Ultrasound, shortwave, microwave, superficial heat and cold in the treatment of pain. *Textbook of Pain* **20**(2): 932–941.
Low J, Reed A (2000) *Electrotherapy Explained: Principles And Practice*, 3rd edn. Oxford, Butterworth–Heinemann.
Michlovitz S (1996) *Thermal Agents in Rehabilitation*. Philadelphia, FA Davis.
Nadler SF, Prybicien M, Malanga GA et al (2003) Complications from therapeutic modalities: results of a national survey of athletic trainers. *Arch Phys Med Rehab* **84**(6): 849–853.

7.7 LASER THERAPY

Read in conjunction with the generic information in Section 6.

7.7.1 Introduction

This agent is also known as low intensity laser therapy (LILT) or low level laser therapy (LLLT). Terms such as 'cold' laser therapy or 'biostimulation' are confusing and should be avoided. Therapy is based upon irradiation of tissue to accelerate wound healing processes and to relieve pain using laser sources (gaseous or, more commonly, diode-based) and/or so-called superluminous diodes, typically operating in the visible red or near infrared parts of the electromagnetic spectrum (i.e. 600–950 nm). Such units do not exceed radiant power outputs of 500 mW per single source, but may incorporate multidiode arrays with total radiant outputs well in excess of this. Regardless of the total power output, laser therapy units are essentially athermic and irradiation should normally cause no discernible rise in tissue temperature.

7.7.2 Contraindications

	Reference
• Increased sensitivity to light.	Expert opinion

7.7.3 Precautions

	Reference
None agent specific	Expert opinion

7.7.4 Hazards

None agent specific.

7.7.5 Application and mandatory warnings

● Appropriate eye protection (e.g. goggles) is used at all times during treatment to prevent potential ocular damage to both patients and practitioners from accidental intrabeam viewing.

● Patient should not feel discomfort or heating.

● Patient should not look directly at output from treatment head.

7.7.6 Treatment record

See 'Application for all agents' – *Recording.*

Supplementary reading

Baxter D (1994) *Therapeutic Lasers: Theory and Practice.* Edinburgh, Churchill Livingstone.
Bissell JH (1999) Therapeutic modalities in hand surgery. *J Hand Surg (Am)* **24**(3): 435–448.
Karu T (1998) *The Science of Low-Power Laser Therapy.* Amsterdam, Gordon & Breach.
Kitchen S (ed) (2002) *Electrotherapy: Evidence-based Practice.* Edinburgh, Churchill Livingstone.
Lampe KE (1998) Electrotherapy in tissue repair. *J Hand Ther* **11**(2): 131–139.
Low J, Reed A (2000) *Electrotherapy Explained: Principles and Practice,* 3rd edn. Oxford, Butterworth–Heinemann.
Nussbaum EL, Baxter GD, Lilge L (2003) A review of laser technology and light-tissue interactions as a background to therapeutic applications of low intensity lasers and other light sources. *Phys Ther Rev* **8**: 31–44.
Peterson HA, Wood MB (2001) Physeal arrest due to laser beam damage in a growing child. *J Pediatr Orthop* **21**(3): 335–337.
Pukach LP (1993) [The indications and contraindications for laser therapy]. *Voen Med Zh* **2**(23): 25–26.
Santana-Blank L (2004) Contraindications in noninvasive laser therapy: truth and fiction. *Photomed Laser Surg* **22**(5): 442.
Tuner J, Hode L (2002) *Laser Therapy: Clinical Practice & Scientific Background.* Grangesberg, Sweden, Prima Books.

7.8 ULTRASOUND (US)

Read in conjunction with the generic information in Section 6.

7.8.1 Introduction

Ultrasound is a mechanical vibration that results in the molecules of a material through which it can pass, such as biological tissues, oscillating or vibrating. This occurs at a frequency above the upper limit of human hearing, generally taken as being in excess of 20 kHz. Most therapeutic machines utilize frequencies in the low megahertz (MHZ) range, i.e. 0.5–3 MHz. The guidance in this document is applicable to MHz therapeutic ultrasound.

7.8.2 Contraindications

None agent specific.

7.8.3 Precautions

None agent specific.

7.8.4 Hazards

	Reference
● Reversible blood cell stasis can occur in small blood vessels if a standing wave field is produced while treating over a reflector such as an air/soft tissue interface, soft tissue/bone or soft tissue/metal interface while using a stationary applicator; continuous movement of the applicator removes this hazard.	016*

*016 Fry FJ, Sanghvi NT, Foster RS et al (1995). Ultrasound and microbubbles: their generation, detection and potential utilization in tissue and organ therapy – experimental. *Ultrasound Med Biol* 21(9): 1227–1237.

7.8.5 Application and mandatory warnings

Safety:

● The treatment applicator should be kept in motion throughout the treatment.

● If the patient feels any pain, reduce the treatment intensity, and if the sensation persists, terminate the treatment.

Preparation:

An appropriate coupling medium should be employed in order to ensure energy transmission to the tissue

7.8.6 Treatment record

See 'Application for all agents' – *Recording.*

Supplementary reading

Barnett SB, Rott HD, ter Haar GR et al (1997) The sensitivity of biological tissue to ultrasound. *Ultrasound Med Biol* **23**(6): 805–812.

Carnes KI, Drewniak JL, Dunn F (1991) In utero measurement of ultrasonically induced fetal mouse temperature increases. *Ultrasound Med Biol* **17**(4): 373–382.

Fry FJ, Sanghvi NT, Foster RS et al (1995) Ultrasound and microbubbles: their generation, detection and potential utilization in tissue and organ therapy – experimental. *Ultrasound Med Biol* **21**(9): 1227–1237.

Goodfriend R (1984) Ultrasonic and electrohydraulic lithotripsy of ureteral calculi. *Urology* **23**(1): 5–8.

Guo Y, Zhou L (1993) [The effect of high energy shock waves on growth and metastasis of implanted tumors of nude mice in vivo]. *Chung Hua I Hsueh Tsa Chih* **73**(7): 420–423.

Harrison GH, Balcer-Kubiczek EK, Eddy A et al (1991) Potentiation of chemotherapy by low-level ultrasound. *Int J Radiat Biol* **59**(6): 1453–1466.

Hay-Smith EJ (2000) Therapeutic ultrasound for postpartum perineal pain and dyspareunia. Cochrane Database Syst Rev(2): CD000495.

Hekkenberg R (1998) Characterising ultrasonic physiotherapy systems by performance and safety now internationally agreed. *Ultrasonics* **36**: 713–720.

Hekkenberg R, Oosterbaan W, van Beekum W (1986) Evaluation of ultrasound therapy devices: TNO test: radiation safety and dose accuracy often leave something to be desired. *Physiotherapy* **72**(8): 390–394.

Hekkenberg RT, Reibold R, Zeqiri B (1994) Development of standard measurement methods for essential properties of ultrasound therapy equipment. *Ultrasound Med Biol* **20**(1): 83–98.

Kerr CL, Gregory DW, Chan KK et al (1989) Ultrasound induced damage of veins in pig ears as revealed by scanning electron microscopy. *Ultrasound Med Biol* **15**(1): 45–52.

Lejbkowicz F, Zwiran M, Salzberg S (1993) The response of normal and malignant cells to ultrasound in vitro. *Ultrasound Med Biol* **19**(1): 75–82.

Lyon R, Liu XC, Meier J (2003) The effects of therapeutic vs. high intensity ultrasound on the rabbit growth plate. *J Orthop Res* **21**: 865–871.

McCabe M, Pye S (1997) Therapeutic Ultrasound: Risk associated with poor calibration. *Physiotherapy* **83**(5): 228.

Merrick MA, Bernard KD, Devor ST et al (2003) Identical 3-MHz ultrasound treatments with different devices produce different intramuscular temperatures. *J Orthop Sports Phys Ther* **33**(7): 379–385.

Miller MW, Nyborg WL, Dewey WC et al (2002) Hyperthermic teratogenicity, thermal dose and diagnostic ultrasound during pregnancy: implications of new standards on tissue heating. *Int J Hypertherm* **18**(5): 361–384.

Mohamed MM, Mohamed MA, Fikry M (2003) Enhancement of antitumor effects of 5-fluorouracil combined with ultrasound on Ehrlich ascites tumor in vivo. *Ultrasound Med Biol* **29**(11): 1635–1643.

Nacitarhan V, Elden H, Kisa M et al (2005) The effects of therapeutic ultrasound on heart rate variability, a placebo controlled trial. *Biology* **31**(5): 643–648.

Nolte PA, Klein-Nulend J, Albers GHR et al (2001) Low intensity ultrasound stimulates endochondral ossification in vitro. *J Orthop Res* **19**: 301–307.

Oakley EM (1978) Dangers and contra-indications of therapeutic ultrasound. *Physiotherapy* **64**(6): 173.

Ogurtan Z, Celik I, Izci C et al (2002) Effect of experimental therapeutic ultrasound on the distal antebrachial growth plates in one-month-old rabbits. *Vet J* **164**(3): 280–7.

Oosterhof GO, Cornel EB, Smits GA et al (1996) The influence of high-energy shock waves on the development of metastases. *Ultrasound Med Biol* **22**(3): 339–344.

Pye S (1996) Ultrasound therapy equipment – does it perform? *Physiotherapy* **82**(1): 39–44.

Pye S, Milford C (1994) The performance of ultrasound physiotherapy machines in Lothian region. *Ultrasound Med Biol* **4**: 347–359.

Reher P, Elbeshire NI, Harvey W et al (1997) The stimulation of bone formation in vitro by therapeutic ultrasound. *Ultrasound Med Biol* **23**(8): 1251–1258.

Sicard-Rosenbaum L, Danoff JV, Guthrie JA et al (1998) Effects of energy matched pulsed and continuous ultrasound on tumor growth in mice. *Phys Ther* **78**(3): 271–277.

Sicard-Rosenbaum L, Lord D, Danoff JV et al (1995) Effects of continuous therapeutic ultrasound on growth and metastasis of subcutaneous murine tumors. *Phys Ther* **75**(1): 3–13.

Spadaro JA, Albanese SA (1998) Application of low-intensity ultrasound to growing bone in rats. *Ultrasound Med Biol* **24**(4): 567–573.

Taskinen H, Kyyronen P, Hemminki K (1990) Effects of ultrasound, shortwaves and physical exertion on pregnancy outcome in physiotherapists. *J Epidemiol Commun Health* **44**: 196–201.

ter Haar G, Rivens I, Chen L et al (1991) High intensity focused ultrasound for the treatment of rat tumours. *Phys Med Biol* **36**(11): 1495–1501.

Wiltink A, Nijweide PJ, Oosterbaan WA et al (1995) Effect of therapeutic ultrasound on endochondral ossification. *Ultrasound Med Biol* **21**(1): 121–127.

7.9 ULTRAVIOLET RADIATION (UVR)

Read in conjunction with the generic information in Section 6.

7.9.1 Introduction

Ultraviolet radiation (UVR) covers a small part of the electromagnetic spectrum and spans the wavelength region from 400 to 100 nanometres (nm). The biological effects of UVR vary enormously with wavelength and for this reason the ultraviolet spectrum is further subdivided into three regions.

UVA	400–315 nm	Black light, will provide fluorescence in many substances and may encourage healing
UVB	315–280 nm	Will produce an erythema in skin
UVC	280–180 nm	Germicidal region

National Radiological Protection Board, 2004 figures; it is worth noting that bands are not fixed and other, albeit similar, values may be found in the literature.

Treatment of skin disease by exposure to UVR is termed *phototherapy*. When treatment with UVR is combined with a photosensitizing agent (for example *psoralen plus UVA* exposure – PUVA), the term *photochemotherapy* is used.

7.9.2 Contraindications

	Reference
In deciding which treatment to use, the diagnosis, extent or severity of the skin disorder, and the contraindications listed below (adapted from the British Photodermatology Group guidelines for PUVA) [*British Journal of Dermatology*, 1994], should be taken into account.	017*
• Photoallergy	018*
• Previous exposure to arsenic or ionizing radiation	018*
• Concomitant immunosuppressive therapy	018*

7.9.3 Precautions

• Those aged less than 16 years should be treated at the therapist's discretion	018* Expert opinion
• Previous or concomitant treatment with methotrexate	019*
• Check patient is not taking photosensitizing medication	019*
• Avoid unnecessary exposure to sunlight on treatment days	019*
• Avoid exposure of the male genitalia	020*
• Patient wears UV-opaque eye protection during treatment (and for remainder of day in case of PUVA)	Expert opinion
• Female patients, and male patients' female partners, should preferably avoid conception during treatment*	Expert opinion
• Cataracts*	Expert opinion
• Significant hepatic dysfunction*	Expert opinion

* Apply to PUVA only due to drug component of treatment.

*017 British Photodermatology Group (1994) Guidelines for PUVA. *Br J Dermatol* **130**: 246–255.

*018 Walker S, Hawk J, Young A (2003) Acute and chronic effects of UVR on the skin. In Freedberg I, Fison A, Wolff K et al (eds) *Fitzpatrick's Dermatology in General Medicine,* 6th edn, vol 1. New York, McGraw-Hill: 1275–1282.

*019 Low J, Bazin S, et al (1994) Guidelines for the safe use of ultraviolet therapy equipment. *Physiotherapy* **80**(2): 89–90.

*020 Stern RS (1990) Genital tumors among men with psoriasis exposed to psoralens and ultraviolet A radiation (PUVA) and ultraviolet B radiation. The Photochemotherapy Follow-up Study. *N Engl J Med* **322**(16): 1093–1097.

7.9.4 Hazards

• Excessive erythema	• Blistering
• Burns	• Acute eye damage if eye protection not worn
• Severe itching	• Local skin pain (puva only)
• Nausea (if oral psoralen used)	• Skin cancer

7.9.5 Application and mandatory warnings

Safety:

● Staff using UVR must wear eye protection and cover exposed skin.

● UV treatment cabinets should be safe and comfortable, for example non-slip flooring, the door will open from inside, and a safety alarm should be present.

Preparation:

● The ultraviolet treatment area is screened from other people.

● Patient sensitivity to UVR, previous exposure and medication must be ascertained.

● An erythema test dose must precede treatment.

● The treatment should be carried out with the lamp previously used on patient.

● The distance of application is accurately measured.

● Exposure is confined to the area being treated and is replicable.

- The patient should:
  - maintain adequate eye protection throughout the exposure.
  - keep still.

7.9.6 Treatment record

See 'Application for all agents' – *Recording.*

Supplementary reading – ultraviolet radiation

Goldsmith L, Katz S (eds) *Fitzpatrick's Dermatology in General Medicine*, 6th edn, vol 1. New York, McGraw-Hill: 1275–1282.

7.10 WAX

Read in conjunction with the generic information in Section 6.

7.10.1 Introduction

Paraffin wax, when melted, can be applied to the extremities to produce mild superficial heating of the tissues. Mineral oil is added to paraffin wax in order to lower its melting point to between 42°C and 50°C, for therapeutic use.

7.10.2 Contraindications

	Reference
• Unstable, fragile early-stage skin grafts	Expert opinion
• Open wounds/lesions	Expert opinion
• Local infection	Expert opinion

7.10.3 Precautions

	Reference
The dip and re-immerse method should be avoided in patients with oedema	Expert opinion
Cooler wax temperatures are required for the foot than the hand	Expert opinion

7.10.4 Hazards

- Thermal burns
- Blistering

7.10.5 Application and mandatory warnings

Preparation:

- The body part to be treated is washed and dried.

- The patient's clothes are protected from accidental spillage of wax.

Application:

- The patient should feel only a mild warmth. Any sensation greater than mild warmth could cause a burn.

7.10.6 Treatment record

See 'Application for all agents' – *Recording.*

Supplementary reading

Lehmann J (1982) *Therapeutic Heat and Cold.* Baltimore, MD, Williams & Wilkins.
Lehmann JF, de Lateur BJ (1989). Ultrasound, shortwave, microwave, superficial heat and cold in the treatment of pain. *Textbook of Pain* **20**(2): 932–941.
Low J, Reed A (2000). *Electrotherapy Explained: Principles and Practice*, 3rd edn. Oxford, Butterworth–Heinemann.
Michlovitz S (1996) *Thermal Agents in Rehabilitation.* Philadelphia, FA Davis.

SECTION 8: NOVEL AGENTS AND EQUIPMENT

Increasingly, physiotherapists find themselves in the position of trialling or using a 'novel' piece of equipment; essentially, such situations can usefully be considered as falling into two types:

- Use or trial of a new model of an existing agent e.g. ultrasound, TENS.

- Trial of a new agent.

8.1 USE OR TRIAL OF A NEW MODEL OF AN EXISTING AGENT

In these cases, the position of the physiotherapist is relatively straightforward, in that the biophysical principles, parameter specification and safety aspects will already be established for the agent (and thus the device in question), and appropriate recommendations, guidelines or standards for use (such as this document) will already be available. In such situations, the physiotherapist should ensure that:

- Necessary measures have been taken by the manufacturer or supplier to comply with appropriate legislative requirements e.g. in terms of electromagnetic compatibility, labelling e.g. kite-mark.

● The position surrounding product liability has been clarified, i.e. where equipment is loaned for a demonstration period. In this case, the majority of trusts or similar bodies will typically require some written undertaking from the manufacturer concerning indemnity for such loaned equipment, and physiotherapists in private practice should consider instituting similar arrangements in these circumstances.

In all such cases, the physiotherapist:

● Should insist on a full and detailed demonstration on the operation of the apparatus, including identifying and recording the output parameters of the particular machine to be used.

● Must take all reasonable steps to confirm its safe operation before instituting patient treatments.

Finally, whether the equipment is specifically loaned at the instigation of the manufacturer or distributor, or at the request of the physiotherapist, the physiotherapist's role should be clearly defined at the outset. Specifically, is this a loan to allow an extended trial of the apparatus prior to purchase or lease, or is the purpose to undertake market-based or field-testing on behalf of the company? In the latter case, the physiotherapist may need to consider potential requirements in terms of extension of indemnity cover, ethical permission and informed consent.

In these cases, regardless of any assurances regarding indemnity received in respect of the apparatus, the physiotherapist remains ultimately and solely responsible for any treatments performed, and should therefore take all reasonable steps to ensure the safety of the patient.

8.2 TRIAL OF A NEW AGENT

This situation would arise where a physiotherapist is approached, normally by a developer or manufacturer, to perform trials or tests on patients, or on healthy human volunteers, of agents which are not already in routine clinical practice. Such agents could be based upon the use of novel ranges or combinations of electrophysical parameters, or novel methods of application. In all such cases, while the biophysical principles underlying the new therapy may be well described and documented, e.g. in the literature provided by the developer or manufacturer, the biological, physiological and clinical effects will typically be unclear.

As a consequence, the safety of the agent, and particularly the contraindications to application, are likely to be poorly understood. All such work will therefore need to comply with current research governance procedures, including full written ethical permission and valid consent from patients and volunteers. NB: Private practitioners will need to identify an equivalent group responsible for research ethics with whom to seek approval. There may also be specific requirements or arrangements, for example in terms of payment, indemnity, etc., concerning what may be regarded as 'contracted research' by trusts or other similar bodies.

In these cases, it is specifically recommended that physiotherapists should not undertake any such trial work without prior consultation with relevant *independent* experts, for example in terms of trial design, biophysics, safety, etc. In these situations, advice is available through the Chartered Society of Physiotherapy, or through the Association of Chartered Physiotherapists Interested in Electrotherapy. This not withstanding, physiotherapists are explicitly reminded of the provisions of the Rules of Professional Conduct, which apply in all cases.

It is essential that physiotherapists consult the recent literature for a particular agent. Up to date literature can be accessed through a local library, or the Society's Information Resource Centre (telephone number 0207 306 6666).

SECTION 9: BIBLIOGRAPHY

GENERAL LITERATURE

Chartered Society of Physiotherapy (CSP) (2005) *Standards of Physiotherapy Practice*. London, CSP.

Chartered Society of Physiotherapy (CSP) (2003) *Policy statement on continuing professional development*. London, CSP.

Chartered Society of Physiotherapy (CSP) (2002) *Rules of Professional Conduct*. London, CSP.

Chartered Society of Physiotherapy (CSP) (2006) *Information Paper 6 – The Delegation of Tasks to Physiotherapy Assistants and Other Support Workers*. London, CSP.

Chartered Society of Physiotherapy (CSP) (1997) *Safe Practice with Electrotherapy (Shortwave Therapies)*. Health and Safety Briefing pack, No 4. London, CSP.

Consumer Protection Act, 1987. HMSO, London.

Goldsmith L, Katz S (eds) *Fitzpatrick's Dermatology in General Medicine*, 6th edn, vol 1. New York, McGraw-Hill: 1275–1282.

Health and Safety at Work Act 1974. HMSO, London.

Kitchen S (ed) (2002) *Electrotherapy: Evidence-based Practice*. Edinburgh, Churchill Livingstone.

Lehmann J (1990) *Therapeutic Heat and Cold*, 4th edn. Williams and Wilkins, MD, Baltimore.

Low J, Reed A (2000). *Electrotherapy Explained: Principles and Practice*, 3rd edn. Oxford, Butterworth–Heinemann.

Robertson V, Ward A, Low J, Reed A (2006) *Electrotherapy Explained: Principles and Practice*, 4th edn. Edinburgh, Butterworth–Heinemann.

ACKNOWLEDGEMENTS

The following contributed to the development of this publication:

● David Baxter, University of Otago, New Zealand

● Sarah Bazin, Heart of England NHS Foundation Trust

● Brian Diffy, Royal Victoria Infirmary, Newcastle-upon-Tyne

● Melvyn Docker, Retired

● Mary Dyson, Emeritus Reader in the Biology of Tissue Repair, King's College, London

● Sheila Kitchen, King's College, London

● David Maskill, Brunel University

● Suzanne McDonaugh, University of Ulster

● Ann Reed, University of East London

● Alison Skinner, University College, London

● Deirdre Walsh, University of Ulster

● Tim Watson, University of Hertfordshire

● Secretariat: Sue Finley, Heart of England NHS Foundation Trust

SECTION 10: APPENDIX 1: INFORMATION SHEET: ELECTROPHYSICAL AGENTS TREATMENT RECORD OF UNEXPECTED EFFECTS

INTRODUCTION

Current safety guidance provides clear criteria for the use of electrophysical agents, as well as providing information about possible dangers and contraindications. It is essential that the physiotherapy profession monitors all unexpected effects so that information can be provided to practitioners about the incidence and prevalence of both good and bad unexpected effects with the different agents. Such effects do arise; they are often fairly minor, but occasionally can be more serious.

DEFINITION

For the purpose of this reporting system *unexpected effects* will be defined as:

'an unexpected or unusual reaction, over and above the normal physiological or psychological effects expected'.

The following are examples of the types of incidence you might need to report:

Skin:	rash	Cardiorespiratory:	breathlessness
	irritation		
	unexpected reddening	Neurological:	numbness
	burns		pins and needles
	blisters		changes in muscle tone
	break down		
	peeling	Attitude:	not like
			scared
Eyes:	aching		waste of time
	conjunctivitis		
		Musculoskeletal:	joint aching
Symptoms:	pain		muscle aching
	nausea		pain
	headaches		
	dizziness		
	fainting		
	aching		
	vomiting		
	diarrhoea		

This list is not exhaustive – please report any others you encounter.

CONFIDENTIALITY

● No patient will be identified by name at any time.

● The practitioner may remain anonymous.

The form does ask for a contact name on an optional basis. This is to allow a limited group of no more that two individuals involved with auditing incidences to request additional information in order to clarify specific issues.

WHAT WILL HAPPEN TO THE INFORMATION:

Reports will be retained by the CSP. It will be analysed regularly to look for trends, which may be important for clinical practice and research. Data will be available to members via the CSP website.

ELECTROPHYSICAL AGENTS TREATMENT
RECORD OF UNEXPECTED EFFECTS

Please complete as much of this form as possible, inserting ticks [✓] in the boxes as appropriate or fill in your own answers.

Section I: The patient

1. Male ☐   Female ☐

2. Age of patient   _____ years

3. Condition being treated: _____

4. Other diagnosed conditions: _____

5. For what reason(s) were you using the agent?   _____

Section II: The treatment

6. What treatment agent(s) were you using?   _____

    _____

7. Was this the first time you used this agent with this patient?   Yes ☐   No ☐

8. List any other physiotherapy treatment(s) you were giving: _____

    _____

9. List any drugs you know your patient was receiving at the same time: _____

    _____

10. List any other treatments you know your patient was receiving at the same time: _____

    _____

11. What treatment dosage were you using?
    Machine settings   _____
    Length of treatment   _____
    Area of the body being treated   _____

12. What make/model of machine were you using?   _____

    _____

Section III: The unexpected effect

13.   Describe the unexpected effect that occurred: _____

_____

_____

14.   In your opinion, was this effect: mild ☐   moderate ☐   severe ☐

15.   How soon after the treatment did the effect occur? _____

16.   How long did the effect last for? _____

17.   Did the patient require treatment for the effect: Yes ☐   No ☐

18.   Did you repeat the same treatment for this patient?   Yes ☐   No ☐

      If yes, did the same effect occur?   Yes ☐   No ☐

Section IV: The therapist

19.   Have you used this type of treatment for this   Yes ☐   No ☐
      type of clinical problem before?

20.   Please list any unusual effects you have noted with this type of treatment with **ANY** patient before:

EFFECT	CONDITION
1)	
2)	
3)	
4)	

21.   Please list any thoughts you have on why the effect(s) occurred:

_____

_____

_____

22.   Can you be contacted for further information?   Yes ☐   No ☐

      If yes, please provide a contact name, telephone number and/or email address:

      Name: _____

      Telephone no. _____

      Email address: _____

      This form may be returned by email to enquires@csp.org.uk

                    or posted to: Clinical Effectiveness Unit
                                    Chartered Society of Physiotherapy
                                    14 Bedford Row
                                    LONDON WC1R 4ED

Index

Please note that page references to non textual matter such as Boxes, Figures or Tables are in *italic* print